THINKING OUTSIDE

THE PILL BOX

A consumer's guide to integrative medicine and comprehensive wellness

TY VINCENT, MD

authorHOUSE®

AuthorHouse™
1663 Liberty Drive
Bloomington, IN 47403
www.authorhouse.com
Phone: 1-800-839-8640

Published by AuthorHouse 8/15/12

ISBN: 978-1-4772-5514-8 (sc)
ISBN: 978-1-4772-5515-5 (dj)
ISBN: 978-1-4772-5513-1 (e)

Library of Congress Control Number: 2012914245

To my wife, Brandilyn, who has never made me doubt my own self worth.
And, to anyone who may find something useful in this book.

PREFACE

Welcome to my rant!

Hopefully this book will find you well, or possibly ill, and be of some use to you in either case.

My goal is to educate people, in the optimal care of their body, and to promote health for both themselves and their family. A second goal, which will become obvious in Section II, is to encourage every individual to take charge of the world in which we live. I would like everyone to realize that we all have the power, and the responsibility to steer our collective future toward a healthier one.

I would like to offer some guidance as to the structure of this book, so that you may get what you want from it, and not waste your precious time reading sections you care nothing about.

There is a rather long "About the Author" passage. It reads more as an autobiography of sorts, with far more personal detail than one would expect in a book like this. I felt it important for the reader to understand the source of opinions and information offered in this book. If you don't care about my personal story, feel free to skip it.

The Introduction provides an overview of the purpose and ideas within the book. No surprises. If you tend to skip introductions in nonfiction books, intending to read the rest of the text, feel free to skip this as well. You have my blessing.

Section I is largely a glossary. It offers my own definitions and explanations for some terms used in integrative medicine. It also may introduce the reader to some new concepts in health and science. It may be important for most to read this because some terms used later in the book can then be better understood. It may also be useful to understand the relevant philosophies in integrative medicine at the outset.

Section II is a fairly long, somewhat ranting, account of my view on how American medicine got to the place it is, and what I feel is wrong with it. It admittedly gets fairly opinionated and somewhat inflammatory at times. I am very passionate about this. I tried to tone it down, but likely failed to be diplomatic here and there. If the history of modern medical evolution or dealing with potential socio-political conflict is of no interest, just skip this entire section. It is not critical to improving one's health.

Section III finally gets to the meat of this text. It is a large portion of this book, devoted to all the things I think are important for people to achieve optimal health. It involves understanding the "inputs" to our bodies. This includes food, fluid, mineral, vitamin, the air we breathe, as well as concepts related to psychology and energy. This section should be useful to every reader, in its entirety.

Section IV is the largest section of the book, and may not all be relevant to a given reader. This is where my particular experience in medicine comes into play. It is a section where I discuss what I feel are the real underlying "causes" of most chronic medical problems seen in our society. It is going to be the most important section of the book for anyone suffering from chronic medical illness, and may be of some interest as well to those currently enjoying good health. I suggest reviewing the chapters within the Table of Contents and then choosing which material to read first; this section does not need to be read in order, nor completely, to find what is needed.

The last section is my attempt at a brief summary of the book, the meat of what I think should be understood. Feel free to read this section first if you wish, and then go back to read the relevant parts of the book for anything you would like more information about. In a way this is your final checklist for optimal health, so feel free to copy it or write it out as a "To Do" list for yourself, and post it somewhere that will be in your face.

Last is a bibliography that includes sources of information for my writing. I encourage reading any of the books I've mentioned here, or that are suggested in the text. There is a mountain of information out there, funneled through many different minds and opinions. Don't take what I have to say, or any of these authors I've mentioned and respect, as the "gospel" in this field. I encourage all of you to read as much as you can, broaden your experience and form your own opinions.

CONTENTS

ABOUT THE AUTHOR

Who am I, and why should you listen to me?

Well, that's a very fair question and one that should be asked more often of all health care professionals. I imagine that very few of you have ever asked your doctor what their test scores were like through school, just as people rarely seem to question why a celebrity spokesperson should be trusted regarding a scientific topic. It's also quite striking how differently the same news can be reported between any two news channels, such as MSNBC and Fox News, for example. Always consider the source and the motives behind it.

So, I'll tell you a little bit about myself, where I'm coming from, and where I hope we can all get to with the information in this book.

My name is Ty Robert Vincent. I was born in Anchorage, Alaska, on July 6, 1973, to Dennis and Mary Vincent. They were living in a small trailer in the Spenard area (if you don't know Anchorage, this is not a nice part of town) when I was born. By age two, we had moved, out of the city, to a much smaller community, called Wasilla (yes, that's where former Governor Sarah Palin is from, and no, we are not related). When we made the move, less than 1,500 people lived there at the time. I actually still live and work in Wasilla (as of 2009-11, when this was written), but now, more than ten times that many people live in the community.

My father worked as a correctional officer and my mother stayed home until I was in elementary school. A few years later, they went into real estate, which seemed like a good idea at the time. There was a point, in the early 1980s, when the housing bubble burst and it looked like we might have to run from bill collectors. Luckily, my father found another job back with the state correctional system that allowed us to stay where we were and maintain a basic standard of living.

I was a Caucasian, lower middle class, left-handed, extremely nearsighted, socially awkward, mildly asthmatic boy. I guess this is relevant because my wife learned, in her psychology training, how people, with that particular set of demographics, tend to do better in school. The theory is that we aren't very good at sports and probably have access to, and prefer, books. It wasn't much fun for me at the time, but I guess things turned out well enough in the end.

We lived in a fairly rural area, so I spent a lot of time in my youth running around in the woods with my dogs. There were no guns or methamphetamines involved; that's more consistent with the reputation of modern-day Wasilla. I guess I had decent interpersonal skills but was socially somewhat shy. It wasn't until I worked as a waiter at Denny's in Anchorage for a couple years during college that I began to develop what would later become a blunt and sarcastic bedside manner.

We had fairly small schools, but, academically, I always seemed to be in the top of my class. This was true, even in first grade, despite the fact that we discovered toward the end of that year how extremely nearsighted I was. I had somehow made it into the advanced classes without ever being able to see a damn thing on the board. My mother also tells me that I used to put together complicated jigsaw puzzles upside down (with the cardboard side facing up). You would think that might have been a clue to get my vision (or something) checked a little sooner. I like to think these experiences in the first six years of my life helped me become a better listener.

Based on my SAT scores, I qualified as a National Merit Scholar in high school, one of only a few such students ever to have come out of Wasilla at that time. They made a big deal out of this and led me to believe that it would take me places. Sadly, I never seemed to qualify for any big scholarships, possibly because affirmative action was in full swing at the time.

This problem continued later on when I was trying to get funding for medical school. I was not eligible for a scholarship through the Coast Guard because I was not a member of a minority. I missed out on scholarships to the National Health Service Corps, in part, because of a female preference at the time, and I was disqualified from all branches of the armed forces due to my poor eyesight. I flunked the physical, even though I could bench press well over 300 pounds and had less than 8% body fat. Oh, the irony!

Later, I came to feel extremely relieved that I did not owe any of these organizations any time of service. I have since come to realize that things work out very well for me even if it doesn't seem like it at the time. If something seems negative at first, I now just wait to see what the true, positive, outcome will be in the long run.

My parents made me an offer to pay for college if I stayed in Alaska, close to home, for the first two years, and then give me further assistance to go out of state if I needed to. However, like so many young men, I was not thinking logically of my future, at the time. My girlfriend, from high school, had just moved to New Mexico with her family so, of course, I applied to a small college in Durango, Colorado which was within an hour's drive of her.

This worked out well in retrospect because we were later married (after having a child out of wedlock, a standard tradition in Wasilla, apparently) and eventually had two more beautiful children together.

It was a small liberal arts college in Durango, and I completed my first two years there towards a degree in biology. What I really wanted to study was marine biology and had wanted to since about eighth grade. Colorado seemed to have strikingly little coastline so, at that point, I applied and was accepted to a program in Hawaii. It just so happened that my girlfriend and her family moved back to Alaska during my second year in Colorado. We split up temporarily after that, but got back together over the summer. I think it was Robin Williams who once said "men have two brains, but only enough blood to run one of them at a time". I have to agree because, by the end of that summer, I had canceled my plans to go to Hawaii and was going to stay in Anchorage so I could be near my girlfriend again.

The University of Alaska in Anchorage did not have a marine biology program either, so I was forced to change my mind about my future plans for that career. For some reason, the obvious choice seemed to be going to medical school and becoming a doctor. I'm still not really clear on how I came to that decision, other than, I thought "I'm a pretty smart guy; I could probably go to medical school". This lack of deeper thought on the subject probably kept me from getting accepted the first time I applied.

I had been living on campus and not working while I was in Colorado and had accrued about $10,000 worth of debt in student loans. The week I turned twenty, I moved into Anchorage and found my own apartment and full-time job as a dishwasher at the Denny's restaurant in mid-town (my older sister already worked there, and put in a good word for me). I continued to work about thirty hours per week while I took sixteen or more credit hours, each semester, through three more years at UAA. I supported myself completely and had my first child in the summer before my last year of college. I continued to work hard to support my young family and, eventually, graduated magna cum laude in May of 1996 with a degree in biological sciences.

I had taken the MCAT (the aptitude test for entry into medical school) and scored in the 99th percentile, which is where I've scored on virtually every national exam in my life.

I think I was overconfident about my chances of getting accepted into medical school because my grades and test scores were so high. It seemed, however, that they were interested more in volunteer work and some experience actually doing something in the medical field. I wasn't sure where I was supposed to fit in the volunteer work with working, going to school and having an infant at home. It's my feeling that this bias tends to favor those from wealthier households.

I think what really sunk me that first year applying to the University of Washington, which has a special student exchange agreement with Alaska, was my answer to one particular unusual interview question. One of the senior faculty members from Alaska asked the question: "Who do you think is the most admirable person from the 20th century?" This question caught me off guard because it didn't seem relevant and, as I may have mentioned before, by this point in my life I had a somewhat sarcastic attitude. I thought I should answer somewhat quickly and give an answer that perhaps no one else would have given. So, of course, I said: "Arnold Schwarzenegger." Mind you, this was 1996 (it would be a much better answer now) and, at that point in time, Arnold Schwarzenegger was mainly known worldwide for bodybuilding and being an action movie star.

After the "shock and awe" reaction I received from my three interviewers, I went on to explain that he had come to America as a teenager with nothing, not even speaking English, and now was known worldwide. I explained that he had been awarded an honorary Ph.D. from a prestigious American university and, at one point, had been named the President's Council on Physical Fitness. None of this really seemed to impress them, and I think they just saw images of me sitting and watching *Conan* or *The Terminator* movies over and over. Suddenly my good grades and high-test scores didn't mean so much.

In my ignorance and arrogance, at the time, I was still surprised when I got my rejection letter. In retrospect, this was one of the best things that ever happened to me, especially regarding my career as a physician.

It forced me to look at my true motives and to first seek out medical experience at a different level. I moved into a trailer that my parents owned with my young family. (Oh yeah, it may not have helped that I was still not married at the time of my interview, but had an infant; some people had more traditional family values, I guess. Oh, and I forgot to mention that I also wore earrings that I refused to take out for my interview even though my father suggested it. I had figured if they didn't want me the way I was, then I didn't want to go). I worked for eight dollars an hour, doing minor construction and labor for a general contractor who was a friend of the family.

I found a local training course for certified nursing assistants, and my father graciously gave me the $2000 I needed to attend. I finished the twelve weeks of training at the top of my class and managed to get an ideal position at Providence Hospital in Anchorage. I worked in a sub-critical care section with fairly ill patients, and I was able to see a wide variety of medical problems and practitioners. I took vital signs, checked blood sugars, emptied bedpans, bathed the more debilitated patients, emptied colostomy bags, and performed other duties that involved experiencing humanity in a way most people never do.

This is where I really developed my interpersonal skills and learned how to talk to patients and their loved ones. If you have ever been in the hospital, you may have noted that the nursing staff spends hours with you, while the doctors spend often just a few minutes per day with each patient. Above all I think I learned how to hear, rather than just listen.

My first son Isaac was born in July of 1997, almost two years after Alexandria had come along. I didn't make quite enough money working as a nurse's aide, so I worked a second job waiting tables at another restaurant (Village Inn this time). Between the two jobs, I earned enough to buy our first home in November of that year. Somehow I've always been very responsible and good with money, which I don't find to be a great strength of most physicians and, in a financial sense, this may relate in some way to our current health care problem.

When I again applied to medical school in 1998, I was readily accepted because of this experience (and not mentioning Arnold). I always kept the humanity I had developed during my experience as a nurse's aide. I would frequently lag behind the group on rounds at the university hospitals to make sure the patient we had just mobbed had their bedside table within reach and the door closed if they wanted. The surgical residents, in particular, always looked at me like I was from another planet. I took that as a compliment.

My first year of medical school was in Anchorage, starting on my daughter's third birthday, with a class size of only ten students. It was part of what's called the WWAMI program, a cooperative type of agreement through which the University of Washington supports surrounding states that have no medical school of their own. There was one other person with children in my class, but he was significantly older than me and he had only one to care for. My third child, Olivia, was born right after the end of that first year, giving me a distinct two-child lead on my Alaskan classmate.

After the first year, all of the satellite sites within the WWAMI program converged on Seattle at the UWSOM campus. There were now about 180 of us, and the boy who grew up in small-town Alaska was suddenly living in a city with millions of people. We seemed to adjust fine, actually, and found some other families within my medical school class with children also; even another family with three kids (new competition). I had always been the smartest kid in school, but now I expected I was going to be a small fish in a big pond.

I tried to prepare myself psychologically for being in the middle of the class rather than the top. To my surprise, I found myself still in the top of the class. Even in my first-year class of ten, I was, initially, a bit intimidated by the fact that two students had graduated from Princeton and one from Harvard. Somehow, I had still made it to the top of my small group. I was even chosen for our annual class award given to the best student in anatomy. This entailed a $3,000 cash prize, which I desperately needed, and was spent right away because the transmission had gone out in our car.

I had a wife and small children that were the true focus of my life. I couldn't play most of the time and then expect to cram for tests the weekend before like most of do in college. I disciplined myself to stay up late and study every night, even if there was no test for a month. I would study until I couldn't stay awake anymore, then go to the 24 hour gym and work out, so I had the energy to study, for another 30 minutes or so, when I got back home. My trick was to study standing up in the kitchen with my books raised up to my level on a box or laundry basket. After falling asleep standing up a couple of times and nearly falling, I would go to bed. This was usually around 1 a.m. Then I would get up with my oldest daughter, always an early riser, around seven.

Most people would expect that having a family would be a major hindrance through medical school, but my experience was completely the opposite. It seems that being consistent and disciplined helped me learn and retain the information better. I learned to function on much less sleep so, other than the time spent in classrooms, my medical studying rarely had to intrude on my family time.

I managed to achieve "honors" designation in 22 out of 27 courses in basic sciences and systems biology during the first two years of study. We were told that anything greater than ten such designations was considered outstanding. I scored higher on the first part of the USMLE (United States Medical Licensing Exam) than anyone I have ever encountered (a '261' for those of you who care). I later scored in the top 1% on the rest of the sections of the USMLE as well. I also scored in the 99th percentile on our practice board exam in all three years of residency, which is extremely rare for an intern.

I'm not citing this to brag, just trying to give you some reason to consider listening to my ideas based on my ability to think things through and master medical knowledge. You certainly don't want to listen to someone just because he/she is a doctor. You know what they call the person who finishes dead last in their medical school class? "Doctor."

Ironically, I did not graduate from medical school with an overall "honors" designation despite achieving honors level in the majority of my classes and clinical rotations and scoring extremely high on the national exams. It turns out "honors" is a designation at graduation that is chosen by the department chairs in the medical school and is not based purely on merit. I had completed many of my clinical rotations in Alaska rather than staying in Seattle, and many of the department chairs didn't even know who I was.

It was a little bit annoying when my family acted like there was something wrong with me for not getting honors. They were used to me achieving the highest standard every step of the way. When you set the bar that high there is nowhere to go but down. In reality, all of this was fine with me because at this point in my life, I was no stranger to disappointment and had learned that I really needed to find approval within myself more than anyone else's. I also knew by then that I was somewhat different-minded than my fellow physicians and really didn't care about being "in the club" so to speak.

So on to residency! Residency is generally accepted as the absolute worst time of your life. It's like medical boot camp, but it goes on for a minimum of three years depending on your specialty. I had chosen to go into family medicine because I loved the variety, the chance to be the first person to try and solve a problem, and the degree of interpersonal relationship you get with your patients. It seemed like every specialty rotation I had been on, the residents and physicians would ask me why I wanted to go into family medicine and "waste my talent and intelligence". My reply was usually, "wouldn't you like to have a good family doctor?" I was always a bit annoyed that they felt so damn superior to primary care physicians who solve most patients' problems without specialist referral and are relatively underpaid.

I was accepted to the residency program in family medicine back home in Anchorage even though the residency director was, apparently, suspicious of my extremely high test scores and wondered whether I was going to be able to communicate like a normal human (I found this out later). I guess I did better during my interviews this time. I suppose it also helped that they had a preference for Alaskans.

I was just as nervous about residency as everyone else I think. There is a certain amount of terror in the knowledge that you will now have the power to kill someone through your own mistakes. This really hit home with me on the first day of orientation when I saw a prescription pad with my name on it. Shortly before the end of medical school, I had *"Primum Non Nocere"* (meaning "first, do no harm") tattooed around my right arm because I take that concept very seriously every day in practice. To this day, I'm pretty sure I've not killed anyone. Side note: Just so all of you know, July 1st is when each training year begins in medical residency. That means you may not want to be in a teaching hospital in July or August if you can help it.

Many interns start out with sweaty palms, shaky hands, and that "deer in the headlights" look in their eyes. I seemed to hit the ground running. I'm sure this was due, in large part, to my time spent working in hospitals as a nurse's aide. I was more afraid of the stress that residency could place on my family, and I worked extremely hard, fast, and efficiently, to try to make sure I had adequate time at home. This was particularly important because, at the time, my wife and I didn't have the greatest relationship. We were married young and, seemingly, grew in different directions as people. All we had in common was our children and that proved insufficient. It was, statistically, no surprise when we separated two-thirds of the way through my first year of residency.

The medical training had been surprisingly easy and enjoyable for me but, for a while, my intern year ended up being the worst time of my life. Since then, my ex-wife and I have a congenial, co-parenting relationship and have both gone on to have more children with new partners. We have shared the kids equally since my graduation from residency; they are all wonderful, well-adjusted kids. Lexi, Isaac, and Olivia are all straight-A students, talented athletes, and have defiant sarcastic attitudes. I couldn't be prouder of them.

I was extremely lucky to have an absolutely wonderful and talented group of fellow interns and also very competent, compassionate, and understanding faculty and senior residents. Years before this, I had developed a policy of never needing help from anyone, but going through a divorce (as many of you know) is also one of the worst times in your life. So, going through a divorce during my intern year was especially no picnic, and it really changed me, for the better, to find that I could rely on others to give me support. One of my classmates gave me a room to rent in his house and one of my faculty organized a "guys' night out" every month for a while.

Towards the end of that first year I met my soul mate (if I don't put it that way I'll never hear the end of it; plus, it's true). Brandilyn and I were married at the end of my second year, have gone on to have three beautiful children together and are blissfully happy (Sage in February of 2006, Maya in September of 2007 and Bodhi in January 2011). In our house, we are a family of five, half the time, and a family of eight, the other half, week on/ week off. As a result of my experiences, I've come to understand that the path through life can be very erratic and unpredictable, but you can get to a much better place when you keep your head up and maintain a positive attitude. This is also very true in the field of medicine.

I know that's a lot of "sharing", but I think it's really important for you to understand who it is that's giving you their opinion. I was not born with a silver spoon or raised in a 'medical' family. I'm the first and only medical doctor in my family anywhere as far as I know. My parents studied only to an associate's degree level, but have been very successful people. My father is a war hero with the emotional battle scars to prove it, but he managed to hold it all together for his family and always provide whatever was needed. My mother is one of the hardest working and emotionally strong people I know. I like to think I got the best they both had to offer, except on the days I like to think I'm actually adopted. My older sister Gina achieved her doctorate in forensic psychology shortly after I graduated with my MD.

My parents must have done something right with their kids because we're both doctors.

I know what it's like to be poor and to work extremely hard to get ahead. For years we were on various forms of public assistance while my children were young, and I seldom had health insurance of my own until I was in residency. I think what is most important about my development is that I learned to think for myself, to problem solve and come up with creative solutions. Along with this came what you might call a 'respectful disagreement' with authority; especially when that authority was at odds with what made sense to me. This became more and more evident in me and important for my patients, as I progressed through medical training and practice. The medical "Box" is somewhat stifling, but you can't tell that until you get out of it. As Dr. Jonathan Wright, one of the founders of modern integrative medicine in the U.S., likes to say: "Does a fish know it's wet?" I've learned a lot through my own experience and frequently tell my children: "being the only person in the room who thinks what you think doesn't make you wrong".

Now I want to talk about my philosophies of medicine a bit and how they formed.

Before I got into medical school, I was under the impression they were going to teach me about how the body worked and how to promote its ideal functioning. I was reading books on natural medicine by Dr. Andrew Weil, and they made a lot of sense to me. The summer before I started medical school, I bought a biochemistry textbook and began researching vitamin structures, the functions of minerals in the body and other things I expected to learn about.

Boy, was I surprised that none of this stuff was ever discussed in my medical school (the number one primary care medical school in the country, no less). I focused, intently, on understanding the basic sciences through the first year of medical school because I thought that would be the most useful information for me to be able to figure out how to fix what was going wrong with people. The second year of medical school, we expanded basic science information to the understanding of how the different organs and systems in the body function physiologically. This also seemed extremely useful to me. In that year we also studied pharmacology to a great extent, which becomes (unfortunately) exceedingly important in American medical practice. The first part of the USMLE, as I mentioned before, was all based on these basic science concepts and I scored extremely high; I guess my disciplined approach worked.

The next two years were devoted to clinical medical practice (hands-on and observational learning). Suddenly, the majority of that information I had so carefully studied seemed to have been somewhat forgotten by most everyone else. The way we were taught to treat patients often made no sense based on the physiology of their problem. When I would ask questions and point this out to my supervising residents or attending physicians, I would usually get the reply: "This is the *standard of care*." I never really accepted that as a useful answer and in my mind it gave me the freedom to look for my own answers because, it seemed to me, that the authorities clearly didn't really know what was going on. Since then my own standards have risen far above the *standard of care*, and I've come to realize that "standard" practice is heavily influenced by drug companies and other capitalist healthcare industries.

Once I was out of medical school and in residency, I (and every other resident) was considered a "doctor" in my own right, though, under what is supposed to be constant supervision. I was lucky enough to be in a program that was somewhat open-minded with some excellent faculty members who did not seem threatened by an independent thinker. After I proved myself to be quite competent in the first half of my intern year, I was largely left alone in terms of my decision-making. My developing knowledge of nutrition, and its application in medicine, was fairly well received. In my final year, I was even allowed to study acupuncture and do clinical rotations with naturopaths. In addition, I also spent time with dentists and veterinarians.

I was chosen to be one of our two chief residents in the third year, a position elected by fellow residents and faculty. In terms of the academic aspect and workload, residency was easy for me. I did things a bit differently from others, but since I had excellent outcomes there was no negative feedback (also, family medicine tends to be more open-minded). I still asked a lot of questions to which nobody, including the specialists in a number of fields, gave me good answers. I thoroughly enjoyed teaching the newer residents and interns and getting them to think more. Later, at graduation, I was chosen for the national teaching award designated by our faculty.

What's ironic about this is that after graduating from this residency program, where I was held in an apparently high regard, I have now become some kind of feared outsider because of my nonconventional practice. Whatever.

After residency, I went back to my home town, about an hour away, and worked in a large group practice for the first eighteen months before feeling the need to set up my own practice with a much more integrative approach. I had several residents come out and spend time with me and most of them said it was one of the best and most useful experiences of their training. After some of them went back to the residency program and tried to implement some of the different approaches that they learned from me, it caused a stir with some of the local specialists and residency faculty. The program director even decided not to let residents spend time with me anymore. The rationale he gave was that "the residents would have to study too hard or read too much in order to validate the things I was telling them."

That's very interesting to me, but just goes to show that we are expected to swallow, without question, the bad information that is fed to us by the pharmaceutical industry and is propagated through our medical education system. Using techniques that are safer, cheaper, and make more biological sense would apparently "require too much time to learn". Wow! That really scares me, and it should scare you too.

This is pitiful in my opinion, but exemplifies one of the huge problems in our country's health care system: that our medical education involves a lot of propaganda from special interests and is more like a vocational curriculum on how to sell drugs than it is an intellectual healing art. I will rant more about this in a later section. I have come to realize that part of what makes me able to practice with better focus on the goal of human health is the fact that I never wanted to be a doctor for the sake of the title, and don't care at all about the perceived prestige or self-importance that most of my colleagues seem to crave by being in the "club".

I practice based on what makes the most sense biochemically and scientifically, what gets results, and what improves the health of my patients. The standard of care in American medicine is not an acceptable standard, and I can see that more clearly because I don't have my identity or ego wrapped up in it. I don't care if the other kids think I'm strange or an outsider; I got over that in high school.

As I mentioned before, in my third year of residency, I was able to learn acupuncture. As a physician, the greatest amount of educational time required, by any State is only 300 hours to become a certified medical acupuncturist. One gross injustice in our country's medical system is that an insurance company is far more likely to pay for a physician acupuncturist with my level of training to treat a patient with acupuncture than to pay for a licensed acupuncturist (L.Ac.) who has had three to five years of training in the discipline. Even more laughable, Medicare considers acupuncture to be "experimental". I guess a 3000-year experiment in several diverse cultures on the planet isn't good enough for them.

I attended what is probably the oldest and best medical acupuncture training course in the country, which was at the time put on by UCLA and run by Joseph Helms, MD. I learned a new approach to medical diagnosis and treatment that was incredible, both in its difference from Western medical philosophy, as well as its effectiveness for many conditions.

This experience in Chinese medicine was my first solid evidence that my conventional medical training was extremely limited and incomplete. I suppose the first evidence was really the fact that most of my patients in residency just kept returning for medication refills without their problems ever getting any better (that would be the *standard of care* in our country). I found I could often treat pain without medications and could correct diverse functional problems such as digestive complaints, anxiety or even bedwetting.

I was so intrigued by Chinese medical theory, I went on to further training in Chinese Herbal Medicine through the same organization. Again, this was a very limited level of training in the field, entailing just fifty hours of home study. Naturopaths and Oriental Medical Doctors have several years of training in herbal medicines, gaining the knowledge and skill needed to mix individualized formulas. My training was restricted to the use of several dozen premade manufactured herbal mixtures for specific indications. It still required an understanding of Chinese medical theory which is, again, extremely different from Western theory.

I saw further increased success treating patients with herbal remedies where I had found no prior success using pharmaceuticals. Of course, in some cases, the herbs did not work at all, but they never had any significant toxic effects either. I still found that some patients did well with pharmaceuticals, while others did extremely well with acupuncture and/or herbs. I did know something about nutritional therapies at this point as well, many of which I found extremely successful for various problems.

This sort of evolution of practice, where you continue to include aspects of every type of medicine you've learned, is the essence of "integrative medicine". This separates it from "alternative medicine", which can become just as dogmatic in its opposition to "conventional" medicine as conventional medicine is with its own stance. The term alternative medicine does not apply at all to what I do because I don't believe there is any alternative to truly *good* medical practice. I will continue to look at each patient in terms of the unique situation, desires and needs of that individual.

"Complementary medicine" is a more favorable term, implying a more collegial feel and a sense of working together with conventional medical therapies. However, the term tends to separate providers into their own specialties, whereas the term "integrative medicine" suggests a single provider with diverse training and approach. That's where I fit, and it is a rapidly growing type of practice in American medicine today.

After delving into Eastern medicine, I decided the next obvious thing to explore in more depth was nutrition. I found a graduate level nutrition textbook and read most of it. I also read a small toxicology textbook from the 1960s, published in Great Britain, which was very interesting and more than a little useful. I found conference syllabi from *the American College for Advancement in Medicine (ACAM)* in heavy metals toxicology and chelation, as well as intravenous nutrition therapy. I eventually stumbled across an excellent textbook in clinical nutrition, compiled and published by the *Institute for Functional Medicine.* This textbook was extremely user friendly and informative. Finding this resource then led me to the large and comprehensive *Textbook of Functional Medicine,* published in 2005 by the same organization. I urge any interested health practitioners out there to acquire (and read) this text.

When I began to read this book, it was like an orphan meeting their real family for the first time. The scientific information presented in this book was geared towards understanding the causes of illness and treatments based on biological and physiological principles. Here was the information I had hoped and expected to gain in my conventional medical education. It was so refreshing to know that there were groups of other healers who thought like I did and, even more refreshing, to find that they had already done much of the work without me.

I blazed through the first five hundred pages of this textbook, word for word, and attended my first scientific symposium put on by the Institute, in October 2006. There were hundreds of attendees at this conference and not just MDs, but also osteopaths, chiropractors, naturopaths, dentists, psychologists, veterinarians, and many other health practitioners. Everyone there seemed happy to interact and share knowledge. In fact, they seemed fundamentally happy and content with the world in general which, as you may have noticed, is not the typical feeling you get from conventional physicians.

Since becoming involved with the Institute, I've also found and learned more from other organizations, including *ACAM* and *The American Academy of Environmental Medicine (AAEM)*, a national organization for which I currently serve on the board of directors. Through these organizations, independent study, as well as my own clinical experience, I have gained skills in advanced nutrition including intravenous nutrition therapies, heavy metals toxicology and chelation therapy, bio-identical hormone therapy (via *The International Hormone Society*), identification and treatment of environmental and food allergies, chemical sensitivities, and detoxification.

I decided, at some point, that spirituality and energy medicine were extremely important and also missing from my training. I found a local master in the art of Reiki and have been "attuned" to the practitioner level. I find that this works extremely well in combination with acupuncture treatments and have, at times, been able to heal people with the energetic treatment alone. That may sound somewhat bizarre or hokey to some of you and, believe me, I understand completely since I was a hard-core Western scientist for most of my life. While in residency, I had the opportunity to read two complete textbooks on energy medicine (*Energy Medicine*, by Oschmann is a good place to start for those who are interested). These sorts of treatments have been scientifically explained and validated believe it or not. They aren't in the coding books put out by the AMA for billing purposes, but they work somehow in spite of that.

In practice for myself now, since January 1st of 2007, my style has continued to develop and grow. I learn more every week, often from my own patients, because I take time to listen to them. My new patient visits are all an hour long, and no one gets less than thirty minutes in follow up visits. I would say roughly 80% or more of my patients improve their chronic health issues significantly, as opposed to the 20% or so that probably improved when I practiced conventionally (there's that *standard of care* again).

I love seeing patients with what appear to be complicated, diverse medical issues or unsolved mysteries, especially if they have been to some ivory tower medical establishment like the Mayo Clinic, Virginia Mason or a major university. They frequently return from those places being told there is no answer, no solution, or maybe given some diagnostic label that doesn't really mean anything or is totally noncommittal. Common examples include "fibromyalgia", "irritable bowel syndrome", "viral syndrome", "hormonal imbalance", "psychosomatic disorder", or "idiopathic" condition. It's incredibly gratifying to actually find an answer for these people and, often, a solution.

Of course, I have failures too, and they eat at me; but it occurred to me one day that this is what drives me. I am perpetually driven by my failures to learn more and climb over the walls in my path. Regarding many of today's chronic medical problems, conventional medicine seems to have sunk into complacency and "learned helplessness". This will be further discussed later in the book, but now I believe it's time to stop talking about me.

INTRODUCTION

Why this book, at this time

The health of Americans in this second decade of the 21st century is deteriorating despite the incredible sums of money that are thrown at our medical care. For example, death from infectious disease has been replaced with escalating numbers of chronic diseases in new variations; sperm counts are dropping and infertility is on the rise; childhood diseases of a chronic nature are increasing. These include cancers and neurological problems such as ADHD, allergies, asthma and autism. Obesity has become a serious issue in our society afflicting children at younger and younger ages. In addition, we are now finding teenagers with higher rates of adult diseases such as Type 2 diabetes, high blood pressure, and high cholesterol.

Our life expectancy is decreasing for the first time in over a century and conventional medicine seems to be confused as to why this is happening. The extremely high and ever increasing cost of our health care system in the United States is not only a testament to the deterioration of our health as a population, but also implicates our health care system itself as being part of the problem.

It is becoming obvious, to those of us who are paying attention, that big business controls our health care and is largely responsible for its decline. This is not only true in the case of the pharmaceutical companies and the insurance industry, but it also includes our transportation systems, our food and manufacturing industries, as well as everything else affecting our environment.

It is apparent to me, and many other like-minded physicians with similar training and views, that the conventional approach to medical care is failing to deal with modern problems and modern causes of illness. Some of us suggest that the roots of many of today's chronic diseases lie far upstream and are related to such issues as poor food quality and environmental pollution. This book is my effort to try and spread awareness of the causes of these current health problems. I will also attempt to offer some ideas and recommendations addressing this subject that I believe we can all embrace and act upon.

Elaboration of the problems

Decreasing life expectancy

A little over a hundred years ago, the most common causes of early death in the U.S. were various infections including smallpox, influenza, tuberculosis, pneumonia, measles, meningitis, diarrheal illness and other such diseases. Advances in basic sanitation and the development of vaccines and antibiotics were the main factors responsible for changing that trend. As a result of those developments in medical care and environmental safety, the causes of death shifted more to chronic illnesses such as cardiovascular disease, cancer and other degenerative conditions.

These diseases are still our leading causes of death, but now they are beginning to have effects at younger and younger ages in the population. This is what brings down our "average" life expectancy. Changes in infant mortality make a tremendous impact on this average. An infant that dies is passing away 75 years early (before the "average age" of death) rather than just five years early, for example, if a person dies at 70. Therefore, a single case of death in infancy drags the "average life expectancy" down significantly.

Infant mortality is what separates many of the world's populations in terms of this statistical marker. For example, an article published in *Time* magazine (December 2008) shows the infant mortality rate in the United States to be 6.9 out of 1000 live births; while in Afghanistan that number is 165 out of 1000 live births. Correspondingly, the average life expectancy is 77.9 years in the United States and only 42 in Afghanistan.

This does not mean people tend to die at age 42 in Afghanistan, it merely reflects their high rate of deaths at extremely young ages. It is likely that for every newborn that dies, there is someone who lives to be 84; that is the nature of averages. You could be just as likely to see 100-year-old people in Afghanistan as in the United States, or even more of them per capita. Average life expectancy doesn't truly describe how long people are expected to live if they make it to adulthood. Numbers don't always mean what they seem to indicate on first glance.

In the aforementioned survey of 165 nations, the United States ranked only 34th in terms of life expectancy and 29th in infant mortality rates. Japan topped the list with an average life expectancy of 83 years of age and an infant mortality rate of only 2.8 per 1000 live births. Statistics also inform us that Okinawa, Japan has the highest proportion of individuals who are 100 years of age or older. This is particularly curious in light of the facts that the Japanese are thought to smoke more and drink more alcohol than the average person in the United States; but I'll get into more of those details later.

What makes these numbers even more disturbing for us in the United States are the financial numbers. We spend an astounding 16% of our gross domestic product on health care, an average of $7,026 per individual per year. Canada spends only 10% of its GNP on health care, and only $3,912 per individual. The number one country, Japan spends only 7.9% and a corresponding $2,690 per person.

So, exactly what the hell are we spending their money on?

Increasing rates of chronic disease

I suspect most everyone is acutely aware of the obesity epidemic that is occurring, and how the size of Americans has grown over recent decades. All you have to do is watch a movie from the '60s or '70s and compare the sizes of those people to the sizes of the people you see in the aisles at the store today. Or you can just look at the difference in John Travolta between *Saturday Night Fever* and *Wild Hogs*. Something is definitely happening to us, and it can't be just due to human behavior; after all, people have always enjoyed eating.

Obesity is just one chronic medical condition, but it is somewhat of a sentinel condition in that it reflects an underlying metabolic derangement on multiple levels with multiple causative factors. The fact that we're seeing it in our children at dramatically increasing rates shows that these metabolic changes are now occurring very early in life. These same types of metabolic changes also contribute to the formation of cancer and cardiovascular disease; neurodegenerative diseases like dementia or Parkinson's, arthritis and osteoporosis; as well as other inflammatory conditions later on in life.

Japan has recognized the obesity problem as such an important factor that they have recently levied financial penalties against companies and local governments where individuals' waistlines grow too large and stay that way. It may surprise you to know that their waistline cut-off for a man is only 33.5 inches, and 35.4 inches for women (*The New York Times*, reported in *The North County [CA] Times*, June 13, 2008).

Type 2 diabetes is clearly linked with obesity to some degree. Increases in obesity itself somewhat explain the rise we've seen in diabetes. Sadly, we are seeing type 2 diabetes at an increasing rate in our teenagers, paralleling the rise in obesity found in that population as well. Obesity cannot completely explain type 2 diabetes however, because we find people who have increased their weight to over four hundred pounds and are not diabetic.

Recent research has suggested that a number of environmental pollutants are the causes for this illness in many people. Common chemicals have been shown to cause insulin resistance and pancreatic beta-cell (the cells that produce insulin) dysfunction, the physiologic processes leading to type 2 diabetes. Examples of such chemicals include many common pesticides from nonorganic food and bisphenol A, a very common chemical additive in plastics (Alonso-Magdalena, 2011). Bisphenol A is ingested by most Americans on a near-daily basis; it is obtained from plastic water or beverage bottles, sauce bottles, cans with plastic liners, other types of food containers, and most frightening of all, virtually every type of baby bottle made prior to the past few years (some manufacturers have realized this danger and voluntarily removed the chemical, while the government has still to date done nothing to regulate its use). Practitioners of environmental medicine understand it is these chemicals and many others causing the metabolic derangement in individual cells leading to type 2 diabetes and obesity.

We are also seeing dramatic increases in other conditions such as cancers. Pancreatic cancer is certainly more prominent now than it was fifty years ago, and thyroid cancer has increased more so than any other single cancer in the last three or four decades. These two cancers in particular are clearly linked to nutritional conditions to some degree. A review by the *World Cancer Research Fund* (2008) determined the rise in pancreatic cancer is somewhat attributable to the presence of nitrites in our foods such as hot dogs, lunchmeat, sausage and bacon. I watched a report on the national news in 2011 suggesting the chemical used as "caramel coloring" in processed foods has also been implicated in pancreatic cancer specifically (but it isn't being removed from foods by the FDA, and neither are nitrites). It appears that thyroid cancer may be linked to deficiencies of nutrients such as iodine, selenium and zinc; and it is also likely linked somewhat to the presence of bromine in our bread products and some beverages.

But we have drugs for diabetes, right? We have drugs for cardiovascular disease, and surgery as well, right? We have chemotherapy and radiation for cancer, as well as screening tests for some of them, right?

Yes, we do; but apparently that approach is not working, is it?

The failure of conventional treatment approaches

Almost all of the drug therapies for diabetes cause increased weight gain and a worsening of their underlying metabolic condition. Some may contribute to other dangerous diseases as well; some have been shown to cause fluid retention and heart failure, while others may cause pancreatitis or other life-threatening reactions. Even more frightening is the fact that the vast majority of these drugs offer absolutely no decrease in death rates for patients with diabetes (the most common cause of death in diabetics being cardiovascular disease). Given the weight gain and other side effects of most of these pharmaceuticals I suspect that if someone impartial looked at the data they would probably see *increases* in death rates. Further disturbing is the fact that many of these drugs cost well over $100 per month (in the U.S.).

Similarly, the drug therapies we use for cardiovascular disease show very limited improvements in death rates and other outcomes. The cholesterol-lowering drugs, the highest selling drugs in the U.S. and worldwide right now, actually exhibit no real decrease in mortality (this is why it is not a claim that they make in their numerous TV commercials). Coronary bypass surgery actually has the same ten-year mortality rate that purely medication-based management does for patients with stable coronary artery disease and angina (McGee, 2007).

Overall cancer rates have been increasing despite our screening efforts. The obvious reason for this is that "screening" only *finds* cancer at an earlier stage; it does not *prevent* cancer. The best hope for screening efforts is that we find cancers early enough to treat them more effectively; and these efforts have in fact led to decreases in death rates from cancers of various types including cervical cancer and, at least to some degree, breast and colon cancers. Our screening efforts for prostate cancer have recently come under scrutiny and are of unclear benefit in general. Screening doesn't seem to work for the more aggressive or difficult to treat cancers such as lung and pancreatic; which is why there are no recommended screening efforts for those cancers.

Chemotherapy and radiation do have positive results with certain specific cancers; but each type of cancer is actually somewhat distinct and is its own unique disease. The same treatments do not work for different cancers, and some cancers are not amenable to any conventional therapies. Besides that, it is well known that both chemotherapy and radiation have significant toxic effects to the human body. These toxicities are deemed acceptable when there is some documented success of treatment and the perceived alternative is death from cancer. There are complementary therapies that may decrease the toxicity and risk from these treatments, but they are sadly underutilized in conventional American medicine.

From the above discussion we can get an idea of what we are spending our money on in our efforts to treat some of our most important causes of chronic disease and death. Some efforts appear useless and wasteful, while others do seem to be effective and worthwhile.

So, why don't we get rid of the stuff that doesn't work? Well, the blunt answer is: someone's making lots of money from the way things are currently done.

Solutions?

Is there anything we can do about these issues? Of course there is. And obviously it will entail things that people don't like; otherwise, they likely would have done it already. That's just human nature.

There are possible solutions involving actions of the general public, driven by consumer behavior and awareness. There are huge potential solutions to be brought about by Industry, possibly forced by government regulation.

There are considerable discrepancies in medical education and training in this country. This may be a more difficult issue to address; but this is one specific area that is key to solving our problems. It may sound overly obvious, but we need medical practitioners who actually know how to prevent and cure disease.

Identifying and correcting many of the causes of our systemic problems is the main premise of this book. These topics will be fleshed out more as I proceed with this writing.

Goals for this book

I admit my main goals in writing this book are selfish in nature. Not in terms of financial gain mind you, but in terms of preserving a life for my own family in the future. The problems with our healthcare system affect everyone in our culture; and similar problems are pervasive throughout other parts of the world. America often sets global trends in lifestyle, and we can see a "trickle-down effect" of our decadence in other parts of the world.

Much of this book will discuss what one can do as an individual to promote his/her own health, but I will also discuss what can be done on a local and global level to improve the health of our society and the entire planet. This requires a more ecological perspective and appreciation of the big picture.

My hope is that in sorting out your own health problems you can achieve a greater appreciation for the bigger picture, and we can then work together in the growing movement towards a more sensible existence on this planet.

There are so many people in our society now that we have a tendency to feel we can make no difference on an individual level. But we just need to realize that it is the power of consumerism that drives things. Consumer habits can really be altered only on an individual scale, and one of my goals is to motivate every reader of this book to make positive changes in those habits.

This book will focus on creating awareness as to the causes of illness in our selves and in our loved ones, as well as explaining the roots of major medical trends in our society. I will emphasize education: a big key in moving forward. As G.I. Joe used to say, *Knowing* is half the battle", which means the other half is *Doing*. Talk is cheap, and the importance of actually doing things cannot be overstated.

The first parts of this book will discuss some important definitions, then further analyze and discuss the causes of our current predicaments. Later I will present information to help clarify the underlying aspects of health for the individual and the population, and then relate things that can be done to promote health for each individual as well as changes that can be made to promote health on a broader scale.

I will try to explain things succinctly and clearly as I am able, rather than using medical lingo that may be confusing. Any medical folk reading this book (and I hope there will be at least a few who will investigate these pages) may take this as a negative, but this book is really not designed for them. I spent years trying to convince my colleagues that their training was limited and then I tried to get them enthused about some of the things I have become excited about; but I gave up on that quite some time ago. I do welcome, though, those individuals who approach me with genuine interest.

I think most of us have come to realize that people tend to cling to their ideas, and it is very difficult to change someone's ingrained opinion. This is why it generally takes fifty years or more to affect significant positive change in medicine or other industries. Basically, the "old guard" has to move on and make way for the new, with hopes that the young grow up holding new ideas as "normal" and with greater acceptance for alternative solutions in general.

Unfortunately the world is still "flat" for many of our doctors. This book is my attempt to make it appear "rounder" for as many people as possible.

SECTION I

INTEGRATIVE MEDICINE: CONCEPTS AND PRACTICE

Having all the pieces of a puzzle is critical to seeing the whole picture. Putting them together in the proper way takes time and patience. In this first section, I describe some terms and concepts that are important in understanding integrative medicine and health. I explain some important principles guiding integrative practice, and I outline the goals and priorities representing key differences between integrative medicine and conventional medical practice. Changing the paradigm for medical education and medical practice is very important to changing the health of our population for the future; this is also the first step in changing one's own individual health.

CHAPTER 1 – DEFINITIONS

In order to communicate with someone it certainly helps to speak the same language and, at least, have a similar understanding of what words mean. There have been many terms used in nonconventional fields of medicine that have not necessarily been well defined for the general population. I will go through some of them and offer my definitions and explanations so that it will be easier to understand what I'm talking about when they appear in this text. Perhaps, eventually, our culture will have more familiarity with these concepts, and they may even acquire totally different definitions than what I am about to suggest; after all, a "cell phone" is not something a prison inmate uses to call home, and "surfing the web" is not how a spider gets around his home. These terms have new meaning in a modern context.

Conventional, or Allopathic Medicine

I use the term "conventional medicine" quite a bit and, to me, it refers to the current type of mainstream medical practice in the U.S. that leans toward reductionist diagnoses and has a preference for pharmacological or surgical therapies. I use it to describe the system of medicine taught in our medical schools in this country. This is the form we are all most familiar with from TV shows and personal experience seeing a modern MD or DO. The term "allopathic" is more correct, basically meaning it is a system of medicine that attempts to relieve suffering. This generally translates to a focus on symptomatic relief only.

The strengths of conventional/allopathic medicine are a strong foundation in basic science; the technological and scientific advances made in urgent and emergency medical care, surgery, radiology, intensive care,

11

pharmacology and other more modern-science based aspects of medical care we have in developed countries. Our mainstream medicine has made some incredible achievements in terms of saving lives in acute situations, treating serious problems in many cases, and making diagnoses through laboratory or radiological testing.

I make some negative comments about conventional medicine throughout this book, but this is because this book concerns the areas where conventional medicine fails us. I want to make it very clear that what we have achieved in conventional medical practice in this country and other technologically-advanced nations is nothing short of amazing and, it seems, advances continue to be made every day. I use my conventional training constantly, and I am vastly more effective as a healer because of it.

The problem lies with the fact that conventional medicine possesses a very narrow perspective on human disease and complaints. Conventional practitioners are not taught enough theory and philosophy outside the narrow conventional principles. It's a lot like Newtonian physics versus quantum physics. The scientific community believed so deeply in the concrete principles and rules identified by Sir Isaac Newton that when Einstein and others began to reveal these other guiding forces and principles in the universe which conflict terribly with some of Newton's principles, they just couldn't handle the discord and cognitive dissonance that resulted.

Both sets of principles just happen to coexist in the same world it seems, and one doesn't have to replace the other. In fact, it is most beneficial to understand both systems and sets of principles. We have a similar situation in medicine. Conventional training is much like Newtonian physics where there are sets of defined concrete principles from our current accepted basic science principles and treatment algorithms that tell us what to do. The problem is there are many other truths about our health and living in the human condition, many of which lie outside the understanding of conventional principles, but are no less real or important.

Conventional medicine, in my opinion, is an important part of integrative medicine overall, but one really needs to incorporate many other types of knowledge and practice to be an effective practitioner and healer.

Complementary and Alternative Medicine

These terms are used to describe those nonconventional aspects of health and healing I mentioned above. They are terms, I believe, coined by conventional providers with the term "alternative" coming first. That term suggests those types of practices are outside the norm and has a negative connotation in my opinion. It was usually used in a negative way through my medical training, and I don't use that term to describe the way I practice medicine today. I generally believe there is no alternative to good medicine, and I practice the best medicine I can. This includes the best aspects of conventional medicine in addition to various other styles and approaches.

There is also a large community of practitioners who do refer to themselves as alternative practitioners, and they see that distinction as being important. I think this is because they want to be seen as totally separate and different from conventional medicine. This may include people practicing acupuncture, herbalism, iridology, energy medicine of various types, chiropractic, massage, reflexology or many other forms of healing.

These practitioners are often people who think conventional medicine is inherently or even totally bad medicine in principle and practice, and they attract patients who agree with this stance. I don't agree with this attitude, which is why I use the term "integrative" for my style of practice. I think we should use all these skills for what they do best because each has something beneficial to offer.

The term "complementary" is much more recent and, as the name suggests, it is used to denote a more inclusive feel. It suggests that nonconventional medical practices may be used in harmony with conventional medicine and complement or enhance the benefits for the patient. Psychiatry is one area this has been fairly well accepted. Patients are offered training in meditation, hypnosis, guided imagery or other mind-body therapies along with their conventional psychiatric care which may include medications and mainstream counseling and therapy. Harvard even has their school of mind-body medicine within the medical school.

Complementary medicine is catching on in this country to be sure. The federal government has a division of complementary and alternative medicine (often referred to as "CAM") within the NIH (National Institute of Health), but it is grossly underfunded relative to the conventional areas of study (e.g. drugs, surgery, radiology), and they somehow manage to report negative results for CAM therapies much more often than positive ones. This is because the funding they do receive comes from the pharmaceutical company-controlled government and comes with a serious bias attached.

More than a third of U.S. medical schools now actually have some form of CAM curriculum, which may be a very positive step. I would be more excited about this if it weren't for the fact the general attitude of the allopathic medical institutions may remain somewhat negative and the teaching may actually focus only on awareness of these therapies, rather than meaningful skills training. "Awareness" often just entails teaching about what these therapies are and showing how they are ineffective or harmful. Doctors may come out of their training with a more informed view but still a very negative one; even more negative possibly, because they could have been shown only a negative perspective rather than leaving them with a general ignorance which would have allowed the more open-minded among them to still at least tolerate the use of these therapies for their patients.

I'll try to be optimistic, but I'll be much happier when our medical schools actually begin to incorporate effective complementary medical theories and skills into the formal curriculum. They should begin to offer electives related to skill sets such as acupuncture, musculoskeletal manipulation, clinical nutrition, bio-identical hormone therapy, energy medicine practices and other practices that show promise. I fear this sort of educational curriculum is still a long way off.

Traditional Medicine

I don't like the typical use of this term in our culture. I don't know what it is supposed to mean in this country, and it annoys me when people use it to refer to the way we generally practice medicine in this country today. That's the way it is usually used when I hear it, and I prefer the term "conventional medicine" to describe our modern mainstream way of doing things.

The term "tradition" to me suggests something that has been done for a really long time, like when you say "it was a culture steeped in tradition". When Americans use it to describe our modern medicine it just reminds me of how little cultural identity and tradition this country really has.

I could see using the term "traditional Chinese medicine" to refer to the use of herbs and acupuncture in their healing system, rather than their modern one which has incorporated much of Western civilization's current technology. I could see saying the traditional medicine of India is Ayurveda, or using the term to describe shamanistic and indigenous medical practices from more primitive cultures of the world.

It bugs me, though, when the term is used to refer to America's modern style of medicine, when our practices have changed tremendously over just the last fifty years. Our modern medical knowledge and practice grows and changes on a continuous basis. This is the complete opposite of tradition, isn't it? Tradition should indicate something that hasn't changed in a really long time, don't you think? I suggest we just avoid this term, unless we're talking about something that has been done for at least a hundred years or so.

Holistic Medicine

I want to make it clear this is not at all an actual system of healing or a type of medical training. It is just a concept of medical practice, suggesting it involves a more comprehensive way of looking at the patient. Holism in medicine involves understanding not just the physical and physiological, but also the psychological, emotional and spiritual aspects of the person in question and how these factors play into their illness. Most nonconventional types of practitioners have a relatively holistic view in my experience; and those concepts are typical in the training for things like naturopathy, chiropractic, acupuncture, herbalism and other common complementary and alternative practices.

There is an American Board of Integrative and Holistic Medicine in the U.S., which offers medical providers a broad perspective on other systems of healing and nonconventional methods in medicine. It is a good organization, in that it gives like-minded practitioners a forum in which to meet others with an interest in providing better medical care with more attention to the diverse interests of the American patient. They offer a "board certification" that is recognized among the integrative medical community but not by the conventional medical world at this point. The testing for this board certification is based on greater knowledge in a broad array of integrative and alternative medical topics, but it is not currently based on new procedural training or intensive study in any particular area.

In my opinion one should be wary of people who advertise themselves as simply "holistic medical providers" or something similar. It is important to find out what sort of formal training or credentials these people have by looking them up on the internet or researching them in some other way, as well as interviewing them thoroughly during the course of your first interaction. There are certainly some extremely knowledgeable folks out there with no formal training who can do a lot of good for you, but there are also some people advertising their services who are frankly being grandiose or dishonest.

This is not to say you should place your complete trust in any medical provider at all just because they do have some kind of certification or training. Goodness knows I've met some medical doctors whom I would not trust with anyone's care, and conventional medical providers are responsible for many thousands of injuries and deaths every year due to medical mistakes. I'm just suggesting you be wary of this term "holistic", because it really doesn't mean anything specific or concrete when it comes to medical providers.

Homeopathic Medicine or Homeopathy

I have many people ask me if I am a homeopathic type of provider or they tell others that I am "homeopathic". I believe the term they are really looking for is "holistic", as discussed above. People in this country frequently seem to confuse these two terms. I've described the term holistic above as referring to an inclusive, broad sort of practice in medicine that tends to focus on natural and non-pharmacologic treatments, and this is how most Americans seem to use the term homeopathic as well. This is completely wrong.

Homeopathy is actually a distinct system of medical philosophy, diagnosis and treatment that was founded in Germany well over one hundred years ago. So it could actually be referred to as a "traditional" type of German medicine I suppose. Its development is credited to Samuel Hahnemann, circa 1796. The name means "same suffering" in Greek, and the practice involves using substances which evoke certain symptoms in people to treat those same symptoms or an illness exhibiting those symptoms. This follows the concept of a "law of similars". A good example is to use the diluted essence of red onion (*allium cepa*) to correct allergy symptoms; real red onion will cause irritated eyes and a runny nose, so the treatment is supposed to negate those same symptoms.

Homeopathy works by using extremely diluted solutions of those substances with no real detectable substance in them any longer (this is where most Americans say "huh?"). The diluted extracts are then bottled as liquid or made into little white sugar pills, or possibly mixed into creams or lotions for topical use. Labels on these treatments show such ingredients like *arnica montana*, which is used for bruises and minor trauma; or magnesium, which is used for relaxation and decreasing muscle tension (the real substance of Mg does those things also, so it seems to me these treatments don't always work in an opposite manner). Harmful substances such as mercury and arsenic may be represented, which I suspect are there to reverse the symptoms seen from poisoning with those toxic metals.

Many other sorts of substances can be found listed in these products as well. You have to be careful about some products listed as homeopathic here in the U.S. now. Some manufacturers are putting measurable, therapeutic amounts of various substances into products, in combination with some truly homeopathically diluted items. They are most likely doing this to capture the more "naturally" inclined consumer, but it is a clear case of fraud in my opinion. A person may experience some adverse effects from the pharmacologically-dosed items in these products; this is not really possible with a truly homeopathic agent.

The whole system of homeopathic medicine is extremely complicated and takes its own long course of training over periods of years to master. A true homeopathic provider, similar to an herbalist, should make specific remedies for patients based on their problems and other specific circumstances for them as an individual. There are also some standard starting mixtures for typical common medical problems, and these are widely effective as well. I'm sure many of you have seen these sorts of remedies at the store for things like teething, anxiety and nerves, sleep aid, headache, colic, allergies and other conditions.

The idea behind it is the essence of that substance being used is still in the water, even after the substance itself has been diluted into oblivion; and your body will recognize that energetic essence or resonance and react to it in such a way as to correct the symptoms or imbalances it would have caused in the body. The expected result is therefore resolution of illness symptoms, resulting from the human body making the necessary corrections.

Homeopathy is therefore a form of energy medicine with an oral, topical or injected physical delivery system. This is a very tough concept for many Americans to get their heads around, and I think most people assume that they are more like herbal remedies. When I explain to people there is actually no real detectable substance within most of these remedies, I generally get the standard Western-minded skeptical "well then how do they work?" response. The answer is a complicated one involving quantum mechanics, bioenergetics and vibrational harmonics, but I assure you there is a sound scientific basis. There have also been numerous clinical studies of different homeopathic remedies for various clinical conditions showing a positive effect of treatment, so many of them are becoming accepted by conventional practitioners as well (though they usually don't know how they are supposed to work either, and are just as confused when I try to explain it to them).

I would assert that health care practitioners should not be described as "homeopathic" unless they have truly had training in the field of homeopathy. A true homeopath is a skilled provider trained for years in a specific system of healing. An understanding of these concepts and the use of some common homeopathic preparations are important and common among integrative practitioners, but it is quite rare to find someone with true homeopathic training. I am certainly not a homeopathic practitioner myself; not yet, that is.

Osteopathic Medicine

An osteopath is a doctor who completed the same amount of schooling and training as an MD including an undergraduate bachelor's degree and then four years of medical school, in this case an osteopathic medical school, achieving the "DO" degree, then going on to internship and residency training just like an MD physician. There is the same level of education and very similar content these days. An osteopath is, for the most part, a conventional medical practitioner with some additional training and a traditionally different philosophy.

Many people think of osteopathy as just a form of skeletal manipulation similar to chiropractic medicine, but it is more than that (as is chiropractic practice, to be fair). A doctor from Missouri, Andrew Taylor Still, developed osteopathy in the late 1800's. He trained as an MD under his father, and later at a medical university in Kansas. After three of his children died of meningitis he decided the conventional way of practice of the day was very flawed, and he pioneered a new way of thinking and practicing medicine (this is all available on Wikipedia, if you want to read about it). He founded the first school for osteopathic medicine in Kirksville, MO in 1892, and it is still there, going strong. I actually applied to this school myself and wanted to be an osteopath more than an MD because of their philosophy and training. But I went the MD route instead to stay closer to home.

The philosophies of osteopathy involve the practice of correcting musculoskeletal and non-skeletal systemic problems through spinal, cranial and joint manipulation. It also involves the philosophy of treating the patient as a whole person with attention to other aspects of their overall health and being. This was certainly an attempt at a more holistic approach to medical care than the standard practice of the day in the 1800's (and today as well), which was overly problem-focused in Dr. Still's opinion.

The manipulation aspect, like chiropractic theory, is founded on the principle that the nervous system controls the function of organs to some extent, and if proper alignment of the spine is maintained, the signals will keep traveling from the central nervous system to the periphery flowing like they are supposed to. There are also systems of blood, lymphatic, cerebrospinal fluid, and possibly energy that flow around the body, which need to be kept in proper working order through alignment of the skeletal system as well. It is a way of relating body structure to body function.

Osteopathy, as well as other types of treatment termed "manual" therapies, involves the practitioner actually putting his/her hands on the patient in a therapeutic way (i.e. chiropractic, massage, acupuncture). It is a very useful adjunct to other aspects of clinical medicine and has been shown to work very well for a wide range of issues both skeletal and non-skeletal medical complaints. There are also visceral osteopaths who attempt to directly manipulate your internal organs. Osteopathy is another excellent tool to have in one's medical toolbox. The practice seems to be very provider-dependent, however; some people will never be good at it no matter how hard they train while others seem to be able to heal people almost effortlessly (these are the ones, of course, that a patient should seek out).

In the beginning osteopathic medicine was not accepted at all by conventional medical practitioners (I know, shocking, right?). It took decades before it gained respect and began being accepted into conventional residency training programs alongside MD graduates. Until then, osteopaths had their own postgraduate training at their own institutions, which were very few in number. The process of integration was slow and gradual but is pretty complete now, and there is really little or no distinction between an MD and a DO (doctor of osteopathy) these days in terms of education and practice. Osteopathic students currently still learn about musculoskeletal manipulation, but they don't have to master it or use it in practice.

Unfortunately, in my experience, the majority of modern osteopaths do not utilize manipulation in their practices. For some prospective medical students it seems an osteopathic school became their fallback option when they couldn't get into a more competitive MD program. I hate to propagate this unfair stereotype of osteopaths because many of them truly have a passion for manipulation and the osteopathic philosophies of practice. Again, these are the ones to seek out. I know many osteopathic graduates who have gone into very specialized medical fields when the whole tradition holds comprehensive primary care at its core. Most DO's are now indistinguishable from MD's in attitude and practice, with the same narrow-minded views on medicine. It seems that the AMA has now gotten a grip on them too.

Again, if looking for a true osteopath, I suggest calling around and finding someone who utilizes manipulation as a significant part of their practice. This doesn't mean they practice in a nonconventional way in general. They may still just prescribe drugs for symptoms otherwise; but it does define the difference between an MD and a DO and would therefore be the typical reason why a person would seek out the DO over the MD.

Naturopathic Medicine

The concept of naturopathic medicine involves using only "natural" methods for the treatment of illnesses. This typically includes diet and lifestyle interventions, nutritional items as therapies, lots of herbs, possibly homeopathic remedies, and certain types of manipulation like massage and craniosacral therapy. In some states it can also entail the use of prescription drugs, though this may seem like heresy to some.

Some naturopaths incorporate acupuncture and some Eastern herbals like those found in traditional Chinese or Ayurvedic medicine. Some states license naturopathic physicians for limited prescriptive authority, and they may prescribe pharmaceuticals based on natural substances, or otherwise depending on individual state rules. There are currently about a dozen states allowing this.

I urge caution in selecting a naturopathic practitioner because there is a large group of people calling themselves naturopaths who have obtained a more limited degree based on home study courses, but they still may use the designation "ND" after their name. These people have done extensive study into the science and book knowledge of nutrition and natural medicine but have not had clinical instruction. They will not be licensed for prescription capacity anywhere and should not be using the designation "naturopathic physician". This term is reserved for those who attended a four-year naturopathic college with clinical training (or an even longer program if they trained in acupuncture as well).

Naturopathic physicians do not have to attend a residency program after graduation like a DO or an MD, so they still don't have hospital-based medical knowledge or skills in emergency procedures, intensive care, surgery or obstetrics. Some do receive training in basic office procedures including minor skin-level excisions, biopsies and gynecological procedures.

As in other medical disciplines, there is a wide range of attitude, skill level and practice philosophy among naturopaths. Some are totally about using herbs and nutrition, some use a lot of homeopathic remedies, some do acupuncture, and some have training in hormonal therapies. Still others, for example, may prescribe loads of narcotics for chronic pain patients. Most are very committed to correcting medical problems without reliance on drugs. It is a very eclectic group, and it is important to figure out what scope of training a given naturopath has, rather than assuming they are all practicing the same.

Some naturopaths work well with allopathic physicians in their community or even within the same medical practice or organization. Cancer therapy is one area where this type of collegial relationship is increasingly common, much to the benefit of the cancer patients receiving this integrated care. Most naturopaths, however, operate quite separate from the conventional providers in their community. This is not because they don't want to associate with allopathic physicians. In most cases it is due to disdain and scorn from the conventional side. Unfortunately most of my conventionally trained colleagues are not open-minded about naturopathy and remain very ignorant of its benefits.

Positive community relationships are frequently found between naturopaths and other local complementary providers such as massage therapists, acupuncturists and chiropractors. There are also growing numbers of conventionally trained physicians like myself, "recovering allopaths" if you will, who seek out professional relationships and cross-refer with their local naturopaths and other complementary providers. In my opinion this type of networking tremendously improves patient care and health outcomes.

I think the basic training common to naturopathic programs should be taught to all medical providers. A solid understanding of diet and nutrition physiology is essential to any successful mode of healing. Without a doubt, their teaching on these issues is far superior to what is taught in conventional MD and DO programs. I have met a lot of naturopaths at integrative medicine conferences and many of them are fantastic healers and clinicians. Of course, as with conventional doctors or any other professional occupation, there are some who are incompetent.

I suggest seeing a naturopathic physician every couple years for a physical and wellness counseling. Their knowledge is essential to maintaining proper health and avoidance of chronic medical problems. I also suggest seeing a naturopath for any chronic internal medicine problem or mental disorder, high blood pressure, diabetes, high cholesterol, fibromyalgia and other chronic fatigue syndromes, dementia, hormonal disorders, autism, ADHD, obesity and many other issues. Their approach can often fix some of these problems without drugs or decrease the need for drug therapy to some extent. Their expertise is a very useful adjunct to allopathic care for any chronic problem.

Functional Medicine

This is a modern scientific medical system that also has a very holistic approach and comprehensive individualized view of the patient. The Institute for Functional Medicine (IFM) originated in the 1980's and, it seems, has grown tremendously in recent years. Dr. Jeff Bland, an extremely bright and scientifically knowledgeable man, who is a pharmacologist by training and not a clinician, founded this system. Functional medicine is firmly grounded in biochemistry and science. Bland was joined by many others from various fields including MD, DO, and naturopathic physicians, chiropractors and others who believe in the principles of treating medical problems based on addressing the causative factors rather than just treating symptoms.

Functional medicine, as the name implies, involves understanding and manipulating how we truly function on a molecular and physiological level as well as addressing psychological and structural function issues. This is a group of practitioners who have come up with an effective and sensible model of medicine that pays attention to a "matrix" of biochemical, structural, environmental and mind-body issues affecting one's health. This approach allows an IFM practitioner to treat or even cure medical problems by identifying and addressing the causative factors.

These ideas in my opinion are at the essence of what I think integrative medicine is and all good medicine should be. I have belonged to the organization as a member and have grown tremendously in my clinical practice as a result. Functional medicine is not really its own system of healing or a distinct specialty in medicine at this point, but at the time of this writing, the IFM has started a "fellowship" training program and certification which may catch on and achieve wide recognition at some point. For now, any provider listed as an IFM trainee on his/her website is probably someone to be trusted and, I suspect, should yield better results.

Any provider who has completed certification is likely to be an effective healer and clinician.

Dr. Mark Hyman and other members of the IFM have recently (2009-10) spoken to congress in an attempt to help with our current health care crisis. They have outlined a number of points where following a functional medicine model could cut the cost and improve the quality of health care in this country. It makes complete sense to me. I have seen these principles improve the health of my own patients and decrease their individual health costs for sure. I know it can work.

Orthomolecular Medicine

This is more of a philosophical and scientific principle in medicine rather than a system of healing or type of practice. It is not a common term, and because of this, it is difficult to find any medical providers practicing "orthomolecular medicine". It is founded on the idea that clinical changes in a patient's medical condition can be affected by using large doses of specific nutrients, vitamins, minerals, or other internally present biological molecules in a manner that makes sense given the individual's problems and the known physiology of the situation.

This concept is built upon the work of pioneering individuals like Linus Pauling and Abram Hoffer. I mention it here simply because I may use the term later in the book. It is here, rather than in the chapter on guiding principles that follows, because there is an actual organization for these types of practitioners with their own conferences and publications.

Environmental Medicine

This field of medicine has been around formally since the 1960's. Prior to the formation of the American Academy of Environmental Medicine (AAEM) there was the Society for Clinical Ecology founded by Theron Randolph, MD and others with similar interest and expertise in environmental factors behind illness conditions. Environmental medicine involves understanding and modifying the causes of illness that come from our environment, as well as treating the resulting disease states. It does not directly deal with the healing of our world or the cleaning up of our environment itself. This is truly a crucial part of our own healing I believe, and I will address this topic later in this book in greater detail. It is a subject that has been sadly neglected in conventional medical training.

The AAEM is currently a relatively small organization of physicians and other medical practitioners who learn skills needed to effectively treat problems related to allergies, environmental toxicity and chemical sensitivities. There are components of diet and nutrition, hormonal balance and other general integrative topics as well, but the organization focuses on issues of detoxification, allergy identification and elimination (including chemical allergies or sensitivities), and nutritional support for chronic conditions.

This is a field of growing importance as our world becomes more and more toxic and dangerous to live in. Currently, allergy problems are the most common reasons for visits to primary care physicians in the U.S. Allergy is a classic environmental illness. Other organizations have also begun to focus some conferences on the role of the environment in health and disease as well. I may be a bit biased because I currently sit on the board, but I feel the AAEM has the best training and treatment methods available for chemical toxicity issues, sensitivities and allergies to foods or inhaled antigens.

To anyone suffering from problems with environmental illness such as allergy, mold sensitivity or toxicity, chemical toxicity or sensitivity, I suggest looking at the AAEM website (aaemonline.org) for a practitioner nearby.

Integrative Medicine

This is my preferred term for the type of medicine I practice. This term I hope will eventually catch on and become the new paradigm for medical practice in this country and the world. If so, I suppose it will become "conventional" medicine (but still not "allopathic") and then I'll have to stop badmouthing conventional medicine, as long as it continues to breed an attitude of learning and discovery, rather than getting mired in its own dogma like every other generation seems to.

My idea of integrative medicine, as the name implies, involves blending every aspect of medical knowledge and understanding a practitioner can, in order to reach a diagnosis based on upstream concepts and a treatment plan using a very wide range of different therapies, tailored to the individual patient. The concept of a toolbox is widely used among medical practitioners. With integrative medicine, the clinician has the largest and most diverse toolbox imaginable because, in theory, the tools of every other system of medicine and healing are included. At this point, this requires lots of training from a variety of sources to obtain such diverse skills. As I mentioned, there is not a defined integrative medicine specialty available yet with its own curriculum or compiled knowledge.

There are some guiding principles I find vital to the process of integrative medicine. These include, for example, such items as thinking upstream to find the underlying causes, understanding of individual differences and needs, practicing individualized medicine rather than following rigid algorithms and protocols, and understanding the diverse array of possible causes of disease. Integrative medicine also includes the principles of holistic medicine because it necessitates a view of the whole person and all their aspects of health. I will describe certain aspects of integrative medicine in more detail shortly.

In my opinion integrative medicine has to involve an understanding of current conventional medical practice, since there is great power in those therapies and it is the most common system of treatment in our population right now. Therefore I still consider an acupuncturist who also has herbal training to be a complementary provider, and not an integrative provider per se. I also think an integrative provider should have training in clinical and medical nutrition, detoxification, hormone therapies and, ideally, some form of manual therapy or energetic healing modality.

Again, manual therapies include musculoskeletal manipulation (i.e. chiropractic or osteopathic sorts of treatments), reflexology, acupuncture or acupressure, massage, and perhaps some other skills. Basically, they involve a practitioner getting his/her hands on the patient in a therapeutic fashion. Energetic treatments include acupuncture as well as homeopathy, reiki, healing touch, thoughtfield therapy, the use of bioenergetic machines and various other approaches.

I am somewhat particular about whom I think should be allowed to call themselves an integrative medicine practitioner. I think some have realized the term is attractive to a growing number of prospective patients; they may label themselves as such just to attract patients who would typically be looking for complementary and alternative medical practitioners, but want the security of a conventionally-trained physician as well. Some may term themselves integrative because, for example, they give B-12 shots and have a massage therapist in their office, or because they perform hypnosis and teach their patients to do guided imagery.

I'm not sure what the field is going to entail when it is finally defined more officially, but there will likely be some basic requirements and lots of "elective" expertise. Just like family doctors may or may not do obstetrics, hospital care, endoscopy or certain types of surgery; they are required to have a certain understanding of these things even if they do not perform them regularly in practice. Integrative medicine is a similar multidimensional situation, and the provider should at least have the understanding to refer patients appropriately for those other therapies when they do not perform them themselves.

At the time of the writing of this book, there are some diverse groups attempting to create a national standard for integrative medicine. The goal is a nationally recognized board certification and educational standard. There are groups from the academic realm, as well as practitioner-based groups, trying to collaborate in this endeavor. I am not sure how it will turn out, but I am concerned the academic world will have too much influence over the process. This is concerning to me because the university-based integrative medicine programs, in my opinion, are far too conservative in their practice; they don't go nearly far enough "outside the box". Those of us in practitioner-based integrative medicine groups often refer to the academic curriculum as integrative medicine "lite", and view their approach as only part way to the goal.

Whatever comes next for healthcare in the U.S., I hope integrative medicine plays an increasing role and gains more formal recognition. Biased as my opinion might be, I feel this concept is definitely something everyone should watch out for and throw their support behind. Integrative medicine certainly represents progressive thinking and an ever-improving approach to health and medicine. This is something we need, now more than ever.

Chapter 2 – Guiding Principles of Integrative Medicine

This section addresses some of the philosophical and intellectual principles important to the practice of integrative medicine and effective medicine in general. I will try to explain these ideas in plain English without using an excessive amount scientific terminology or boring research. This background will make it easier to understand terms and concepts that are presented later in this book.

Holism

As I mentioned earlier, holism refers to making an effort to look at the comprehensive picture and all aspects of the person's health and being. Perhaps it should be spelled with a "w" to reflect the appreciation of the whole. It is a very important philosophy shared by most complementary medical and integrative medicine fields. It suggests to me that if I have not been successful yet in my treatment plan, then perhaps there is some component I have missed. I suppose this could also be seen as "hole-ism", suggesting there is a hole in my theory somewhere if I'm not successful. Maybe that's why there's no "w".

Balance and "homeostasis"

This is an extremely important concept and seems obvious and intuitive. We have all heard the adage "you can have too much of a good thing", and this is true. The term homeostasis refers to that dynamic balance in the body's physiology operating normally in a healthy individual. It is important to understand that this is not at all the same meaning as "equilibrium", which refers to equality on both sides of the scale. That would be the classic general concept of balance with things being equal on both sides of the equation. An example may be that a man has maintained his equilibrium because he is still standing up straight.

Inside our bodies, things are certainly NOT equal on both sides of the equation in many cases. We keep about thirty times more sodium outside our cells than inside and thirty times more potassium inside the cells than there is outside. We have to maintain these steep gradients (differences on one side from the other) in order to have dynamic movement across the cell membrane and resulting electrical signaling that makes so many of our cellular processes work. Great amounts of energy are used constantly to maintain this distinct IM-balance, which is essential to homeostasis. This is a technical example, but it is one that is extremely important to life.

Easier examples of our necessary imbalances are the observation that there is far more water under our skin than outside our skin (an advantage we have over amphibians), and the body's temperature is often maintained very different from the surrounding ambient temperature (an advantage we have over reptiles). If one's body temperature was to fall to meet room temperature (from your typical 98 degrees down to 70) then it would truly be at equilibrium, but that person would be dead.

So much about remaining alive in a biological sense depends upon the maintenance of biochemical imbalance rather than equilibrium. The human body is constantly expending energy and struggling to maintain its necessary biochemical gradients and metabolic processes. This includes simultaneously breaking down and building up of organs and tissues. The result is sort of an overall balanced dynamic disequilibrium needed to keep cycles moving and cells dying and regenerating; we call all this "homeostasis".

Good examples of where balance is a problem in clinical medicine involve therapies like nutrients, hormones and, of course, prescription drugs. We need to keep salt and water intake within a certain balance. Relative levels of testosterone and estrogen are very important, but very different, for both sexes. We are all quite familiar with the practice of prescribing a new drug to deal with the side effects caused by the first one, and so on and so forth. Each drug, it seems, does more to push the body's physiology out of balance, and the problem often gets worse rather than better with the addition of more drugs.

Toxins and toxicity

A toxin is any substance that causes biochemical damage in some fashion to our cells and tissues. These can come from the body's own processes in the form of metabolic byproducts or products of digestion, bacteria or other organisms which are living in or infecting the body. They can come from the environment in sources like food, water or air. Common sources of toxins today involve most man-made items, from food and cosmetics (items marketed for use in or on your body) to paint and other industrial chemicals within household products.

Other, more unusual, toxic influences, may include electromagnetic radiation from appliances, cell phones and electrical power lines, even negative emotions coming from others or originating within one's self. This may sound hokey now, but stay tuned.

Many of us willingly put various toxins into and onto ourselves every day. An obvious one is cigarette smoke, but also think of the engine exhaust inhaled in traffic or at work during the day. You know that alcohol is a toxin, I would hope, since the term for having too much is "in-*toxic*-ated". Makeup, perfume and fragrances, fluoride from toothpaste, artificial sweeteners (which become formaldehyde inside the body), plastic residues, pesticides, nitrites, and other food additives are just a few which people are likely exposed to daily. There's much more to say on this topic later.

Biochemical individuality

This is a critical concept to understand, and once understood, a patient will be way ahead of most of doctors in terms of appreciating why a person needs to be treated as an individual and not just like everyone else. It is a key principle in integrative medicine, and every clinician needs to have a grasp of it to be truly effective. This idea was developed by early thinkers on the subject including Bruce Ames, Roger Williams, and Linus Pauling.

Basically it means that each of us has specific needs in terms of nutrient intake and certain other environmental factors. Good examples are phenylketonuria (PKU) and Wilson's disease (not to be confused with "Wilson's Syndrome" which involves thyroid and adrenal problems). These are examples of the conditions we term "inborn errors of metabolism", suggesting they are genetic conditions which make some physiologic process or processes work incorrectly.

In PKU, individuals cannot properly metabolize the amino acid phenylalanine; if they consume too much of it, there may be a toxic accumulation leading to brain damage and mental retardation. The problem is that phenylalanine is an "essential amino acid" which means it is necessary for human life and must be obtained from food; the body can't make it on its own like it can with most amino acids. The treatment for this condition is a special diet that confers just the right amount of phenylalanine and prevents overload in the brain with its toxic effects (too much of a good thing it might be said, which is apparently different for everyone).

Wilson's disease is another example; it involves a toxic accumulation of copper in the body. The patient assimilates copper too avidly and cannot seem to excrete it properly. The end result of the excess copper is brain injury, mental retardation, and possibly other neurological or immune problems. The excess copper can be cleared out with chelating medications such as penicillamine; further accumulation can then be prevented by watching copper intake in the diet and taking extra supplementation of zinc, which competes for absorption with copper. So, this is again something that can be controlled largely through diet, as long as the proper diagnosis is made and the biochemistry is adequately understood.

Conventional medical training suggests these types of conditions are rare, but they are just considering the ones with these dramatic manifestations. Each discrete disorder may be quite rare in and of itself, but these types of problems are very common when taken as a whole concept. Each of the aforementioned conditions, along with many others like sickle cell anemia, cystic fibrosis and many others, only requires a single DNA base pair mistake. We call these "point mutations" or "single nucleotide polymorphisms" (SNP's, or "snips"), and there are an estimated 30,000-plus possible SNP's in humans causing a wide spectrum of differences in us metabolically. Being different is the rule rather than the exception.

In his book *Nutrition Against Disease,* Roger Williams details a number of such individual biochemical differences he identified in humans and other animals, even many-fold differences in specific physiologic functions or nutrient needs between genetically identical individuals (i.e. twins, quadruplets). Many of them do not cause noticeable disease, and some of them may in fact confer some sort of advantage.

A clinical example that has been extensively studied in recent years involves folic acid metabolism and a point mutation in the MTHFR gene (methylene tetrahydrofolate reductase) which codes for the enzyme that helps recycle folic acid so it can perform the process of methylation.

Methylation is important for many metabolic functions including detoxification, gene expression, and the clearance of the harmful metabolite homocysteine. It has been shown that people with a mutation here may be prone to cardiovascular disease, heart attacks, and chronic depression as well as other problems.

The MTHFR mutation is a good example because somewhere between ten and thirty percent of us have a variation in this gene! I bet you'll look it up now won't you? It is suspected that an individual with this type of mutation may help to significantly prevent negative complications such as cardiovascular disease and depression by supplementing with large amounts of methylated folic acid, vitamin B-12 and maybe some other nutrients. We don't know for sure yet, and you can bet that no drug company will be funding a large enough study to properly validate this idea.

Biochemical individuality is the rule and an extremely important concept in medicine. Attention to this phenomenon is imperative in providing the best medical care possible. Following some once-size-fits-nobody standard of medical practice ignores these critical, unique differences among us.

Genetics and Epigenetics

I touched on the idea of genetics in the preceding paragraphs, and I suspect this is not a new concept for most people. In addition to DNA mutation, genetic problems can also involve having the wrong number of chromosomes such as in Turner Syndrome. This is when a female has just one X chromosome and no second sex chromosome; we term them "XO" rather than XY (male) or XX (female). They tend to be small individuals, with other subtle structural differences, and are infertile. Other types of sex chromosome imbalances result in Klinefelter's syndrome (XXY) or perhaps the "super male" syndrome (XYY). Down's Syndrome is a well-known case of having an extra autosomal (non-sex related) chromosome, more appropriately called "trisomy 21", to describe the presence of the extra chromosome number 21.

Molecular genetics also involves the more complex details of DNA being copied properly when cells divide, being read to generate RNA and then expressed as proteins, transfer RNA or ribosomal RNA (the last two versions are used in the "reading" of the "messenger RNA" to generate proteins in a process called translation). When the DNA is misread, a mutation results that can be propagated on to every future cell.

Genetics is a very complicated field of study these days, much more so than when Gregor Mendel was cross-pollinating his pea plants long ago. Now we have molecular genetics showing us the vast expanse of our DNA strands and all their potential information and, more recently, the field of "epigenetics".

Epigenetics is a new philosophy or field of understanding that involves a deeper understanding of gene *expression*. We have discovered through the Human Genome Project and other studies that most of our genes are not actually used at all times in any given cell type, and they are used to varying degrees at various times. Every cell in an individual's body supposedly holds the same chromosomes, genes and set of instructions. However, there is a very different set of genes activated in a brain cell from a bladder cell for example; all the unnecessary genes are turned off and lying dormant. The manner in which genes get turned on and off involves, in some cases, nutritional factors spanning multiple generations.

Some of the genes that get turned off include the ones for continued growth and replication. After all we don't want the liver to just keep growing in size until it no longer fits in the abdomen; nor do we want our arms and legs to keep getting longer. If a mutation occurs in one of these genes due to nutritional deficiency (because it takes certain nutrients to keep them turned off), or toxin exposure (i.e. benzene, nitrites, fluoride, UV light, etc.) cancer may result if the mutation allows the transformed cells to start growing beyond their normal boundaries.

Since some of us have a genetically stronger need for certain nutrients, some of us are more genetically prone to cancer and other diseases if we don't get our own individually required amounts of those nutrients. If we knew what our specific individual needs were, we could just adjust our diet or take the necessary supplements and conceivably prevent some diseases and live longer. I believe that was the goal of the Human Genome Project, which was supposed to be completed around 2005. What happened to that anyway? I personally think that drug companies and other medical industries probably paid to keep the results quiet. But maybe that's just me being overly paranoid.

So we don't know exactly what we need, and we don't always have specific tests to figure it out either. To make things more complicated, our need for various nutrients will change as our circumstances and environment change. For example, when a person is stressed out, drinks alcohol or caffeine, takes diuretics for blood pressure or other toxins or substances, magnesium will be wasted in the urine. Magnesium is involved in over three hundred different enzyme reactions in the body and with any sort of muscle function in the body including the muscle within the bowel wall and blood vessels. So, when particularly stressed, exercising a lot, drinking caffeine or alcohol, or taking diuretics, more than the normal amount of magnesium is needed. These same general issues apply to many other nutrients in many other situations, making nutritional medicine extremely complicated. I will discuss this concept more in the nutrition chapters.

I mentioned above that sometimes the modulation of gene expression spans generations, and I want to expand on that. An excellent short book to read on this subject (from before the concept was really understood) is *Pottenger's Cats* by Francis Pottenger, MD. He was using cats for research in the 1930's and 1940's and found they did much better on a certain diet. He removed their adrenal glands surgically and found that the cats fed raw meat scraps from a local butcher survived the surgery much more easily and more often than cats fed cooked meat scraps from the kitchen at their facility.

He began to study the cats more directly and found if he fed them a diet of raw meat, raw milk (not pasteurized or homogenized) and cod liver oil, the cats fared extremely well and were apparently in optimal health. They were uniform in size, good-natured, had distinct gender features (the males were physically distinct from the females without looking at the genitalia), had easy pregnancies and healthy litters, and they had virtually no health problems.

Then he changed just one variable. He took a group of cats and gave them cooked meat scraps rather than raw, keeping the raw milk and cod liver oil the same. Another group received pasteurized milk (which means cooking it at high heat) rather than raw milk, but had cod liver oil and raw meat. What he found in both groups was pretty much the same; they began to deteriorate more and more every generation. The cats fed cooked foods began to develop health problems, had miscarriages and more difficulty getting pregnant. The offspring exhibited notable diversity in size and shape rather than the uniformity seen before. There was less visible difference between genders (sounds like some humans today right?); they had bad dispositions and were no longer playful. They had tremors and trouble landing on their feet. They developed all sorts of health problems from allergies and arthritis to kidney problems and cancers, and they had more and more trouble getting pregnant and carrying litters to full term.

These issues became more and more pronounced every generation on the cooked food diets. After four to five generations the cats were no longer fertile at all and basically went extinct as a subpopulation. What made this even more interesting and elegant is that Pottenger at one point decided to take some individuals from a few generations into the cooked-food diet groups and fed them the ideal raw-food diet again. The overall health of those particular individuals improved only a little, but they had stronger offspring with fewer health problems. They did not have "normal" offspring in the first generation, though, which is the scary part. It took about four generations of feeding the ideal diet again before he saw individuals with the fitness and characteristics of the original healthy population.

Why is this scary? The way I see it is that our modern population in the industrialized world is at least a few generations into eating a diet that is highly processed and devitalized. The encouraging part is that there is hope for reversal of our current inexorable decline in fitness as a species. But it just doesn't seem likely to occur, given what I've observed in human behavior.

To extrapolate Pottenger's work to our human population, we've probably only got a couple more generations (forty to sixty years maybe) before the curtain comes down on our little show. In order to stop this possible progression we would have to get rid of all our processed food and start eating a purely natural whole-food diet again and be willing to keep this up for several generations before we get back to true health. It's hard enough for me to convince anyone to eat right for their own health, much less the health of their great, great, grandchildren!

"Well, we're not cats!" someone might declare. Though this is true, it always baffles me how so many people fail to acknowledge that we are just another animal species and many of the same rules apply to us. The point is we need to eat a natural diet appropriate to our particular species. Cats happen to be obligate carnivores, eating only meat and animal foods, while humans are omnivores and can have a much more diverse diet. It is the quality of our foods that is truly critical here. That said, there are more similarities than differences between humans and many other animals.

We use lots of other animal species for test subjects prior to experimenting on humans. Scientists take advantage of the similarities in our physiologies. Pottenger was originally using his cats to test adrenal cortex extracts derived from cows that he was going to use medically in people with adrenal failure. The same cortisol derived from a cow works in a cat, and also works in us. Similarly, I routinely prescribe a thyroid hormone made directly from pig thyroids for use in humans, and it works extremely well. So how different are we really?

At this point, if someone is not able to see the epigenetic deterioration of our human population, then that person has on some really dark, rose-colored glasses. The scope and severity of human disease in our culture is increasing dramatically. The rates of infertility and miscarriage are currently quite high, and they are getting worse. Sperm counts and testosterone levels in young men are half what they were a generation or two ago. And our population is becoming more diverse at the same time it's becoming more androgynous.

Look at films or photographs of a group of villagers from some remote place in the jungle, and the people look like clones of each other to some extent. They are all about the same height and weight; skin tone and facial features are very similar. The landmark work of Dr. Weston Price from the 1920's encourages us to appreciate just how much healthier humans were prior to the introduction of processed food.

Dr. Price was a dentist, and he showed how the people raised on their indigenous diets had completely straight teeth that all fit perfectly in their faces without cavities or gum disease even though they had never seen a toothbrush. He documented the incredible differences in dental and medical health between those primitive individuals and their offspring after just one or two generations of eating processed food. Back then this just meant ground flour and white sugar, not the toxic onslaught of food extracts and chemical additives we've been eating the past fifty years or so. How many kids or even adults today need braces or their wisdom teeth pulled out because they do not fit in their mouths? I have seen a growing number of people who never even developed their wisdom teeth. This is a notable example of epigenetic change over time.

I know I've really gone on about this subject, but it is a very important concept to grasp if we have any hope of maintaining the health of our species. We are nearing the crisis point in terms of our health and epigenetic expression is a big part of that. If we are to steer the ship away from a potential iceberg, we must ditch our toxic, devitalized food and go back to natural whole-foods for good. We have to clean up and limit the exposure to chemicals from our environment and in our everyday lives.

This may sound extreme now, but pull this book out in 2050 when the rates of infertility are around 50% or greater and our average life expectancy is in the mid-sixties or younger. Maybe that's overly pessimistic though. Maybe we will wake up and start eating the way we should, maybe we'll stop polluting the world, or maybe we'll make a drug that fixes it all. That last one was a joke by the way. We really need to ditch our acceptance and complacency on this subject and start paying attention to the future of our species if we want to be around in another thousand years.

Mutation and evolution

Above, I presented a long tirade about epigenetics and how we are changing ourselves through nutritional influences. The big difference between that and evolution is that those epigenetic changes are reversible over generations. Mutations involve specific changes in the DNA sequence, which are going to be passed on from generation to generation with virtually no chance of ever reverting back to the original. Mutations that confer a survival advantage become more persistent in the population, causing an evolution in that species or a divergence into an entirely new species.

Our DNA speaks a pretty simple language, with only four different letters to play with; however, changing just one character in a string of thousands or millions can result in a devastating disease like sickle cell anemia, cystic fibrosis, or many others that are not even compatible with life. Mutation isn't all bad; it is the stuff of progress as well. Mutations in genes can confer a greater advantage to an organism like resistance to illness or certain infections (there are people who are genetically immune to HIV infection, malaria and other infectious diseases). Mutations can bring forth greater size or strength, better fertility, or the potential for longer life expectancy.

Many mutations we are familiar with like eye color, ear lobe shape or blood type, do not confer any real advantage or disadvantage under usual circumstances. Some may confer a social and environmental disadvantage; examples include albinism, which allows individuals to burn terribly in the sun and often leads to social mistreatment, or Fragile X syndrome, the most common genetic cause of mental retardation.

A good example of the contrast between genetic mutation and epigenetic drift is to compare the albino mouse to the "agouti" mouse. We have all seen albino animals; they have pure white skin or fur and pink eyes. They cannot make any pigment in their outer layer, and this is due to a change in their DNA sequence. It is not reversible and their offspring will either have the same trait or not, depending on whether they inherit the altered gene from their parent. It is not influenced in expression by anything in the environment.

The agouti mouse is an individual with reddish-brown fur that is somewhat ratty (no pun intended). They gain weight readily and develop obesity much more easily than their typical counterparts. These traits get passed on through the generations. Initially they can be born from thinner, dark colored mice with smoother fur, and the condition looks very much like the result of a DNA mutation. Modern research has shown that this manifestation is actually just a change in gene "expression" rather than the DNA sequence per se, and it is modifiable with dietary change.

If you supplement a female agouti mouse with high amounts of nutrients like folic acid during her adult life and through her pregnancy, her offspring will revert to the original type with dark smooth fur and no tendency toward obesity. If the mice are supplemented through every generation they remain "normal" or wild type. If their diet is reverted back to the typical, unfortified sort they will begin to have agouti babies again with persistence through generations until the diet is fortified once again. This is a perfect example of epigenetics rather than pure genetics.

Evolution is a term that may bother some, but it really shouldn't. One does not have to participate in the indefatigable argument about creation vs. evolution in terms of the origin of man in order to appreciate the fact that evolution as a principle is occurring all around us on an ongoing basis. It merely means that there is acquired genetic variation between individuals of a species over multiple generations and that some of those variations confer some kind of advantage in terms of reproduction and the resulting ability to pass on their traits. Over time this equates to persistent differences in the population as compared to their ancestors and, eventually, this may result in two very different species. This process is termed "adaptation" by some Christian groups, instead of "evolution", because they find the latter term offensive. Whatever.

Evolution/adaptation explains how the average height of people has gone up, perhaps because taller people were more likely to breed with other tall people and their mutually tall genes created even taller offspring. It is the process that explains the significant differences between groups of people living in very different climates. People living in colder latitudes generally having larger torsos and shorter limbs compared with people in tropical zones (Holmes, 2008).

Drug resistance among bacteria is a very good example of evolution in real-time because they "reproduce" every thirty minutes or so. We can, therefore, witness the effects of many generations of change in a single day rather than the centuries it would take a human population. In a population with billions of bacteria it is likely that, just by chance, a few of them will spontaneously mutate in some way that confers resistance to a given antibiotic. This mutation may actually make those individuals weaker under typical circumstances, perhaps because that gene, for example, was used in the production of a tougher cell wall in the normal type and now their cell wall forms 40% slower.

If the entire population is suddenly exposed to the antibiotic in question, perhaps all the "normal" individuals will be killed, leaving only those resistant mutants to reproduce and repopulate. Within a few days, rather than just 1% in the population having this new mutation, greater than 90% will have it because most of the others have been killed. The longer the antibiotic is present, the greater percentage of the residual bacterial population will be resistant to it. In the example of a child with an ear infection, it is possible the next time they get the same antibiotic it will not work as well. This is because their bacterial population will have evolved or adapted to that particular environmental pressure; it has nothing to do with the child himself.

One of the tenets of evolutionary theory is that genetic mutations occur all the time in a spontaneous fashion and with significant frequency. This has to occur for the species to continually adapt to the changing environment, which is always changing to some extent. What I want to emphasize is that these mutations also occur due to environmental influences that drive evolution or adaptation at a faster rate. We know that certain chemicals, drugs (e.g. chemotherapy agents), and even sunlight will cause mutations in our DNA. This is how adults get cancer much of the time; some of their cells acquire a mutation through one of these forces and those cells "forget" they are supposed to stop dividing or behaving in a certain way.

Consider the possibility that some of these mutations triggered by our environment may affect our eggs and sperm, causing higher rates of mutations in our offspring. Some would say "no, because the DNA in our eggs and sperm is formed before we are born." This is true, but those gametes (eggs and sperm) do have to undergo a final process of division before they are used during our adult life (meiosis, for those who recall their high school biology). What is to stop the DNA from being influenced and mutated during that division by environmental factors in the adult?

Even more frightening is to ponder what the effects on those eggs and sperm are from all the environmental chemicals, toxins and adverse nutritional factors our babies are currently exposed to at the time of conception through gestation and birth? There are now toxins in the father's semen, the mother's blood stream and uterine tissue. Our children are often born today with thousands of different foreign chemicals in their umbilical cord blood. Consider how this may drive the forces of evolution/adaptation in our population similarly to treating a bacterial infection with an antibiotic.

Perhaps a positive evolution is occurring right now in our human population. Perhaps people are gaining genetic traits that enable us to effectively utilize high fructose corn syrup as a fuel without causing inflammation and obesity. Perhaps we will somehow turn Yellow Dye #5 into a defensive chemical against bacteria and viruses. Maybe we will use more regions of our brain as a result of Mercury contamination (I do think that's actually manifesting in some kids with autism and Asperger's) or adapt in such a way as to thrive in an atmosphere containing less oxygen and more carbon dioxide. That's great for our species in the future in terms of still having humans in a progressively more toxic world, but it may mean over 90% of us dying off and only the "strong" few persisting. After all, that's what happens in other animal populations within the ecosystem all the time.

So, maybe we should just keep feeding our kids highly processed foods full of chemicals, inject them with more mercury and aluminum from vaccines, keep building more industrial machines that pollute our world, and see which kids survive. It's possible that some will, and they are likely to become somewhat different than we are today in various ways. If we look back at film or photos of people just 50 to 100 years ago we may see some striking differences already. They are likely to appear a little shorter, quite a bit thinner, have straighter teeth and possess smoother skin. There aren't as many with dark circles under their eyes or with that persistently tired expression we often see today. Back then there weren't nearly as many people with asthma, allergies, autism, autoimmune diseases or cancer. But maybe we are evolving in the right direction after all. Sure.

Xenobiotics and Xenohormesis ("zee-no-hor-mee-sis")

These are strange-sounding words I'm sure, and they are not likely to be found in any home dictionary as of yet. Break them down, and they mean something like alien or foreign biological compounds and hormonal effects. They refer to something that is disturbingly common in the modern industrial world; processes which are likely going on inside each of us, and especially in our children, right now.

A xenobiotic is the term for a chemical made by man and not found in nature that has a biological effect inside our bodies. Many of these man-made chemicals in our new environment behave like hormones in some ways when they get into our body. These chemicals are "new to nature" (a term frequently used by Dr. Jeff Bland, founder of the Institute for Functional Medicine), and have no actual role in our body's physiology. When they are consumed via our food or water, or absorbed through the skin, they are there interacting with all of our cells, whether we like it or not.

Many people assume substances like these either leave the body peacefully or just accumulate in our fat tissue without any biological effect. I wish that were true. Unfortunately many of these chemicals have very potent biological effects, and they are often negative. This should not seem unrealistic to any of us since the drug companies make billions of dollars selling chemicals which are foreign to our body but have powerful, and sometimes deadly, physiological effects.

Take into account the some 8,000 chemicals present in our processed and packaged foods, as well as the additional chemicals in our air, clothing and household goods. At least some of them are bound to have effects on our physiology. Some of them block normal chemicals from binding to their receptors, prevent normal enzyme function, mimic or interfere with neurotransmitters, disrupt detoxification systems, cause severe inflammation and oxidative stress, or cause other types of adverse chemical responses.

The term xenohormesis refers to those that behave like hormones or disrupt normal hormone systems ("endocrine disrupters"). A well-known recent example is the plasticizer Bisphenol A. This is a chemical added into plastic in order to make it more pliable and less brittle. This stuff is now proven to cause significant estrogen-like effects in the body and was removed from many types of water bottles and baby bottles after this all became clear. That's great, but how many people were irreversibly affected prior to that?

How many other plasticizers have similar effects and just haven't been studied? You can bet many of them do and, in my opinion, they probably all have these effects to some degree because they all have the same effects in plastic. What happens to the fetus if the mother consumes these chemicals when the brain or sex organs are forming?

Other chemicals with proven hormonal effects include flame-retardant chemicals like PBDE's (polybrominated diphenyl ethers, which were made to replace PCB's after they were banned in the 1970's), some pesticides, herbicides and fungicides.

I saw an article on MSN.com once titled something like *"Could the chemicals in your car's dashboard be shrinking your unborn son's penis?"* This was referring to PBDE's. I have heard of remote areas where water is generally consumed from large plastic jugs (left out in the heat), and the plasticizers have caused the men to develop enlarged, feminine breasts. There were researchers studying breast cancer whose cell cultures began to grow out of control when the plastic in their test tubes was changed (Colborn, 1997). I have seen more than one obese teenager or pre-teen male in my practice with enlarged breasts, and they usually had consumed lots of manufactured beverages from plastic bottles.

Xenohormesis is a concept that is new in understanding but has been already affecting us all for more than a generation. It is something we should all be aware of, as well as other general adverse effects environmental chemicals may be having on us. It is not something considered in the usual "toxicity" testing the FDA requires before a chemical is allowed in food and, therefore, many approved food additives may possess these properties. Integrative practitioners should be able to speak intelligently about these issues and counsel patients as to avoidance of these substances and their attendant problems.

Root causes

I have discussed this to some extent previously, but it is a very key concept in integrative medicine and bears repeated mention. The goal of every medical provider should be to identify treatable or removable causes of illness and symptoms, thereby, effectively "curing" the condition if at all possible. Directly addressing symptoms is helpful, as in allopathic medicine, but should not be the sole means of treatment. Practitioners should all have the education to understand physiologic causes of illness and address them progressively with the safest interventions possible.

The alternative to this is what we already have in conventional medical practice in the U.S. and many other developed countries; that being merely the treatment of disease symptoms with pharmaceuticals or other substances in order to alleviate suffering. I would include herbal remedies with drugs in this concept, as I feel they are often used the same way and without attention to underlying causes. It is not just conventional practitioners that are guilty of this ignorance and shortsightedness. Naturopaths may keep using herbs for a patient's symptoms without ever identifying and fixing underlying conditions. Chiropractors may keep people coming back for manipulation twice a week for years without more definitively correcting the underlying muscular and structural issues.

This philosophy relies on the concept and belief that the condition in question actually has a cause, which logically it must, and that the cause is something that can, in fact, be determined and fixed. The latter, of course, may not be true, such as in the case of pure genetic conditions like Down Syndrome or some instances of severe tissue or organ dysfunction. Sometimes chronic problems really have no permanent solution and chronic symptomatic management is the best we can do.

There are far too many diagnoses in conventional medicine that are just symptoms or syndromes comprised of multiple symptoms and are not truly descriptive of the actual causes. Obvious examples include pure symptoms such as cough, fever, diarrhea or pain. More complex examples include conditions such as type 2 diabetes, depression, obesity, fibromyalgia, migraine, asthma, lupus and many other disorders.

In my opinion there are actually only a handful of general true causes of disease. Some of them are: deficiency of essential nutrients, neurotransmitters, hormones or other metabolic substances; excesses of hormones, chemical messengers or other internally-produced biological substances; genetic mutation and epigenetic changes; toxins derived from man-made processes, plants, microbes or other places in the environment; infections with bacteria, yeast, viruses, prions or parasites; immune system imbalance such as allergy or immune deficiency (though admittedly these immune problems often stem from the nutrient deficiency and environmental toxicity problems); structural abnormalities such as skeletal deformity or spinal misalignment; psychological stress and spiritual imbalance or discord; or energetic imbalance and other mind/body problems.

Looking at every complaint or chronic disease in terms of these and other possible upstream causes, in many cases, makes things much simpler. I can often find a single unifying cause of multiple symptoms or problems in an individual. Alternatively, I may find there are multiple causes for a single symptom, such as Vitamin D deficiency, hypothyroidism, mercury toxicity and job stress all contributing to a person's fatigue. An integrative practitioner needs to be able to sort through the causes of illness in order to truly cure the problem.

Triggers, perpetuating or propagating factors

These are similar to root causes but involve factors that may not be the true upstream causes; but they clearly do make the symptom or disease condition worse. It is important to identify what they are and help the patient alter their exposure if possible. These are key concepts in functional medicine, and environmental medicine especially, and an essential component of the management of allergies and environmental problems.

It's pretty obvious if an individual has red itchy eyes and a runny nose around cats that the person is probably allergic to cats. It may be less obvious to some if it is the MSG in their ranch dressing that triggers their migraines, or the artificial sweetener in their chewing gum perpetuating their "lupus". Some people will look like they have multiple sclerosis because of their allergy to wheat, and they may never figure it out until someone suggests they do an elimination diet. It is arguably their immune sensitivity that is the actual root cause, but it is the wheat that is the trigger. It may be possible to address the root cause through allergy desensitization (to be discussed later) but avoiding the trigger will certainly help in the meantime.

Other perpetuating factors or triggers may come from within, such as stress and anxiety. Some people can experience skin problems like acne or hives from emotional stress. Some will have digestive problems like heartburn or diarrhea and many of us will have muscle tension or headaches. Temperature can contribute to symptoms like arthritis, rashes and other conditions. Other internal and external forces may alter a person's symptoms as well, and it must all be sorted out to help some people completely.

Relevance in research rather than "surrogate markers"

This is the counterpoint to addressing root causes and leads back to a discussion of one of the characteristics I find terribly wrong with our current medical system. I previously gave examples such as high cholesterol and high blood pressure as being surrogate markers for cardiovascular disease because they have been identified as risk factors for those disease conditions, yet they don't appear to directly cause the disease. One huge problem in our modern "evidence-based" culture is the bulk of research that pays attention to risk factors and encourages treatment of them as if they were diseases themselves, rather than focusing on outcomes that are truly important to the individual. Sadly, this is typically driven by the desire for pharmaceutical profits rather than human health.

Taking hypertension (high blood pressure) as an example again, it is true that sometimes your blood pressure can get so high it is its own acute problem. If it gets up around 220/120 or so without intense exercise (when you are exercising vigorously it may be functionally normal to reach this range) many of us will have a headache, get vision changes, dizziness, chest pain or some other problems. For some it runs the risk of causing kidney damage and brain injury. In those cases it is important to treat this aggressively and get the numbers down, because one can have "malignant hypertension", an acutely dangerous condition.

In this example there is likely to be another underlying cause such as drug use or certain endocrine tumors, but it is imperative to treat the symptom also. This is a good example of why an integrative medical approach is important; the patient can benefit in the short term from conventional medical methods while using a broader approach to find the long-term solutions.

In the case of milder chronic hypertension, the drug companies want us to believe that people should control their blood pressure with drugs to numbers below 125/75 pretty much all the time. They base this on huge studies with large numbers of people showing what amounts to only very small differences in outcomes. There are some blood pressure drugs that do seem to effectively decrease death rates from cardiovascular disease by a small amount; however, many drugs that effectively lower blood pressure somewhat have no apparent benefit at all in lowering death rates.

This means that blood pressure itself is probably not a true cause of cardiovascular death in most cases and may not even really directly contribute in many instances. This suggests there are likely underlying causes for hypertension that also cause the eventual heart attacks or strokes if left unchecked. It is more imperative to figure out the underlying causes and address them in order to extend life and improve health.

In the case of elevated blood lipids, although statin drugs may lower cholesterol dramatically, they actually improve cardiovascular outcomes only by a very small margin in men and not at all in women (this is in those who do not have known cardiovascular disease). There is an even worse example of this principle within the field of lipid chemistry involving the treatment of high triglycerides.

Elevated blood triglycerides has been found in large epidemiological studies to be a risk factor for heart attack and stroke even without other concurrently elevated bad cholesterol. Triglycerides are a type of fat used to store energy. Triglycerides are usually made in our bodies by the liver from sugar consumed in amounts that could not be burned off right away. The theory is these elevated fats may contribute to the deposits within our arteries. Extremely elevated triglycerides have also been seen to trigger acute pancreatitis in some people, a condition that can be fatal in the short term.

So it makes some sense that finding a drug to decrease one's blood triglycerides may decrease the risk of heart attack or stroke. This is a good target for research for sure. In 2009 I read the research cited in a drug advertisement printed in a national family practice journal for a new lipid drug, Trilipix™. The pharmaceutical company did not do outcomes research on this drug itself because it takes years to get that data, so they instead just cited fundamental past research for the older drugs in the class such as Lopid™ and Tricor™. The studies cited showed that these drugs do lower blood triglyceride levels effectively. So, that's great, right?

The problem is that no studies (*none at all* apparently, or I assume they would have been cited in the ad) showed any decrease in the risk of heart attack, stroke or pancreatitis. There were no decreases in death from cardiovascular disease or any other cause reported. An even bigger problem is that these drugs seemed to actually cause increases in death from cancer and neurological diseases and, in some studies, they even increased pancreatitis episodes. The analysis done by the World Health Organization actually showed an increase in death from *cardiovascular disease* using these drugs! You can read this data yourself in a printed Trilipix™ ad if you wish.

So, why the Hell are we prescribing these drugs? Why are they approved, on the market, and promoted to patients on television? Well, because they *do* lower one's triglycerides. That's *all* the FDA was approving the drugs for; it doesn't matter that they actually don't do anything important like lowering one's chances of death or disability.

The FDA doesn't seem to care that the drug may actually kill a person in the effort to achieve a meaningless surrogate endpoint! I mean, these studies should have been suppressed or hidden away somewhere shouldn't they? People who produce these drugs should be totally ashamed and the drugs immediately taken off the market. But no, the studies are quoted right in the advertisements. It's embarrassing!

I guess they are sitting there amused, knowing that doctors rarely ever read this information and most will go right on prescribing the drugs according to the pathetic standard of care and thinking that they are doing the right thing. In my opinion it could easily be considered malpractice to prescribe one of these drugs for some people. Now, I tell my patients to stop them immediately if I see they have been placed on one by another provider. I must confess, I only recently discovered this particular injustice in 2009 when I read that drug advertisement; prior to that I had prescribed these drugs a number of times myself. So I completely understand how it happens.

In reality the solution to high blood triglycerides lies in reducing sugar and alcohol intake, avoiding processed grains, starches and, especially, corn syrup. Exercise helps tremendously as well. Therapeutically, natural substances like niacin, fish oil supplements and lecithin can be used to improve the body's metabolism of fats in a natural way. As I mentioned, in the past I used the aforementioned prescription drugs in patients who maintained persistently high triglycerides in spite of the natural measures taken. Now I don't use them at all, in anyone. The science suggests one is still better off without them.

The cholesterol and blood pressure issues are prominent examples of the treatment of surrogate markers and misuse or misguidance of modern research. There are many more. This whole thing really pisses me off, more than most of the problems in our modern medical system – hence the long rant. What makes me most angry is I'm sure I still use things myself that, in reality, don't help and may even cause more harm than good. Whoever markets them may know it, but these sellers may be too corrupt to pay heed to the evidence and stop doing so for the sake of what is right, instead of for the money.

An integrative medicine provider should know the difference between an actual disease problem, its true causes, and the surrogate markers that can be used for tracking progress but should not be treated directly as diseases. They should know how to critically analyze the available literature (with a healthy skepticism of pharmaceutical research) and make good decisions about patient care and not just follow the purported "standard" of practice when it makes no sense for the actual patient.

SECTION II
ANALYZING THE PROBLEM

If you don't understand the problem, how are you supposed to fix it?

If you don't ask the right questions you may never get the right answers.

CHAPTER 1 – THE FAILINGS OF
OUR HEALTHCARE SYSTEM–

In this book's introduction, I briefly discussed the results published in a December 1, 2008 *Time* Magazine article that evaluated the U.S. healthcare system as it compares to 164 other countries in the world (Park, 2008). You may recall that we ranked number one only in terms of spending: a landslide victory to be sure. We spent nearly twice as much as the second-place country on the health of our citizens. That shouldn't really surprise anyone familiar with America's general consumer habits and lifestyle choices.

The surprise comes when you look at our 34th place finish in life expectancy and our 29th place finish in infant mortality. This is, of course, in spite of the fact that we have the "best hospitals" with the newest technology and the most advanced methods in neonatal intensive care. To be sure, our medical professionals also fancy themselves the best in the world.

Unlike the housing crisis and impending collapse of the economy at the time of the writing of this book, health is not a problem that can be fixed by simply throwing money at it. We can't "buy off" cancer, heart disease, diabetes, or obesity. We can't bribe autism and ADHD, or influence our allergies with creative advertising or smear campaigns. I know these analogies seem a little farcical, but I use them in order to try and question our society's way of doing some things. We have gotten used to throwing our influence around and expecting to get what we want. Let's explore, in more depth, some of the fundamental problems in our thinking and our implementation of America's health care system.

ACCESS TO CARE

Access to care could be our biggest failing in the U.S. medical system. What good is the world's best technology, if you can't afford to use it? What use are the best hospitals if a three-night stay is going to bankrupt you? What's the use of having the best physicians if you can't afford to see them?

The news frequently reports there are now more than 50 million Americans without health insurance; most of whom are in the lower middle class and certainly can't afford the $500+ monthly premiums required for even very limited health insurance with a very high deductible. This means they are also unlikely to be able to afford our extremely expensive medical care when they need it. The December 2008 *Time* article reports an estimated 110 deaths per 100,000 people every year in the U.S. could have been prevented with better access to care This pretty much puts us behind every other industrialized nation.

Medical costs are the number one cause of bankruptcy for Americans – which, by the way, entails a large cost to all of us. In 1981 only 8% of those filing for bankruptcy cited the costs of a medical illness as the reason. But a Harvard study from 2007 showed that number had risen dramatically to 62%. That was just prior to the recession; and 78% of those filers in the Harvard study even had medical insurance at the time of their illness, 60.3% with private insurance (Arnst, 2009).

Of course, once bankruptcy is declared and a person is sufficiently destitute, he/she may qualify for Medicaid. If a patient lives to become old enough or becomes totally disabled, that person may qualify for Medicare. These federal programs reimburse doctors and hospitals quite poorly, though I think they pay full-price for medications - gosh, I wonder who influenced THAT policy?

As a result of the poor payment and difficult regulations, many doctors refuse to see Medicaid and Medicare patients, or they drastically limit the numbers in their practice. Furthermore, this poor level of reimbursement leads to what is called 'cost shifting'. Cost shifting means that doctors and hospitals charge more money to those who can or will pay in order to make up for the money lost on those federal payer systems and the poor patients who can't pay the balance at all. So, if a patient has no insurance and a little money, that person may pay much more than someone with no money and no job. Therefore, the burden of cost-shifting is mainly carried by the middle class. And who pays for most of the cost for the health care doled out by the government? Oh, it's the working middle class again!

The poor status of our federal insurance systems is often used as an argument against a more comprehensive government-run health care plan, but there is no reason we couldn't do it better. Another common argument I hear is that patients would have to wait a long time to get the care they need, such as cancer treatment. I keep hearing arguments against nationalized health care like "patients in Canada with breast cancer will sometimes die while they are on the waiting list for treatment". My answer to this argument is: "At least they can get care." Many people die in the U.S. every year of treatable diseases for which they cannot afford care, and are not even on a waiting list. Rationing of resources is a biological reality on this planet; at least the health care ramifications of that are more explicit in other countries.

There are millions of people here in the United States who don't have access to care at all because they can't afford it. Recall the 110 unnecessary deaths per 100,000 people in the U.S. every year? Well, in that same study Canada only had 77 per 100,000! We can talk negatively about their system all we want, but the statistics clearly show that ours sucks much worse. And don't forget we spend nearly twice as much per capita. Are they so much smarter than us they can spend less than half the amount and put out a better product? That should be a major blow to America's ego. But, as with most egotists, we are oblivious to the reality of our own shortcomings and failings.

Also, in regards to the "dying while on the waiting list for cancer treatment" issue, if someone dies of cancer within several months while on a waiting list, they were probably beyond treatment anyway and may have just been spared some toxicity and decreased quality of life in their final days. This is likely why that particular perceived "flaw" has not apparently impacted the bottom line of overall unnecessary mortality or life expectancy.

The fact is that resource utilization is likely to become a reality for all of us with the current economic direction the country is taking. The healthcare pie, enormous as it is in this country, will ultimately have to be rationed in some fashion. This is no different from the budgeting we do in our own household. For example, we have to make decisions about what to spend our limited money on every day, I imagine, and I suspect some people's own health needs may take a backseat to their house payment or to their children's needs.

At some point the fantasy of limitless wealth and supply needs to be dispelled for the American public. We can print meaningless money only for so long until the bottom falls out of the system. We need to find ways to make more people healthier with less expense. This is where integrative medicine comes in.

We have plenty of smart people in this country as well as the experience of many other nations from which to learn. I suspect that, if we wanted to, we could come up with a universal health care plan that worked well. It just wouldn't make as much money for those who currently benefit from the system the way it is. *That* is why we don't have a national health care system.

This brings us to the insurance industry again which, somehow, manages to continue making millions for CEO's despite our extremely expensive medical care. If you were an insurance company, could you still make millions in profit if you charged affordable premiums to people with chronic medical problems and then covered their necessary services at a good rate? Of course not, so that's not what they do. They charge high, ever-increasing, rates to everyone; and in most cases don't offer coverage to those with "pre-existing conditions". They routinely change a person's coverage, usually cutting services rather than adding them, while raising premiums at the same time.

It seems to me insurance companies hire claims adjusters and investigators primarily to:

- deny payments
- make rules that are difficult to understand and follow
- argue with doctor's offices about the coding of services and fee schedules (I know this from personal experience)
- try to stick the patient with a bill as high as possible

The health insurance system is somewhat immune to our nation's racketeering laws, so it has been permitted to fix high prices. Specifically refer to the McCarran-Ferguson Act of 1945, which was a bipartisan congressional bill between Pat McCarran (D-Nev) and Homer Ferguson (R-Mich); it serves to partially exempt insurance companies from the federal anti-trust legislation that applies to most businesses. This "M-F" Act has been used repeatedly in state courts to refute racketeering lawsuits against insurance companies and has consistently been cited to overrule the federal RICO law.

The M-F Act was the result of a U.S. Supreme Court case in 1944 (*United States v. South-Eastern Underwriters Association*, 322 U.S. 533) wherein this insurance agency (South-Eastern) that controlled 90% of the home insurance policies for six southern states had set rates higher than competitive levels and was accused of using intimidation, boycotts and other coercive tactics to maintain a monopoly (allegedly, mind you). The court ruled that the insurance business was not technically "commerce" and, therefore, not subject to the commerce clause of the U.S. Constitution or the Sherman Anti-Trust Act.

This is one of the reasons insurance executives can still make huge sums of money while those in need of their help get less and less. I hear people complain about this all the time and my standard response is: "Welcome to America".

HIGH COSTS

High cost is a healthcare problem that ties directly into the access issue. As I mentioned before, health care expenses are the number one reason for families to go into bankruptcy in the United States. The cost of health insurance is expected to rise by more than 8% again in 2011. This will mean a full doubling of cost since 2001 (*Reuters* Washington report – Sept 27, 2010). This is, of course, while insurance company profits have reportedly soared by far greater margins than that year after year (actual stats for corporate profits are available online as a matter of public record, if you want to look up your particular insurance company). Therefore, the biggest single budget item accounting for absolute insurance premium increases is probably corporate profits.

Probably every aspect of medical care is far more expensive in this country than in most others. Actually, doctors' visits themselves may be the most similar. It seems that doctors in many other countries earn a similarly good standard of living, comparatively speaking, as they do here in the U.S. I do have a physician friend in Canada, though, who gets paid only $40-50 for an office visit that would pay well over $100 where I practice. He is a general practitioner; and my understanding is that doctors in specialty fields there make far more, more in line with the earnings in America. This lack of "support" for primary care physicians creates a whole other problem for the health care system because everyone wants to become a specialist and very few are left to try and look at the whole person. A similar situation exists in the U.S.

The things that are far more expensive and account for a far greater share of health care expenses than physician office visits include medications, tests, hospital fees, and overall procedure costs. It is well known that the same medications can be found in other countries for a fraction of the cost that paid here in the United States. These are typically the exact same medications, made by the exact same pharmaceutical factories. So how does this happen?

Well, you can rest assured that the pharmaceutical companies still make a profit in those other countries even while selling their medications at such decreased cost. It does not cost much to make a pill. The reason they sell their drugs for so much more here in our country, is that WE PAY IT! The pharmaceutical giants control much of our government policy and there is no regulation on how much they can mark up the cost of drugs (that would be "socialist"!). They have used their influence to ensure that the federal government does not attempt to negotiate lower prices for their medications. Evidence of this influence is within the legislation during the last Bush administration, creating Medicare Part D. The bill includes language that specifically prohibits the federal government from directly negotiating drug costs.

A Harvard-sponsored study in 2008 suggested there could be annual savings of nearly $22 billion nationally if the government were to just negotiate the prices of the top 200 medications dispensed to seniors back down the level of the 2006 Federal Supply Schedule. This would be legally permissible under federal law (Gellad, 2008). Since costs have continued to rise since then, one would expect those savings to be potentially even greater now. In my opinion, this should have been a primary component of the healthcare reform pushed through by the Obama administration, but there was nary a whisper about this sort of thing.

The pharmaceutical companies are allowed to patent a new drug for many years and sell it at an extremely high rate during that time. We are led to believe they need to do this in order to cover the high cost of research and development but I have heard that drug companies spend four times as much on advertising as they do on research and development. Advertising encourages doctors to prescribe a company's particular drug and for patients to ask their doctor for it by name even when it doesn't really work any better than the cheaper and older alternatives. To complement the direct-to-consumer advertising, they apparently have four or five drug reps for every doctor in America. These minions provide samples and severely biased literature to as many clinics and hospitals as possible.

To compare the cost of medications and physician fees, consider this: a patient may see their internist four times a year and, even if they spend $1000 total for those visits, this is nothing compared to the cost of the four medications their doctor prescribes. A cholesterol drug will often cost $150 per month, an acid-reducing pill about the same. A blood pressure medication might cost $100 per month and the latest diabetes drug may be in excess of $150. Add up all of these costs, and it is easy to see spending over $6,000 per year on medications. This is five or six times as much as what is spent on the physician. Therefore, if you can find a physician who may provide care effectively without expensive drugs, they are worth their weight in gold (well, maybe not at the current price of gold).

Hospital care is the single greatest total expense portion. It accounts for $.31 out of every dollar spent on health costs according to that *Time* article (Park, 2008). This is very interesting considering only a small minority of us end up in the hospital each year. Again, hospital expenses in our country are extremely high because it's a big business. The CEOs of hospital organizations and pharmaceutical giants individually make millions of dollars every year, and the CEOs of the insurance companies manage to do so as well (actual numbers are a matter of public record). These industries make billions of dollars every year, while the costs to the consumer skyrocket.

So, how can the people paying the money (insurance companies), and the people collecting money (hospitals, drug companies, and laboratories perhaps), all make billions? It's simply by them screwing over the rest of us. This includes the physicians who often, inappropriately, get the blame for the high costs. I hope I've established that this isn't the case, especially since the vast majority of our physicians make under $500,000 per year rather than millions. This isn't to say our physicians don't make a good living. There is a very wide range though; a pediatrician may earn under $100,000 per year while a specialist surgeon (i.e. orthopedist or neurosurgeon) may earn a million dollars or more annually.

One relevant difference lies in the duration of education and training. A pediatrician needs four years of medical school and then three years of residency. An orthopedic surgeon requires a few additional years of residency beyond that. I'm not sure how long the average pharmaceutical CEO goes to school, but I imagine a master's degree in business administration is likely to be enough. That may be six total years after high school then;

compare that to the eleven years a pediatrician endures. The other huge difference is that it is the doctor who carries all the risk of malpractice if something goes wrong; it is not the pharmaceutical company, insurance company, or hospital organization CEO's.

It isn't just the pharmaceutical companies and hospitals making all the money. There is also a tremendous markup in radiological and laboratory testing. I don't think it uses $1000 worth of electricity to perform a CT scan or MRI. Some radiological tests cost several thousand dollars or more. This is another huge expense the physician may order up with the stroke of a pen. I've noticed some labs charge only $25 for a particular blood test while another lab charges $100 for the same thing. Laboratory costs are another expense that far exceeds the physician fees. It's easy to order $1500 worth of blood tests during a $150 office visit. Again, if a patient finds the right doctor a lot of money may be saved by ordering fewer and more selective tests and finding ways to cure ailments without expensive prescription drugs or procedures.

This is free market justice at work in medicine; not much of a "trickle-down effect", just people getting pissed on. Treating medicine as a business and allowing capitalism to steer its behavior has been, in many ways, directly responsible for the increasing cost and decreasing quality of our health care. Doctors are not innocent in this either. It was the physicians themselves who, in the past, freely increased their prices just to see what they might be able to earn. This eventually stimulated the creation of HMO's (health management organizations), which were meant to control these costs. I'm not sure what the entire solution is, but what we are currently doing is unsustainable.

LOW STANDARDS

O.K. this one really bugs me, largely because people themselves are responsible as well. We have become extremely lazy and complacent about our own health. People have started to just accept, as a fact, that they're going to get fat, tired and sick as they age. The problem is that people ARE getting fat, at an alarming rate and at earlier ages, and we are "aging" far more rapidly than we used to.

This has occurred gradually over time, but instead of recognizing it and taking steps to change, we have just lowered our personal standards. To accommodate our growing backsides, we make our chairs bigger and our clothing larger. Clothing manufacturers have, since about the 1980's (according to Wikipedia), largely abandoned the convention of listing actual dimensions on their garments in favor of providing catalog sizes. These can be numerical (2, 4, 6, etc.) or word-based (small, medium, large, etc.) and allow for what is called "vanity sizing" in the industry. This means they can mark a larger garment as being a smaller size than that same garment used to be. This causes the buyer to be happier in thinking they are purchasing a more trim size (numerous discussions of this controversy can be found online).

Using this same logic, if our kids are getting dumber, we should just make the standardized tests easier and teach the more difficult material later on in school for those who make it that far. Meanwhile, kids from other countries are running intellectual circles around ours. "No child left behind" may as well mean: "*Every* child left behind." If everyone's dumb, then nobody's dumb, right? This is an example of lowering expectations until everyone can meet them. This was not likely the goal for those who created that program. (note—No Child Left Behind was created by Ted Kennedy and another Democrat and was signed into law by Bush as one of his first efforts to "cross the aisle" and show bipartisanship when he became president—this fact has been long forgotten by educators who blame Bush for the debacle)

It seems that, as a culture, we began to take for granted the idea that we were at the top of the heap. But we have forgotten the effort and desire that got us there.

Another good example of this is the fact that two thirds of American adults are now considered overweight or obese. The 2005-6 NHANES (National Health and Nutrition Examination Survey) data reported an estimated 32.7% of U.S. adults (over age 20) were overweight (BMI 25-30 for women and 26-30 for men), 34.3% were obese (BMI>30 for either gender), and about 5.8% morbidly obese (BMI>40). The CDC in 2011 reported these numbers, with perhaps a very mild increase, held pretty steady since then. This should frighten everyone.

Body mass index (BMI) is a number basically calculated by dividing one's weight in kg by one's height in cm squared. A BMI of 19 to 22 is, in fact, ideal in terms of longevity and life expectancy. But in the U.S., we don't consider people "overweight" until a BMI is greater than 25 or 26. We don't consider someone "obese" until their BMI exceeds 30, and we don't consider them "morbidly obese" or "extremely obese" until a BMI is greater than 40. In much of Europe, by contrast, one is considered obese by a BMI of 26 or so and "extremely obese" if greater than 30. As I mentioned earlier, in Japan, they have recently instituted financial penalties when people allow their waist measurement to persistently exceed 33.5 to 34 inches. America has much looser standards to go with our looser waistbands.

Some of our most dangerous low standards are in regards to the quality of our food products, personal care items, and occupational safety from toxin exposures. Food in the United States is allowed to have over 8,000 different chemicals in it, very few of which have been truly proven safe for long-term human consumption. These include bleaching agents, solvents, preservatives, pesticides, emulsifiers, artificial flavors, artificial colors, sprouting inhibitors, and various other chemicals. The nitrites used to cure meats in products such as hot dogs, lunchmeat, jerky, bacon and sausage, have been linked to cancer, however, they somehow remain in our foods (World Cancer Research Fund, 2008).

In contrast to this, the German government and other European governments have much stricter regulations on food safety and labeling. For example, look up "The German Food Law" online (in German called *"Lebensmittel- und Bedarfsgegenstaendegesetz"* or LMBG for short, thankfully). In my opinion, these governments clearly care more about human health than ours does.

These issues tie in directly to our poor outcomes. We don't put enough effort into identifying the causes of chronic disease problems such as obesity and diabetes. We foolishly ignore our food supply as an important factor in human health. We don't ensure that pregnant women have excellent prenatal nutrition with dietary and exercise guidance; measures which would certainly do more to improve our infant mortality rates than just building bigger and more expensive neonatal intensive are units. There is a distinct lack of "upstream" thinking.

Lack Of Appropriate Government Regulation

This topic could spark considerable political debate, but as we've recently seen with Wall Street and the banking industry (2008-2010), lack of regulation can lead to an enormous mess. It's even worse for us when the government policies directly support or protect capitalist interests, such as pharmaceutical and insurance companies. It has improved some, in recent decades, with the passage of laws requiring hospitals to accept any person who is in active labor or has another emergency situation (EMTALA – the Emergency Medical Treatment and Active Labor Act). This includes laws requiring insurance companies to cover at least 48 hours of hospitalization after a vaginal delivery and 96 hours following a Caesarean.

These are fairly obvious examples of where the health care industry was neglecting patient safety in order to maximize profits. But the government stopped these practices. There are many more examples, however, where the government does nothing or even supports the system against its people.

The Eli Lilly Protection Act was an attempt to make it illegal to sue that particular pharmaceutical company over any injury from the injection of thimerosal, the toxic preservative which was in all our vaccinations until around 2005 (now it remains in just a few). In 2002 this bit of legislation was stuck into a homeland security bill by the then senate majority leader Bill Frist, who received $10,000 in campaign contributions from that same pharmaceutical company the following year. That bill was repealed by congress in 2003, and Frist resigned in 2006 due to allegations of stock fraud (this is all a matter of public record). This is not the only instance of governmental protection of the pharmaceutical industry. It's not even the only example relating to vaccines.

A large, federal "vaccine-related injury compensation fund" was created by our government years ago because of the admitted potential harms caused by vaccines. This arrangement makes it so the burden of injury compensation is not carried by the pharmaceutical companies who make the vaccines, but rather by "we, the people", who pay taxes and constitute the injured ourselves. Interesting. It's also interesting that autism was exceedingly rare prior to the placement of thimerosal in childhood vaccines around 1930. It later surged in incidence after 1991 (from 1 in 2,500 births to 1 in 166) when three new infant vaccines were instituted (Jepson, 2007).

Furthermore, the UK removed thimerosal from all of their vaccines years before we did, and publicly stated that it was due to concerns regarding a possible connection to autism. Our government allowed it to persist in our vaccines for years later and then eventually removed it citing reasons related to concerns for the "environment" (Jepson, 2007). I guess we don't want that mercury to leak out of our children into the water supply. Fortunately for the environment, that mercury tends to stay in the body for several decades.

Our government has consistently denied any possible connection between vaccines and autism. In early 2009, some nearly 5,000 cases of possible vaccine-associated autism were pending settlement through the vaccine-associated injury fund. But the federal courts dismissed these after some "independent" researchers (which is disingenuous, because someone paid them) publicly discredited the work done by Dr. Wakefield in the UK that suggested a link from the MMR vaccine to immune hyper-stimulation in kids with autism. This was a key piece of study that had helped make the MMR-autism connection. But it was just one piece of the whole story. The scientific association does not hinge on this data and the way it was apparently "discredited" in the news made absolutely no sense at all.

In my opinion, this was an example of brushing something terrible that the drug companies have done under the proverbial rug. Our federal government and these same companies avoided having the huge expense of paying hundreds of millions of dollars for the damages presented. This would also have opened up the courts to hundreds or thousands more cases like them.

What is inexcusable, in this instance, is that it has long been known thimerasol is extremely toxic. In early experiments with the preservative test animals kept dying and the dosage had to be repeatedly reduced. There were even a number of immediate deaths when it was first used in humans, and the dosage had to be reduced even further. It was reduced until subjects stopped dying right away from the vaccine, and instead were just more mildly poisoned (Jepson, 2007). Luckily, mercury is one of the most toxic substances known. Therefore this preservative, thimerasol, consisting of 40-50% ethyl mercury, the most toxic form, is able to effectively kill organisms attempting to grow in the vaccine vial even at very trace dosages.

In my opinion, what our government has further done wrong regarding vaccines, is to mandate them for kids attending public schools. A Texas governor even sought to mandate the HPV vaccine for young girls. That vaccine really isn't likely to be all that effective for the overall problems of cervical cancer and genital warts and, in my opinion, it is totally unnecessary in the United States where far fewer women die of cervical cancer now due to very effective screening and treatment.

The CDC reports that cervical cancer was, in fact, the leading cause of cancer death among women prior to the advent of Pap smear screening in the early 1950's. There was then a 74% decline in cases nationally between 1955 and 1992. A further decline in cases and death rates from cervical cancer has continued since then. The most recent CDC data posts only an estimated 4,210 deaths from cervical cancer nationwide in 2010. This is in stark contrast to third world countries (almost entirely devoid of Pap screening programs) where worldwide there are still an estimated 466,000 cases and 225,000 deaths from cervical cancer annually (CDC and WHO data). These third-world countries collectively comprise 88% of the world's incidence.

If anyone's failed to notice, there have been a growing number of deaths directly caused by that vaccine shortly after its administration. In June 2008, *Judicial Watch* reported 9,000 adverse events from the vaccine including at least 18 deaths. This was all in its less than 18 months of use across the country. At my last data check, in the fall of 2010, it was up to 80 or so deaths (if interested, go online and Google "Gardasil deaths"). This number is still climbing. It doesn't even account for the much greater number of patients that just suffer nonfatal neurological injury. Note that this vaccine is "marketed" heavily and given to healthy young women ages 13 to 26. These are young women in the prime of their life, with a lot to lose and very little to gain from this vaccine.

It seems obvious to me why this vaccine is encouraged here in the U.S. where it is not really needed: it sells for at least $120 per dose and three doses are required per the manufacturer guidelines. According to a report I read on the site *Healthcare Global* the manufacturer of the vaccine, Merck, has pledged to provide Gardasil™ for only $5 per dose to many third world countries. They have to push it at high value here in the U.S. to cover the cost (and ensure some *profits*) of this "humanitarian" work where the vaccine is actually needed.

Mind you, I have to agree that vaccines are important and are probably the second or third most effective means of saving children's lives. Basic sanitation and the use of antibiotics are likely numbers one and two. However, it doesn't seem right to *mandate* giving children something potentially very harmful (and if this isn't true, then why have a "vaccine injury" fund or legislation to protect Ely Lily?) when declining vaccination poses no direct risk to anyone else.

I mean, the shots work, right? If they do work, then your immunized kid should be safe from the disease my non-immunized kid may be carrying. If the vaccine doesn't work, then I really don't want it anyway! So if I don't immunize *my* kids, how does that put other immunized kids at risk? Some ignorant celebrities (actors and actresses who are not really authorities on anything, even if they've played a doctor on TV) have even stated that failing to immunize our kids is abusive or irresponsible or even worse (like those parents are "parasites" on society or something). The concept in public health is termed *herd immunity*, whereby if we immunize a large enough chunk of the population the whole burden of disease will go down and everyone will be at greatly decreased risk of ever encountering the particular disease. That makes some sense, but doesn't entail a global mandate in my view, especially for diseases that are rare in our population at this point (we no longer require the smallpox vaccine, for example).

In my experience, the parents I've seen who have chosen to not immunize their kids or have chosen just a select few shots, have more in-depth knowledge of the vaccines than most doctors I know (including me, until I started listening to them and doing more research). It should be within our rights, as parents, to decide what gets injected into our kids, wouldn't you agree? I sign vaccination waivers for parents as long as they can demonstrate to me an understanding of the risks and benefits of the vaccines. I also support them in choosing full immunization of their kids if that's what they want.

Sorry to drag on this discussion about vaccinations and thimerosal, but it has to appear somewhere in this book. I will discuss vaccinations more later on and propose a safer way of doing things as well. Now, let's move on to other items in this list of government failures or acts of commission.

We pay such high drug costs in the U.S. it's ridiculous. Again, everyone knows that the same medications can be obtained just over either our Northern or Southern border for a fraction of the cost. Why does our government allow this? Why do Medicare and Medicaid also pay full price for drugs when the prices could clearly be negotiated downward? They cut the doctors' fees without any negotiation or recourse on our part and, as I discussed earlier, the medication costs far exceed the amount paid to doctors.

Further annoying is the Medicaid "preferred drug" list that first came out while I was in residency. The drugs on the list to be covered by Medicaid seemed to change every 2-3 months. This made it very difficult to keep up with. I had to constantly rewrite prescriptions for these patients, switching back and forth to the drug *du jour*. It became very clear that the drugs were being chosen based on lobbying efforts by the manufacturers, and not what made the most sense medically or financially for our system. It is possible to get a different drug for a patient, but the physician must report that the patient is allergic to the listed drug or must prove the patient tried the listed drug and it failed for them; it created unnecessary excess work for practitioners and staff. This is one way all those drug lobbyists earn their keep, and it's even more annoying than when drug reps try to come into the office (they are not allowed in my office at all, and I have no drug samples whatsoever).

There is no government protection for our citizens against the immoral behaviors of insurance companies. We can be turned down for "pre-existing" conditions or be denied coverage for specific services, seemingly, at random. When the new health care reform We may be forced to go to a hospital over an hour's drive away, even in an emergency, if we want the costs to be covered, depending upon which hospital our insurance company has bargained with. We continue to see our premiums increase and our care coverage decrease to the point where even a "catastrophic" policy is not affordable for most people.

Our government acknowledges this is a huge problem for our people and the economy but nothing is done about it. The CEO's of insurance companies continue to make millions by effectively *not* paying for necessary care. They do it by employing armies of claims adjusters to systematically deny payment and lobbyists to make sure our politicians look the other way. As I frequently say to my patients: "Insurance companies don't make money by actually paying for things." Perhaps there should be some medical care available to everyone that is not driven by capitalism?

The pharmaceutical industry, of course, has a great deal of influence over our government as well. This leads to serious health and financial consequences. The industry has over 1,200 lobbyists in D.C. (Drinkard, 2005), also a number within each individual state; and the drug companies spend more than any other industry lobbying our government (Smith, 2007). It must be working in their favor or they wouldn't keep doing it. There is good evidence it is paying off for them. The Medicare Prescription Drug Improvement and Modernization Act of 2003, for example, prevented the government from negotiating drug prices and resulted in 61% of Medicare drug spending being direct profits for pharmaceutical companies (Sager, 2003). According to Marcia Angell, former head of the New England Journal of Medicine, "The United States is the only advanced country that permits the pharmaceutical industry to charge exactly what the market will bear." (Angell, 2002)

If our government really wanted to dispense with the current corrupt system and provide or mandate an affordable, basic level of medical care for everyone, it would be easy to do. After all, it's already been done by virtually every other industrialized nation on the planet and, somehow, they seem to do it better and cheaper (though I appreciate that many people feel the *better* part is debatable). All the arguments against government-provided health care in this country are essentially groundless in my opinion. There is no reason the intellectual power that we have in this country can't analyze the systems in other countries and devise strategies to incorporate their successes and avoid the mistakes they've made. Pointing to another system that isn't working perfectly and concluding that it can't be done at all is ridiculous. That's like saying the Commodore 64 was a lousy computer, so we shouldn't have bothered trying to make better ones. It's just about money and, the fact is, capitalist interests are consistently favored in the United States at the ever-growing expense of human health and safety.

Okay, I'll get off this particular soapbox – for now.

Lack Of Regulation Of The Food Industry

I'm going to look at this concern as an entirely new soapbox, but a potentially taller one. The food industry is not a direct part of the health care system, but I hope everyone will acknowledge the fact that food quality and safety are extremely important factors in one's health. I will discuss how food relates to health in much more detail in the later sections of this book but, for now, I will address the failings of the public and our government in regards to this important aspect of human health and safety.

Our food supply has not only been steadily devitalized by repeatedly growing the same monoculture crops on the same land, excessive processing and heating practices but, as I mentioned before, it is also polluted with over 8000 different chemical additives that are not truly safe for human consumption (Rea, 1992). In contrast, European governments have extensive, strict regulations on food additives. The British government doesn't even allow the addition of any sweeteners to foods intended for consumption by infants or children under age 3 (UK Food Standards Agency, Council Directive 89/398/EEC).

Are chemicals in our food a problem? Well, people in those other countries believe so, and there is a mounting body of research out there demonstrating or suggesting direct harm from a number of these substances. The nitrites in cured meats (lunch meat, sausage, bacon, hot dogs etc.) and caramel coloring have been linked to pancreatic cancers. Pesticides have been shown to cause neurological diseases and hormonal disruption (after all, they are chemicals designed to kill living organisms right?). Many of us already know we get sick from additives such as MSG and sulfites.

Artificial sweeteners trigger headaches for many people (I hear these things from patients frequently). There are many other examples.

So why are these poisons allowed in our food? It's partly because we have a national and even global food economy in this country, rather than a regionalized one that could provide clean, natural foods transported over only short distances. This makes it necessary for our manufactured foods to have longer shelf lives. We feel the need to have fresh fruit during the winter, thus we expend huge amounts of fossil fuels shipping items from all over. The distance that food is shipped is not a direct threat to human health. But it definitely indirectly affects us in terms of the true cost of that produce and the effects on the environment we all live in. There is excellent attention paid to this problem throughout Barbara Kingsolver's book, *Animal, Vegetable, Miracle.* I encourage everyone to read that book as well as Michael Polan's *Omnivore's Dilemma.* It also contains a great deal of important information about our polluted and dangerous food supply.

Direct harm from our produce comes in the forms of pesticides, herbicides, sprouting inhibitors, and chemicals to induce color changes. Humans are attracted to the color and appearance of produce. A large percentage of the chemicals polluting our produce are there simply to improve the color of the product, and are not adequately proven safe for consumption. Of course, "organic" produce is not supposed to have these chemicals, but the definition of that word has been revised under influence by the food production industry, with progressively loosened restrictions of course. Publication of the rules in 2000 allowed the term "100% organic" to be used if something contained all organic ingredients with the exception of only added water and salt, "organic" to be used if 95% or greater of the ingredients were truly organic (which means up to 5% *non*-organic), and "made with organic ingredients" if at least 70% of the ingredients are organic (which allows for up to 30% *non*-organic ingredients!).

Preservatives, artificial fragrances, flavors, and colors are also dangerous chemicals. Preservatives are basically chemicals that kill microorganisms and "preserve" the food for our own consumption instead. Some preservatives are natural substances and pose no threat to humans at all. Some artificial flavors and fragrances are byproducts of the petroleum industry, which happen to be perceived as certain tastes and smells by our sense organs. Industries would have to pay for proper disposal of these chemical byproducts if they weren't allowed to stick them into our foods and other products for humans. Just read the list of ingredients (the ones they actually choose to list on the label anyway) on most processed foods and count the substances that aren't really food at all.

Another dangerous food production process is "cold pasteurization". This is also called "electronic pasteurization". The standard way of pasteurizing or sterilizing liquid foods, such as milk or juices, is by heating them to the point where potentially harmful organisms are killed. "Cold" or "electronic" methods utilize radioactive waste to kill any organisms in the food. They pass the containers of milk, juices, or other foods by some dangerous waste material that is giving off harmful radiation. This is expected to kill anything living in the food. Unfortunately, there has not been a thorough attempt to find out if this practice is dangerous to the humans consuming these irradiated products. It is reasonable to suspect there could be changes in the foods themselves or perhaps small amounts of retained radiation present. Maybe that is harmless to us, but maybe it's not.

Why do they do this rather than heat the products? It just might be cheaper to buy radioactive waste material than to pay for the energy to heat a large amount of liquid; especially since those industries selling radioactive waste would otherwise have to pay large amounts of money to dispose of it properly. It's probably a win-win for the industries, and this often leads to a loss for consumers. I suspect we will see more and more of these products in stores if we go to more nuclear power generation in this country. After all, they have to do something with all that waste.

I will discuss more of the specific problems associated with various groups of chemicals as they relate to our health later on in this book. For now, suffice it to say, our government allows them in our food without evidence of their safety and with mounting evidence to the contrary. Our government willingly sacrifices our health for the almighty dollar. I know that sounds harsh, but it's absolutely true. Our government agencies, such as the EPA and FDA, are saddled with the task of "proving" that unnatural chemicals may be harmful to us rather than government requiring that the industries prove their products and practices are safe. This seems totally backwards. I will discuss our own guilt in regards to this problem later on as well. Don't think we have no responsibility ourselves regarding this matter.

Chapter 2 – Problems with Health Care Delivery

In addition to the system-wide philosophical problems, there are some major shortcomings in the way health care is administered to patients in the United States. I'm going to focus on practice habits of doctors themselves mostly, both in terms of practice philosophy and format. Some of these problems actually stem from issues involving medical education. That will be discussed in the next chapter.

SHORT VISITS

How much can a patient truly accomplish in a ten or fifteen minute office visit with a physician? It takes a few minutes just to say hello, be cordial, and for the doctor to figure out the reason for the visit in the first place. At best, really only one or two issues can be reviewed, and yet there are typically more problems than that to discuss. Even more importantly, multiple diverse issues may have just a single cause; but if the practitioner doesn't get the big picture, he/she is likely to miss the overriding upstream causes. Every primary care physician I know feels this is not an ideal way to practice. They feel rushed and stressed. So why do we operate in this manner?

Well-meaning doctors feel that they do the best job if they see as many people in the day as possible. They also feel that their bottom line depends upon this. What results is ineffective care, excessive testing (because it's faster to order a bunch of laboratory and radiological tests, in lieu of talking to the patient and examining them), and excessive use of prescription drugs for reported symptoms (again, it is much more time-efficient to start writing prescriptions specific to the symptoms you're complaining of, rather than seek out the underlying causes).

I have had numerous patients complain to me that their other doctor just immediately whips out the prescription pad and starts ordering drugs for them as soon as they begin to talk about their issues. In my experience, most patients don't want this type of care. Statistically, a large percentage of these prescriptions never get filled because the patient doesn't want them, can't afford them, or doesn't understand why they got the prescription in the first place. What too often results is an increase in side effects from taking unnecessary drugs. More importantly is the failure to truly identify the cause of the patient's problems and potentially "cure" them. In addition, we get an extremely expensive health-care system with relatively poor outcomes.

So is it really necessary to see so many patients in one day in order to provide "good care"? No, it's not.

Integrative physicians, such as myself, have found that if we take more time with each individual patient, we may actually begin to solve their problems. If we give ourselves enough time and information to make good decisions and figure out what the underlying issues truly are we can guide the patients to change their behavior, address underlying disease mechanisms, supplement their deficiencies, or otherwise find the ideal treatment to eliminate the causes of their problems. This eventually results in fewer visits by each individual patient over the course of the year, improved overall outcomes and health of our patient population which significantly lowers costs overall. Cost savings of integrative medical care also result from ordering fewer tests and prescribing fewer drugs.

So can this be cost-effective for a physician? Yes. I typically see only about ten patients per day. Those visits are either thirty minutes or a full hour in length. The difference is I speak-to multiple concerns at each visit. I often find that many of these seemingly-diverse issues are linked together and cannot be adequately addressed if taken separately. The financial result is billing a higher amount for each individual patient visit. This does not equate to a greater overall cost for the patient because they require fewer visits over time, and I generate fewer tests and drugs.

I currently have over 2,000 patients under my care, and I can usually see an established patient within a week or two. In residency training, I was seeing eighteen to twenty patients per day, had only a few hundred patients, and it took over three weeks for someone to get in to see me.

Granted, I only had 2 1/2 days of clinic per week, but this amounted to forty-five to fifty patient visits per week. This is about the same as I see now.

The biggest difference between then and now is that, before, my patients kept returning with the same problems over and over again. Their laboratory results rarely improved, their weight rarely went down, and their symptoms rarely alleviated. This occurred even though I was following the standard of care and prescribing all the right drugs. Their drug doses and the number of drugs they took just went up over time. Therefore, so did the salaries of CEOs for pharmaceutical companies and the cost of insurance premiums. Unfortunately, there was no similar benefit for their individual health or circumstance. In fairness, I also saw a generally more ill patient population with poor social and financial resources in residency.

Throughout later sections of this book, I will detail what I see as a better way to approach medicine and health care in general. Much of this relies on individual behavior and lifestyle habits, but there are also things doctors can prescribe other than pharmaceuticals. Prominent examples include nutrients, hormones and herbs. These things can affect positive changes in one's physiology and usually without adverse effects and with much lower expense.

Crowded Waiting Rooms And Sterile Environments

The fifteen-minute visit duration might not be so bad if the patient didn't have to wait an hour just to get in for that visit. Since it is virtually impossible to truly conduct many office visits in a ten to fifteen minute period, doctors tend to run perpetually behind schedule. I frequently run five to ten minutes late by the end of my clinic morning or afternoon, and this is with thirty or sixty minute appointments.

What results from doctors with perpetually behind schedules is a very crowded waiting room filled with not-so-thrilled patients looking at outdated magazines. To compound this problem, the front desk staff in most medical offices experiences a high rate of employee turnover and is therefore often staffed with irritable, grumpy individuals. It doesn't help that they field most of the complaints from unhappy patients. My office is not run this way.

Once a patient gets past the crowded "corral" and down the cattle chute, the exam rooms are likely to be cold and sterile in appearance. It isn't very often that a doctor's office has warm and inviting examination rooms with comfortable furniture or a pleasing decor. Personally, I have a couch and a couple of relatively comfortable chairs for patients and visitors, books and toys for children to play with, and lots of interesting decorations around my office. This is also my only exam room (that's right, nobody has to wait alone in a cold exam room after they already waited forever in the lobby).

If society is going to treat medicine as a consumer-driven "industry", we need to realize at some point that customer appeal is important. It does not cost very much nor take much time to dress up a waiting room a little bit and make it more comfortable and inviting. Paying an extra employee to staff the desk and answer the phone improves customer service dramatically as well as the general efficiency through the office. People hate it when nobody answers the phone at the doctor's office. Making exam rooms more comforting improves patients' experiences, increasing the likelihood they will remember what the doctor says to them as well as increasing their willingness to return. It reduces the stress of a medical visit, which is a huge barrier to successful therapy and healing in my opinion. The days of white lab coats, white or odd-green walls, and cold hard chairs are over. At least they should be.

Aside from the customer service aspect of all this, there is the humanity factor. This seems to be ignored too often. It may be just another day at the office for those who work there, but some patients come in with issues that are truly life or death matters. They may have fears of some horrible illness, are enduring debilitating symptoms, or are experiencing severe depression and sadness. They may feel incredible financial stress by coming to a physician's office (after all, medical care is the number one reason to go bankrupt in the United States), and this makes it all the more important to ensure that their experience is a positive one.

Focus On Diagnosis And Symptomatic Treatments

The concept of a "diagnosis" in modern medicine is a peculiar one. Most of our diagnoses are just a description of the symptoms, and do not reflect the true cause of the problem. Common examples include high blood pressure, obesity, diabetes, anxiety or depression, fibromyalgia, allergic rhinitis, insomnia, congestive heart failure, anemia, and many others.

There's this big book of 'ICD-9 codes' (international classification of diseases). This book contains thousands of "diagnoses", each having a corresponding code number. These codes are used for billing purposes and are the language of insurance companies. Many of these codes correspond to just pure symptoms such as cough, nausea, dizziness, and pain of all sorts. These are the numbers to use when a doctor doesn't have a better diagnosis. The tendency in medical practice is to find a "diagnosis" and then prescribe the appropriate treatment. This treatment is almost always a drug. This may involve anti-inflammatories for arthritis, blood pressure pills for hypertension, statin drugs for elevated cholesterol readings, antidepressants for irritability and sadness, acid reducing drugs for heartburn or narcotics for pain.

The problem is that these "diagnoses" usually have real treatable causes. Therefore, the diagnosis should not be the end, but rather the beginning. Once doctors have determined the full constellation of everything the patient is experiencing, it then behooves them to try and figure out *WHY*. The '*WHY*' is the really important part, don't you think? The *WHY* is often the reason a person goes to the doctor in the first place; people want answers and real solutions.

If you're depressed because you have vitamin D deficiency, don't you just need vitamin D? If you are hypertensive because you drink too much coffee and you are magnesium deficient, don't you just need to stop the coffee and take some magnesium? If someone is obese and has diabetes mainly because the individual is genetically intolerant of corn syrup, then doesn't he or she just need to stop consuming corn syrup?

Those examples may sound far-fetched, but I have seen them proven true time and time again. I could offer many more examples where there are simple non-drug solutions to common medical problems. In most cases though, things admittedly aren't that simple; there are often multiple causes for a problem. All need to be identified and addressed.

One of my mentors in my first year of medical school used the term "looking upstream". He described how this was so much more important than just treating symptoms. I also heard, numerous times, how it was most important to get a good history from the patient, and how this provided the diagnosis more than 80% of the time. It seems that our typical modern medical practice completely disregards these simple truisms. Quick symptomatic relief is too often favored over real long-term solutions. Quickly ordering expensive tests frequently occurs instead of spending more time getting the right information from the patient.

So how did medical practice end up this way? Why do so many doctors focus on treating symptoms rather than investigating for causes?

When did physicians start ordering so many unnecessary and expensive tests instead of talking and thinking adequately?

Well, we have these things called "algorithms". These algorithms are guidelines or protocols for treating our established diagnoses. So where do these algorithms come from? Too often, they come from the people who are making money off of the symptomatic treatments: drug companies, of course. Copies of medical treatment algorithms can be downloaded that often even have a drug company logo on them. Otherwise, they have some national medical association name on them. This is basically the same thing in my view, because they are all heavily funded and controlled by drug companies. These algorithms almost never contain nutritional or herbal interventions even if there is evidence those therapies work equally well or better. I will discuss more the concept of "evidence" a little later because this is a key element to the current problem.

Poor Approach To Prevention

Do smoke alarms prevent fires? Do seatbelts and airbags prevent car collisions? No, of course not, but they do reduce the consequences of these occurrences, and no one would say they are bad ideas.

Do mammograms prevent breast cancer? Do Pap smears prevent cervical cancer? Do colonoscopies prevent colon cancer? Does lowering one's cholesterol artificially with a drug reduce the risk of death from heart attack? Does using insulin for a type 2 diabetic prevent early death from cardiovascular disease? Do any of these things actually address the true cause of disease or prevent poor outcomes?

Firstly, mammograms do NOT prevent breast cancer from occurring. Mammograms are only an effort at "early detection". This can theoretically decrease death rates from breast cancer, and is therefore thought to be of significant value; however, it does not reduce the occurrence rate. Reducing the occurrence would depend upon understanding why it happens in the first place and intervening earlier. A "thermogram" is a test that can alert a physician to potentially precancerous metabolic changes in the breast and spark intervention before there is any cancer. This hasn't caught on very well yet because most doctors in this country, unfortunately, do not know what to do with the information. If conventional doctors were taught more about breast physiology, hormonal effects, natural anti-cancer concepts, and other aspects, then more practitioners would know how to intervene before there was full-blown cancer.

71

In actuality, the poor efficacy of conventional treatments for such cancers as lung and pancreatic cancers is why, in many cases, these diseases are not screened for at all. Finding cancer early doesn't help prevent death unless it can effectively be treated when it is discovered. Screening for such forms of cancer statistically appears to help at first because people live longer after diagnosis than if the diagnosis was made later on after symptoms develop.

Over time, though, the death rate looks just as bad as it did before and all that occurred was what is called "lead-time bias". This means that things were made to look better in terms of survival duration only because the diagnosis was made earlier. For example, if you find stage IV terminal pancreatic cancer on a screening CT scan (which we don't do) while you have no symptoms, it is likely to kill you at exactly the same time it was going to end your life in the first place, because it's not treatable; but, you may have the diagnosis documented perhaps six months earlier than when it would have been found once it had caused symptoms that drove you to the doctor for diagnosis. Finding it early therefore does not truly benefit you because it does not result in longer actual survival; but on paper it looks like you survived "with the diagnosis" six months longer than it would have.

The reality for the patient is just that they know about their cancer and impending death longer than they otherwise would have. This is not a true success. This is why we don't routinely screen smokers for lung cancer with annual chest x-rays; that was attempted in the past and did not result in people living longer (but they knew about their impending death longer). If we aren't likely to change the outcome, there is no reason to look for the disease.

Some authorities, such as the U.S. Preventive and Screening Task Force, are also starting to say this about prostate cancer, suggesting that screening with rectal exams and PSA levels is possibly not worthwhile because after years of doing that we haven't seen a decline in overall death rates from prostate cancer. I still screen people, however, because there are harmless and effective natural treatments that help reduce death from prostate cancer. Also, the prostate can be surgically removed and, if the cancer is caught early enough, the patient can truly be cured. These things should be considered on an individual basis, not just based on overall population statistics.

Pap smears and colonoscopies, on the other hand, can in fact reduce the occurrence of the cancers themselves. These tests can find *pre*-cancerous changes. Cervical changes on a Pap smear can be identified and intervention can then take place with effective natural therapies like folic acid, iodine, DIM, olive leaf extract, and vitamin D. Also, conventional treatments can be used such as cryotherapy or LEEP. These prevent the formation of true cervical cancer. Polyps can be found during a colonoscopy, and they can be removed. This prevents true cancer formation within the colon. These interventions are clearly more upstream and of much greater benefit, but they still don't address the true underlying causes of cancer.

Cholesterol drugs have not been similarly shown to reduce death rates from cardiovascular disease. Just listen very carefully to the next Lipitor™ or Crestor™ commercial; they don't claim that their drug is going to save or extend your life, but only lower cholesterol numbers. Who really cares about that if it doesn't mean being able to live longer? In fact, most lipid-lowering drugs have actually shown increases in death rates from a variety of causes outside of cardiovascular disease (CVD) (McGee, 2007), or even from CVD itself in the case of the fibric acid drugs used to lower triglycerides (World Health Organization study, cited in the drug information ad for the medication Trilipix™. They even admit this in their own drug information!).

Using insulin for type 2 diabetics has not led to any decrease in mortality from their number one killer: cardiovascular diseases. Insulin use often leads to persistent weight gain, which may have the consequence of worsening the underlying condition. Many other medications used for type 2 diabetes such as Actos™ and Avandia™ do the same thing: cause weight gain and increase the real problem. Avandia™ has been all over the news in recent years due to studies showing it increased the incidence of heart failure. Yet, as of mid-2011, there has not yet been a drug recall. It looks like it will be taken off the market soon at least, and the other drug in it's class should be removed at some point as well in my view. I stopped prescribing these drugs years ago because of how they work; it made no sense that they would really be good for someone.

Type 2 diabetes is completely preventable and even reversible through dietary and lifestyle measures. Most drugs marketed for diabetes make the underlying problems worse or cause other problems. Understanding the condition from a basic science and physiology perspective allows a practitioner to truly help the patient control and even reverse the disease. Prescribing only the *standard of care* therapy offers a false sense of security and typically just makes things worse.

Other failed attempts at prevention involve our usual wellness care.

This includes physical exams, well-child checks, and prenatal visits. If these visits were truly effective, we should not be seeing the increases in obesity, diabetes, cancers and other chronic diseases. We should not be seeing so many pregnancy complications leading to emergency c-sections and a persistently high infant mortality either. Doctors are generally not educated well enough to counsel patients effectively in preventing chronic disease. It takes a long time to provide the education to patients that may truly benefit their long-term health. Most of these visits simply generate a list of screening tests, only a few of which are helpful, as discussed above.

Most effective prevention involves changing lifestyle and dietary habits. The understanding of these issues is very poor or nonexistent in mainstream medicine. Rates of obesity, diabetes, and cardiovascular diseases continue to rise despite the encouragement and increased provision of routine physical exams and a steady diet of prescription drugs for our population. I recall when studying for my medical boards, the literature I read stated the odds of finding something important on routine physical exam were only three out of one thousand. Maybe we weren't taught to look for the right things?

The approach to our problem with infant mortality and poor pregnancy outcomes has involved increasing the number of recommended prenatal visits throughout pregnancy. I've noted how poorly we still rank amongst other nations, despite the U.S. having an average number of prenatal visits of about twelve to thirteen per pregnancy. Many other countries with better pregnancy outcomes than ours, average less than eight prenatal visits (Strong, 2002).

Going to the doctor more often doesn't help if the doctor doesn't know how to provide proper preventive care and advice. What is accomplished with this approach is that some serious problems are discovered early. This is a good thing but results in hospitalizing moms, possibly inducing labor, or delivering babies early by c-section when needed. There is some value to this, but it increases the complication rate as well because of all the intervention. In my world it is far from perfect. The c-section rate in American hospitals is now roughly one-third of births. I delivered our last two babies myself, at home in the bathtub.

Attendance at all suggested well-child visits is not likely to decrease a child's risk of obesity, ADHD, cancer, or autism. This is because the causes of these problems are poorly understood by mainstream physicians and are often in place prior to birth. It is unlikely those wellness visits will help reduce a child's risk of heart disease later in life. This is despite new recommendations by the American Heart Association and the American Academy of Pediatrics that cholesterol drugs be prescribed for kids as young as eight (their recommendations are available on their websites and are material of public record). I've already mentioned the failure of these drugs to prevent deaths and disease. The real solution is to change the kids' diets and get them exercising more; but taking a pill every day is far easier.

These problems all come down to the fact that our doctors, and our population in general, have no idea how to actually promote health and prevent most of our chronic disease problems. A better understanding of the causative factors behind our illnesses is needed. This information is available in most cases, but it is not directly taught to medical practitioners because those in charge of medical education want drugs to be used instead. Much of this book is dedicated towards educating the reader about those underlying causes, as well as providing strategies for fixing some of them on a large scale.

Antiquated Doctor-Patient Relationships

This could be placed in the next chapter because it relates to physician attitudes and philosophies. I placed it here because it is also a key part of health care delivery and involves cultural attitudes, just as much as physician attitudes.

Most doctors and health-care providers in this country still have a "paternalistic" attitude toward healthcare. This means that they feel patients should just do what they are told, preferably without asking many questions. Many mainstream physicians get quite annoyed if asked a lot of questions, and certainly irritated at a patient referring to medical information they read on the internet.

Many people, usually from older generations, actually feel most comfortable with the paternalistic style of physician-patient relationship. They were taught to hold doctors in high regard and feel they should be given extreme respect. The attitude of the older generations was that the doctors knew best and the patient should just do what they were told. This was probably a much safer attitude to have in the past, before doctors had such a vast armamentarium of toxic drugs to prescribe and when the causes of illness were more straightforward. In my opinion, as the patient/consumer, you should really double-check everything for yourself.

Most people don't really go for the paternalistic thing these days. The large proportion of prescriptions that never get filled is evidence of this. This traditional type of practice also seems to lead to a juvenile kind of behavior from the patient, one where they lie to hide things from their doctor. Probably the most common lie is to assure the doctor they are taking the prescribed medication when, in fact, they are not and may have never taken it. Most are also likely to deny drug use or excessive alcohol use when their doctor inquires.

The National Health Interview Survey in 2007 found that the use of complementary and alternative medical (CAM) therapies by American adults was up to 38.3%, from 36.0% in 2002. I have seen other surveys in the past revealing that a large percentage of such patients do not tell their (conventional) doctors about their use of CAM therapies. Many of my own patients have told me they would even lie about it when their prior doctors asked directly.

I know many of these things, not just because of studies and surveys, but because my patients tell me. They will admit to me things about their drug use and other sensitive things, saying: "I've never told another doctor this…" They will talk freely with me about all the different and unusual treatments they've tried because they know I'm open-minded about the subject. Some think that I may even have an educated opinion about it. It's less and less common for me to hear something new as the years go by, and my knowledge base is far greater because of the information patients themselves share with me. I have received many books, articles, product pamphlets, and internet printouts from my patients over the years; it's like having my own huge research team.

Many of my patients see various specialists as well seeing me. Some have other primary care doctors and will often tell me they don't tell their other doctors about the things we are doing; some will even lie to their other providers when directly asked about it, just to avoid the conflict. This may be because they've gotten into arguments with their doctors who have become angry with them for trying different approaches. Why should anyone have to worry about a doctor being mad at them? Aren't we, as medical providers, just supposed to be helping people? Shouldn't we be offering positive guidance, information, and education?

In my experience, most people really want to know *WHY* I am prescribing a particular test, treatment, or course of action. Correspondingly, I have found that if I take the time to explain everything to them, they're much more likely to follow through with it. Also, if I present multiple options to a patient, they get the feeling they are in charge of their own health decisions. This is as it should be, and it's a big reason why my patients tend to do better; they are engaged and empowered in their own care.

My style follows what is termed the "collaborative" model of medical care. This acknowledges the extremely vital role patients themselves play in their own health. A doctor can prescribe all the drugs they want, but the patient has to swallow them in order for them to work. Doctors can tell people to eat better and exercise, but if they don't explain what that means in practical terms, the patient won't be successful. Even better, if physicians can offer specific solutions and options for their patients, they will improve their success rate even further.

The word "doctor" is Greek for "teacher". This is why Ph.D.'s are called "doctor"; the "D" stands for *doctor*, and the "Ph" for *philosophy*, the designation meaning "doctor of philosophy" in whatever field. In fact, they are more aptly named doctor than a physician is, with that definition in mind. A "doctor" of some academic or professional field is generally one who teaches that material to others.

I take this to mean that my true job lies in explaining to the patients before me, why I believe what I do, and what I think they should do accordingly. My real job is to educate them about their own health and help guide their own decision-making about treatment choices. It is not my job to tell them what to do, as if my plan were the only option.

I still run into people, typically from older generations, who want me to do just that: tell them what to do. In these instances, I still explain multiple options and why I'm choosing one in particular. I also try to explain what the next step is likely to be in the event the first option doesn't work out.

In my experience, and corroborated by every integrative practitioner I know, this collaborative model of healthcare relationship works much better than the paternalistic, traditional style. Patients are far more successful in maintaining and improving their health if they take a personal role in the decision-making and implementation of their care.

On a personal level, it is better for me as well: I don't feel I "own" everyone's problems. I act as consultant, not dictator. Patients will often return to my office and apologize for not doing what I suggested they do (and I mean *often*). I usually reply, "That's okay, *I* still feel great!" This is to make it clear that the responsibility for their health and implementation of their care plan is truly *theirs*; therefore, I am not offended by their lack of adherence to our plan. I try to keep my own ego out of it.

My job is to continually encourage them and help them find strategies for success, not chastise them when they've gone against my advice. On the other side of that coin lies the personal responsibility on the part of the individual. I can't make someone eat right, exercise, or swallow a pill. I've found that seeing certain people as patients is frankly a waste of my time; they cannot benefit from my particular style of care until they are self-motivated to improve their own health. I end up prescribing symptomatic drugs for them, just like my conventional colleagues would, sometimes for years, until such time as they are ready to take charge of their health. This is annoying to me, but I do it when I am hopeful they will come around eventually.

Throughout the later parts of this book, I hope the reader will come to realize how important one's own behavior truly is in being healthy, and how limited it is what a doctor can really directly do for a person. Individuals must be proactive in regards to their health if being truly fit and successful is what is desired.

It is important to realize medical care itself is one of the leading causes of death in our society. I have seen it on various lists, sometimes ranking it as high as third or fourth (Starfield, 2000), just behind cardiovascular diseases, cancer, and autoimmune diseases. A recent CDC list, looking at more specific causes of death, listed hospital-acquired infections (related to the way we do medical care) as the fourth leading cause of death overall (that's up from sixth place some years back). Caused by "medical care" doesn't just refer to medical mistakes mind you; it includes the fatal adverse effects of treatments prescribed "appropriately" according to the standard of care, misdiagnosis, and failure to identify the true cause of the problem.

Therefore, if patients are at all unsure, I strongly encourage them to do lots of their own research and to question anything I say that they may feel uncertain about. I also encourage people to consult multiple practitioners and physicians until they get answers that make sense to them. It is important for each individual to realize that he/she is the most important member of his/her health care team, and the medical providers are just consultants or facilitators. We are not bosses or parents, and patients/consumers shouldn't just blindly do what we say. That being said, we the practitioners do not have to order any tests or prescribe any particular treatments just because a patient wants them; we are still liable for anything bad that may happen as a result, and we need to feel that what is happening is acceptable. It is truly a collaborative effort.

Research And Development

I know this doesn't directly address healthcare delivery, but it does help guide the way doctors do things and dictate what type of care gets paid for. It has become increasingly obvious that the money controlling most research and development comes, either directly or indirectly, from pharmaceutical companies or other big industry involved in health care. This is true even when the research comes from some government-funded or supposedly "independent" organization; the money ultimately comes from somewhere. Of course, this inappropriately tends to direct medical research towards the utilization of those strategies and technologies.

It is true that some fraction of research is being done in clinical nutrition and other more biological methods of healthcare. The problem is that most of the money to pay for these studies also comes from the big industries, too often from industries that have a strong interest in *disproving* those types of treatments. Most of the articles on nutritional therapies published in large mainstream medical journals show failure rather than success; this is an intentional result of studies performed by the very opponents of such therapies in order to show a negative result. It's quite clever actually.

There is also a problem in the medical literature called "publication bias", and it is extremely common on both sides of the table. A journal will have many articles and studies submitted for publication, then editorial preference determines which ones end up in print. Therefore, the editors have control over the "truth" in a sense, dictating what sort of spin medical practitioners will get on the effectiveness of therapies.

Because they are significantly funded by pharmaceutical companies or other special interests, most conventional medical journals and publications are biased toward pharmaceuticals, surgery, and conventional procedures of other sorts. They also tend to publish only studies that reflect negatively on natural therapies, rather than showing the positive results as well. On the other side of this is the fact that most integrative or alternative medical journals tend to publish only positive articles on nutritional and natural therapies. Seldom do they publish failures of natural therapies. This is for the same general reason as the conventional journals: the main source of advertising dollars for the natural journals is nutraceutical companies that produce the therapies in question. This bilateral publication bias results in an even larger divide and an even greater difficulty in finding the "truth", if there is such a thing.

Another annoying theme in drug research is that many or most new drugs are not truly new. Many of the "new" drugs hitting the market each year are actually just a new take on an old theme. They are often what we call "me too" drugs. This is, for example, one company's attempt to create a competitor drug to another popular medication already on the market. For example, if one company produces a great new blood pressure medication in a novel drug class, it kicks off a race for every other drug company to try and produce a similar drug in order to secure their share of that market. These competitor drugs aren't really new in concept or function, but at least they serve to offer financial competition and options for those who may react badly to one or more drugs in a particular class.

Many more new drugs are just a more specific chemical form of a drug that already exists and made by the same company. These "new" drugs are what we call "stereoisomers" in organic chemistry, a concept I won't bore you with here. Suffice it to say that many chemicals exist in a 50/50 mixture of two mirror-image molecules. The "left-handed" version may work far better than the "right-handed" version, or vice-versa. The drug will initially be sold as the 50/50 mixture until its patent runs out, and then the more active stereoisomer will be sold individually as if it were a completely new drug (when the companies know about this from the very beginning). Common examples include: "esomeprazole" after omeprazole went generic, "levalbuterol" instead of plain albuterol, "levocetirizine" after cetirizine, and "escitalopram" instead of citalopram (all generic names – but feel free to look up the brand names so you will better recognize them).

These "new" drug forms are always touted to work better or have fewer side effects than their predecessors. In actuality these differences are either tiny or they are mere statistical tricks in most cases. It is just a sneaky way to extend a patent and make another mountain of money from essentially the same drug. Didn't they know about the most effective form of the drug when they first developed it? Of course they did. These practices do not result in the advancement of medicine. They are just evidence of the unconscionable greed involved in modern health industries.

Drug companies spend far more on advertising for their drugs than they do on research and development (Sufrin, 2008). That gap is even wider for the above types of "new" drugs, since they require very little additional research to gain approval. Pharmaceutical companies like to suggest they need to charge a lot for their drugs in order to cover costs of research and development, but they neglect to mention the much greater costs of mainstream advertising and direct-to-prescriber marketing through drug reps.

There is incredible bias in most medical research because the people who usually fund it have a direct interest in seeing that the new drug, test, or therapy will succeed. They can manipulate patient selection, duration, methods of study, many other variables, as well as their final statistics in order to make the outcome appear in their favor. Also, it has only been in recent years that researchers have been forced to publish all their data and all of their studies, including the negative ones (thank you, Freedom of Information Act). Before that, they could totally suppress any data that reflected badly on their product, and that was regular practice.

It's true that the government funds some research, but who do you think funds our government? Our politicians have to disclose their finances, and it was stated during the 2008 election cycle that more than 60% of our senators were multi-millionaires. Who is making our congressmen into millionaires when their salaries may be $250,000 per year? Or, why would a millionaire take such a large pay cut? Most of them have financial motivators for their decisions, rather than what is truly best for the population, in my opinion. Corruption seems rampant in government regulatory agencies as well.

How is it, for example, after decades of denial, the FDA eventually approved aspartame for use in food? This, just after a new director (apparently a more easily influenced one) was appointed. An excellent timeline of this, by Rich Murray, can be found on *Rense.com*. How is it that Synthroid™ was finally approved for use in hypothyroidism in 2002 after more than forty years of non-approval due to lack of effectiveness data (there are many accounts of this saga on the internet if you Google "*synthroid FDA approval*")? Why did the EPA's own scientists have to publicly speak out against their own organization's stance regarding fluoride in 2005 while the official position still suggests fluoride is safe and beneficial? The 2005 EPA scientists' press release on fluoride may be found online at: http://www.nteu280.org/Issues/Fluoride/Press%20Release.%20Fluoride.htm

Is it because corporate interests control these government-affiliated authorities on multiple levels? It's a reasonable suspicion.

The sad truth, about research and development in medicine in the U.S. is that it is mainly geared toward selling products and maximizing profits for those already in power while very little attention is paid to human health and safety. If this were reversed, there would be far more money spent in studying the benefits of proper food production, environmental toxicity issues, nutrient supplementation, and hormonal therapies in the management of medical problems. These benefits are far more cost-effective and extremely safe interventions. They are also, in my experience, even more effective health-wise than conventional therapies in most cases.

We have to be skeptical when people are quoting "the literature" and making suggestions based on "the best available research". Unfortunately, we cannot often trust the conventional sources of information because the motives are not pure. It is also true that most people only "research" the sources they expect to agree with their own opinions. And, when a commercial says "Nine out of ten doctors agree…", this should immediately cause suspicion because it's very hard to even get two or three doctors to agree on something. I wonder what that tenth doctor knows that the others don't. I'm usually that tenth doctor it seems, rarely agreeing with the mainstream group.

The wrong research conclusions lead the consumer down the wrong path and perpetually farther away from the truth. These dogmatic, but false concepts, dictate much of conventional medical practice. Modern practitioners parrot the things they have heard without really understanding them or knowing where they originated. We are probably all guilty of this to some extent because it's hard to take the time needed to validate everything one hears or is taught. But when it's our job to help people get better, and they're not improving, we should do some more looking and learning, rather than just "walking the dogma".

Chapter 3 – Problems with Medical Education and Philosophy

In my opinion, the current state of medical education is one of the most important problems with our health care system. If our doctors were better educated regarding the ultimate causes of illness and the use of therapies that are less harmful, less expensive, and offer more long-term success, there would be significantly improved health outcomes in our society.

Going to the doctor more often will not help you if the doctor doesn't know how to help. Even worse, going to the doctor can be dangerous, if the doctor only prescribes therapies that can cause harm. In my experience, physicians and other conventional medical providers are very good people with the best intentions for their patients; we are just fed a lot of garbage and propaganda during our education and training, as we are led unwittingly into "the box." Health practitioners come out of training wanting to do a good job, but are not given the proper tools and are too brainwashed to see it. This chapter will cover some of the glaring shortcomings in medical education on both a formal and informal basis.

Content Deficiencies

What medical students and residents are *NOT* being taught is possibly a bigger problem than what they are actually being told to do.

<u>Nutrition</u>

An obviously glaring deficiency in our medical education is the subject of nutrition. I would be surprised if any American-trained M.D. or D.O. (osteopath) currently working in this country had more than twenty hours of total nutritional training, during medical school and residency combined. I believe my own experience, at the University of Washington, consisted of one two-hour session per week, for eight weeks; and this is, supposedly, the number one primary care school in the U.S. During that time, the training mainly focused on blood cholesterol levels, instructing patients to avoid saturated fat (not really a good idea by the way), how to count calories, and how to calculate intravenous nutrition.

There was also some limited discussion on protein and carbohydrate metabolism. Nothing was covered about vitamins and minerals, phytonutrients, essential fatty acids, or many of the other things I've learned about since which are indispensible for good health and medical care.

This was a serious disappointment to me personally. I had expected to learn a lot about vitamins and minerals, as well as proper food sources for the right macronutrients (protein, fat, carbohydrates). I always thought the old adage "you are what you eat" was one of the few clear truths we had. This critical concept was really not seriously discussed. Throughout later medical training, it was frankly sort of ridiculed or, at best, deemed unimportant.

I hate to break it to all the conventional medical folk out there, but every single part of our body, from your brain to your toenails and all the little chemical molecules in between, is made from *FOOD*. That is, everything which isn't currently made out of petroleum waste products or other chemical agents in our body. I guess I should say we are <u>supposed to be</u> made from food. Unfortunately, when we truly are what we eat, we have to take the good with the bad these days.

I have since learned that the most critical thing I can do regarding bettering patients' health, is to educate them about nutrition and encourage them to begin rebuilding their body with proper materials. If a person weighs roughly 100 pounds, he/she eats about a pound of food material per day and has a few pounds of water per day; the individual will easily consume his/her body weight in materials every month. If a small portion of that material is retained as new tissue, to replace that which is broken down on a regular basis, a person gets practically a whole new body, in terms of raw materials turnover, probably every 6 to 12 months.

There is, of course, wide debate on this and some would argue that certain cells of our body don't turnover at all in our lifetime (like brain cells), while others turnover extremely slowly (like cardiac muscle cells) – but I'm not talking about the individual cells as entities. I'm talking about the materials from which they are made; that "stuff" does get constantly cycled through us like the water of a river. It appears there is always the same river in front of you; but the water molecules you see at any given moment are different from the last, and they came from all over the world in the past. The benefit of this constant nutrient cycling is that, if people start eating extremely healthy and take care of themselves, they can make tremendous improvements in health within that first six to twelve months.

What makes the nutrition deficiency in our education even worse is that much of the prevailing dogma in our society regarding nutrition is just plain wrong. Examples of this errant information include the avoidance of cholesterol and saturated fat, with resulting demonization of eggs and butter, avoidance of salt, the suggestion that grain and cereal products should be the bulk of our diet, suggested limitations of meat products, and the idea that it is necessary to eat dairy products or drink milk for optimal health. I'll discuss why these assertions are false later in the book.

The medical community itself propagates a lot of this nonsense, as we are supposed to be the authority on the matter. The suggested American Heart Association (AHA) diet is really *not* the best way to reduce cardiovascular risk through food. They ascribe to the low-fat diet concept, but there is not true validation for this. They tend to follow the work of Dr. Pritikin mainly, but Dr. Pritikin himself eventually developed cancer and committed suicide. It is very possible that these events are directly attributable to his low-fat diet because other studies into this concept have demonstrated increased cancer rates and neurological problems, which include mood disorders and suicides (Fallon, 2001). The AHA diet is also at opposition with the Mediterranean diet, which *has* in fact been shown to reduce cardiovascular disease, cancer and death (Mitrou, 2007).

The AHA also strongly encourages low salt intake, a recommendation based on fairly poor research. There was an epidemiologic study into other cultures on the planet, looking at the question of salt intake, and how it related to blood pressure. One particular group's diet, which lived in the jungles of South America, had very low amounts of salt and low blood pressure in general. What wasn't emphasized was the fact that this population rarely lived past their thirties, so we don't really know if it led to a decrease in mortality from cardiovascular causes or not. The vast majority of other populations showed no correlation at all between salt intake and blood pressure (Brownstein, 2006).

The reality of this subject is that some individuals truly are inherently sensitive to salt, while others actually see reduced blood pressure with intentional sea salt intake, myself included. There will be a thorough discussion of salt and how it relates to your health in Section III.

I don't want to sound too much like a conspiracy theorist (though it's probably too late for that), but it is very likely that the American food and pharmaceutical industries intentionally foster our poor education regarding nutrition. How else are they going to sell us all of their hydrogenated oils, genetically modified corn, and heavily processed packaged foods riddled with chemical agents? What better way to keep our population sick, than to feed them bad food? The last thing they want is a doctor who actually knows something about nutrition.

Nutrition as medicine

To take this issue a step further, it is often possible to use basic nutrients in place of many medications. This concept includes a medical philosophy called orthomolecular medicine. This is a field founded largely by Linus Pauling, and others, who discovered that large amounts of particular essential nutrients could correct disease processes.

This practice is far safer than using pharmaceuticals and frequently just as effective. Some nutrients actually are part of conventional medical training. One example is N-Acetyl Cysteine (marketed as the brand name Mucomyst™). This is a modified amino acid that is key in producing your body's most potent antioxidant, called glutathione. It is given orally in the emergency setting as the sole effective treatment for acetaminophen (Tylenol™) overdose. It is also given intravenously to protect the kidneys from the effects of IV contrast administered during CT scans, and it is administered in an inhaled form to help break up mucous in the lungs.

Magnesium is another excellent example. It is first-line for many obstetricians in the management of preeclampsia (toxemia of pregnancy) or preterm labor, and it is still the "drug" of choice to correct a potentially fatal heart rhythm disturbance called torsades de pointes. Magnesium can be used intravenously to treat many other acute problems as well, but it is seldom chosen as the first-line therapy because there are no drug reps going around encouraging doctors to use it.

Our medical schools may touch on using nutrients to replace a severe deficiency condition (i.e. iron for anemia, vitamin B12 for pernicious anemia, thiamine for beriberi, vitamin C for scurvy, and so on), but they do not usually emphasize the use of nutrients as therapeutic agents in the absence of such proven deficiency. Some exceptions include the use of vitamin D for osteoporosis, niacin for high cholesterol, and the use of fish oil to treat high triglycerides or cardiac arrhythmias. There are many other places where nutritional therapies should be used as the first choice of treatment but, due to our biased training, it takes much more convincing to get conventional doctors to use a natural or nutritional therapy before a prescription drug in most instances.

As I mentioned before, it's my opinion that we should always, if possible, use something that actually belongs in the human body first. I think we should try to use items that are safer and less expensive before reaching for pharmaceuticals. I don't know why this isn't the prevailing opinion among my colleagues who seem to prefer dogmatically following the standard of care, even when it makes no scientific sense.

Herbal medicines

I don't recall many particular herbs being discussed in my medical school training except, perhaps, to note the origins of some of our common drugs. Modern American medical training may touch on the use of such things as Echinacea, St. John's Wort, milk thistle, saw palmetto, or others. However, herbal medicines are seldom suggested as the first line therapy over a pharmaceutical agent. Herbs are often discussed only in respect to negative studies attempting to discredit them. Milk thistle may be the one exception to this because it has shown significant promise in aiding liver detoxification. There are no drugs that do so, since they are generally toxic chemicals themselves after all.

Many other cultures have utilized herbal medicines for millennia with success. Many third world countries still rely heavily on this type of medicine because, if they know where to look, it is available to everyone. Some industrialized nations, notably Germany, have numerous herbal medications on their national formulary (the German "E Commission") as first-line treatment choices.

Conventional medical training is virtually devoid of education in the proper preparation or use of herbs. Naturopathic physicians, however, have extensive training in this. Oriental Medical Doctors and licensed acupuncturists do as well. Naturopaths typically focus more on western herbs, while the other two study eastern herbs. Ayurveda is an East Indian system of healing that heavily relies on herbs as well, with its own particular varieties. There are strong herbal traditions practiced by indigenous peoples on every populated continent and island. People in the past instinctively knew, or learned through generations of experimentation, how to heal themselves and others with the plants and other substances around them. As I mentioned before, many of our common medications are initially derived from herbal substances. Examples include digitalis from foxglove, aspirin from willow, and Taxol™ (a chemotherapy drug) from the yew tree. There are many others.

We have numerous examples demonstrating that, if the whole herb itself is used, better efficacy and reduced side effects result compared to extracting the single chemical and giving it at a higher dose. One excellent example of this is the original active agent in our first "statin" drug used to lower cholesterol. "Lovastatin" is the active chemical agent within red yeast rice. This is an herb (specifically a fungus) used for lowering cholesterol levels today, apparently used for other health issues beginning more than one thousand years ago in China. Lovastatin is also now the generic name of the drug Mevacor™. This was the first so-called "statin" to hit the market. Studies have shown that the cholesterol-lowering effects of Lovastatin are much greater when used in the whole herb form. Typical prescription doses of Mevacor™ range from 20 to 40 mg per day, but usually only 7 to 15 mg of the active chemical within red yeast rice extract is needed to achieve similar results (derived from 600-1200mg of the whole herb). Also, this entails a greatly decreased risk of side effects, with only rare and mild adverse reactions being reported from use of the herbal form (Hendler, *PDR for Nutritional Supplements*, 2001).

The company that produced Mevacor™, of course, tried to sue nutraceutical manufacturers who produced red yeast rice extract on the grounds of patent infringement. A judge appropriately threw the case out (the drug company didn't even change the chemical name, and the herbal medicine had been around for a long time). Meanwhile, we all know that the pharmaceutical version can cause liver failure, muscle breakdown, kidney failure, and other devastating consequences (just read the drug package insert). In spite of all this, Lipitor™, a newer statin, eventually became the number one selling drug worldwide for a time (listings of current best-selling drugs, complied from various sources, can be found online; but who knows how they keep track?).

I would like to propose some cautions in dealing with herbal medications. Some of the concerns that the conventional medical community has about herbal medicines are, in fact, appropriate. There is significant concern regarding the standardization and quality of herbal medicines in this country and others because the manufacturing practices are not very well regulated. When an herbal preparation is bought off the shelf, there may be no assurance on the label that it's potency is what it should be, whether it contains contaminants such as solvents or heavy metals, or if it might contain other herbs or substances that could interact in a harmful manner.

Also, there is a vast difference between indigenous herbalism and modern herbal supplements. If an herb is obtained in its natural environment, at the appropriate time in its growth cycle, at the right time of year and the right time of day, then it should have all of its power and potency to offer. This is an extremely different situation than an herb that was farm-raised under ideal conditions, possibly treated with pesticides or irrigated with water containing arsenic or lead, picked at the wrong time because of convenience or manufacturing demands. The wild herb would be expected to have far greater medicinal potency because it had to fight for survival, thereby inducing the production of those health-promoting compounds for its own use (plants don't make those chemicals specifically for *us,* after all).

In this country, most of our published research is based on the mass-produced version of herbal therapies and often shows poor efficacy. Mainstream medicine points to this as an argument against using herbs. I would have to agree that using typical herbs off the shelf at the grocery store is less likely to benefit most people. Real indigenous herbalism, however, is something close to nature, which offers some of the true healing power of the Earth. This sort of thing, I believe, is taught in naturopathic training and the other systems of healing mentioned previously. Many of these practitioners get their bulk herbs from carefully selected providers and produce combination remedies their selves. That's what is ideally desired in an herbal therapy.

I personally put most herbal therapies a little way down the list in my toolbox, after lifestyle change, nutrition, hormone replacement, and possibly even acupuncture. This is because, to me, an herb is often just a kind of "green pharmacology". They offer chemicals that manipulate one's physiology in abnormal ways, rather than replacing something that is missing in order to achieve improved symptoms or function. It is always better to replace that which is missing, and remove that which is damaging, first. Granted, herbs are much safer than prescription drugs in general. I would prefer to use them first, if possible, before writing a prescription.

Exercise

"Eat right and exercise." That's typically the extent of the nutrition and activity advice given by most doctors in this country. I haven't seen this sort of flat, limited advice work very well. This approach is clearly lacking in substance, mainly because our medical education on the topic is also lacking in substance.

We do get training in physiology and how it relates to physical activity. We do know how sugar and fat are burned to make energy. We do understand the concept that increasing one's activity level burns more calories, and eating less puts fewer calories in. Unfortunately, there are problems with this oversimplified view.

Weight loss is not nearly as simple as just calories out versus calories in. A calorie is just a unit of energy measurement, and we all get different "gas mileage" so to speak. Telling a patient to count calories in their diet is often not a very useful thing to do. This is because a person really has no way of determining how many calories they are going to expend on any given day. The Olympic swimming star, Michael Phelps, claimed to eat 10,000 calories per day while he trained; and he looked pretty darn skinny to me. I have had many obese women tell me they are eating 1000 calories or less per day. Though I was trained to disbelieve them, I've come to find this is often the truth.

The fact is that the vast majority of your daily energy expenditure is dependent mainly upon your resting or "basal" metabolism, and not so much on your level of physical activity. We can probably manipulate only about 15% of our daily energy expenditure through exercise activities, unless we go to an extreme. This is why the typical advice from doctors, telling people to just walk or do some moderate aerobic activity for exercise, is usually ineffective.

Studies have demonstrated that when patients walk for exercise, they usually have to walk more than a total of five hours per week to begin losing weight (Hyman, 2008). What really happens here is that people may burn an extra 200 to 500 calories with an hour of walking, but then they tend to sit more during the rest of the day, leading to no net increase in total caloric expenditure for the day. To make matters worse, most people will eat more because now they have worked up an appetite. They often give themselves some sort of treat for their effort, eliminating any potential benefit in terms of calorie balance. It must be realized that it is far easier to put in 500 calories than to burn it off.

I think this is why I see a lot of obese people walking, and walking, and walking, and staying obese. Poor advice usually yields poor results and leads to major discouragement. I will go over this again and further discuss exercise for various health issues later on in this book.

Environmental medicine and detoxification

It should be obvious to anyone who's paying attention that our changing environment and the increases in pollution have a lot to do with human health and the dramatic increases we have seen in chronic diseases. Unfortunately, these concepts do not enter into conventional medical training very often, if at all. Therefore, these environmental factors don't even exist to most practitioners. If a doctor is asked about it, they may just completely blow off the question. At best they will suggest there may be an issue, but they don't know much about it. At worst, they may act like you're an idiot for asking.

We do get some limited training in "toxicology", but this typically relates to massive short-term exposures and is under the rubric of emergency medicine; it is not at all the same idea as *environmental medicine*. The concepts of chronic, heavy metal poisoning, long-term accumulation of pesticide residues, the effects of ingested plastics and related chemicals on hormone systems and childhood development are never really discussed in conventional medical training. And yet, we have mounting data to suggest that these, and other environmental toxicity issues, are at the root of many of today's rapidly increasing chronic medical problems (Christiani, 2011).

Notable conditions that have a clear relationship to increases in environmental toxicity include autism, infertility, hypertension, cardiovascular disease, fibromyalgia, hypothyroidism, PMS, cancer, diabetes (type 2, or adult onset), Parkinson's disease, as well as many others. Simply treating the symptoms of these conditions, without addressing the underlying toxic causes, is an utter failure of modern medicine.

Doctors trained in our conventional medical system still think that those of us doing heavy metals testing and detoxification are "quacks" or maybe some less favorable term. And yet, if you look at the environmental protection agency website, it will tell you lead is an extremely pervasive toxic metal in our environment, and we are all likely to have some level built up within our tissues at this point. It lists an extensive array of symptoms and medical conditions that may arise from accumulated lead toxicity, then (laughably) suggests that if you believe you may have a problem with lead, talk to your doctor about it. Unfortunately most doctors won't believe you, and if they did, they generally lack the knowledge to assist you properly. It's just not part of our conventional training.

We have evidence linking the nitrites in our cured meats to the development of pancreatic cancer (World Cancer Research Fund, 2008), the pesticides in some of our foods to the development of Parkinson's disease (Le Couteur, 1999), and the fluoride in our water supplies to increased rates of bone cancers in children (DeNoon, 2006). In spite of the data, these poisonous chemicals are still pervasive in our food and water; and these are just three examples. The fact that our medical providers are not trained properly in regards to environmental toxicity helps perpetuate this problem.

Luckily, there are teaching organizations for health care providers in this country such as The American Academy of Environmental Medicine and The American College for Advancement in Medicine. These organizations train physicians and other medical providers in ways of testing and treating these toxicity issues. I will provide more details about this in the sections on environmental toxicity and detoxification.

Energy medicine and spirituality

To some extent, these topics have in fact gained some ground in conventional medical circles. Harvard Medical School has their Center for Mind-Body Medicine; Andrew Weil, MD, has his integrative fellowship in Arizona; and Deepak Chopra is a popular writer and speaker on the subject (though I don't know how often he is invited to lecture at conventional medical schools).

Some related concepts during my own training, involved the respect of and the suggestion that we pay attention to the spiritual beliefs and practices of our patients. This was discussed in both my medical school and residency curricula, and I see that as a positive thing. There is also a strong belief that the psychological state of the patient influences their health. Unfortunately, this is usually used in a negative sense to declare that a patients' problems are "all in their head", rather than identifying the underlying physiological causes that typically exist.

Some common energy-based therapies that I feel are neglected include acupuncture, Reiki and other energy healing techniques, kinesiology, and electro-diagnostic machines for identifying energetic imbalances in the body. In addition, just the general understanding of the energy fields our human body possesses and the role they have in our overall health is neglected.

Conventionally trained physicians readily accept the concepts of the EKG (electrocardiogram) and EEG (electroencephalogram). Notice both tests have "electro" in them, since they work by evaluating the electromagnetic energy fields given off by the body. These are both frequently used as diagnostic tools but, for some reason, practitioners won't accept the similar technology of the EAV machine (electro-acupuncture according to Voll) or newer versions, such as the *Indigo*™ machine. These devices involve attaching electrodes at various places and running a diagnostic study on the body's energy fields. This is similar to what the mechanic might do with a car. Most of the early machines were developed in Germany, which as I've already mentioned, has what seems like a more integrative and effective health care system.

The problem is that our medical providers are not taught about the basic energetic systems in the body. They aren't taught about the meridians, the chakras, the kundalini, or the different layers of subtle energy fields all about our bodies. They aren't taught about the microcrystalline structure and microtubule system that runs through every tissue of the body, which has been identified structurally by Korean scientists and corresponds to the acupuncture meridians demonstrated by ancient Chinese medicine.

They don't even wonder how a small, spherical human embryo "knows" how to turn into a four-limbed, bilaterally symmetrical shape instead of a worm or fish. Neither do they understand how a drug such as thalidomide can interfere with that development, causing a child to grow one arm but not the other. Scientists have shown that a round salamander egg has a measurable energy field in the shape of the adult salamander. This field and the electrical polarity at the limb (which is different from ours) is how that salamander can actually re-grow a severed limb in the appropriate shape and size (Oschmann, 2000). Why couldn't we do that for people if we figured out how to create the same circumstances energetically? First, we have to actually take notice of the possibility.

Medical providers aren't taught how an individual practitioner can learn to manipulate energy and stimulate the healing process in someone. Nurses have developed the practice of "healing touch", but I don't believe this is taught in medical school like it should be. For centuries, many other cultures have had energy healers, people who could help with symptoms or the healing of tissue merely with their intention and focus.

I have had training in Reiki, a system of Japanese energy healing that translates to English as "universal love". Having been trained in conventional medicine, I was skeptical about this myself at first. But I have since had many occasions where I was able to alleviate someone's pain and affect other types of healing using these techniques without even touching them. One could easily suspect it is a "placebo effect", but I don't think it is. It seems to work just as well on skeptics as on true believers. It has also worked on people when I did not tell them what I was doing.

Why would an energy healer's hand, hovering above a person's skin, provide a better placebo effect than a prescription painkiller or muscle relaxer? More importantly, does this even matter? A big part of our problem here is just plain lack of acceptance of what we do not understand. Luckily, books have been written on these topics with significant amounts of basic science to back it up. The two key books that I've read in this area are *Energy Medicine* by Oschmann and *Vibrational Medicine* by Gerber. I highly recommend the first one to everyone, and the second to those who want more information.

Holistic health concepts

This isn't a specific educational content issue, but more of a philosophical one. It is, however, an approach to the patient that is not formally taught. The drive to make a diagnosis then jump to symptomatic treatment is more the standard teaching.

Conventional medical providers are not taught to evaluate how various medical issues interact with each other, how much patients' lifestyle and environment truly impact their health, or how severely ongoing stressors in their life might be directly influencing their physiology. We are taught that diet has a little something to do with one's health but nothing more specific about nutrition. We are taught that one's mental state influences a person's health, but mainly just so we can put people on antidepressants for just about any chronic complaint. Conventional doctors are taught about the effects of stress, but we are not typically taught stress reduction techniques to offer our patients.

Much of the later parts of this book will be devoted to discussing this complexity of human health, and how we need to address all of its parts in order to be successful.

Other missing subjects

There are many other areas where our conventional medical education is deficient, such as the use of therapeutic and bio-identical hormone therapy or a thorough understanding of drug interactions and their long-term effects on physiology. I believe I learned more useful clinical material in the first five years after finishing my formal medical training than I did in five years of conventional clinical medical training. I have spent hundreds of hours and thousands of dollars doing additional training and education in integrative medicine topics. I firmly believe much of what I've learned should be required study in all medical schools.

Errant medical philosophies and practices

Some of these philosophies and practices are true medical education content issues, but many are more commonly related to habitual practices of physicians that arise from underlying principles we are taught and attitudes acquired through working with other practitioners. I can perceive the roots of some of these issues, but I have no idea where the others originated.

This category involves what I call medical dogma. It is a compilation of some of the attitudes and philosophies that the general medical community seems to hold true in rigid fashion. In my opinion, the conventional medical community is very much like a cult. We are expected to believe and do certain things, and anyone deviating from those typical behaviors is deemed inappropriate or even unsafe. There is both formal and informal "excommunication", if you will, from the conventional medical community for practitioners who opt for some unconventional therapies.

We are at risk of being professionally or socially ostracized by our medical colleagues, and even investigated by our state medical boards. These investigations are often instituted even when there have been no patient complaints or harm whatsoever. It is ironic that most practitioners being scrutinized and persecuted are actually trying to develop or utilize methods that are safer or more effective than conventional therapies; or, in some instances, where no conventional treatment even exists (see, for example, the recent case of the Texas state medical board versus Dr. William Rae, a founder of modern environmental medicine. Doctor Rae finally prevailed, but only after years of distress and lots of money spent on lawyers).

<u>The roots of some "medical evil"</u>

It is very interesting to learn how our conventional medical model came to rely so heavily on pharmaceutical therapies and became so set against "alternative therapies". The roots of this major swing can be, at least partially, traced back just 100 years or so to something called the "Flexner Report".

Abraham Flexner was a secondary school teacher. He was not a doctor or medical person of any sort. In 1910 he published an extensive report as to the state of medical schools and education throughout the United States and Canada. He had reviewed the status and curriculum in all 155 such schools. He had German roots in education, having attended a university in Berlin. He felt that medical education should have its most firm grounding in biomedical science and formal analytic reasoning, but with a stronger clinical teaching element as well (Cooke, 2006).

He felt a doctor's decisions should be firmly rooted in basic science concepts, but they should also have a very good social and humanistic aspect to their delivery of medical care. He believed that careful research was extremely important, but only as a tool for providing better health to the patient. He was of the attitude "think much, publish little" (Cooke, 2006). This sounds like a great idea, but as with so many other great ideas, the people involved tend to screw things up.

As a result of Flexner's report and the recommendations of the AMA that followed, many of the medical schools at the time were shut down or went out of business. It just so happened that most of these failed schools still taught primarily nutrition and natural medicine rather than delving into more biochemical and pharmaceutical research. It was those latter institutions to which the AMA then threw its support.

Interestingly, Flexner was employed in this effort and funded by the Carnegie Foundation for the Advancement of Teaching. The request for this particular project originally came from the American Medical Association in 1908. So the AMA later took part in the final formulation and enactment of the Flexner Report. If we look back to the roots of the AMA, this organization arose in the mid-1800s with the formation of the modern AMA around the 1880s.

The AMA was an organization of white male doctors only, until well into the 20th century, and it has a long history of heavily supporting the pharmaceutical industry. This is evident by looking at any copy of their publication, *The Journal of the American Medical Association* (JAMA), and finding that drug ads comprise more than half its weight. The AMA also has willingly taken financial support from purveyors of ill health. The tobacco industry was one of the biggest sources of advertising dollars for JAMA and other medical journals until cigarettes were finally prohibited from advertising by federal law. This was long after the scientific evidence had made it abundantly clear that smoking was bad for a person's health (Blum, 2010).

The AMA has a well-documented history of attack against alternative medical practitioners and groups. Spokesmen for the AMA in the early to mid 20th century openly condemned the use of herbs and nutritional therapies in medicine. They founded their own "Bureau of Investigation" which looked into the practices of individual practitioners and healers and identified those who didn't comply with their idea of conventional medicine as "quacks". Their "quack file" eventually grew to contain over 300,000 names. I don't believe this designation or condemnation was based on any documented harm to patients at all, just as the majority of cases against perceived alternative or integrative providers today are not based on any such issues. Search "Quack Watch" on the internet over time– maybe my name will be there one day (I would be honored!).

It is well documented that the AMA basically tried to stamp out the entire practice of chiropractic medicine in an organized fashion through most of the 20th century. Finally, in August of 1987, the District Judge Susan Getzendanner found the AMA guilty of waging a conspiracy against the practice of chiropractic medicine in an attempt to eliminate them. This was seen as a violation of the Sherman antitrust law (this history is a matter of public record). After that, the attacks finally had to stop, and chiropractic medicine has been allowed to exist relatively peacefully ever since.

For many years, osteopaths (D.O.) experienced similar discrimination problems until conventional medicine pretty much assimilated them (if you can't beat them, *convert them*, I guess). Nowadays, a D.O. is virtually the same as an M.D. in practice. Most D.O.s these days though do not continue to perform osteopathic manipulation after training. Osteopathic education is now basically controlled by pharmaceutical companies, just like M.D. programs are. The majority of them practice typical conventional medicine or they go into subspecialty fields rather than primary care, upon which the whole field is based (Johnson, 2001).

If there is any doubt that pharmaceutical companies control American medical education, look at the front page of the *New York Times* from March 3, 2009. There is an article by Duff Wilson, detailing a four-year controversy within Harvard Medical School regarding investigations into the financial ties between many of their medical faculty and pharmaceutical companies or other medical industries. This all started when medical students (and you know they only accept the really smart ones at Harvard, right?) began asking critical questions about the cholesterol lowering "statin" drugs. Their professor at the time began to ridicule these students and belittle them because of their comments and foolish notions. Some of the students decided to look into this professor and found that he had extensive ties to, and received a large degree of funding directly from, the manufacturer of a major cholesterol drug. This sparked further investigation and led to the requirement that all professors fully disclose any ties to pharmaceutical companies or medical businesses.

Since then, one Harvard professor's disclosure in class listed forty-seven different company affiliations. Sixteen hundred of Harvard's professors and lecturers have disclosed industry ties, including 149 with financial ties to Pfizer and 130 with ties to Merck. Incidentally, just a week after the publication of the March 3rd *New York Times* article, these two companies merged.

Harvard students have spoken out saying that they believe Harvard needs to live up to its name as a respectable institution, and that they feel they are being indoctrinated into a field of medicine that is becoming more and more commercialized. Harvard representatives say that industrial funds are an entirely appropriate source, if done properly. I think the word "appropriate" really means "lucrative" in this case.

According to Wilson's article, pharmaceutical companies contributed $8.6 million for basic science research and $3 million for continuing education classes to Harvard in 2008. These numbers do not count dollars that were paid directly to individual professors and lecturers. Many professors reported "over $30,000" as their industry dollars received the prior year because the university only required that they report actual amounts up to $30,000. One professor was paid $270,000 in 2007 for sitting on the board of Bristol-Myers Squibb (all from Wilson, 2009). But I'm sure their teaching isn't influenced by these relationships or money at all. Sure.

Again, I'm pretty sure most health practitioners of all types are truly trying to make people better. I'm not sure where the crime is in that unless people are getting hurt, or real fraud can be proven such as with the proverbial "snake oil salesman." Well, I've seen a lot of modern-day drugs come out of the pharmaceutical companies and kill patients, just to be recalled within the first two or three years. Does anyone remember Vioxx™, Baycol™, Omniflox™, Bextra™ and many others? The recalls of those drugs were national news at the time, but quickly forgotten by the public in many cases. Even worse, there are many other drugs that remain on the market even though we know they cause devastating consequences including death by various means (cholesterol drugs, antidepressants, antipsychotics, blood thinners, painkillers, cardiac or diabetes drugs, etc.). If you read the package inserts for many drugs, the serious risks, including death, are written very plainly but often ignored or not treated seriously.

Some estimates suggest that every year well over 100,000 deaths in America are directly attributable to the negative effects of prescription drugs. Based on the FDA's reported data, which is often felt to be very conservative in it's publicly-reported numbers in this regard, have posted a 61% increase in drug-related deaths from the 2000-2004 period (141,715 "summary" deaths reported) to the 2005-2009 period (228,341 total drug deaths). These stats are posted on the FDA site and recanted by a myriad of news agencies or other reporting agencies.

If you go to the FDA website, www.fda.gov, and search for the "Adverse Events Reporting System", you can find the actual raw data the FDA has had reported from health practitioners around the country. They don't make this easy to access, but it is there, as mandated by the freedom of information act (so noted at the top of the document I found). This data posts 183,567 suspected drug-related deaths from just the last quarter, October to December, of 2010. If this is consistent throughout the year, it amounts to a possible drug-related death count of over 734,000 per year! Somehow the FDA whittles this number down to less than 100,000 deaths per year for their official reporting. Granted, not all the reported cases will be truly related to the drugs in question since doctors are supposed to report all "suspected" cases; but it seems like a huge proportion of cases reported are found to be "unrelated".

Those drugs stay around because they are part of our "standard of care" as determined by the illustrious AMA. It's unfortunate that the standard of care does not start with basic lifestyle and nutritional modification; nutritional supplementation to fix deficiencies; high-dose nutrients in an orthomolecular medicine fashion; herbal remedies that achieve the same effects as pharmaceuticals but with fewer side effects; hormones or other substances that actually belong in the human body and achieve physiological effects while promoting health and alleviating symptoms at the same time; and many other so-called "alternative" therapies. My response to physicians and others when they suggest that my practice is "alternative" is to say: "there is no alternative to good medicine."

It is evident that money is perhaps the root of all evil in medicine, as it is in many other areas of our society. Let's look more into some of the belief systems and philosophies of modern conventional medicine, in an effort to try and understand this disconnect many of us perceive between conventional medicine and integrative medicine.

The Brainwashing

I'm sure that Harvard is not the exception, but the rule, in regards to pharmaceutical and other industry influence of medical education in this country. What results is a very insidious control over the minds of our medical doctors. They have forged an unwitting army of pawns to do their bidding, which is lined out in the practice standards and treatment algorithms brought to us directly from companies like Pfizer and Merck. What makes this even more effective is how doctors are repeatedly ridiculed during training if they try to think outside this "box". In my opinion, only self-confident, open-minded, dedicated, and bright students manage to make it through medical education without being thoroughly brainwashed. Many are brainwashed in spite of meeting those criteria.

I once asked another integrative colleague of mine why it was that so many doctors don't seem to "hear" what we tell them, when explaining aspects of biochemical medicine such as he and I practice. After all, it's based solidly in science, unlike much of conventional medicine. His response was that medical school admission tends to select for "rule followers." I realized that this was true; the application process involves a lot of hoops to jump through, and they like to see students who do the volunteer work and get the right letters from the right people. Students who stand out as having their own unique opinions (like I did the first go-round) are not as well received. Once a candidate is in the medical education system there are more "rules of practice" to learn, rather than learning basic information and applying it creatively. Original thought is discouraged, while following conventional practice standards is expected.

So what has resulted is very insidious and heavily favors the drug companies. Our medical education system has fostered numerous errant philosophies, some of which propagate the nearly singular use of prescription drugs to treat symptoms rather than the search for actual causes of illness and treatment based on addressing those causes. We don't teach our doctors to use nutrition, herbs or other natural forms of healing. We have them convinced that those things are worthless, or even dangerous, even though most other developed countries, and virtually all third-world countries, utilize these therapies extensively. We have a medical system that seeks to extinguish other types of healers and practitioners, through formal and informal means, such as medical board investigations or public scrutiny, rumors, or community ostracizing.

The conventional medical reliance on drugs is so apparent that I repeatedly have patients tell me they think their previous doctors are "getting kickbacks" from drug companies. I explain to them how it is even worse than that. The doctors actually believe they are practicing the best medicine; hell, most of them even take the prescription drugs themselves and give them to their spouses and children. That is the degree of brainwashing we endure through conventional medical education. Sometimes, I think it's akin to a suicide bomber for the mujahidin. When some of us are able to still think for ourselves, which is strongly discouraged in conventional medicine, we cannot fathom how we ever used to think that way and believed all the nonsense at one point.

I would like to go a little deeper into some of these nonsense philosophies, and how they came to be so prevalent.

The pharmaceutical age

Following the dramatic shift in overall medical education that resulted from the Flexner report, medical schools, teaching predominantly natural and nutritional therapies, were basically shut down. The institutions that remained were those focusing more on biochemical science and more interested in pharmaceutical research. Even though Flexner had suggested doctors research things for themselves and apply knowledge directly to patient care, what resulted was very different.

The remaining medical schools began looking for grant money to do more research and publish more articles. The largest sources of money available were from chemical and pharmaceutical companies, which were far smaller and fewer in number then than they are today. There logically began a major publication bias toward writings that demonstrated positive effects of drugs rather than the negative ones, in order to stay in the favor of those with the money. This bias seems to be at least a hundred years old.

The bias is particularly glaring when a drug company is funding the study, as the vast majority of pharmaceutical studies are. Sometimes a study claims to be from a government agency or alleged "independent" research group, but if you trace the roots, they usually lead right to "big pharma" (the pharmaceutical industry as a whole). You have to look at the authors listed for the study and research their funding sources and professional affiliations, because this information is not presented explicitly. I would contend that identifying the funding source of a study is just as important, if not more important, than evaluating the statistics and conclusions that are published.

What resulted from this new focus on drug research was an explosion of pharmaceutical companies, along with vast sums of money dumped into research and development toward this cause. The increase in wealth rapidly strengthened the pharmaceutical companies' hold on the medical system, and eventually on our government and regulatory bodies. I believe, along with many others, that pharmaceutical companies have a frightening death grip on our medical education, health care system, and government. The pharmaceutical industry, as a whole, had 1,274 registered lobbyists in Washington D.C in 2005 (Drinkard). Big pharma spends on average over $120 million per year on federal lobbying, more than any other industry (Senate Office of Public Records, lobbying data), and donates more than $12 million per year to political candidates, giving approximately three times as much to Republicans as to Democrats (Smith, 2007).

Basic marketing strategy says that in order to sell a product, the message must get out. That's why we have a drug rep (traveling salesmen) for roughly every seven doctors in this country (Sufrin, 2008), and multiple pharmaceutical company lobbyists for every congressman and major government official. Pharmaceutical companies spend far more on advertising than they do on research, with estimates ranging from $30 billion to $57 billion in the year 2005 alone. As of 2008, New Zealand was the only other country allowing direct-to-consumer advertising of drugs (Sufrin, 2008); the rest must have figured out that it's a bad idea.

Recently, drug companies began advertising their products on television, which I personally feel should never have been allowed. It must be an effective tool, because the ads have clearly increased in number. The public media is an excellent tool to convince the masses that they need drugs to be healthy. And, of course, our conventionally trained doctors will certainly agree. It's easy to find medical experts for public product support, especially if they are well paid.

The flipside of this is that along the road to making more drugs, we also left behind many safer and effective therapies. We forgot about basic nutrition. We forgot about stressing exercise and lifestyle interventions. We forgot about herbs and have paid little or no attention to mind-body therapies. We have ignored the environment as a major cause of disease, and learned nothing about detoxification. We have attributed way too many symptoms to depression or other mental illness, and therefore frequently just toss psychotropic drugs at people. Conventional doctors tend to throw drugs at folks for just about everything, and then more drugs to treat the ill effects from the first round of drugs. We've got to stop this insanity at some point.

Pharmaceuticals as the "best" treatments

My first-year physiology course in medical school primarily discussed the effects of drugs on human physiology, which was actually quite instructional since many of our pharmaceutical agents disrupt human physiology significantly. However, there was virtually no discussion of any vitamins, minerals, phytonutrients, or herbs and their effects on physiology. From the very beginning it was more about pharmacology than it was about understanding how the body works on its own, with solely natural and internal influences. It was never explained how all those amazing natural chemicals reacting in our body are all derived from nutrients in food.

In the second year, there was a full year course in pharmacology that was very time-intensive and thorough. As I have mentioned previously, there were about twelve total hours dedicated to nutrition, which in my opinion was not really about nutrition at all.

In the third and fourth years of medical school, we focus on *clinical* training, which entails following around residents and faculty physicians, learning how to actually *practice* medicine. I'm not sure I ever heard anyone give dietary advice, suggest vitamins, minerals, or other nutritional agents (other than a prenatal vitamin for pregnant women), much less any herbal remedies, during those two years. There were lots of prescriptions written however.

These are the years when we begin to attend those wonderful drug representative sponsored luncheons as well. We might even get clipboards, pens or other trinkets with drug names on them. The most expensive thing I ever received from a drug rep was a textbook, which I was allowed to choose myself, valued up to $150.

It turns out that medical students are very influenced by food, hence the sponsored lunches. It also turns out that mere name recognition is an extremely powerful advertising tool, hence the free pens and other items. This is also why corporate advertising time on TV is so valuable, and even negative press is good advertising for a product. If we want to prescribe a certain type of drug and there are five to choose from, we are probably going to choose the one we happen to have printed on our pen, merely because we see it out of the corner of our eye all day and it therefore seems familiar.

In residency, the training focuses quite a bit on standards of practice and treatment algorithms, both of which, as I've mentioned before, heavily favor pharmaceutical treatments in the United States. Again, there's no real formal training regarding nutritional therapies, herbs, or any other natural practice in most residencies.

I should mention, however, alternative and complementary therapies do seem to be gaining more interest in conventional medical training. Many U.S. medical schools now have a CAM (Complementary and Alternative Medicine) interest group, or even elective courses in later years. Some residencies, including the one I attended in Alaska, offer formal training to some extent broaden our perspectives and understanding of trans-cultural and holistic practices.

As far as I've seen, however, these forms of training focus mainly on just a rudimentary understanding of what those other practitioners are doing. This does not mean the students come away with any sort of useful skill in these areas, or necessarily a positive appreciation for what those practitioners are doing. This training seems to be geared toward giving our medical doctors the ability to have an educated discussion with their patients regarding those therapies. Similarly, it seems to me that many of them still feel just as negatively towards those therapies, and now they present a more convincing argument against them because they feel like they know what they are talking about (but, of course, they don't really).

Our current medical training system benefits the drug companies in at least five major ways. First, drugs are the primary tools our doctors reach for as therapy. Second, they tend to directly discourage their patients from using other forms of therapy such as herbs, vitamins, chiropractic, acupuncture and other therapies. Third, with our treatments focused mainly upon symptom management, patients tend to (conveniently) stay ill, which means they will need more drugs. Fourth, many of these drugs have side effects, requiring (also very conveniently) other drugs to control them. Fifth, in most cases, the general public doesn't know differently, so they usually follow the recommendations of their doctors and, thereby, adopt the same attitude in favor of drugs.

So basically, our medical training is focused on drugs, drugs, and more drugs. Even astute clinicians who identify a cause of a patient's symptoms are still likely to just prescribe the recommended drugs for alleviating those symptoms. This is our training, and this is what we're good at. It's fast and easy from the doctor's perspective; we can see someone every ten to fifteen minutes using this model.

As my former residency director put it to his residents, "It would take too much time reading and researching to validate the new things Dr. Vincent is suggesting and doing" (paraphrase); that's why they aren't allowed to spend time with me any longer – we wouldn't want them "thinking" too much outside the dogma. Meanwhile we are expected to happily swallow what information the drug companies feed us, without even chewing. There was no required reading or research to validate the formal teaching in my residency. I, during my time as chief resident, proposed reading assignments and formal testing to ensure accountability for learning the material in each rotation during residency; this idea was summarily put down by the faculty because it would be "asking too much" of the residents.

Evidence-Based Medicine

As I've mentioned, I often compare modern, conventional medicine to a religious cult, and every religion has its scripture. There is a need to describe what "truth" is, and what it looks like. This concept in medicine has evolved over the centuries. Early on, one man's observation about something was passed on by word of mouth; medical education was largely in the form of apprenticeships. Examples of these traditional healing methods include native herbalism and folk medicine. Shamanistic types of medicine even involved observations using senses that the rest of us don't seem to readily possess (maybe with a little help from some peyote or mushrooms, smoking some herbs, licking a frog or something – possibly similar to how congress comes up with some of its ideas).

As science and the written word began to develop, information was more readily disseminated; knowledge was eventually put into textbooks and medicine began to have more standardization. As more and more people enter a given field, more and more diverse ideas result, which logically beget more and more arguments. Therefore, we developed the concept of "peer-reviewed" information and research in our literature.

Medical information used to primarily consist of laboratory science and case reports or observations based on single encounters or a handful of cases. Primary laboratory research is basic science and is still considered highly valid, although most clinical practitioners don't read that stuff because it's too technical and difficult for us to understand. Clinical research articles contain intentionally complex language and statistics as well, which causes most physicians to spend little time reading them. Instead, most of my colleagues rely on the drug representatives to provide the highlights and tell them what they should do.

What we have progressed to in modern medical research are larger and larger "clinical trials" evaluating the effects of a given therapy on a given problem. This type of research is extremely easy to manipulate and generates the "expected" results far more often than is legitimate.

Epidemiological research attempts to identify risk factors for disease or characteristics of how something infectious is perhaps spread. It involves looking at large groups of people and trying to find common factors that seem to relate to a given condition. A good example of this is the Framingham, Massachusetts study on heart disease (usually simply referred to as "Framingham"). This study involved thousands of people, in the same town, and tracked them for more than a couple of decades. The study evaluated a number of factors thought to be related to cardiovascular disease and then used statistical analyses to decide which ones truly seemed related to the outcomes of interest.

Through this landmark study, we developed some of our parameters for cholesterol and blood pressure. It was discovered that smoking was a major problem, found that males had higher heart disease risk than females as well as other important conclusions. The problem with epidemiological research is the way that those with special interests twist the statistics and report false conclusions to suit their own goals. Drug companies have convinced most of America, and more than 90% of our doctors, that the Framingham study identified high cholesterol as a major risk factor for cardiovascular disease. If the data is interpreted logically, however, it is evident that this isn't a valid conclusion. Analysis of this data can be found in many sources, most of them biased (in one direction or the other, depending upon the source). Explanations arguing my point here can be read in books such as *Heart Frauds*, by Charles McGee, MD, and *Overdosed America*, by John Abramson, MD.

The data actually showed those with the lowest levels of cholesterol had just as high a risk for cardiovascular disease, if not worse, than those with the highest levels. Also, epidemiological research has shown that half of people having heart attacks have completely normal cholesterol levels.

The connection is really not there, but the cholesterol drug ads on TV all day convince many people otherwise. Doctors don't often take the time to read the actual research or investigate all sides of an argument; that would take way too much time. Instead they mostly go with the dogma and follow the herd like good worker bees.

"Observational" research involves looking at people with a certain condition versus people of similar makeup, who don't have the condition to see which factors are more prevalent in one group or another or perhaps how the condition progresses. This gives further clues into what habits or lifestyle factors, even medical interventions, may be related to the development, prevention or treatment of a given problem.

Epidemiological or observational studies don't adequately help us evaluate treatments and their successes according to modern medical dogma, but they may provide clues about which treatments to investigate further. Those "clues" used to be good enough to pattern treatments after, or at least strongly encourage certain lifestyle behaviors. These days these types of study are rarely respected enough by themselves. For example, epidemiologic population studies have repeatedly suggested a decrease in heart attack rates with greater magnesium intake from drinking water (Catling, 2008), but this does not get incorporated into formal practice or even garner further study.

Observations by clinicians as far back as Hippocrates have shown that gum disease or gingivitis is a strong risk factor for heart attacks, and more recent studies have again confirmed that association (Andriankaja, 2011). Furthermore, multiple recent epidemiologic or observational studies have suggested a clear correlation between higher vitamin D levels in the blood and lower rates of heart attacks, stroke, heart failure and various cardiovascular risk factors (Anderson, 2010).

Based on these studies, one would hope for cardiologists to tell their patients to supplement with magnesium, brush their teeth and use a WaterPik™ twice daily to keep their gums healthy, and take a therapeutic dose of vitamin D on an ongoing basis in order to help prevent heart attacks. Those interventions are all exceedingly safe and inexpensive. Unfortunately I don't think many, if any, cardiologists do this. However, I'm sure they regularly suggest aspirin, blood pressure pills, and cholesterol drugs. Unfortunately, these drugs have shown inconsistent benefits at best, and they have all caused numerous deaths.

So, why is there such a disconnect between logic and practice?

The search for better truth, specifically the "truth" pharmaceutical companies want us to believe, has led to the development of larger and larger "clinical trials" to evaluate the effects of a specific therapy for a specific problem. It is not deemed valid to base our medical decision-making on epidemiological or observational research, and we certainly don't try to claim a given treatment works based on just a handful of successful cases. That's called "anecdotal" research, and even though it's what healing systems all over the planet were founded on, it is now considered worthless under the current dogma.

Our current "truths" come from extremely large and expensive research trials that generally involve one drug being used to treat one condition or symptom. Under the current intellectual regime in medicine, this is the only real way to "prove" something really works. We have to take thousands of individuals and give groups of them different therapies, such as aspirin for one group and a sugar pill or "placebo" for the other group. Placebos are in fact very powerful medicines themselves. They can cause (mild) side effects and actually help treat the condition of interest, often 30% of the time or more across a myriad of different studies, depending upon the condition being treated. This is suspected to be a psychological effect and prescribing placebos is not common practice any more, as it was in the past, even though they are cheap and virtually harmless.

Anyway, back to the idea of the big expensive studies. After choosing two treatment groups, the subjects must be followed over time, sometimes many years if the event in question is a fairly rare one, such as heart attacks. Something interesting about research is that it relies upon statistics, and then how someone chooses to interpret those statistics. I like to say: "statistics don't lie, but statisticians do."

A good example of this is the top-selling drug, Lipitor™. They have done many enormous studies with drugs like this. A prominent example is the Anglo-Scandinavian Cardiac Outcomes Trial, called the "ASCOT" study for short. It looked at more than 10,000 people over a three to five year period These were people who had mild to moderately elevated cholesterol plus three or more risk factors for cardiovascular disease. They gave half of the group the drug and the other half a placebo pill. They found that, within about three years, the men in the placebo group had a 3% rate of nonfatal heart attacks and a much lower (than 3%) rate of heart attack-related death. The men treated daily with 10 mg of Lipitor™ had no significant decrease in death rates overall, or death by heart attack specifically, but showed only a 1.9% rate of nonfatal heart attack.

Incidentally, I mentioned these results for men specifically, because there was no such decrease seen in women as a subgroup. This implies the drug is not at all helpful in women who have not had a previous heart attack, even if they have three or more risk factors plus mildly high cholesterol, right? Results of the ASCOT study are available on the Lipitor™ website, with analyses of the study's data found in numerous articles, usually biased in one direction or another. I encourage you to read the actual study data and form your own conclusions, rather than accept any biased analysis.

Now, do you think the headline of this study's article read: "Lipitor™ slightly decreases heart attack rates but doesn't save anyone's life and doesn't work at all in women"? No, of course not. For Pfizer, this translated to a "36.7% decrease in heart attacks!" because 1.1 divided by 3.0 is 36.666. Well, that sounds pretty darn good, doesn't it? Unfortunately, it is misleading to the general public. Average people, hearing those statistics, may think that if they take Lipitor™, they will have a 36% lowered risk of having a heart attack, even if they are female. This isn't what it means at all.

A more useful way to interpret such data is to calculate what's called a "number needed to treat", or NNT. To get this, you take the absolute reduction in occurrence rates and divide it into 100% (because <u>everyone</u> in the study took the pill, not just the people who would have had heart attacks). So, if you divide 100 by 1.1, you get 90.9. This means in practical terms, you have to treat roughly 91 of these high-risk men with 10 mg of Lipitor™ daily, for three years or so, in order to prevent one nonfatal heart attack. The other 90 men will have no apparent benefit, but will have the risks of adverse effects from the drug (which are extensive). The data also suggests that you will not see decreased death rates from use the drug, no matter how many people like this are treated.

Suddenly, the odds of truly benefiting from this drug don't look so good, do they? Especially for women, right? Based on the available evidence overall, you're a lot better off drinking more water, exercising, eating healthier (e.g. the Mediterranean diet), using a water-pik, having a glass of red wine here and there, taking some magnesium and vitamin D. But Lipitor™ is the number one selling drug in the world, so what the heck is going on?

This brings up the problems of "publication bias", advertising, and relevancy. As I mentioned previously, the major medical journals are full of pharmaceutical advertising. This means that not only are the drugs constantly waved in our faces with misleading statistics, but also the drug companies have powerful influence over the information that is published in those journals. Is an editor going to publish negative results for a drug, or even critically review a study with obviously skewed conclusions, when they have come to rely on the advertising dollars from that drug's manufacturer? Probably not, when that editor and his/her journal benefit thousands, or even millions of dollars by remaining in the drug company's favor (Smith, R., 2005).

In my opinion, advertising for drugs shouldn't be allowed, especially direct advertising to the consumer, such as television ads for drugs. If we truly want our medical care to be based on "solid evidence", then we should rid ourselves of these psychological influences and statistical shenanigans. I've seen hundreds of women who have been prescribed these cholesterol drugs without proven benefit to them. I was even responsible for a number of these prescriptions myself before I read the research for myself. Prior to that, I think I just believed what I was told by my peers and the pharmaceutical reps, just like everyone else.

The issue of *relevancy* in our evidence and research is here in this example as well, because people will argue, "I take those drugs, and they definitely make my cholesterol levels go down". The commercials on TV for Lipitor™ talk about how effectively the drug lowers cholesterol, but who cares? Listen closely, they do not claim to prevent death because that would be a lie and yet, that's the outcome a person probably cares most about. Our previous epidemiological studies (e.g. the Framingham Study) were not really clear whether cholesterol has some causal association with heart attack risk. The drug may effectively lower your blood cholesterol levels, but you have to ask yourself why that matters to you at all.

It has to be proven the drug "works" in clinical trials. In this case, and in my opinion, they failed. High cholesterol is, at most, just an associated factor and not a true "cause" of cardiovascular disease. For these drugs to have relevance in my practice, they should decrease death or disease as well. They do apparently reduce heart attacks to a small degree for men with multiple risk factors, diabetics, and those with established cardiovascular disease. They have even better data in those who have already had a cardiovascular event, such as a heart attack or stroke. So their use should, in my view, be limited to those groups.

The relevancy issue goes back to the "so what?" regarding cholesterol. Looking at the first twenty years of using various drugs to artificially lower cholesterol levels (because we've been trying to do this for over thirty years now), it can be seen that none of the medications worked at all to improve cardiovascular events, and many of the studies actually showed worse outcomes when this was done (McGee, 2007). No cholesterol-lowering medications showed cardiovascular benefits until the statin drugs came on the scene.

A modern example of cholesterol drug failure is drug ezetimibe (the brand name is Zetia™). The 2008 study called the "ENHANCE Trial", evaluating simvastatin versus the combination drug Vytorin™, which is simvastatin plus the new drug ezetimibe, it showed that plaques inside patients' coronary arteries actually *increased* in size when using the combination with this newer drug. The study suggested, to anyone reading with objectivity, that ezitimibe was probably not a good thing to use (Toth, 2008). This information was noted in the news all over the country and has stirred up significant controversy. As of this writing, the drugs Vytorin™ and Zetia™ remain on the market and continue to be prescribed by many of my colleagues, who apparently believe drug reps over obvious scientific evidence to the contrary.

The available "evidence" would lead me to conclude that cholesterol levels are just a "surrogate marker" for cardiovascular disease. It is just another *symptom* of some underlying metabolic process, which leads to higher cholesterol and/or cardiovascular disease in some people. There is an "association", but clearly not a cause and effect relationship. So why are we still trying to artificially lower cholesterol levels with drugs? Well, ask conventional medical doctors and they will claim that it's because "the evidence supports it", or "it's the standard of care." I don't think the evidence supports it very well at all, and I think the standards suck frankly. As I've said before, my standards are much higher.

The practice of prescribing cholesterol drugs is a good example of the ingrained corruption we have in our medical system. Antidepressants, antipsychotics, acid reducing medications, and numerous other substances are grossly overused without adequate data to support their long-term use. There are many other examples in other drug categories, I assure you.

The fact is, even if only one out of ninety-one men is going to benefit from their Lipitor™ prescription (but won't necessarily live any longer, mind you), the manufacturers are going to benefit a lot. Multiply $100 per month for the drug, times twelve months per year, times three years (because remember, that's how long it took to see this difference), times the ninety-one men given the drug; the resulting sum is $327,600. Wow, that is one expensive heart attack! But this drug is not prescribed for just ninety-one men. It's prescribed for millions of men, as well as millions of women who do not apparently benefit at all.

In defense of statin drugs like Lipitor™, they do at least show some measurable benefit. Those benefits are definitely greater when considering patients who are much higher risk, have already have had a heart attack or stroke, or have known cardiovascular disease. But these numbers still aren't very impressive. Maybe one person in 30-40 benefits, though, instead of 90 or more.

There is research suggesting the same cholesterol-lowering benefits can be achieved taking a statin drug just once per week, rather than daily, and this is much better tolerated (Backes, 2007). This is how I have now taken to prescribing them for the high-risk patients who want to use a statin, though I have to say long-term studies have not yet been done to see whether weekly dosing has similar effects on cardiovascular risk. Drug companies certainly do not advertise this information, and have no motivation to study the idea further, because it would eat dramatically into their profit margin.

So what we have with our modern, evidence-based medicine is a very successful tool for control over our physicians in terms of treatment and prescribing habits. The only people with enough money to fund "adequate research", as they define it, are pharmaceutical companies; other wealthy medical industry corporations; or possibly the government, which is heavily lobbied by said corporations. Those who control the "truth" and the "evidence", dictate how physicians practice and where the money goes in terms of medical care.

Physicians themselves are certainly not free of guilt on this subject. There have been many cases of fraudulent research and reporting by physicians and physician groups themselves over the years. The most recent case I've heard of is in regard to a spine surgery product called Infuse™, designed to stimulate new bone growth. The product is made by Medtronic Corporation and is used by many surgeons during spinal surgery. Its use netted Medtronic nearly one billion dollars in 2010 alone. The product causes certain side effects, including some residual nerve and spinal pain after surgery, but some physicians were publishing studies that exaggerated the drug's benefits and notably underreported the adverse effects. The authors of those biased studies, doctors, were found to have financial ties to Medtronic. In this case, another group of spine surgeons, from the North American Spine Society, publicly spoke out against this extremely biased research and made the country aware of it (Broder, 2011).

There is a wide range of ethical fabric and behavior among doctors, just as with any other profession; we have to be careful what we choose to believe. I imagine that those biased studies were repeatedly cited by the company to promote their product.

Again, I can't help but equate modern conventional medical training to a religious cult, and in this case, the scripture is handed down to us by the devil (pardon the hyperbole). Well, I'm not drinking the Kool-Aid, eating the pudding, or believing the dogma anymore, and I suggest the public doesn't either. I frequently find that I have to look towards the past in the literature to find more legitimate information or truth. It is hard to believe the conclusions reported in most research today, when you truly read the studies with a critical eye. This includes studies evaluating natural remedies, too, not just drugs. I practice much better medicine when I focus on basic physiology and metabolic processes, things that haven't changed in thousands or millions of years.

The powers-that-be have certainly done an excellent job with their medical disciples. I can try to explain to my conventional colleagues how I've seen oral magnesium supplementation reduce headaches for the clear majority of people suffering from chronic tension headaches or migraines, and I will give intravenous magnesium injections in my office for people with acutely severe headaches with 80% or better success. Some of them may just scoff outright, while others will say something like "show me some studies and I'll believe it". A rare few may say, "Wow, maybe I'll try that." It is further annoying that there is a great deal of research showing this positive effect of magnesium (Sun-Edelstein, 2009); but the dissenters aren't really interested in looking it up. They would rather just cling to their current beliefs and practices. This is just one example of my peers' narrow-mindedness, but it has frustrated me to the point that I've almost just stopped trying to convince other physicians of anything.

"Reductionist" research

Further problems with the quality of our "evidence" involve the way in which the research is conducted on a philosophical level. People are biological organisms with very complex and interrelated molecular and physiological systems. Modern research seeks to assess the effect of one single variable change on this complex system. To put it plainly, this is completely impossible.

There are a great many different factors in your life that influence your health and every other aspect of your being. Reductionist science works fine in a laboratory when playing with chemical reactions in a beaker, but it does not work when dealing with a complex biological system, even one as simple as a species of bacteria.

If a culture of Staph bacteria is exposed to a particular antibiotic, some of them will die at very low concentrations, but other individuals within the population will endure much higher concentrations of the drug before they are killed. If mercury is given to a population of 1000 rats, there may be a greater than 10 fold difference in the amount it takes to kill the first rat, versus the last or "toughest" rat. This is why "survival of the fittest" depends greatly upon the environmental challenges confronting the population. Antibiotic-resistant bacteria, for example, may not have been the most rapidly-multiplying individuals in the group to begin with, but when an environmental stress (the antibiotic in this case) kills off all the competition, they suddenly become the "fittest" ones around.

These are examples of what's called "biochemical individuality". In the study of human health and medicine, it is just one of the factors that make reductionist science very limiting. In some way, every one of us is an exception to a rule. This makes us all exceptional, and none truly average. There is no population of uniformly similar animals. Even among genetically identical individuals, there can be drastic differences in physiological parameters because of differences in their nutritional status and other aspects of their environment during development. For example, armadillos often have genetically identical quadruplets and it has been shown there can still be as much as a 10-fold difference in the adrenal gland content of cortisol between them even just after birth (Williams, 1971).

You can try to find a thousand people who all eat the same diet, work in the same job environment, have similar degrees of marital stress, have similar exercise habits, have the same colored eyes and hair, smoke the same number of cigarettes, drink the same amount of alcohol, eat the same amount of sugar, and had equally abusive parents (I think you get the point), but that's not possible. It is also not possible to make sure they all have the same genetics, but, even if we could, we would find significant differences in the way they respond.

The problem in trying to isolate one variable in a group of people is they would have all grown up in a different environment, which would have altered their biochemical responses. Among other factors, they all would have had differences in nutrition and toxicity that altered their own tolerance to stress and chemicals. The armadillo research, noted above, suggests that even small differences in the prenatal environment can incur dramatic differences.

When best efforts are made to find this mythical homogenous group, and then just one variable is changed, we are trying to determine how much difference that one change makes. But this is essentially impossible. If there is a really large difference observed, we may be somewhat confident that the intervention is of value. If, however, there is only a small difference, such as the 1.1% decrease in nonfatal heart attacks as seen in the ASCOT study, it could possibly be explained away by some of the other myriad of differences between the real people in the two groups.

So how do we know which results are significant? Well, the word "significant" is a very particular one in statistics. To the public, this word suggests the results are large in magnitude and decisive. But in statistical terms, *significant* only means the results are not likely explained by mere chance alone. It has nothing at all to do with how important the result is, or how large the result is. It just means specifically that a given result was probably "real" and had only a very small possibility of occurring due to random chance.

Therefore, the statement "10mg of atorvastatin daily significantly reduces heart attack rates in men" is true. However, the reality from the ASCOT study data shows it's only likely to benefit one man out of 91. And this is only true in men with three or more risk factors. If this concerns a man with moderately high cholesterol and no additional risk factors, the odds of this drug benefiting them are going to be even lower.

Another interesting thing about statistical significance is that the larger the population of subjects in the study, the easier it is to declare a tiny difference to be significant. This is why the study I repeatedly quoted on Lipitor™ had enrolled over 10,000 subjects. These studies are extremely expensive, and they wouldn't enroll so many subjects unless they truly needed to. They needed to get that large a number of people involved in order to report such a small difference as being "significant". In fairness to the researchers, the event in question is a fairly rare one, so it does take a large number of people over a long time to see a measurable difference.

What we really need is for our physicians to critically analyze the available "evidence"; to interpret statistics in a more meaningful fashion; to look at various sources of information rather than just the pharmaceutical-ad-ridden peer-reviewed journals; and, also, for society to demand that medical studies are of good quality and based on solid ethics. We need our doctors to take their jobs seriously and look hard for what is truly best for their patients, not just what is easy.

Unfortunately, our current medical "gospel" is the prospective, randomized, placebo-controlled trial. This is a study design that must start with two similar groups of people, randomly assigning half of them to placebos or standard care, half to the treatment in question, and then follow them over time (years in some cases, just a few weeks in others). The results of this are then used to establish cause and effect relationships, effective treatment suggestions, and gain FDA approval for drug prescribing. This type of study is supposed to be as pure as possible, but the important factors are fairly easy to manipulate. Bias can enter into the selection process for the subjects, the randomization process, the quality of product used, the methods of study, statistical analysis, selective reporting of results, and other ways.

The unfortunate fact is the drug companies control most of the "truth" in American of medicine and, therefore, the practice. They are the only entities with the money and resources to conduct the sort of research that they themselves have set as the new standard for acceptable information. They aren't legally allowed to give doctors expensive gifts, money, or trips to Fiji anymore (though they used to), but they certainly still have influence over medical practice. Perhaps that wouldn't be such a bad thing if they weren't purely motivated by profit.

CHAPTER 4 – PROBLEMS WITH MEDICAL PROVIDERS' HABITS AND ATTITUDES

Some of these habits-and-attitudes issues are secondary to market pressures and the rules of the health care payment system, some to educational biases, some to individual practitioner biases and beliefs; and some have evolved for unclear reasons. In my opinion, they all serve to impede optimal care to some extent.

The 15-minute "hour"

I use that oxymoronic statement as the title for this section because there is actually a book with that title directed at medical students, residents, and psychology trainees (book by Stuart and Lieberman, now in its fourth edition). It explains how a practitioner can try to get an hour's worth of patient interaction in just fifteen minutes. This involves actively steering the interview to get what the doctor feels is the most useful information out of the patient, in as little time as possible. We learn how to redirect the patient when they begin to ramble about what we see as unnecessary information.

The belief is that patients don't really know what is important and, if they are just allowed to talk, they will lead the care provider all over the place rather than focus on key symptoms like we want them to. We want to know what symptoms they having specifically, how long they've had them, their character (stabbing, burning, sharp or throbbing pain, for example), the location of their symptoms, and other associated factors. We also care about when those symptoms occur, if they aren't constant. We may additionally ask what makes it better or worse, but not much else.

This is basic medical history taking which, as I mentioned before, is supposed to yield 80% of our diagnoses without requiring any testing or even physical examination in most cases. There was a great figure in Western medicine named Sir William Osler. He is often quoted and one of his more famous lines is, "If you listen to the patient long enough, they will give you the diagnosis." I'm not sure when that was lost in our medical practice but, perhaps, it was somewhere around the inception of HMOs. One modern study evaluating medical visits found that primary care residents (doctors in training for either family practice or general internal medicine) interrupted their patient 25% of the time and averaging only twelve seconds into the patient telling their story. The average interview time was only eleven minutes, with the patient speaking for only four minutes total (Rhoades, 2001). This is probably not what Osler had in mind.

It isn't that doctors are taught to believe that a ten to fifteen minute office visit is the ideal length; this is just a consequence of other aspects of our medical philosophy. We think it is the best approach to serving as many people as possible, in a given period of time, while also maximizing profit. The fact is, doctors get paid based on the "complexity" of their visits, rather than on the time spent, unlike a lawyer or counselor does. This means that a doctor can have a few low-complexity visits, or one high-complexity visit, in the same amount of time. Most practitioners will, therefore, make more money by seeing the greater number of people in their workday.

Unfortunately, our brief and expedient office visits typically allow us time to focus on only one problem at a time. The patient has time to ask the questions above about one specific issue, but will not have time to delve into other issues, which may actually be related and help point to an upstream cause. There is just enough time to make a single diagnosis or review a couple prior problems, then prescribe the appropriate treatment. That treatment is most likely to be a drug because it takes very little time to write a prescription. It takes far more time to describe a diet plan, write out a list of supplements and explain why each of them is important, describe an exercise program, or do other counseling regarding therapies that require more patient involvement and understanding.

Many patients complain about this aspect of medical care to me, and express great appreciation for the fact that I actually try to listen to all of their complaints. They are further impressed if I can make sense out of multiple complaints together, unifying them as one problem, in the setting of their overall health. I've discussed previously how a practitioner can actually provide much better care with longer visit times, even in terms of the long-term quality of care and diminishing the patients' total costs and need for future care.

Reductionism in medical care delivery

Unfortunately, the tendency to examine just one variable at a time in our research carries over into the clinical encounter. Our doctors are trained to focus on individual problems, rather than unifying concepts and upstream factors. This reductionism can be viewed as the opposite of holism, and conventional medicine differs greatly in this way from holistic medicine. The term holistic really refers to a philosophically different approach, rather than the kinds of treatments that are used. If we just look at one problem in isolation, we are likely to stick with symptomatic treatments for that problem, because the actual causes aren't evident. This approach does work to help alleviate short-term suffering for many people, but I would contend it is not ideal medical care for chronic problems at all.

Let's look at the example of adult acne. If the patient is a thirty-year-old man who is also obese, fatigued, has mild psoriasis or eczema, irritable bowel symptoms, joint pains, frequent headaches, or other various symptoms, then it is likely this person's acne is caused by food allergy. Therefore, if we test him and identify the triggering foods, we may make his acne and all his other problems go away. That same patient may have his symptoms due to yeast overgrowth or sensitivity; therefore, the problems may all clear up with a couple weeks of antifungal medication.

If it's a relatively thin thirty-year-old woman, whose acne started in her early teen years, tends to get worse during the two weeks prior to her period, and she also has PMS symptoms and migraines during that period, then her acne is probably related, at least in part, to progesterone deficiency or estrogen/progesterone imbalance. Therefore, if she uses a little over-the-counter progesterone cream during the two-week period prior to her menses, all of these problems are likely to get better.

Contrast this simple approach (those other problems only take five minutes to inquire about) with the standard internal medicine or dermatology approach. Typically, they will ask the patient how long the acne has been there, whether pustules or deep cysts are formed, if it occurs on the back as well as the face, and other such questions. In reality, most practitioners don't even really care about those answers, because they are already planning to prescribe the typical treatments in the typical order. Such providers generally start with topical benzoyl peroxide and a good face washing program, then progress to topical antibiotics, perhaps use oral antibiotics if that doesn't work. If the patient has deep cystic acne that tends to scar the face, he or she may be a candidate for Accutane™, a very powerful and potentially toxic drug that only certain physicians are allowed to prescribe.

This approach may clear the acne during active therapy, but does not get to the root of the problem. Those treatments do not clear up any other issues, the problem at hand returns as soon as therapy is stopped, and it is very likely new problems will develop as a result of treatments such as oral antibiotics and Accutane™. For example, people will often develop problems with yeast overgrowth and gut dysregulation because of oral antibiotics; and then they may return later with a myriad of new complaints.

There are many other examples I could offer, where common problems are addressed in obviously inappropriate fashion under the standard of care. What baffles me the most about this particular example is that dermatologists are trained in *internal* medicine first, but then it seems that they mostly practice *external* medicine. They just start gooping stuff on the skin, when we all know one's skin is being actively made from the inside. The real key to almost every dermatological problem is addressing what's going on inside the body physiologically, not just putting stuff on topically.

Again, I repeatedly have patients complain to me about the fact that other doctors won't let them discuss more than one problem at a time. Sometimes these complaints are based on practical concerns, such as the fact that the patient had to take time off of work and pay for an office visit, and so they want to get their money's worth. Getting to the doctor may be difficult, not to mention expensive, and they would like to address all of their issues while there. Some astute patients also realize that some of their problems seem related or linked to some extent, and are frustrated that their provider does not seem to be interested in that.

My own idea of "reductionism" is to reduce the number of prescription drugs my patients are taking, and find other ways of reducing their complaints. That way, in the long run, my patients may reduce the number of doctor visits they have, while also reducing the amount of money they have to spend on health care.

Failing the masses

Our current approach to medicine, based on large studies showing small differences, isolating small variations in people, and disregarding the inherent biochemical differences between us, tends to fail the individual patient in front of us the majority of the time.

For example, if a drug only really benefits 1 man out of 91, then it fails the remaining 90, right? And, it fails all 100 out of 100 women, if it has shown no benefit at all for them. If a drug is stated to reduce a given symptom by 30%, that could mean that everyone will have a 30% improvement in their symptoms, but it doesn't. It means that some small number had complete resolution, a larger (but still minority fraction) had partial improvement, and a larger group still (probably the majority) had no improvement at all.

Our treatment algorithms are an approach to "one size fits all" medicine, even though practitioners acknowledge they are just a starting point. Astute clinicians realize that when a patient fails the first-line therapy, they should look at other factors in that individual's case and vary their treatment accordingly. In my experience, this is the rule rather than the exception, so I try to look at the big picture from the very beginning, and in as much detail as possible. Individualized medicine is far more effective and, in the long run, saves time and money for everyone.

Similar problems are seen with lifestyle issues such as diet. The same diet does not benefit everyone equally. There are differences in cultural heritage and race, environmental factors, and individual biological differences. Global recommendations and treatment algorithms should just be seen as a starting point because, in most cases, the most ideal treatment lies further upstream. This problem should be obvious to everyone with the problems of increasing chronic disease burden and decreasing life expectancy as mentioned previously.

Overall, our current system does not seem interested in truly solving the problems of the individual. Instead, we are trained to treat everyone with the same apparent problem in the same manner. Then, if they don't get better, we either blame them, tell them their problem can't be solved, or send them to a specialist, who may order more expensive tests and more invasive or toxic interventions. Too often, at the end of this line lies a useless, made-up diagnosis (psychiatric or otherwise) that only serves to push the patient down a path to overmedication and disability.

Diagnosis-based treatment and billing

I've mentioned how basing decisions on an end-of-the-stream diagnosis, like "Fibromyalgia", "Depression" or "Hypertension", fails to address cause and precludes any hope of actually curing the condition. So, let's examine how our medical billing and payment system influences this.

There is this great big book of code numbers called the "ICD-9" coding system. It stands for *International Classification of Diseases* (not "Idiotic Compendium of Diagnoses", but it should); and we'll be up to version 10 sometime soon, which will change everything. The code list is updated every year because new conditions are being discovered or described, or there is a new classification of previously recognized conditions. An example of the latter is the some twenty individual classifications for headache in the 2009 edition because just plain "headache" is no longer specific enough. There are a dozen or so different types of migraine listed separately as well.

New categories in the book are sometimes real and newly discovered, such as HIV infection in the 1980's, or are sometimes an attempt to describe a seemingly related group of symptoms that acquire a unifying title such as "Fibromyalgia" or "Metabolic Syndrome". Some diagnoses that can be heard about on TV are not in the book because they were made up by drug companies to try and sell their product. A good example of this is "PMDD" (premenstrual dysphoric disorder), which is purported to be a more severe version of PMS, which itself is another example of a nonsense diagnosis based on a related group of symptoms.

The makers of Prozac™ "created" the devastating condition *PMDD* because they are seeking to market the identical drug under the new name of Sarafem™ for this new indication, and thereby acquire a new patent with a higher price tag for several more years. *PMDD* is not a real, accepted diagnosis in the medical field or in the ICD-9 code book; and Sarafem™ is just the drug fluoxetine, the same generic drug in Prozac™, stamped with a new name and marked way up in price. You can get generic fluoxetine at most pharmacies for just four dollars per month; while Sarafem™sells (according to www.drugstore.com) for $66.99 per box of just seven pills. That means they are selling the exact same drug for roughly seventy-one times as much money based on this newly manufactured diagnosis.

A doctor gets paid by an insurance company only if the diagnostic code or codes (numbers only please, no words – they don't understand words it seems) reported for the visit are on the approved list and seem to warrant the visit level indicated. It's a big game to some extent. For example, if a person gets food poisoning, I could report all the different codes for nausea, vomiting, diarrhea and dehydration, making it look like there are four different diagnoses. This means that I could bill for a much higher visit because I covered several problems instead of just one which would have bundled all those other things together and not been nearly as impressive.

This seems like a ridiculous example, but to me it's not really that much different from billing for depression, fatigue, back pain, and insomnia when they are all just symptoms of that individual's Vitamin D deficiency. Basically, this billing and payment system does not benefit the patient at all and does nothing to improve health care delivery or quality. Quite to the contrary and, in my opinion, it impairs the quality of care because the practitioner has no added motivation to find one single upstream diagnosis. They just go on treating disparate symptoms as separate conditions. We are, in a way, rewarded for failure in this regard.

It is also a clever and covert way for insurance companies to deny payment of claims. They will each have certain diagnostic codes they do not cover, which may include important common conditions like depression, obesity, or erectile dysfunction (almost all insurance companies deny claims for those last two). They will never tell in advance what they do or do not pay for; only after filing the claim do we find out, by being denied. We may then try rebilling with a different code, if possible, and then just hope for the best.

The system is confusing and cumbersome to almost everyone involved. It unnecessarily takes up provider time and requires the hiring of additional staff trained in dealing with the ever-changing rules of medical coding and billing. Meanwhile, the patients suffer under the burden of their diagnostic codes which offer no effective treatment strategies, but do serve to get them denied future insurance coverage because of what will later become "pre-existing conditions".

Symptomatic treatment and forgetting to "first do no harm"

The Hippocratic oath is actually quite long and has multiple facets, but the one line people tend to remember is the one about *doing no harm*. Many medical schools have modified the oath to meet their modern perspectives, and some no longer utilize any oath at graduation. I think that's too bad and, with studies suggesting that conventional medical care is a common cause of death in the United States, perhaps we need to reinforce this idea.

Certainly, many medical mistakes could have been avoided and were based on sloppiness or inattentiveness. Many deaths and harms are caused by things done in "appropriate" standard-of-care fashion. Every year, there are hundreds of thousands of people in this country harmed by drugs prescribed using accepted indications and according to the current standards of practice (recall the more than 183,000 adverse drug events reported to the FDA in just the last quarter of 2010 alone). There are people who are unexpectedly harmed by surgical operations or other procedures performed with the best intentions and for well-accepted reasons.

Many of the harmful medications are prescribed for symptomatic management and many of these procedures are performed when disease processes continue unchecked because the underlying causes weren't addressed. If we improve the quality of our practitioners' education, their understanding of causation of illness and prevention of disease may avoid many future such occurrences.

How many colonoscopies are done on young adults with symptoms of "irritable bowel syndrome" (IBS), when the vast majority of these individuals just have food allergies or abnormal gut organisms which, in most cases, can be addressed and dealt with easily? Usually nothing useful is seen when doing a colonoscopy on one of these patients. But the diagnosis justifies the procedure to insurance companies and it's a roughly $4,000 undertaking – so one might think the gastroenterologists are motivated to do one on every IBS patient. In defense of the specialists, they don't actually understand what causes IBS symptoms; so I guess, in a way, they are doing the best they can and trying to rule-out serious conditions.

How many people undergo joint replacement surgery for crippling arthritis when, if implemented early enough, a proper diet, exercise regimen, MSM (methylsulfonylmethane) and glucosamine supplementation, vitamin D, reduction of inflammatory factors, and possibly acupuncture may have alleviated, or at least delayed, the need for surgery? An orthopedic surgeon makes thousands of dollars for one of these surgeries, and the hospital charges far more than they do. Of course, the surgeons don't understand why arthritis happens or how to deal with it metabolically and they are not usually consulted until the condition is so severe that surgery is inevitable. Also, many severe arthritis cases are caused by past trauma or other uncontrollable problems. In addition, the surgery is effective and dramatically improves the patients' quality of life in most cases. The point is we definitely do need joint replacement surgeries. We should just do a better job of treating these problems with safe, effective, nutritional and functional therapies much earlier before proceeding to surgery.

How many kids have tubes put in their ears for their recurring ear infections, when most of them merely need to stop consuming milk products? How many people suffer kidney disease, heart attacks or stomach ulcers from anti-inflammatory drugs when there are a variety of safe and effective alternatives for pain control in most people? And the list goes on.

These problems go back to our medical philosophies and the way conventional practitioners are trained. The conventional therapies are thought to be far superior when, in truth, they often are not. They are considered perfectly safe at best, or at least to have "acceptable risk". I think our healthcare outcomes overall are unacceptable, and many of our treatments have too high a risk. Acetaminophen is thought to be so safe it is used for pain and fever in people of all ages with impunity and is available over the counter. Yet, it is absolutely lethal even in mild overdose for some people, and it is a common cause of poisoning death in our country every year. The CDC reports that in 2009 alone (available on their website) there were over 700,000 ER visits for unintentional poisoning with over 30,000 deaths. The most common agents are prescription or OTC medications.

This is why I have *primum non nocere* ("first do no harm", in Latin) tattooed around my right arm. As far as I know, I haven't actually killed anyone yet, and hopefully my current practice style makes it far less likely for me to do so than my conventional colleagues. Luckily for us, most people seem pretty difficult to kill. That's what I used to jokingly tell the interns in residency. I meant to reassure them and calm their anxiety but in fact, I wasn't really joking.

I don't mean to suggest that we should get rid of all the drugs and stop teaching surgery. Rather, that we should use them more judiciously and save them for later down the decision tree. In my opinion, we should always start with the safest treatment options possible. I would expect most rational people to agree with that. The problem is that, most of the time, our practitioners are not aware of these safer treatments, and they don't believe those things are effective enough to use. Often, the safest thing to do in acute conditions is to do nothing and just wait a while, but many practitioners (and the patients themselves) get too impatient and feel the need to intervene anyway. Ironically, it is just the opposite with chronic disease problems; conventional medicine fails to recognize and intervene at the very early stages, waiting until things are much worse and require more aggressive therapies.

Confusing *"Normal"* with *"Common"*

Can anyone here tell me what "normal" really means?

Okay, you in the back.

"Normal means it's the most common."

Wrong!

This one really chaps me, I tell you. It exemplifies the lack of original thought and the lowering of standards that we have in today's medicine. When something occurs really often we start to see it as normal and completely forget what the proper or optimal state of things really is.

With this attitude, we should soon feel it is normal to be obese, have high cholesterol, and diabetes. It will become normal to die by age sixty. It's pretty normal now for kids to have allergies of some kind. It's almost normal now for boys to have ADHD or even autism.

In medical training, I was taught that it is normal to gain weight as we age, have our blood pressure increase, and begin showing signs of senility. That's all a load of crap! I was told this about weight gain, because it had been *observed* that people in our society gain one to two pounds per year after age twenty-five or so. That doesn't make it normal! Actually, we should naturally LOSE weight as we age past forty or so, due to loss of muscle mass as our anabolic hormones begin to drop. Gaining fat steadily over the years is the result of an overfed, sedentary society and is not *normal* in any way! It sure is common though, and it's very comforting to the average person to think the way their body is morphing and enlarging in all the wrong ways is normal. In fact, my patients don't like it very much when I explain to them that they should actually lose weight as they age, rather than gain it. I'm pretty sure most choose to keep believing the opposite.

I've already discussed how our concept of a normal body mass index in the U.S. ranges up to 25 or 26 even though solid research suggests increased risk of earlier death as BMI increases from levels far below that. The best study I have found on this subject is one looking at nonsmoking, nondrinking, vegetarian/vegan, Seventh-Day-Adventist men (as "standardized" a population as can be found) published in 1991 from the Loma Linda University School of Public Health. This research clearly showed a linear relationship between BMI and mortality rate, starting from the lowest BMI's (<20) all the way up (Lindsted, 1991). Numerous, more recent studies, have instead suggested a J-shaped or even U-shaped curve in this relationship. These suggest a low BMI is just as bad as a high one and usually find the lowest mortality in those with BMI between 24 and 26 (I reviewed several, and this is where they tended to fall). The problem with these results is that the populations have less healthy lifestyles in general, and the reasons the lighter individuals are thin are much more likely to be related to illness problems than improved fitness.

Our normal range for blood pressure is based on noting when it starts to be associated with increased cardiovascular disease events, so why shouldn't our body weight be rated the same way? If our parameters were really geared toward ideal human health, our suggested ideal BMI range might be from 19.5 to 22. We should really replace the word "normal" with "optimal" or "ideal" and adjust our thinking accordingly.

Laboratory data is one area where this concept is a huge problem in medicine. Our reference range for blood sugar is based on disease outcomes, such as diabetes, and lots of study looking at healthy individuals. Our normal ranges for sodium and potassium are based on when we start to see clinical problems such as seizures and cardiac arrhythmias, and they have fairly tight ranges. These are examples of laboratory ranges that make sense clinically.

Many other lab tests, however, do not come with this sort of scientific analysis guiding the determination of the reference range. I use the term "reference range" because that is what's actually printed on the lab report, not the word "normal" or "optimal". In fact, many of our lab results come with a posted reference range that is merely a statistical range, capturing 90-95% of the measured values from some early group of patients who had the test in the past.

These don't represent any sort of scientific study or clinical relevance.

They are just statistical constructs based on observations from *unhealthy* people! I'm sure the labs probably used a lot of data from the general public, so-called "healthy volunteers", to get their reference ranges. But, as I've alluded to, most of our society is *NOT* healthy, and many who seem fine are, in my opinion, chronically ill. Personally, I would rather be compared to some sort of ideal parameters for human health, not the average American's parameters.

Some prominent examples of this annoying problem that I deal with commonly are the reference ranges for vitamin D, testosterone, and thyroid hormone levels. Many labs report the reference range for 25-OH vitamin D as low as 20ng/mL, but now we realize that we need much more than that to have optimal calcium absorption, not to mention all the other things vitamin D does for us. Most people will have symptoms of some sort if they are below 60ng/mL. Also, on most labs, the upper range only goes to 100ng/mL even though there has never been true toxicity seen below a level of 150ng/mL or anywhere close to that level. The benefits of vitamin D are so vast and important that I consider this a huge failing of education for our practitioners, who mainly don't know any better than to go by the reference range on a lab report.

Testosterone levels are definitely supposed to be different at different ages, highest around age eighteen to twenty-five, then stable but in the high-range for a few decades, gradually declining after age fifty or so. What we've seen in recent decades, which I will discuss in the hormone section later on in the book, is a fairly dramatic decline in testosterone levels in teenagers and men of all ages. Unfortunately, lab reference ranges have been modified to lower levels over time, in keeping with this decline. They have posted reference levels for young adult men ranging all the way down to 240pcg/dL even though, historically, we probably should not be hitting levels that low until many decades later.

Thyroid levels are a special case for people. The reference ranges are perhaps based on some science, but a big problem is the individual variation between different people. Some people really need to be at or just above the high end of the range in order to feel good and function optimally, while others seem to be just fine sitting in the lower end of the range. If a practitioner is just trying to get their patient into the lab reference range and does not use the eradication of symptoms as their primary goal, they will usually fail the patient to some extent.

The reference range for TSH (thyroid stimulating hormone) has been modified over the years, bringing the upper range level down from twelve to below five now, and is widely thought to be in need of downward adjustment again. To make matters worse, practitioners have been trained to pay attention to the TSH level and little else, when that test frequently offers poor guidance about what the patient actually needs. I have an extensive discussion of thyroid problems later in the book. It will be relevant to most women over forty, as well as to a great many others.

My favorite hormonal reference range to point out is that posted for a twenty-four hour urine cortisol collection. Cortisol is an adrenal steroid and is extremely important for normal cardiovascular function, blood sugar regulation, immune system function and other things. People who develop Addison's disease suffer destruction of the cortisol-producing portion of their adrenal glands and will die without daily cortisol supplementation. What is ridiculous about the lab range for the urine test is the posted range goes from "zero" to fifty. Zero cortisol is not compatible with life; it's absurd.

Sometimes, I often think we would be better off if the labs did not come with any posted range at all. Then the ordering practitioners themselves would actually have to know how to interpret the levels. After all, it is not the laboratory's job to interpret results and decide what is best for the particular patient; that is the job of the medical practitioner. Our goal of "normal" should be based on what is <u>optimal</u> and not what is <u>common</u>. My goal is always to help my patients achieve the best health they can, not just minimally adequate health. You wouldn't want your employer to pay you just what you need to cover all your bills, would you? The road to optimal health care starts with setting optimal goals.

Preventing death rather than promoting health

This is really a difficult issue, and it falls more into the realm of biomedical ethics than health care and medicine. It is a philosophical attitude that is responsible for a great deal of the high expenses in our health care system. A man may live to age sixty without spending more than $1000 in medical care, and then go into bankruptcy from the costs related to a heart attack, only to die a month later anyway. There are many more examples of patients living with chronic disease problems, which persist for years under medical management that only slows the progression of their disease a little bit, but does not stop it. People tend to work extremely hard all their lives, saving for a retirement they hope to enjoy. Too many of these people end up spending their life savings on medical bills and medications, which may only slightly delay the inevitable. A lot less money, focused on promoting health much earlier, could have saved them many years of life and their life savings.

In integrative medicine philosophy, there is the concept of "compression of morbidity." This idea entails living a healthy and vibrant life until a ripe old age, then passing away peacefully over a fairly short period of time. This would be "dying of old age", so to speak. According to this philosophy, this is how we are all meant to go out, and the expected age of death should be well past one hundred years. It should be much cheaper for the system because we would go quickly, from basically "untreatable" processes, and at ages where we feel more comfortable about this life ending.

As I mentioned previously, in our modern society, people are now expected to die at younger ages than the previous generation. A Harvard School of Public Health study published in 2008 showed increasing mortality rates in women and certain other segments of the population. The overall projection is that today's children will be the first generation in recorded history to live a shorter life span, in general, than the preceding one (Ezzati, 2008). We are contracting more chronic and debilitating illnesses at younger ages. We are going bankrupt over our health care costs that are at higher rates than ever before. And sadly, in spite of our modern healthcare system and its high expense, overall there are apparently no years of life being saved.

If we were to focus more on promotion of health, rather than the treatment of disease after-the-fact, I believe we would see the cost of our health care system drop dramatically. In addition, our life expectancy would likely climb again, rather than decrease. It is certainly cheaper to be healthy than to be sick. Of course, if our population were to start commonly living past one hundred years of age, it may bankrupt Medicare and Social Security in no time, right? Maybe not, if that population were healthy and productive right up to the end.

Another, more emotional aspect of this philosophical issue is end-of-life care. We tend to string our human loved ones along for quite a while, often just prolonging their misery and discomfort. We do have the option of hospice care, but it's often wrongfully perceived as a distasteful option. Many terminally ill patients themselves decline this service, presumably because they feel it would be admitting defeat or acknowledging the fact that they are going to die.

The prolongation of suffering is typically a result of the wishes of the patient and/or, quite often, their family. Most physicians, in my opinion, are quick to point out the futility of continued treatment for those who appear terminally ill. This is not always true, of course; some physicians routinely press onward with every intervention they can think of, even encouraging the family to let them try something else. I think those practitioners are at times projecting fear of their *own* mortality onto the situation. Hospitals are typically quick to encourage discharge to home or hospice when things appear to have gone beyond the point of no return, which is the most cost-effective idea certainly (and that is their motivation). It seems it is the nature of our culture to fear our own death and the deaths of our loved ones. We will fight death tooth and nail, at times going beyond heroic measures, and certainly paying heroic prices. I'm not saying this is "wrong", it's just our tendency, and may have some unintended consequences.

In some other cultures, my specific experience is with East Asian cultures or subcultures; it is customary not to tell the patients when they have a potentially fatal illness. The family will be aware, but not trouble the individual with the knowledge that their end is approaching. That way they don't have to deal with the fear and anxiety. They instead get to focus on living, rather than dying.

Some feel that in American society, we treat our pets more humanely than our human loved ones because we will euthanize our animals when they are severely ill, rather than allow them to suffer. Typically, the closest thing we offer our sick or elderly is hospice care. This service tries to keep them comfortable when they are declining and will likely soon pass on. Oregon has had a "Death With Dignity" law (ORS 127.800-995). This allows many terminally ill individuals to take a fatal dose of medication that is prescribed by a physician, after confirmation of the terminal condition and a thorough psychiatric evaluation (we wouldn't want any clinically depressed or insane terminally ill people taking their own lives, I guess). This seems to me to be the most progressive system we have in this country.

I realize this is mainly a cultural issue as well as a serious moral and philosophical dilemma, and it doesn't necessarily belong to the "physician attitudes" section. It is probably only in a minority of cases that the physician is the one pushing for continued futile treatment, though it does happen. I think our doctors, nurses, social workers and our medical system, most often do a good job with this one. I think what we could do better as practitioners is focus more on the promotion of life and health early on, and less on the prevention of death at the end.

The medical community does have some responsibility here, in regards to the development of life-prolonging technologies. These are, of course, a good idea in general and are often used to save lives in acute situations and get younger patients through major illnesses so they can live many years more. To many people, it would not seem appropriate to deny older patients these therapies even when it seems somewhat futile. When we come up against the eventual, harsh reality of limited resource utilization, we will have to make tough decisions about who gets treatment and who doesn't. This is an ethical issue that currently exists only with organ transplant lists as far as I know. When we, as a society, start to run short on funding and resources, it will be in increasingly real problem.

Inattention to diet, nutrition and lifestyle

I have already mentioned how nutrition education is notably lacking in our modern medical education, but I think it is very remiss to ignore its importance in our overall health. Our medical training does discuss lifestyle issues such as TV watching and our general lack of exercise as being risk factors for obesity and chronic disease. In spite of this, doctors do a poor job of actually guiding patients to a more successful lifestyle.

Also, as a profession, we do a lousy job of educating our patients about nutrition. Much of the advice we give is erroneous and not founded on good science. Later, I will discuss some of the specific instances where this is true and attempt to debunk some of the pervasive myths in our culture regarding diet and exercise. For now, I will just suggest that the lack of effective nutrition education for our providers and patients, the weak attempts at using lifestyle and diet modifications as first-line therapy for health problems, and the poor advice we propagate are part of the problem with our health as a nation.

Much of this blame rests on the health care practitioners and their attitudes or biases. I heard repeatedly throughout my medical training that diet has no major effect on health and medical problems. The "you are what you eat" adage seemed to be completely disregarded. In cases where diet was an indisputable causative factor such as obesity, atherosclerotic heart disease, and diabetes, I was typically given the sense that discussing diet and nutrition with my patients was a waste of time. It was hinted that this is because the patients weren't likely to adopt good habits, and drugs were more effective interventions anyway.

The belief that people get everything they could possibly need from the typical American diet, false as that obviously is, was held nearly universally by medical school professors. Anyone who tried to disagree was usually openly ridiculed. I guess they don't read population health and nutrition surveys like the NHANES (National Health and Nutrition Examination Survey) reports that come out every several years or so. Very clearly they show the rising rates of various nutrient deficiencies in our country. Many conventional doctors still tell patients they only need to get ten minutes of sun exposure to their hands and face in order to acquire adequate vitamin D for the day – even in Alaska!

They don't seem to read studies that show less than half of pregnant women in Boston are getting even the (pathetically low and inadequate) RDA for iodine (NHANES data). Nor do they seem aware of the link between iodine deficiency and low IQ or mental retardation in children. I was told that vitamin D deficiency caused rickets and vitamin C deficiency caused scurvy. But nobody mentioned that vitamin D supplementation has also been shown to reduce the incidences of heart attacks, type I diabetes, MS, schizophrenia, and other important medical problems. Nobody seems to be aware of the long-observed link between severe vitamin C deficiencies and heart attacks (Libby, 2002).

The fact is, for a few bucks per month per person, we could make tremendous reductions in chronic diseases and improve human health in the process. I think the problem is there's not much profit in that for anyone, so it's not waved in front of practitioners' faces like pharmaceuticals are. We have repeated evidence that physical exercise prevents cardiovascular disease, decreases obesity, and is one of the most effective treatments for depression. But it's so much quicker and simpler to just prescribe the appropriate drugs for those problems. There is good clinical evidence that the Mediterranean diet prevents and reduces deaths from cardiovascular disease to a significant degree, as well as other ailments (Kushi, 1995), but doctors still just prescribe cholesterol drugs, which have no such documented impact.

Some well-meaning practitioners do mention lifestyle issues to their patients, but most of them do not really know what advice to give and just suggest to the patient: "eat right and get some exercise". Well, our general population clearly doesn't know what this means, in practical terms, so that sort of generic advice is essentially useless.

Willful mistrust of nutritional supplements

There is a very strong attitude in conventional medical training and practice that nutritional supplements are at best a waste of money and, at worst, are extremely dangerous. Many of my patients say they just stopped telling their other providers about the supplements they take. They got tired of the eye-rolling and other disparaging reactions, or the lectures they received about the supplements being worthless or bad for them. It is very curious to me how so many reasonably intelligent people can think the natural substances, which may actually help a body function more normally, might be bad, while foreign chemicals (i.e. pharmaceuticals) are better. It's baffling!

Given that there is virtually no formal teaching regarding nutrients and their role in human health in conventional medical training, I'm not certain where all these doctors gained their eminent knowledge on the subject, other than the occasional negative study published in the large conventional journals. These studies serve to keep us firmly skeptical about nutritional supplements, if not adamantly opposed to them. The negative studies are seldom scrutinized or questioned by conventional practitioners, because their posted results are in line with the preexisting attitudes of the practitioners themselves.

A classic example of such a study is the one evaluating the use of beta carotene (a vitamin A precursor and antioxidant) for the prevention of lung cancer in smokers. This study used just one antioxidant nutrient alone, in the lowest-quality form available, resulting in a slightly higher rate of lung cancer development in people taking the beta carotene. This study has been quoted repeatedly over the years to demonstrate that vitamin supplements are a very bad idea. But the results have been analyzed and investigated extensively since then, illuminating some peculiar interactions between beta-carotene and some chemicals from cigarette smoke (Goralczyk, 2009). Beta carotene comes from colored fruits and vegetables (like carrots, kale, tomatoes, and the like), and consumption of greater amounts of carotenes through these *foods* has clearly been shown to decrease the incidence of lung and other cancers in prior studies (Shekelle, 1981).

For some reason, conventional practitioners don't typically seem interested in the paradox between the results of that study and the results of a high intake of natural carotenes. People who understand antioxidants know there is actually a chain of reactions involved here, using multiple nutrients and other antioxidants (vitamin C, vitamin E, selenium, zinc) to deactivate free radicals in a multi-step process. If just one of the antioxidants is used in isolation, toxic intermediate compounds may accumulate, rather than seeing the process through to the complete eradication of the free radicals.

There is a valid biological explanation for why that study showed a negative result, and it should serve to educate everyone that a balanced mix of multiple nutrients must be taken for optimal health, rather than just isolated ones. There are major important teaching points here for sure. Instead, the negative study is presented to medical students all across the country, presumably in the effort to harden us against the idea of using vitamins for health. This is reductionist thinking at work. I previously mentioned the publication bias promoting dissemination of these negative, out-of-context ideas. This is an example of a similar *education* bias in our formal training.

A more recent example of this willing bias against nutritional supplements is the study supposedly linking the trace mineral selenium to the development of type 2 diabetes. Negative reports on this study were sent to me by multiple doctors I know. I assume they were trying to show me the error of my ways. I mean, how dare I suggest that essential nutrients could be good for my patients? There was a study by the National Cancer Institute where around 35,000 male subjects were given various combinations of vitamin E, selenium, or a placebo (it's called "the SELECT trial"). When they ended the study there were a *non*-significant greater number of selenium-taking people who had developed type 2 diabetes during the study, which had gone on for an average of around 5-6 years (Lippman, 2009). On the surface that sounds bad for selenium and, of course, providers with pre-existing biases will not bother to look into the matter any deeper because it jives perfectly with their current view of things.

That reported "result" is not even relevant of course, because it was not a statistically significant finding. Also, if anyone were to look even a little more closely, they would find that the study in question was looking for the outcome of *prostate cancer*, not diabetes! The diabetes thing was an incidental finding that they chose to report on, for some reason, even though the study for cancer would not have randomized subjects based on important diabetes-relevant characteristics like obesity, baseline fasting glucose readings, family history or other factors. They may, just as easily, have noted that the treatment group incidentally had more parking tickets by the end of the study and declared selenium guilty of causing parking violations.

It makes no physiological sense that selenium could increase the development of type 2 diabetes. In fact, it is quite a bit more likely to be the opposite, given my understanding of the biochemistry. It would make sense to perform a follow-up study, and appropriate biochemical research. This would specifically look at this question, given this incidental finding, as was done after the surprising results with beta-carotene and lung cancer; something truly useful may be gleaned from that. But the research has not yet been done to my knowledge. Unfortunately, already-biased physicians might now be propagating the false, or at least as yet unproven, idea that selenium causes diabetes. Just for the record, in prior studies, selenium had been convincingly suggested to reduce the incidence of prostate and other cancers. The SELECT trial was an attempt to further evaluate that possible effect on prostate cancer in a large-scale trial (Lippman, 2009).

Interestingly, the researchers stopped that trial after five or six years because they were worried both supplements (selenium and vitamin E) may actually increase the cancer rates. That's interesting because, if you look up the study, the relative risk "increase" was not statistically significant in either case, meaning the confidence intervals (for those statisticians out there) all crossed 1.0 (Lippman, 2009). It is also interesting that the study was stopped so soon and without real cause. The cancer being studied is known to be slow growing and slow to develop. In real terms, the SELECT study neither proves nor disproves the effect of vitamin E or selenium on prostate cancer. It is an "insignificant" study all around in my opinion; but the published results are framed in an intentionally negative light in regards to nutritional supplements.

Another good example involves the herb St. John's Wort, and its use in depression. This herb is supposedly first-line therapy for depression in Germany and other European countries, because it works better and is safer than the prescription drugs we use for mild to moderate depression. Most of the time it has been studied here in the U.S., it has performed similarly. But that is not the usual headline that gets published here. For example, there was a study published about ten years ago with headlines like: "Study shows St. John's Wort ineffective for major depression" (FDA Consumer Magazine, 2002). The original study (which, very interestingly, I could not find listed anywhere now on PubMed; just extensive and very biased-sounding commentary) had compared the herb to the drug Zoloft™ in the treatment of *severe* depression, a condition for which the herb was not typically used anyway. It did not show significant success, no better than a placebo. This was no surprise because those patients usually need something more, for example, electroshock therapy. What the headline did not state, but the results clearly showed, was that Zoloft™ did not work either, and the herb performed slightly better than the drug (Hypericum Depression Trial Study Group, 2002).

The principal investigator for this particular study, carried out through Duke University, was Jonathan R.T. Davidson, M.D., who was the director of the Anxiety and Traumatic Stress Program at Duke. He was quoted as saying: "Rather than self-medicate with an over-the-counter medication or supplement, patients are strongly advised to consult an appropriate healthcare provider to assess the best treatment for a depressive episode". This is not bad advice, really. A co-author stated: "...taking them [products like St. John's Wort] is like playing Russian roulette with your health". Dr. Davidson had disclosures including stock holdings in Pfizer, GlaxoSmithKline, Forest Pharmaceuticals, Eli Lily, Ancile, Roche, Novartis, and other drug companies. In addition he received large amounts of research funding from some of those same companies (*ScienceDaily* report, April 10, 2002).

This is what passes for "scientific evidence" for conventional practitioners. Much of published medical research is blatantly biased toward pharmaceuticals. Even more studies are biased in more subtle and hidden ways. Conventionally trained physicians and practitioners are bred to just believe the headlines; they seldom care to look deeper into the research, since they already agree with the advertised "results". If our practitioners weren't so willing to swallow this nonsense, the pharmaceutical companies and conventional publications might not get away with it so easily.

Over-prescription of antibiotics and other medications

Our lack of adequate understanding of the causes of illness and maintenance of proper health leads to far too many infections. Many of these infections are viral or otherwise don't require antibiotics. But writing a prescription is the typical expectation in encounters for infectious complaints. Apparently, doctors often feel it is their duty and usually the best course of action to prescribe. Medical providers write so many prescriptions for antibiotics, I'm surprised the factories can keep stock on the shelves. Luckily, a great many of them do not get filled.

I remember when MRSA (methicillin resistant *staphylococcus aureus*) was just becoming a problem, and we would isolate patients in the hospital who had infections with this nasty, drug-resistant bacterium. Now, in some populations, it seems more common to have the bug than not to have it. I'm pretty sure that our own hospitals played a key role in disseminating this nasty critter, and my own innocence is in question for sure. Most likely, health-care workers and hospital staff have had a high colonization rate with this organism for many years now. I remember seeing one of the janitors at a local hospital during my residency. He came in to see me in clinic because of skin boils that were showing up spontaneously on his torso. I had to lance one of them, and it was positive for MRSA. He and his whole family were developing the boils and all had to be treated with strong antibiotics.

So how does this happen? How do these "superbugs" come to be? Well, they start out as just typical bacteria, such as the Staphylococcus aureus species. The majority of us carry such bacteria at all times in our nasal passages. Then, some sort of environmental stress causes them to mutate in an adaptive manner and become a little nastier and meaner. In this case, that environmental stressor is an antibiotic.

Human beings and other animals have "co-evolved" with our germs over thousands or millions of years and, in general, we have gotten along just fine with most of them. As long as one maintains a healthy diet and fully functional immune system, infection usually isn't a problem. When you start trying to kill them with chemical warfare, i.e. antibiotics, they can get a little nasty.

There are always a few bacteria in a given population that have spontaneously mutated and become inherently resistant to certain antibiotics. They are typically so few in number their presence is inconsequential. However, if you expose that whole population to an antibiotic, it may kill most or all the others. Even if only 1% of the population has survived, due to this rare inherent antibiotic resistance, it does not take very long for that small group to repopulate to a highly infectious level. This is due to some bacteria being able to divide and double their numbers every fifteen minutes at human body temperature. Then, almost all of the new bacterial population has that gene for drug resistance. You have changed their population genetics on a grand scale.

So, what does this have to do with medical philosophies and practice habits? Well, for example, it's the dogmatic belief that the patient should take a full seven to ten days of an antibiotic for a simple ear infection. Studies have shown that a significant majority of diagnosed childhood ear infections, as well as most respiratory tract infections overall, do not require antibiotics at all. They will take care of themselves just as quickly without treatment. The practice of prescribing so many courses of antibiotics is responsible for a large number of adverse drug events as well as the escalating problem of antibiotic resistant bacteria (Centre for Clinical Practice at NICE, 2008).

In spite of this fact, most doctors will still write the prescriptions. Some will do so because they think it is what the family expects from them.

Others because they just haven't gotten the memo, and still others because they really think the situation warrants an antibiotic. Some ear infections, of course, really do require antibiotics to prevent severe complications. When I see an inconsolable, miserable child, who has a fever and a bulging red eardrum, I typically write them a prescription for an antibiotic too. What I do that is different from the mainstream, however, is prescribe just three to five days worth and give them a refill to use in the event that it doesn't clear the condition adequately. Most infections will start to clear up nicely within just a few days, and then the individual's immune system can take over and finish the job. That way, a patient's entire host of bacterial organisms is exposed to fewer doses of antibiotics, and it decreases the chance of antibiotic resistant bacteria taking over the populations.

This is contrary to the prevailing dogma, which states you should prescribe seven to ten days of medicine and urge the patient to take the full course, even if they feel better after two or three days. The errant belief here is that by taking the antibiotics longer, the drug will more successfully kill all of the bacteria, and have less chance of developing resistant organisms. That doesn't make any damn sense to me at all, and it shouldn't make sense to the scientific medical community either. Repeated studies have shown much higher rates of bacterial antibiotic resistance in areas where there are greater numbers of antibiotic prescriptions handed out (Lai, 2011). The fact is, the longer you expose the bacteria to that environmental stress, the more the population will shift toward antibiotic resistance.

Recognizing this, the guidelines for treatment of simple urinary tract infections have reduced the recommended duration of treatment from five days down to three. This change was stated as being an attempt to reduce the rates of drug-resistant bacteria. Perhaps ear infections in children are just a more emotionally powerful thing. This is an area where the conventional guidelines make sense; similar to when they suggest that antibiotics should be withheld for minor ear infections. But practitioners continue to screw it up. Meanwhile, studies looking at the use of programs to standardize and restrict antibiotic use for community-acquired pneumonia (a potentially fatal condition, unlike ear infections) have shown good success in reducing both antibiotic-resistant organisms and also death from the condition itself (Bosso, 2011).

We need more individual practitioners to practice in a logical manner. Sometimes the conventional protocols have it right, sometimes they have it wrong. Each provider is supposed to think things through and do what makes the most sense scientifically and for the individual case at hand. Sometimes this means following the current standard of care (in spite of my criticism of that through most of this book), and sometimes it means doing something very different from that.

As I will discuss later on, an infection is more about the *host*, "us" in this case, than it is about the infecting organism. Building up host resistance and general health is the real key to success. Allowing the immune system to fight an infection to some extent makes a person stronger in the long run.

I have mentioned the issue of over-prescription of other medications repeatedly now. Most of us are aware of the practice physicians have of prescribing symptomatic drugs, which then cause symptoms of their own. This, in turn, often entails prescribing even more drugs. The dogma tells us that this is a safe practice because each of the drugs has been cleared by the FDA and approved for the conditions being treated.

One problem is that the safety of these drugs is not often assessed over a very long period of time. Yet a doctor may prescribe one for years on end. Another big problem is these drugs are not studied for safety when taken in combination with multiple other drugs. There are some known dangerous drug interactions, but most interactions are probably not yet known or fully appreciated.

In geriatric medicine, people commonly use the term "polypharmacy" to suggest that it is unnecessarily harmful for an elderly individual to be on too many prescription drugs. Astute geriatric practitioners frequently trim down an individual's medication list as one of the first therapeutic interventions. Often, things improve dramatically for the patient when the chemical onslaught is lessened. Basically, we've got way too many people sitting around way too medicated.

Inattention to costs

This is one aspect of our informal education that I too bought into early on. It made sense to me that we should not let financial considerations cloud our judgment as to the best diagnostic approach or treatment option for the patient. It seemed to make sense to provide the best care for everyone, and that cost should not really be a deciding factor in that. This belief lasted until about halfway through residency training for me. When patients tell me they can't afford a drug because it costs over $200 per month, or the MRI I ordered because they don't have $1500 to pay for it, I started to realize that the expense of medical tests and treatment are definitely a deciding factor, whether I like it or not.

When you learn that the World Health Organization ranked 36 other countries above the United States in overall health care system performance, including countries like Colombia, Chile, Saudi Arabia and Singapore (which was 6th overall), we have to wonder what could we be doing better. Even a country like Cuba, at 39th place, was only two positions worse than the U.S. in this 2000 report. What really makes this troubling is the fact that these countries all spend so much less money per capita on their health care (W.H.O., 2000)

When we combine the facts that medical costs are the number one reason to go bankrupt, financial stress is one of the worst stresses to have; and that stress can lead to worsened health, such as ulcers, heart attacks and suicides, we should come to the conclusion that cost must certainly be a consideration in the overall plan of care. It seems to me this pervasive, fiscally irresponsible philosophy is further evidence that capitalist interests control our medical education. Provider attitudes clearly influence the overall cost to each individual patient, and therefore the entire healthcare system.

As I mentioned before, I think we should try to choose the least harmful interventions first. For me, that includes consideration of financial "harms", which medical treatments or tests can impose. It doesn't do any good to prescribe a drug the patient cannot or will not buy. We have to find other ways to diagnose things when the tests are too expensive, and other forms of treatment when the drugs are unaffordable. This doesn't usually occur to doctors, and they may then blame treatment failure on the patient and their "noncompliance" with recommendations.

What makes this even more of a problem, as I've mentioned before, is that our practitioners are not taught how to do things differently. We are not taught how to diagnose things adequately without expensive tests or, if we are, that teaching gets forgotten because we don't take the time to adequately question and examine the patient. It is far quicker to order a long list of blood tests and some radiological studies.

Practitioners are not taught about diet, exercise, nutritional supplements, herbs, and other effective remedies that would be much safer and *cheaper*. We are taught that those alternatives are not really options because they do not work. It is evident how many aspects of our cultural dogma and beliefs in American medicine combine to create major problems.

The cost problem is further compounded by the fact that doctors tend to practice "defensive" medicine. This means ordering lots of tests just for the purpose of ruling-out some sort of serious disease process, even if it is very unlikely in the given situation. It is done largely to try and prevent being sued for malpractice, hence, the term *defensive medicine*. In most cases, the situation can be carefully explained to the patient and testing can be undertaken in a logical, stepwise manner, rather than the extremely cost-ineffective method of ordering what are expensive and, most likely, unhelpful or unnecessary tests up front.

Mistrust of the patient

This problem could also be described as a lack of respect for the patient and their opinions. This is another attitude or philosophy many doctors and practitioners possess that is not a product of direct formal education, but a more informal, collegial belief. Through clinical training, many of us have been told things like "if he says he drinks three beers per night, it's probably a six-pack" or , "if she says that she only eats 1000 calories per day and is still gaining weight then she's lying or really isn't keeping track".

Some of this involves a direct mistrust of the patient as if they are intending to lie to us. Some of it just involves a mistrust of the patient's ability to know what's really going on or keep track of something accurately. I see a major problem here in reconciling the idea that 80% of our medical diagnosis relies on the story we get from our patients with the idea that they are possibly giving us misinformation. This makes it impossible to trust the information we obtain and the conclusions we may reach because of it.

It is true that patients sometimes lie and, even more frequently, unintentionally provide faulty information to us. I know I have had patients lie about their pain to try and get more narcotics, or lie about their functional capacity in order to stay on disability. But to err is human, and I know most patients often get some details of their own history wrong. I see it as my job to sort out all of this, catch people in their lies or errors, and obtain necessary information whenever possible.

It is the job of the medical professional to try and get the most accurate and complete story from the patient. Sometimes this requires asking the same question in various ways, or making more inquiries to get the necessary information. Sometimes based on our intuition we decide a patient is intentionally lying to us, and sometimes we choose to believe the patient's story, even when it doesn't sound reasonable.

It is an interesting problem, when the patient really wants to tell the practitioner the needed information, but doesn't know what it is or how to express it. I must admit it takes much longer to get a thorough and closer-to-accurate story, but it is definitely the most important part of our job. If we choose to believe the patients are a poor source of information, it will not seem important to listen to their stories. We will gladly adopt the brief, targeted type of questioning that prevails in the fifteen-minute visit, and our success will decline. Proper care requires patient participation in almost every aspect of medicine; therefore we must rely on them and trust them to some extent.

Physician arrogance and narrow-mindedness-

In my opinion, this is one of the biggest barriers to proper health care in our culture. I know these are strong words, but I can't think of more moderate ones to use in this case. What else can I call it, when someone is so certain they have the right answers that they cease to hear what is being told to them and openly scoff at anything that may contradict their own theories? And yet, they repeatedly turn out to be wrong or have suboptimal outcomes from their own plan.

Doctors often decide that if they can't find the answer, then the answer *cannot be* found. Even worse, they may blame the patients themselves when things don't go right, or declare the problem to be psychiatric because they can't find a physical cause. In fairness, this isn't just a problem for doctors, nurse practitioners, physician assistants, naturopaths, chiropractors, and every other type of medical practitioner. All sorts of people have this dysfunctional attitude. The difference is that for most professions your ignorance doesn't get people killed. Medicine is really one are where we need to get our ego completely out of the way, in order to see more clearly what is going on.

It may be the minority of practitioners who truly feel themselves to be far smarter and "above" their patients, but many of them tend to come across that way. I frequently hear complaints about other providers that they don't listen or seem to respect the patient's own opinions. Most conventional practitioners scoff at any natural or alternative remedies the patient may mention, while admitting they themselves know essentially nothing about those things. They immediately dismiss anything the patient brings in that they read on the internet or in some non-conventional publication, without even looking at it, because if it wasn't taught to them during their esteemed medical education it must not be valid.

It may be true that you have to be of above-average intelligence to get accepted to medical schools and get through medical training (though I've certainly met examples to the contrary), but that doesn't make any of us omniscient. Probably the greatest possible ignorance is to believe we actually have the answers or know the truth. One of my favorite old proverbs translates into "Follow those who *seek* the truth, and flee from those who have *found* it." When we start to think we've learned everything there is to know and we trust our own opinions too much, it is probably time to retire. This is not because we've won the game, but because we are now a danger to our patients.

It seems like every generation of physicians and medical researchers think they have made major breakthroughs and progress in medicine, and that the previous generation was in the dark ages. I think it's still pretty darn dark in the world of conventional medicine. I don't know that we will ever really know what we are doing or have anywhere near all the answers.

We have set off in directions that, most likely, lead away from truly good medicine. But we are convinced that we are on the path to truth. I mean, most doctors are still prescribing synthetic hormones rather than biologically identical ones, just putting steroid creams on eczema, and doing gastric bypass surgeries on obese individuals. For crying out loud!

Conventional medicine still hasn't figured out where autoimmune diseases come from, or tried to address the reasons for why cancer incidence is increasing. It has forgotten the fact that a goiter requires iodine supplementation (and that's something that almost every lay-person knows)!

One of my favorite things to say to my interns, when I was chief resident, was "The standard of care is always changing. Therefore, it is always wrong." At first, I would usually get on odd look from the more brainwashed among them, and then the harsh truth of that statement would set in. If one believes that we are constantly finding better ways to do things, then one has to realize we aren't doing things that well right now.

It is difficult for truly arrogant persons to admit to themselves that they don't know something, or they may be doing something wrong. Many, possibly most, conventional doctors I've met are so egotistical that these possibilities don't seem to enter their head. I think part of the problem is that we spend so much time and money on our training, it causes a great deal of internal discord to imagine that we received an errant or deficient education.

I used to feel that way myself, early in my brainwashing. I can tell you that the most liberating thing is comfortably saying, "I don't know", and feel like that is truly the best answer to give. "I don't know" is really one of the most common answers I give to my patients' questions. However, I typically follow it with "but I think..." and offer the most likely explanation or expectation I have. I have to constantly admit to myself, and others, that we really can't know what is going to happen when any particular individual tries a new treatment. I have to admit that I only know what I've been told, what I've read, and what I've personally observed in clinical practice. All of this knowledge and experience still does not enable me to accurately predict what will happen with a new individual in a new situation. Heck, it doesn't even enable me to predict what will happen when the *same* individual tries something they tried in the past!

Most clinicians I have encountered, I suspect would agree, that few patients present their problems exactly like what is described in the textbooks. We should learn to set aside our biases and expectations and truly observe what we are hearing, feeling, and seeing. We have to then integrate everything that we know and have learned to the best of our ability and think hard to make the best decision. Then we still have to admit that we really don't know exactly what the hell we're doing or what is going to happen. This enables us to see the actual result of our intervention, rather than blindly "see" the *expected* result even when it did not occur. We must favor *reality* over *belief.*

It is actually very comfortable for me to now admit my own ignorance, but I used to share that strong sense of righteous arrogance that many of my colleagues still seem to possess. I used to listen with disdain when patients would tell me their ideas regarding their symptoms and illness. I would scoff internally at times when a patient would tell me "I know my own body", and I believed that they couldn't possibly understand anything because they didn't have my medical training.

I would follow the standard of care and then blame the patient, either openly or inside my own head, when they didn't improve. I would tell them that their alternative therapies were unproven and probably of no value. I believed in the conventional dogma and thought other types of therapies were sometimes ridiculous. I sometimes wondered where my patients had gone and why they didn't come back. That's my confessional, as a "recovering" allopathic physician, and now integrative practitioner. I've discovered that it's when we manage to drop the "knowing" or "believing" and go back to "seeing" and "thinking" that we have better success.

Now, people often leave their more narrow-minded, arrogant providers (*their* description) and come see me. Many of my patients have seen numerous conventional doctors and have been extremely frustrated by the way they were treated. They often felt they were not listened to, that their own ideas were brushed off or ridiculed, that they were made to feel stupid for asking questions or for bringing up information that they had found on the internet (which is often pretty good stuff that doctors should really know). They were often told to stop doing things that had actually been working for them, simply because these other practitioners thought those alternative therapies were nonsense without truly knowing anything about them. I have many patients come see me and open by telling me, "I generally don't go to doctors, but I heard you were different."

Through my own journey and development, I have discovered that arrogance and ignorance is a terrible combination and, too often, a fatal one in our society. Unfortunately, we are all going to remain somewhat ignorant; so, the best thing we can hope to do, perhaps, is drop the arrogance and struggle to maintain a clear vision and an open mind. In my own journey, I have had the wonderful opportunity to learn volumes of new information from my patients who have encouraged me to seek further research regarding their various concerns. My own practice is constantly evolving because I continue to learn new things, and never for one second do I believe I have all the answers. I try to view my suggestions as possibilities, rather than certainties.

I've sometimes seen patients for years and been up against a professional intellectual wall, not knowing what to do for them. Then I will often later learn something new and finally solve their problems. Practitioners must believe that the answer may be out there somewhere, in order to find it. But in order to believe that, we first have to realize that we don't have the answer right now.

The arrogance and narrow-mindedness of conventional medicine has created words like "idiopathic". This means that we don't know why the condition occurred and often suggests that the answer is not even potentially knowable. It implies that we can't know why the problem occurred and breeds indifference as to the cause. This effectively absolves us of the intellectual responsibility to figure it out (basically, if we don't know it now we probably never will, because we're really damn smart and know practically everything already).

We create terms like "supratentorial". This refers to the tentorium, the membrane in the brain which separates the cerebellum from the cerebral hemispheres with the thinking and emotional parts of the brain sitting on top. This term is used to suggest that a patient is just crazy, and their problems are "all in their head". The term "Somatization Disorder" is the official diagnosis created for this condition. This means the symptoms that a patient is experiencing, which are admittedly real in many cases, are being caused by their own psychological state. Other common examples of diagnoses in this category include fibromyalgia syndrome, chronic fatigue syndrome, and irritable bowel syndrome. They are all "syndromes". a term indicating that these diagnoses are just a collection of symptoms without any clearly identifiable abnormalities, either laboratory or structural. They are also often called "functional" disorders. This means they are a problem with how a patient is *functioning*, not that there is anything truly wrong with that person; this term again implies that the problems are created by their own mind and psychological state.

I get so frustrated and disgusted with this type of thinking in conventional medicine. If we can't figure out what's going on through our wonderful, infallible (and expensive) tests then there must be nothing truly wrong with the patient. Internal medicine physicians and the subspecialists within that field are the champions of this ideal. They will typically order so many blood tests, biopsies, invasive procedures, functional tests, and radiological tests to figure out the symptoms, that patients may well have to refinance their house to pay for evaluation of their cough, diarrhea, abdominal pain or headache.

At the end of it, you may have a laundry list of normal test results and be left with one of our great catch-all, I-don't-know-the-real-cause, diagnostic categories like "viral syndrome", "post-viral syndrome", "hormone imbalance", "idiopathic" condition, "functional" disorder, or maybe "allergy". Allergy would be a great choice if a good attempt followed to then discover what the allergy is and eliminating it, but that usually doesn't happen with conventional doctors.

What this often means, to the conventional practitioner, is that we have ruled-out serious conditions and can now finally just focus on the symptomatic treatments and get on with our lives. For an arrogant-plus-ignorant practitioner, these meaningless diagnoses are just fine. They are an acceptable stopping point. For me, and other integrative or holistic practitioners, they are often just the *beginning*. Most conventional primary care practitioners quickly run out of ideas, because our limited allopathic education provides us with relatively few metaphorical tools in our toolboxes. Most will then refer the patient on to a specialist. The specialist usually orders even more expensive and/or invasive testing, or more aggressive and potentially toxic drugs or other therapies, which perhaps the primary care practitioner was uncomfortable recommending.

I personally really like to get patients who have been to multiple doctors, specialists, and especially the "Ivory Tower" places like big teaching universities, Mayo Clinics, or Virginia Mason, but still no solution has been found for their problem. It seems like I get at least a couple of these people every month. These specialty medical places do a great job of ruling-out many possible causes of the patient's problem before I see them, leaving only those possibilities that conventional medicine remains ignorant of. It makes my job that much easier; and the work they do is vital.

I usually just have to listen to the patient, show respect for their opinions, and come up with something new that makes sense to them, in order to make them feel somewhat happier and more encouraged. When I can actually solve their problem, which happens more and more frequently as the years go by, then I'm a big hero. If I can't figure out what is wrong with them either, I didn't do any worse than the big specialty centers, so there's really no way I can lose. My take on things now is so different from conventional medical "wisdom" that, frequently, the real cause of their problem seems obvious to me. However, I still run into a giant wall of disbelief with conventional practitioners, even if the treatment plan we implement cures the patient! They just can't see it because of their errant, dogmatic beliefs.

If my treatment doesn't pan out, then I didn't do any worse than the big gurus and, at least, didn't do anything damaging or toxic to them. I don't know how many times now, for example, I've seen a woman diagnosed with "fibromyalgia" by some major medical center and given no effective treatment, then, we manage to find the real cause of their symptoms. I often find this condition dramatically improved by my giving them thyroid or adrenal support, Vitamin D, antifungal medications, performing detoxification for mold, chemicals or heavy metals for example. It's a no-lose situation for me, and frequently a winning situation for all concerned. If I can't figure something out at first, I tell folks to come back in six months or so, and I'll probably have something new for them to try.

In residency, and during the first year of my medical career, I would see these patients and just feel relief that "everything possible" had already been investigated and tried; because they had been to the best places and seen the best doctors. Then, I could just follow whatever the sages had recommended, and no thinking on my part was required. Now I love to think, and I relish the challenge of those unsolved mysteries. I've learned that sometimes the person who gets it right is merely the person with a fresh perspective.

One of my favorite inspirational quotes is by Albert Szent-Gyorgyi, the Hungarian scientist who discovered vitamin C. It reads: "Discovery consists of seeing what everybody has seen, and thinking what nobody has thought." I've also come to realize that Einstein was right when he said, "A man should look for what is, and not for what he thinks should be", or "Any man who reads too much and uses his own brain too little falls into lazy habits of thinking." Einstein also said, "Great spirits have often encountered violent opposition from weak minds", a problem which I may have experienced myself.

Those are great quotes, but my favorite quote currently has to be from Mahatma Ghandi, "Be the change you wish to see in the world." I have tried to change my own arrogant, narrow-minded, brainwashed attitudes, and I hope this book can help others do the same. I'm certainly still ignorant to some extent, and likely always will be, but at least I can see that now.

Fear of the unknown or "unproven"-

This was partially addressed under the "mistrust of the patient" heading, and probably discussed quite a bit here and there already. I also discussed the narrow conventional concept of proof and truth in my section on evidence-based medicine. My goal in this section is to speculate a little as to why this attitude exists and persists in medicine.

Again, I can't help but draw parallels between medical dogma and religious dogma. We seem, as a species, to need the comfort of a set of rules or guidelines, a path to walk, and some sort of truth to believe in. We seem to psychologically need the comfort we gain from being in a group that thinks what we think and believes as we do. We typically seem to be extremely uncomfortable with uncertainty or anything that may suggest our current way of thinking is wrong. This sort of collegial belief sharing is also seen in other groups and professions such as politics, the military, law enforcement, education, engineering, and many other occupations.

I have seen Christians (family members of mine included) turn a little pale at the fact that men and women have the same number of ribs, because they have a certain firm concept of one version of Genesis and the *Garden of Eden* story. If your religion teaches that the earth is only five to seven thousand years old, there is a mandatory disbelief of carbon dating as well as a major skepticism regarding concepts of evolution. There is violent opposition to these conflicting ideas, rather than an attempt to *integrate* the new information with the old beliefs as our knowledge and understanding of the world changes and grows.

I have seen similar negative reactions from medical colleagues when I tell them I will give thyroid hormone to patients with "normal-range" blood tests, or prescribe 50,000iu of Vitamin D daily for a month and then continue it a couple times per week long-term. Everyone knows that thyroid deficiency is diagnosed purely based on blood tests (usually the TSH alone in fact) and that Vitamin D is toxic at those doses right?

These ideas are uncomfortable because they shake up our sense of things and make us question our own beliefs. Well, it's important for people to realize that they can edit the more nonsensical or disproven parts of their dogma and beliefs, without the whole system crumbling down around them. It's okay to reinterpret the scripture and stop taking certain things so literally without deciding the whole book must be wrong. We don't have to throw out the baby, just change the bath water once in a while.

It's okay to realize that practitioners treated thyroid deficiency just fine for many decades before blood tests or synthetic thyroid products came on the scene, and that these more "modern" ideas may themselves be somewhat flawed. Progress is not always in the best direction, after all. It's okay to realize that Vitamin D is actually a steroid hormone and not a "vitamin" at all, and that cases of toxicity are exceedingly rare and generally require incredibly high doses over several months. It is okay to think for one's self, even if the religious and medical cults of the world discourage and punish such behavior for fear an individual will leave the flock. Or perhaps a person's different view represents some sort of doubt that they hold within themselves and despise intensely.

In fact, if the flock is leading its members off a cliff, each individual should really want to know about it. If there is security in the unity and camaraderie of the group, then I think individual thought should be welcomed and encouraged. It can lead to better progress. There should be some degree of tolerance for, even interest in, the questioning of one's methods, rather than accusatory interrogation when someone does something differently. After all, if your views and opinions are correct, you should welcome any challenge as another chance to reinforce that, right?

I know some of my former residency colleagues, who openly said I was probably the smartest of the group back then, now tell people I've lost my mind or something, because of the way I do things. They have never bothered to ask me *why* I am doing things differently or what new information and training I may have had to change my practice from the mainstream. Rather than discuss it, they choose to stick with the dogma and feel negatively toward me. I don't worry about it, other than to feel badly for their patients.

If someone is intelligent and open-minded, they often begin to see things more my way, or at least differently, after I talk with them for a little while. They may at least ask good questions and gain more interest. After all, generally, these aren't just *my* ideas. There are thousands of integrative practitioners across the country, who think and practice in a similar way. When someone is more closed-minded, they may just be openly skeptical, or worse, and seem unable to even hear what I have to say. Alternatively, they may just quietly move away from the conversation, clearly troubled by the internal discord caused by hearing ideas that conflict with their own.

In my opinion, we will never make much progress without original thoughts and ideas. Unfortunately for many, that means embracing some ideas that directly conflict with what is currently believed. We have to be careful just how tightly we cling to our beliefs, because it is then all the more painful if they are pried loose. Also, if students are never allowed to question what they are taught or learn outside the dogma, and since they tend to forget a portion of their teaching over time, their knowledge as a group will only get narrower and smaller over time. That's the opposite of progress isn't it? If new ideas are not welcomed and the same old, errant, antiquated notions are not repeatedly challenged, then how can we hope to ever reach anything resembling the *truth*?

If something is true, it should withstand any barrage of questioning or investigation into its validity, and all attempts to find flaw will only strengthen it. If we feel confident in our own beliefs and practices, then we should not feel threatened by questions or challenges. Rather, we should welcome them as an opportunity to educate or indoctrinate someone else. We should also be grateful if anyone proves us *wrong*, because we should always desire to be doing things in the best way possible. Most would agree with this intellectually; and yet it is far from our nature to follow this philosophy.

This goes back to basic ancient Greek Aristotelian and Platonic logic, wherein there is a "thesis" (prevailing view or theory) and an "antithesis" (differing or opposing possibility or theory). They are congenially beat against each other, using mutual logic, until a new theory/thesis is forged that becomes the next accepted version of the "truth" for the time being. Nobody has to get pissed off or accuse the other of being a liar or a fool. Allowing emotion to get involved completely ruins things. This process is necessary to continue the intellectual trek toward progress in knowledge and thought. Sadly, this sort of thinking is absolutely discouraged in medicine. Those who fail to "walk the dogma" are out of the club.

I just don't understand that attitude. We are all trying to achieve the same thing aren't we? I guess it goes back to basic human nature. Luckily for my patients, I never wanted to be in the "club".

There are some attempts made at this in medical research. But now the variables are usually manipulated, statistics twisted, and conclusions reported in such a way as to make us believe, in too many cases, what they want us to believe. There is no such thing as "independent" research, because the money always has to come from somewhere. The closest thing to independent research is that which is conducted every day in practitioners' offices, using an individual as their own personal control group.

Rather than the logic and progress inherent in the model proposed by Aristotle and Plato, we currently have a system that is better represented by Plato's *Allegory of the Cave*. For those who don't know this story, I will end this chapter with a brief synopsis of it.

A man lived in a civilization that existed underground in a large cave. The people there did not know that they were in a cave, and they thought the dark moving images on one large rock face were Gods moving around within their concept of the heavens. One day, an individual from this society found a new passageway that had previously been undiscovered, and he followed it up through the rock. He eventually emerged onto the surface world, and he could there see the sun for the first time. He saw people, much like himself, wearing very different things, in a land very different from his own. He noted that they cast shadows from the sunlight that looked exactly like the images on his people's wall. He also saw crevices in the ground that allowed the light and shadows to cast down into where he and his people lived.

He learned many new things in his short time there and returned, very excitedly, to his people. When he made it back down the hidden passage to his own world, he began enthusiastically telling everyone he could about his experiences. He told them about the other world and the other people that were very much like themselves. He told them that the moving images on the wall were merely shadows cast by people moving about on the surface world and were not gods as they had thought.

Well, as you can imagine, this did not have the effect the man had anticipated. The people he spoke to were extremely disconcerted when hearing his news and, of course, chose not to believe him. They were much more comfortable with their own beliefs, and this new information conflicted with all they had believed in for their entire lives. He offered to lead others up the pathway, so they could see for themselves, but nobody would go.

The more the man ranted about what he had seen, the more agitated the people became and, eventually, they fell upon him and killed him in their attempts to silence this insanity. With that finally ended, they could go back about their usual business and continue believing what was familiar and comforting.

Too many of us live within our own intellectual caves, and I'm hoping to help more practitioners and people climb out into the light, or at least into a new cave for a change. I've discovered that going back to my medical colleagues and enthusiastically preaching any newly-discovered wisdom typically falls on deaf ears or is automatically disregarded because it conflicts with the standard thinking. Many integrative medicine ideas are directly attacked or ridiculed by the establishment, without being adequately investigated for validity. State medical boards have been known to revoke an integrative physician's license without any complaints from, or proof of harm to patients, but merely because the conventional practitioners disagree with the way they are practicing.

Because of this attitude among medical practitioners, I have found much greater yield in talking to my patients and the general public. Non-medical people have not been stuffed into the same cave it seems. They have more fresh air and daylight in which to see new things. It is the general public and their force as consumers that may be better able to force change in our broken medical system.

You, the patient, need to feel empowered to steer your care in the direction that you feel you need. Remember, your medical provider is also just another human being; with their own ignorance and bias. They are truly trying to help you, but their own shortcomings may get in the way of that. You should feel free to find a different practitioner if needed, for your own sake. Find someone who listens to you and seems to make sense. The later parts of this book should help you understand what you need to improve and maintain your own health, and also how to find an appropriate provider if one is needed.

CHAPTER 5 – THE FAILINGS OF OUR SOCIETY

As a society, we cannot feel entirely blameless for our current state of health. We have the power to change things through our influence; this is because everything, to some extent, depends upon our own consumer habits. First, we have to recognize what social behaviors have helped create the problem. Some of these will be relevant to government policy, and others are more directly attributable to population or individual habits.

Consumer-driven decline-

It has been reported that the United States consumes a far greater share of the world's resources than represented by our population. This is certainly true, for example, in regard to energy, manufactured goods, food, and clothing. We know it is also true in terms of health care dollars spent. We are rapidly consuming our way right through the Earth's natural resources, much like an unaware caterpillar eating away at the last leaf on the tree. At least the caterpillar may eventually turn into a butterfly and fly away. I hear they are selling land on the moon, so maybe there's a place for us to go too.

As a culture, we seem to want to have it all. Everyone feels the need to have a car, a big screen TV, brand name clothing, cell phones, and other technological amenities. The welfare system even provides subsidized cell phones for people, as if they were a necessity in our modern society.

To continue with cell phones, as an example of consumerism contributing to our decline, most people don't realize there is a tiny amount of the rare, semiprecious metal called *coltan*, inside every cell phone. Coltan recovery is the main reason the phones are recycled. When I took my kids to the San Diego Zoo in December 2007, we saw a large sign explaining how enormous areas gorilla habitat in Africa is being destroyed in order to mine more of this metal and to make new cell phones, iPhones or Blackberries that we think we need to have. What seems to be a minor, casual purchase here in the U.S., may cause far-reaching destruction to an environment elsewhere on the planet. It may also propagate adverse working or living conditions for humans in a distant country.

I heard in the news once a man declared that having a television set was a necessity of modern life in this country, and he wanted welfare services to provide him with one. To replace analog broadcasts and receive the new digital ones, our government offered coupons, paid for by our tax dollars, to help everyone upgrade their television sets' signals. This is all done in the name of some intangible, unsustainable "standard of living" to which our society feels entitled. Too bad our standard of care in medicine doesn't aim as high!

I believe that a big part of the problem stems from most people having no real clue as to where the stuff they buy comes from. I'm not just talking about the ten-year-old kid, laboring away for five cents a pair in a sweatshop somewhere on the other side of the world so that Americans can pay $120 for their sneakers and corporate profits can soar. I'm talking about the materials that things are actually made from. For instance, where do fiberglass, plastic, and steel come from? The items we take for granted, like airplanes and automobiles, constitute quite a lot of raw material. Much of this has to be mined from the ground or created from other non-renewable resources like petroleum.

Another example is those nifty little compact fluorescent light bulbs that we are all encouraged to buy. Each one contains mercury, one of the most toxic substances known to man. Of course, it's a very small amount, and as long as it's inside the bulb, it poses no risk, right? But what's going to happen when that bulb dies and needs to be replaced? Is it going to given a proper burial inside a metal box or, more likely, just placed in the trash? When it breaks open at the landfill, the small amounts of mercury from millions of those bulbs, will add up to a very real amount that will likely be getting into the ground water. What is more relevant to me is the bigger problem of mining the mercury out of the ground in order to make these bulbs. The mining stirs up tons (yes, literally tons) of toxic material, which, through the wind and water, gets distributed all over.

Currently, for the general public, the main source of mercury exposure comes from consuming fish and sea foods, which are becoming more and more contaminated with mercury and other toxic metals as time goes by. It gets into those animals because they eat the smaller sea creatures that get it in progressively larger doses when they consume algae, which is at the bottom of the ocean food chain. The algae absorb it directly from the ocean water, which contains more and more mercury every year. How does it get into the water? It was safely tucked away in the Earth's crust until humans started digging it up. The biggest natural source of mercury in the environment is volcanic eruption, but humans now contribute much more than that.

Air pollution and ground water run-off lead the way as the main sources of contamination. It ends up in the ground water from mining, landfills, and any place else where we dump our used-up mercury-containing items. Air pollution is the biggest initial human-related problem, and the main source of this is from burning coal to make electricity (there is no such thing as "clean coal" by the way – it is filthy and poisonous, and there is no way around it!). There are hundreds of thousands of tons of mercury spewed into our atmosphere every year through the burning of coal (this information is available through EPA websites and other study). It travels in the winds to land all over the world, two thirds of which happens to be covered with water.

Did you know that China had been building a new, coal-burning (and not "clean" in any way!) power plant, every week, for many years? A BBC News article in June 2007 reported they had stepped it up to two new plants per week! (Harrabin, 2007). In spite of that, it was estimated at that time that the average individual in the UK still generated nearly three times as much pollution as the average Chinese individual, and the average American nearly six times as much (Harrabin, 2007). It seems people in general just don't care how damaging their power generation is, as long as it's a smaller cost on their energy bill every month. China is building these in order to generate the power needed to produce more low-quality crap for us to purchase, brought to you by your friendly neighborhood Wal-Mart, and other peddlers of low-quality, disposable, replace-annually-if-not-sooner junk!

Wal-Mart owes the American public a huge "thank-you" for making it the wealthiest retailer on the planet. This further exemplifies that the pollution problem is the fault of the consumer. And before blaming China for the pollution problem, you'd better run around your house and hide all the stuff that was made there. For example, as I sit here at my desk, I note that my lamp, stapler, mouse, and flash drives are all "Made in China". My coffee cup claims to be made in the USA, so hopefully it doesn't have so much lead or cadmium in the glaze. My laptop refuses to give up its country of origin, despite spending at least three minutes flipping it around and looking for the information. I'm sure it wasn't made in this country, though – I mean when was the last time America made any electronics?

Oh, that's right, our country prefers to buy things made cheaper overseas, sometimes by our own corporations, rather than produce things here for us. These corporations outsource the work, in spite of the fact that, as I write this, our own unemployment rates are approaching 10%. Transporting those items around the world further generates air pollution from the burning of vastly more fossil fuels. That's why this long and convoluted tirade is in the "failings of society" chapter. People seldom consider that sort of collateral damage. Just think of the added pollution generated by our "global" trade habits!

Overconsumption in our country is a huge problem. Our thrift stores are constantly crammed full with donated items that households purchased, apparently unnecessarily in many cases. Granted, it is frequently stuff that our kids outgrew. But couldn't we replace our kids' old toys with other used ones, instead of continuing to buy more and more brand new junk? Couldn't we wear our clothes a bit longer, rather than having to be a slave to the ever-changing fashion trends? The idea of "fashion", in my opinion, is just a way to get people to continually buy more new clothing. The clothing industry has us convinced that we need to constantly update our look to fit in with society. Well, who is this "society", if it isn't you and me? I just don't get it. I will admit that my own household, with six kids, really needs to work on this one too!

These days, there are many cable television shows on home remodeling, house flipping, and selling. Many of these shows suggest that we need to tear out and replace perfectly usable appliances, cabinets, countertops, flooring, and fixtures, so that we can update our home and make it more "modern" presentable. This is another example of incredible waste just to suit the conditioned desires of the American consumer.

Another great example of how we continually throw away perfectly good stuff to get something newer, faster or better involves our electronics products. Software has to be constantly updated for some reason – yes, because they keep making new hardware and software that requires new technology, in order to even use it. Also, in many cases, the poorly made stuff doesn't even work for very long, or the new software version sucks worse than the last one. The makers of electronics technology, automobiles, and other products, already have the ability to make a much more advanced version than they release. This is what I have heard from people working in these industries at least. But, those companies prefer to sell things in phases, so they can make more profit from each step along the way – knowing the American consumer will keep buying/trading/trashing stuff like Dr. Seuss' star-bellied sneeches.

The advance in product manufacturing is labeled as "progress", but it most certainly is not. It is often just a way to make more money for people who already have a ton of it. And in the process, nobody seems to ask about where all the new materials are coming from or where all the old stuff is going. How much of your old stuff do you yourself honestly recycle or donate for someone else to use? How much trash does each of us have at the end of our driveway every week? How much damn packing material does a kid's toy really need to have anyway?

Other countries have clearly envied the "American way of life" in recent decades and, to some extent, many other cultures have followed suit and have begun following our trends in fashion and lifestyle. This just creates more trash and destruction on a global scale. However, these problems aren't just of environmental concern, they cause individual problems as well.

The American food industry contributes to this true "consumer" issue, by finding ways of getting us to eat more than what we actually need. A great way for food producers to continually increase their profits is to somehow increase how much each individual eats (or to increase the number of individuals, but that's much tougher to control). In order to do that, they may use extensive advertising and put additives into food that have addictive properties. The most common addictive substances are added sugar, corn syrup, artificial sweeteners and fat.

The World Health Organization has asked repeatedly for the world's nations to restrict advertising of junk foods and has devised plans to restrict the amount of sugar and fat that could be added to processed foods. This is an effort to help decrease the growing global obesity problem. The food manufacturing industry, with multiple huge, global companies, has argued that there is no scientific proof that higher proportions of those added ingredients leads to weight gain and obesity (this ongoing issue has been followed for years in the Price-Pottenger Nutrition Foundation Newsletter and other health-related publications). After all, people do have to eat, and it's up to them to restrain themselves appropriately, right? Shamefully, this idiotic argument, or the financial influence of our food manufacturers, has succeeded in stalling out plans to make our processed foods a little healthier or reduce their advertising to children.

I could rant much longer about our consumer habits and how they are destroying the planet and our own individual health, but it's time to move on. We will look more closely at specific examples of how these issues directly affect our individual health in the chapters on environmental toxicity.

Environmental inattention-

It would not be an outrageous statement to say that our country is the biggest offender in terms of depleting the world's resources, contributing to planetary destruction, and in the decline of human health. While it's true that many less-developed countries still use chemical pesticides, herbicides, and other chemicals that are banned due to concerns over human safety, here in the U.S., American chemical companies still make many of these chemicals, often in factories within those much poorer countries, where environmental standards are virtually nonexistent. We also ship our garbage out of the country because we produce more of it than we can handle ourselves. There are reports of a "garbage island" floating in the middle of the ocean somewhere (it's difficult to know how much of this stuff to believe though).

I've already gone on and on about the tracking of mercury through the environment and our responsibility for that as consumers, so I won't belabor that point any longer. I bring it up again just to point out that paying attention to the environment doesn't just mean turning off electronics when not in use, taking shorter showers, driving a hybrid vehicle, or recycling beer bottles. It requires an understanding of the global environment and economy in which we live. For example, buying locally-produced items is a simple way to reduce global pollution because those items do not have to be trucked across the country or flown half way around the world. It's worth the extra few cents per pound in many ways. A little more awareness could go a long way for us.

Most of the people I know in Alaska don't recycle because we have to sort, pack, and haul everything to a collection location and then *pay them* when we get there. The whole state stopped recycling glass in early 2009 because it was deemed too expensive to ship out of state to processing plants. The "last frontier" of Alaska seems to take its vast expanses of clean land for granted. Why couldn't the state start its own glass recycling program, producing glass canning jars and bottles for home brewed beer and wine perhaps? That would provide jobs, protect the environment and reduce waste.

Many other places in the country have mandatory recycling, which is usually included with the trash pickup. That is a positive move for our culture. However, we still burn coal or other fossil fuels for energy, rather than really trying to develop clean alternatives. We still ship things all around the country and the world, rather than producing most of what a region needs within a smaller radius. We still largely drive individual cars, rather than developing truly effective and attractive systems of public transportation. And, we still waste huge amounts of power on unnecessary things.

Some of these things may seem a little contrived but, because we have gotten so used to our current way of life, we just expect to have excessive things and pay no attention to the consequences. I'm not suggesting that we all go live in cabins made from recycled tires and live without electricity or running water. I'm sure there are many people out there, who would love to call me a hypocrite for not doing these things myself. Then they would happily go back about their usual habits, feeling even more justified in them, because I've proven it's impossible to change. On the other hand, if I did go live a sort of modern pilgrim lifestyle (which I honestly would love to do, but my wife and kids won't let me), many people would merely find that "interesting" or mock me for my eccentricity. When people don't want to change their minds, or habits, there is no convincing them.

The problem here is our cultural attitudes, and how they've changed over the ages. We have gotten so used to our technological advances that we have completely lost touch with our planet and our environment. People in our modern society usually don't have the first clue where their foods or other goods come from, or even care who may have grown or made them. We have gotten so used to eating out of boxes and cans that we have no concept of how to produce food ourselves, and thereby meet one of our most basic needs. Most of us (myself included) don't know how to make our own clothing or dishes, hunt or gather our own food, build a house or fix our own car or electronics.

Well, why the heck should we have to learn to do any of that, when the grocery stores and restaurants are full of food? There is a Wal-Mart right down the street, and my mechanic is open even on Sundays. Well, what are we going to do when those things aren't there?

The automobile industry could probably make a fleet of electric cars, or cars that run on water and sunlight in a year or two, if the oil all dried up tomorrow. I would bet that, if we tried, almost every community could produce every single thing it needed within a hundred mile radius. We could employ nearly everyone and eliminate incredible amounts of waste previously created by transportation using fossil-fueled vehicles. My own community could probably build a light rail system from Wasilla to Anchorage just using all the old dead cars and major appliances that so many people here keep in their yards, in lieu of lawn gnomes it seems. That would get thousands of cars off the road every day for the work commute.

My kids have been to Disney Land at least four times now, which is admittedly the result of my own decisions. But if it weren't there, I'm sure we could find something else to do that would be much cheaper (and they would get bored again just as fast when we got home, I'm sure). Then there's Las Vegas, an excellent example of waste and depravity.

Everyone would have to agree that education is important and teachers are some of the most important people in our culture, yet how much more money does a professional athlete or movie star make than the typical teacher, policeman or firefighter in our society? How does that happen, and why do we let it continue?

So, why don't we fix these problems, since many people would agree with my assessment (or maybe not, I could be totally alone in my opinions here, I suppose)? Why do we continue to increase our consumption and speed our depletion of the planet rather than find new ways to generate power and turn used things into new things? Why do we keep demanding more when we used to be satisfied with less? Why do we misplace our money and support so drastically? Well, I think the answers lie in our cultural psychology.

If individuals are asked whether or not they worry about the environment, most in our society will likely reply "yes" these days. If asked if they think we consume too much energy, cut down too many trees, pollute the air and water too much, or produce too much waste, the answer is likely to be the same. Of course, there are those who think everything is just fine right now and our environment is not in the slightest bit of trouble.

Unfortunately however, if many of the concerned individuals are asked what they, themselves, are going to change to help fix the problems, very limited or noncommittal replies will be offered. We will readily acknowledge the problems and, when pushed, we will admit to our own role in them, but we will seldom step up and make the individual changes or sacrifices (as if not having a car or a cell phone were the end of the world). I think the feeling we have here (and I admit I can relate) is "It's not going to make any real difference, because everyone else is going to keep trashing the planet", and "why should I go without when everyone else is going to keep doing what they're doing?"

That's right, it just seems pointless to do the right thing when society is going to drag us all down anyway. But who is our "society", if it is not you and I, and a few hundred million others? It's not far removed from the basic mob mentality, where typically good and well-mannered people would run after someone and throw stones at them or burn their house down with torches. When there is a big group behaving badly, there is really no perceived individual responsibility.

Are we just a bunch of furless, two-legged lemmings running off a cliff together? Are we a large flock of bipedal sheep grazing in a pesticide-soaked pasture until we are infertile and have high rates of bipedal-sheep cancer? As a group, why can't we decide to build a guardrail at the edge of that cliff or agree to stop spraying pesticide on our pasture?

I hate to say it, but it seems that, most of the time, people really need to be forced to do the right thing (any other parents of teenagers out there?). Given the option, the typical human will take the easy route almost every time without an eye to the future. Laziness and complacency are the general trends, and necessity is the mother of invention. That really isn't a character flaw of our species, it is just the basic nature of most any organism. It takes big frontal lobes and significant effort, apparently, to change that behavior pattern.

How many of us have crammed for tests the night before, or written a research paper in a single day? How many of us eat bananas from South America, buy electronics from China, and clothing made in Sri Lanka? How many of us drive to work in our own car, when we could carpool or take the bus? On our honeymoon in Mexico, my wife and I saw an entire family of five riding on one little moped – it was the damnedest thing – now that's carpooling to the extreme!

But why shouldn't we relax, make things as easy as possible on ourselves, and take advantage of society's conveniences? Apparently, the answer to that is too complex and depersonalized for many of us to notice.

If we are going to change the direction that the world is going, we have to pay attention to these more subtle aspects of individual and social responsibility. We are going to have to make choices that reach beyond immediate gratification and compliance with social norms.

I'm very sorry to have gone on and on like this about a topic that seems so far from the perceived point of this book, but as I continue, it will be evident that the most important factors in human health involve environmental factors and individual behavior. Also, the solutions to our health problems, which ultimately result from these global environmental factors, will never be found in a convenient pill.

Bigger, faster, easier and cheaper-

I have ranted about this somewhat in the preceding pages, but I will, just briefly, make this point further. We have become a "supersize me" culture. We are convinced that it is better to get more for our money in terms of quantity, while paying little attention to quality. We want bigger burgers and more fries, even when we are full on the smaller portions. We want bigger automobiles, even though it's usually just one or two people in the car (and I happen to know for a fact you can get five people on a moped). We will "buy one, get one free" even though we only need the first one (maybe we'll give the other one to someone else). As a culture we just basically want more for less; and you can't really argue with that natural tendency.

We want faster computers and internet hookups all the time. I recall over twenty years ago hearing my mother complain about how it took several minutes for her fax machine to send a document, and saying to her "but you have to admit, we've come a long way from the pony express." For some reason, she didn't really appreciate my logic at the time (may have even called me a smart-ass or something). We just seem to get used to things and take things for granted very quickly.

We want technology to do more and more things for us, instead of using own effort. The remote control is a notable example, and one that has probably contributed to some of the measurable increase in our waistlines. We have electric can openers, automatic doors, and escalators. These things all consume energy, but not our own physical energy. Couple these conveniences with the super-sized fast foods, and we get a high rate of obesity it seems.

So, in my opinion, the reason we choose these modern conveniences is often the "cheaper" issue. On a personal level, we want more for our money without realizing the greater cost. Unfortunately, when we get our clothing made in China or some third-world country for half the cost, we promote a certain amount of human depravity for those workers. And we are also responsible for the added pollution from the dirty energy they use. Taking into account the added fossil fuels burned to ship it back over here, probably doesn't cross the minds of most people. If there is a similar shirt made right down the road by a local vendor who charges two dollars more, we probably won't buy it. In fairness, most in our culture are unaware of these issues I think; but it seems that more of us are beginning to conscientiously buy locally more often.

Similar issues exist with food and other goods. We may drive an extra few miles in our SUV's, using another fifty cents or more in gas, to a gas station where we can save two cents per gallon to fill a twenty-gallon tank (which, if you do the math, only saves you forty cents, sorry). I realized one day, that I got 10-15% better gas mileage when I used the better grade of gas, which makes it basically the same cost per mile driven, while saving some wear on my car engine, and saving the environment from a little added pollution because it burns cleaner.

We don't even let turkeys have sex any longer in this country, apparently because that process is too slow and inefficient (there is a wonderful account of this in Barbara Kingsolver's book *Animal, Vegetable, Miracle*). Instead, we mechanically harvest sperm from the boys and manually fertilize the hens. We also now need to mechanically fertilize a growing number of our human females due to rising problems with infertility (CDC stats from a 2002 study showed 11.8% of women ages 15-44 had impaired fertility at that time. It is likely steadily getting worse). As a result, we have developed intrauterine insemination and in vitro fertilization with subsequent manual implantation processes. Let me know when they start mechanically harvesting our men's sperm; I'll go hide.

Taste over health, "living to eat"-

In keeping with the above themes, our society demands "destructive luxury" from our food as well. This is a huge issue affecting our health, as I will discuss in greater detail later. Our food culture in the United States is centered mostly on quantity, efficiency and flavor, with almost no attention to food *quality* in terms of nutrition or safety. To some extent this seems innate or instinctive. Just take a child down the cereal aisle at the grocery store. They will beg for the cereals with the most sugar, the brightest colors on the box, and the most interesting pictures. They don't care about what's good for them, only what is good *tasting*.

As adults we consider this sort of behavior to be very childish, and yet, we aren't really any better, are we? How many adults would choose a piece of whole grain toast and a banana over a donut or some pop tarts? How many will only eat a salad when it is smothered with dressing that is full of sugar and unhealthy fat? How many people make a face at their doctor when they suggest drinking water rather than soda or a sports drink?

This last one is what really gets me the most. I see so many adults and children who are hooked on sweet beverages, and to them the idea of drinking just plain water is fairly disgusting. My kids had a friend who lived down the street some years ago. She was quite an obese ten year-old girl. She told me that she was always starving, that there was no food at her house, and no one made any food for her to eat. She spent the night at our house once. She made the most disgusted face when I suggested she drink water for her thirst. She actually requested some sugar to mix into it so she could stand to drink it. In the morning she wanted some cereal, but the sweetest kind we had was Life™ cereal (which I'm sure is still more than 25% sugar). She said she couldn't stand to eat it without several spoonfuls of sugar on top of it.

Sadly, I fear that this little girl is not in the minority of U.S. children. Americans have gotten so used to our processed foods being so crammed full of sugar, added fats, artificial flavors and colors, that we don't even know what real food looks or tastes like anymore. Even my own office staff members typically eat processed food items at lunch. This is either stuff they get from a fast food source or prepackaged foods that they pull out of a freezer and throw in the microwave. I don't nag them about it, nor do I nag my patients. Adults must come to these decisions by themselves; all I can do is educate and give advice.

These foods are not just overly processed and completely stripped of nutrients; it's even worse than that. Generally, they also have excessive additives to improve the taste. This includes sugars and fats (usually from soy or some other bulk source that isn't really good nutrition). On top of this, the little quick meals are generally microwaved in a plastic dish, destroying some of the residual nutrients, while adding new toxic chemicals from the plastic. Yummy!

People eat this garbage because it tastes good and it's quick. If it didn't taste good, we wouldn't eat it; and since the food industry knows that, they make sure to add things that will please our tongues and trick our brains. Part of the problem is that we inherently trust our food manufacturers to provide us with things that are safe and nutritious to eat, rather than just good tasting. Well I'm sorry, but here in the U.S, that is sheer fantasy. Like I mentioned before, our food standards are terrible for an industrialized country. We, allegedly, allow more chemicals, sugar, fats and other additives than European countries for example; and, in terms of nutrition or human safety, our food does not get adequately assessed for quality. We may have tight restrictions on how much aflatoxin is permitted in peanut butter, but there is no restriction on bisphenol A or artificial dye, and there are known carcinogens such as sodium nitrite and caramel coloring allowed in our foods.

More importantly than the individual food quality problem in our culture, people just eat far more than they should. We are, after all, the culture of the buffet restaurant and the supersized fast food choices. We have made gorging ourselves one of our favorite national pastimes. And when someone is going to bring something to the office to share with everyone in the morning, how often is it donuts, cookies, or some other unhealthy food? How often is it a fruit basket, veggie tray, or something else healthy? Why are your coworkers trying to kill you? Maybe they want your job.

The unfortunate fact is that eating the typical American diet is physiologically addicting. The processed foods in this country are geared to play into our natural taste for things that are sweet, fatty, and rich. I think that we inherently like these flavors and substances because the things in nature that are sweet or fatty tend to be very good for us. Examples include fruit, berries, milk (human milk would be best, of course), butter and animal flesh (yes, healthy animal flesh is very good for us).

It's important to note a very important difference between the natural foods and the processed ones. The natural foods have lots of nutrients in them and when you eat those, your body becomes truly satisfied and your overall hunger decreases. Alternatively, when you eat devitalized foods with added sugar and fat, you don't get nourished in the same sense, and your appetite *increases*. This contrast is inherently detrimental, because we eat in order to obtain essential elements and nutrients from our foods; we eat not just energy, and not just for fun.

Recent epidemiologic research has suggested that people who drink diet soft drinks rather than the regular ones may gain weight just as badly as those who consume the sodas with corn syrup (Brown, 2010). Why?

Apparently, the sweet taste triggers a desire for more sweet tasting things that contain real sugars. The taste seems to cause secretion of higher amounts of insulin, which drops blood sugar (by converting available glucose into fat cells rather than using it for energy) and makes a person even hungrier. Generally, that hunger is for *real* sugar or starch, so this leads to greater calorie consumption overall (Yang, 2010).

The overall effect of consuming "diet drinks" with artificial sweeteners is that people eat more than they otherwise would, generate more fat metabolically, and gain weight in the form of fat mass. The "sugar-free" drinks may be better than those with corn syrup or sugar, but the overall effect on weight is not much better it seems; and the artificial sweeteners may have neurotoxic effects on the brain, as I will discuss later on in section IV. All because they refuse to drink water!

Why do some people feel the need to only have tasty beverages, when there are no such things in nature? In my opinion, even fruit juice is an unnatural thing to drink. Eat an apple if you want some apple juice; eat an orange if you want orange juice! There's a reason it's in there. It's to get us to eat the whole fruit with the seeds of the plant in it, which has much more to offer than just the juice. If you drink a cup of juice, it will spike your blood sugar greatly, relative to eating a piece of the whole fruit with the same total amount of sugar in it.

Speaking of fruits and vegetables, our culture has even found a way to make those things unhealthy! I'm not just talking about pesticides and chemicals, but selective breeding and genetic modification. Presumably to increase our liking of them, we have now corn and other plant foods with far higher amounts of sugar than their ancestors. Of course, the chemicals are arguably a bigger problem. Our produce now contains many toxic chemicals in order to make things bigger, brighter, and better looking.

Our animals aren't spared this type of treatment either. Our turkeys are bred and engineered to grow enormous breasts, such that many of them can't even walk around if allowed to grow past six months of age (Kingsolver, 2007). We are developing genetically modified pigs and cows that grow such large muscles they also cannot function normally. In 2010, the first genetically modified fish hit U.S. markets. It originates from Atlantic salmon, and it is labeled only just "Atlantic salmon" because the producers convinced our government regulators that there was no need to label it as a GMO. The animals aren't examples of sacrificing health for taste, but for the size or ease of obtaining the product. Again, we may be giving up what's truly important about our food in favor of cost and convenience, and possibly at some risk.

Of course, other cultures have similar likes in terms of taste but, for many of them, there are huge differences in the food quality. The French are a good example because of the so-called "French Paradox", which comes from observing that the French have notably lower rates of heart disease, despite eating more fat than Americans and other countries with higher rates of heart disease. They even eat loads of real butter! Some believe this is because the French have a higher consumption of red wine, but that's probably not it.

Consuming more than two drinks of alcohol, even red wine, per day has been shown to be detrimental to health rather than beneficial. Also, more recent study has suggested there are many confounding variables involved in the observations that wine drinkers somehow do better than those drinking other forms of alcohol (Holohan, 2012). Therefore, it is really not plausible that the French or anyone else would live longer and have less cardiovascular disease due to drinking more than two glasses of wine per day.

The difference is more likely because the French, famous for their excellent cuisine (so they certainly do not sacrifice taste!), are eating fresh foods, produced on a more local level, using healthier methods. France, and many other nations in Europe, doesn't allow nearly as many chemicals in their foods as the U.S. either. They don't eat nearly as many foods that are processed, have preservatives or other bad things added to them. They buy their foods fresh from the market, pretty much every day. And, as part of the culture, they actually cook and prepare their food on a daily basis. What a concept! Not that eating leftovers from a healthy meal the night before is bad for you; it's more that processing foods to have extended shelf lives likely causes adverse health effects.

The French, and many other cultures, still have wonderful, enjoyable food. They haven't sacrificed any taste or enjoyment in their cuisine, nor have they as often abandoned their health in favor of a quick meal. It is understood that truly good food takes time: time to produce it, prepare it, and to enjoy it. Our culture wants something we can throw in the microwave or eat in the car; and it had better be attractive, large, and yummy! That isn't to say the European countries have "pure" food by any means. They do allow a multitude of organic and chemical additives in processed foods as well these days (read the "Report from the commission on dietary food additive intake in the European Union" online). It just seems they eat far less of those processed foods.

Suckers for advertising-

This is truly a corporate evil. In essence though, our society and culture are at fault. A business can't be blamed for trying to sell its product; that is to be expected. However, I have developed a deep mistrust for advertising, and I don't think I'm alone. I think many of us sit at home and watch a commercial on TV, thinking to ourselves, that the ad is probably all hype and there's probably a lot they aren't telling us. And yet, if we are in the store, and there are three choices for a given product, all other things seeming equal, we are probably going to choose the one we saw on TV.

This is an example of "name recognition", and it supports the fact that even bad press is good advertising. Familiarity is worth a lot to us psychologically, which probably explains why we will stay in a bad relationship or a job we hate for years, rather than change our circumstances. In addition, you may see something on the shelf at the store and decide you want it, but you may not even consciously remember seeing it on TV.

Of course, there are the conscious factors as well, like all the advertising claims of greatness. These are the more obvious methods of subterfuge and trickery. For sure, some advertising for products is honest and straightforward, like when they quote the actual statistics, or provide the Consumer Reports' standings. Some are major twists on the truth, and some are just based on ridiculous distractions. I mean, what does a half-naked woman have to do with the quality of a beer or performance of an automobile?

These same problems not only occur with our food, but with our non-food goods and products as well. This includes drugs being directly marketed to consumers. We have had drug marketing just to doctors for decades, with bad enough consequences. Physicians will often prescribe the newer, more expensive drug on the market, because the pharmaceutical rep showed up to offer samples and tell them how great it is. If one takes the time to make comparisons, the new drugs are rarely any better or safer than the older, generically available medications that have been used for many years and have better established safety records. Providing pharmaceutical samples is a particularly wicked form of advertising and marketing; it is common practice for the purveyors of illicit drugs on the street as well.

The new drugs are tried first because the doctor can provide free samples. Then, if it works, eventually the patient will have to pay for it. When someone nearly chokes to death on the $200-500 per month price tag, the doctor still suggests that it be used, because it has been shown to work for that individual. Ultimately, the patient may go ahead and pay for it, because they don't know there is an alternative. I often save people lots of money just by switching them from their fancy new expensive medications to generic alternatives. It's a greater pleasure to save them even more money by getting them off prescriptions completely, if possible, by using other methods that I'll discuss later on in this book.

Advertising to physicians comes in many forms: free pens, clipboards, office wall posters, calculators, or other little trinkets with the drug name snuck in on them. And, don't forget the fact that nearly half the weight of most mainstream medical journals is comprised of drug advertisements. I figure that if the drugs really worked well, they would sell themselves, like my practice does: by word of mouth. Unfortunately, doctors don't really talk to each other and, due to some personality quirks; a lot of us don't believe each other anyway.

I can tell other doctors that I've seen numerous people relieved of their migraines or high blood pressure, just by taking magnesium. But if they "haven't heard of that", then they think it isn't true. Well, I just told you dammit! So now *you have* "heard of it"! This problem goes back to the earlier discussion about what we consider to be the truth and, unfortunately, we are often more likely to believe what we saw on TV or in a journal advertisement, than what one of our intelligent and honest peers tells us. I suppose that this is the counterpoint to the "word of mouth" phenomenon.

I think physicians arrogantly assume that if something were truly important in their field, they would have heard about it. Well, how many of us even know the names of all our neighbors or what kind of cars they drive – and that's right next door! We can't expect to automatically become aware of everything that is important. The fact is that we are too darn busy to just "notice" things these days. Therefore, whoever spends the money to wave their product under our noses like a fishing lure, is going to get our business. If this weren't true, corporations wouldn't spend millions of dollars every year on advertising (the CEO's would just keep that extra cash for themselves of course).

Failure to control our system or legislate for human health-

Okay, so this is admittedly a political issue, but the problems with our health are not the result of just individual action. Broad solutions to our enormous problems are not going to come from just individual efforts. Politics and public policy are supposed to be tools for improving life for the masses. We need to see where our public policy is failing in order to try and fix it. We also need to get behind those policies that protect us and improve our health.

For a country founded by revolutionaries, we sure have become complacent now. For example, during the George W. Bush administration and since that time, we have let our government tap our phone calls, removed many worker safety regulations, and promoted more pollution of our air, water and food. These phenomena are due to the Patriot Act and some late-term deregulating pieces of legislation. We have become socially impotent as a people and have forgotten our roots. Ironically, we are a society founded by people who tried to escape from, and fought directly against, tyranny.

The tyranny isn't so obvious now, but the effects are still very negative. Our government allows manufacturers and energy producers to terribly pollute the air, spray liberal amounts of dangerous chemicals on our food supply, and stick unknown substances in our food, all in the search for more corporate dollars and at the expense of human health. The problems aren't coming directly from our government. Current legislation is just enabling wealthy corporations to poison us for a buck, while our elected officials line their pockets with sophisticated bribes and payoffs in the forms of "lobbying" and campaign contributions. The smart money buys politicians on *both* sides of the aisle.

Despite my complaining, I do realize that America has far better standards and practices than much of the world. At least our government doesn't allow melamine in baby formula (recall the rash of infant deaths in China in 2008 because of corporate attempts to save money and bulk-up the formula with that toxic substance?); but it does allow "corn syrup solids", emulsifiers, and preservatives. It is frightening to read the ingredients list on most infant formula; medications are even worse. We used to purchase for our toddlers these dissolving cough medicine strips made for kids. I eventually read the label and discovered that the main ingredient was *acetone*, which is what we use for nail polish remover! They were also full of artificial sweeteners and coloring agents. How in the hell does our FDA allow that sort of thing to be given to anyone, much less our small children?

In the processing of our wheat flour we allow chemicals such as bleaching agents, and dough conditioners like bromine, that are proven toxins. They aren't typically listed as ingredients on the bread labels because they weren't added during the making of the bread; thus, the current rules don't require that they be listed there. Unfortunately, the very people who profit from putting dangerous things into our food strongly influence food-labeling rules. That just seems inherently wrong to me.

Every year, we allow millions of tons of pesticides to be used in agricultural production in the U.S. Some of them remain in the food, but far more ends up in the ground water and elsewhere in the environment. We spew millions more tons of other toxins, like mercury, lead, hydrocarbons, and sulfuric acid, into the air from burning fossil fuels within our factories, power plants, and vehicles. This is all considered "acceptable", under our current poor standards, and we are not likely to change our energy sources, until we have earned possible penny from digging those toxic fuels out of the Earth. These practices are already damaging human health and are totally unsustainable.

Of course, it isn't "we", meaning you and I, who are directly profiting from this (well, maybe it is me a little, because of the Permanent Fund Dividend check we Alaskans receive from our oil money every year – oops!), but it is certainly all of us who are at risk of suffering due to the pollution. Our government did not ban thimerosal until several years after it's use was stopped in Europe. Though many countries in Europe have done so years ago, we still here have not banned PBDE's (the fire-retardant chemicals that replaced PCB's in the 70's, and which we now know to be just as bad) or fluoride water treatment (yes, fluoride is a definite toxin!). We keep using these things because of ignorance, advertising, and the fact that industries are making or saving money under current practices. Our government seems far more influenced by that than by the health concerns of its people.

And, there is no such thing as "clean coal"! That's like saying "clean dirt" or "clean oil". It's just not possible. The notion that something inherently filthy can be made clean is total nonsense. Most of the toxins may be captured on their way up the smokestacks, but they are later dumped into the environment elsewhere. These ideas are typical of the nonsense that industry sells us on an ongoing basis. "Biofuels" aren't clean either. Did you ever catch a whiff of the smoke as you've burned your cooking oil? There are obviously much cleaner power sources readily available, but the financial interests of the few in power, keep us from further exploring those options. The "Cap and Trade" bill presented during the Obama administration that would allow industry to pay fees for pollution rather than reduce emissions is, in my opinion, a blatant sale of human health in favor of industry profits.

Solar, wind, hydroelectric, geothermal, and other power sources are truly clean in a real sense. We just need "society" to demand them and steer policy in that direction. Our government could certainly throw more support that way by providing funding or incentives for companies to develop cleaner technologies. We could place higher and higher taxes on companies that produce greater amounts of environmental pollution. We could then put that money toward health care. I think that would be fair. It would be similar to the fines, which most Americans likely supported, that were placed on the tobacco industry.

Even in this day and age, we have poor standards for worker safety. In my practice, I often see men who work in mechanical or construction trades who now have toxicity-related conditions due to exposures in their work environments. It's suggested on the job that they wear protective gear, but it isn't always tightly enforced. The work areas do not have to be adequately ventilated or decontaminated, and some of the substances that they work with are plainly stated as extremely toxic to their health. Is there any one person out there who thinks that our health and safety on the job is not important? I'm sure nobody would ever say that out loud or even claim to believe that. But I suspect it saves companies a great deal of money to have lower safety standards. After all, it costs money to run an air filter, clean up chemicals, redirect or filter machine exhaust, and provide appropriate protective equipment.

We eventually banned advertising for cigarettes after it became abundantly clear that they were harmful, but we still allow their manufacture and sale. This doesn't make sense to me at all. If we know they are lethal, why allow them to be manufactured and sold for profit? We don't allow the production and sale of cocaine or methamphetamine, and yet, we prescribe related, similar substances to people for medical purposes. Doesn't that suggest that those drugs are safer than cigarettes overall? Why don't we make cigarettes only available with a doctor's prescription? (Because there is *no* beneficial indication for use) We even have a pill form of marijuana, and in a growing number of states people can legally use the natural form for medical purposes.

We tried banning alcohol in the past, but we all know how well that worked. There are places in Alaska where, on a local level, alcohol is banned and completely illegal today. These are called "dry" towns or villages. These extreme measures had to be implemented in those areas because of the sheer devastation caused by the use of alcohol in some remote areas of Alaska. This policy makes a huge positive societal difference in those areas, even though it is clearly an infringement on individual rights. So on a smaller scale, it seems to be common sense that the desire to support public safety can at times win out over both corporate profits and arguments for civil liberty.

Many would say that it would be an infringement on personal liberty to ban cigarettes and booze. Isn't it a similar infringement to set a legal drinking age, especially one that sets the limit at five years older than when a person can drive and three years beyond when people can vote or die for our country? Isn't it an infringement on my personal liberty to set speed limits, require that I wear a seat belt in my car or a helmet on my bike? And yet, our government will not put reasonable restrictions on food producers and manufacturers. I guess some personal liberties are more socially important than others, or perhaps it's "corporate liberties" that are more important.

Does it make sense to ban the use of marijuana, which causes far less illness than tobacco and far less dysfunction than alcohol, while having medicinal properties to boot? (No, I don't smoke pot myself, though it's rumored to be the major agricultural export of the Mat-Su Valley where I live) Cocaine is illegal now, but people forget it used to be an ingredient in a bottle of Coke™. Personally, I don't think they should be able to call it "Coca Cola Classic™" unless there's some cocaine in it.

Does anyone else think that these limitations can be somewhat arbitrary and more than a little bit stupid? I mean, don't we all have a dozen things in our house that we could kill ourselves with if we wanted to? You could stab yourself with that knife, so you should need a license to use it. You could get high from that glue, so you should be nineteen years old to purchase it. And you should maybe be arrested for a DUI after making a collage for your kid's elementary school class, or using too much hairspray for example.

Why don't we just allow people to grow their own tobacco or marijuana, brew their own beer, and produce their own meth in their kitchen if they want to? It could still be made illegal to sell it. After all, it's currently illegal to sell milk or meat people raise themselves, unless the government's approval process is followed. It could still be made illegal to drive under the influence of alcohol, glue, marijuana or hair spray. It seems that, without difficulty, the legal industries for tobacco and alcohol manage to buy some privilege with our government, while law enforcement gets a much larger budget to deal with illegal drug enforcement issues.

Granted, there is sarcasm and hyperbole in the preceding paragraphs, but I want to get people thinking again. Think about why we go along with certain ideas and complain about others. Think about what is really important for a change, and what we as individuals can do about it. We create a myriad of ridiculous rules in our society. Can't we start making some that really improve things?

Centralization over regionalization-

This is a concept that will be new to many readers but, hopefully, once I explain what I'm talking about, you will see that it is truly a problem in our society, and one that is fairly new to modern civilization.

What I mean by centralization is that a given product is made at a central location for a very large population area. An example of this might be having just one shoe factory, or one area of corn production for the whole country. These, admittedly, are not real examples because these things aren't truly just produced from one location. However, I think we can all see that, for many of our products, there tends to be a certain area that produces the vast majority of a given thing. For us, that area is increasingly more likely to be a different country altogether (e.g. China or India). With centralized production, we get a few big problems. There are issues surrounding production standards, product quality, transportation, storage, and the effects on local economies.

With centralization, goods must be transported much greater distances; this utilizes far more fossil fuels that cost money and pollute our environment. This is a waste of resources and contributes to the destruction of our planet and deterioration of human health. It must also be assured that the products will withstand the travel and have adequate shelf life (i.e. foods require preservatives). This means more chemical production and consumption, another far-reaching negative influence on our health. This doesn't just involve food either. Most of our furniture, textiles and other manufactured goods contain formaldehyde and other preservative chemicals to prevent mold infestation, breakdown or degradation.

To some extent, when food is shipped from far away, the freshness and nutrient content of foods are somewhat sacrificed. In part, this naturally begins to occur from the time produce is "off the vine". Large centralized operations also often sacrifice some product quality for mass production. In my opinion, a tomato just doesn't taste as good or offer as much nutritional benefit when it is grown under mass-produced circumstances with synthetic fertilizers and depleted soils.

In terms of production costs, local growers usually can't compete with large conglomerates, and most people seem willing to sacrifice some quality for lower costs and greater quantity. A local producer, who has ten acres of production and a smaller, less industrialized operation, will have to pay correspondingly more per pound to produce his crop. The large "agribusinesses", as they are called, can produce greater amounts for cheaper cost, even after paying for the additional transportation. This is how they have become such a large force and our government purportedly adds support by giving more money in subsidies to large corporate farming operations, while offering for less support to small regional farms or organic farmers (Riedl, 2002, and data from the US General Accounting Office 2001-6).

I'm not sure this has happened in many other countries. In most places, I believe food is still primarily produced on a local level. At a local market, 90% or more of the goods are probably grown within a fifty-mile radius. On many levels, this makes the whole community stronger and healthier. Imagine a population that produces everything it needs on a local level, where everyone can rely on each other and feels engaged in the community. Imagine having everything that is needed within walking distance, rather than having to drive ten miles to the nearest big-box store or shopping mall. That is the concept of regionalization.

It doesn't just apply to food either. A factory can make shoes in one's own state or city, rather than people buying ones made on the other side of the planet. Any area could have its own furniture company, automobile factory, clothing producer, or whatever else the community required. Practically everything you need can be made within one hundred miles, or at least within your own hemisphere of the planet. But we don't, and as a result, Wal-Mart™ is a world leader in the retail sale of goods.

I think there is a social factor to this, because we allow this sort of thing on a large scale. But it is clearly something that we can influence through individual consumer behavior. We can't really propose legislation that mandates that our area not import anything from more than whatever distance away. That would never fly. And granted, I live in a place where strict regionalism would severely limit my diet. There would not be much selection for most of the year if I were to only eat things produced within Alaska. (But perhaps this means nobody should live here? Sometimes, usually in January and February, I really think that's the case. Though, one has to acknowledge how the Alaskan Natives did it in the past.)

I encourage everyone, at least those who are interested in this concept, to read Barbara Kingsolver's book, *Animal, Vegetable, Miracle*. The challenge is to try and eat only things produced on a local level, with few exceptions. The more of us who attempt this, the lower our global pollution will be; the cheaper and healthier local produce will become.

CHAPTER 6 – PROBLEMS ON AN INDIVIDUAL LEVEL

Ultimately, the responsibility for our own health and for our children's health falls upon us. It is to some extent a result of individual choices and behaviors. I will describe some of the uncontrollable factors later when we talk about the concepts of genetics and "epigenetics" but, for now, let's take a hard look at what our personal role is in our own health.

Factors working against us on an individual level-

Following social norms
Previously, I discussed our frequent error of considering common conditions to be the "normal" state of things. I mentioned thisusing examples including the attitude that being overweight is now somewhat normal because the majority of our population is overweight or obese. I also mentioned the dangerous assumptions frequently made in laboratory data interpretation based on what values are *common* in the population rather than what would be *optimal*. This problem is even more pervasive within our society on an individual level.

I can't begin to count how many times patients have told me that they figured their complaints were just "normal" because of their age. "I'm just getting older" is not a valid excuse for a fifty year-old person who has obesity, hypertension, high cholesterol, and debilitating back pain or knee arthritis. For starters, fifty is not "old" in human terms. Secondly, it is not "normal" to develop obesity, high blood pressure, or crippling arthritis as a person ages. Today, it may be common to see these things with increasing prevalence as we grow older, but that does not make it "normal". No matter many times I've had this conversation it only seems to make sense to patients about half the time, presumably because my view conflicts with our social beliefs.

I believe this is largely an issue of personal standards, and how we judge ourselves based on what we see in others around us. Gulliver was a giant compared to the Lilliputians, but he may have been just average size in his own society. In terms of health and fitness, what the general public is lacking is a real understanding of what normal/optimal really means and, unfortunately, it cannot be found by looking around at our peers these days.

Behavioral expectations represent another way social norms work against us. If we don't wear the same clothes, talk the same way, listen to the same music, watch the same TV shows, go to the same church, or eat the same way as those around us, then we may be made to feel out of place in some way. Sometimes this is due to direct feedback from others, but more often, it's just a subconscious feeling that we must be doing something wrong if we are doing things differently from others around us. This is a more passive side of the mob mentality concept.

The psychological root of this problem is the natural assumption that what everyone else is doing must be okay. Eating fast food, proudly wearing new brand name clothing, driving SUV's, talking on your cell phone while driving, smoking in public, or pissing on the sidewalk are all much more acceptable when others are doing it. If you have had teenagers at home, you have probably heard these arguments – "But Dad, everyone else is doing it!" "But Mom, Ashley's mother lets her go out until after midnight on weekends!" But you know better than your son's teenage buddies and Ashley's mother, don't you? In reality, you may just have different values, and that's what it all comes down to.

In regard to health, this whole concept relies on the assumption that there is some true ideal out there, some true normal or optimal way to live and exist. There are many different ways to go about things that can provide a good result because, of course, we are not all physiologically the same. Some of us can eat junk food on a daily basis and not seem to gain weight or suffer in any way (don't you just hate people like that?). Others seem to gain a full pound just from licking the beaters after making cookies!

So, it seems to be much easier to agree on ideal or optimal *goals*, rather than on habits. The means and paths will be different for different individuals but, in my opinion, we should all be focusing on similar goals. For starters, as I alluded to above, I think we should all be comparing our own health to some type of optimal health, not some perceived normal based on those around us. I prefer to use the words ideal or optimal rather than normal because I think that is what people actually mean when they say "normal".

This isn't a simple matter since there are surprising variations of individual opinion on what defines good health. My idea of good, or optimal, health is one where the individual has easy fertility (which includes a strong sex drive); is free of degenerative conditions or chronic complaints; does not get recurring illnesses; has all the energy, strength, and stamina an individual their age should have; sleeps well; and has a happy, positive mental attitude and outlook on life.

That may sound like a tall order. I admit that I don't fit it myself because I have a few annoying food allergies, am sensitive to many chemicals, have some sort of arthritis in my left knee, catch colds from one of my kids or patients at least four times per year and, since 2008, I require testosterone replacement because of early gonadal failure. I have also developed alopecia areata in my beard area and have a positive GAD-65 antibody on blood tests; these are both autoimmune disease issues. Well, nobody ever suggested that achieving "ideal" or "optimal" results would be easy. But in my mind, we should all hold these goals as our standard or else we're never going to get anywhere. After all, it's okay to fail if you're really trying.

Contrary to American policy, I don't believe repeated failure should lead to the decline of our goals and standards—we should not lower our standards just because most people don't meet them; that is why so many other countries have pulled ahead of us in education and innovation. In general, a willingness to accept suboptimal things and situations is a big cause of these problems in our culture and in human nature.

To contrast my concept of ideal, I have had many patients tell me they think they are in good health when, in truth, they have a huge burden of medical pathology. Take the following example:

"Doc, I think I'm pretty healthy in general."

"Really sir? You realize that you just had a heart attack, you are 80 lbs overweight, and you have high cholesterol, high blood pressure, chronic headaches, back pain, gout, type 2 diabetes, fatty liver, emphysema, arthritis, and irritable bowel syndrome."

"Well yeah, but I'm hardly ever sick."

This example is admittedly a little exaggerated, but it's not far off from a number of actual patients I've met, usually men. So, for some people, they consider themselves to be "healthy" with a dozen chronic illnesses but are suddenly "unhealthy" when they catch a cold. I guess that's one way to look at it. As long as they aren't in the hospital, can still work the remote control and get to the bathroom on their own, they feel pretty "healthy".

Let me offer a different view: If a young woman can't seem to get pregnant even though she has all her organs and her fallopian tubes are open, then perhaps she is not truly *healthy*. For some reason, her physiology is disturbed to the point that her body will not permit reproduction. The same is true for a man with a low sperm count or who cannot achieve and maintain an erection. If a man is twenty-five pounds overweight, then his life expectancy is going to be shortened even if he "hardly ever gets sick". If you have arthritis in your knees so badly that by age sixty you can't climb stairs, then that is not normal! If you feel tired and unmotivated most of the time, then something is wrong with you!

We have to stop accepting all of our common complaints and maladies as being some form of normal! We have to get our priorities straight again and aim higher, if we are going to start making progress instead of continuing our current downward spiral into potential extinction as a species as well as drastic ongoing decline in individual health. We have to dispense with many of our current social norms and start to think for ourselves again.

Advertising propaganda

To some extent, I have already discussed our social failing of allowing corporate advertising to influence us. Here, I will just point out that it *really works*. If it didn't work so well, they wouldn't spend so much money on blasting our senses with advertisements, product placements and corporate sponsorships everywhere we turn.

On an individual level, this is definitely a force working against our health. We see commercials for fast food, sugar-filled breakfast cereal, soda pop and beer on TV all day. These make us hungry and thirsty for the things we've seen, perhaps through mechanisms that naturally exist in our brains to help us seek out and identify food in our environment.

It is natural for us to be attracted to certain food colors, smells, shapes, and appearances. It is natural for us to be excited by certain proportions of the human form. It is natural for us to want to eat more when we smell or taste something we find delicious. And we now know that just seeing images of something with a known taste or smell will trigger those desires as well.

In addition, clever advertising agents have learned to use the power of humor in selling products to us. We have certain, reinforcing chemicals surge through our brains when we experience pleasure and humor is a true pleasure. We will remember those commercials that made us laugh even though the content may have nothing at all to do with the product being showcased. Nonetheless, we will associate that product with a good feeling.

Advertising companies know all of this and use it to their advantage. If you don't think it works, look around your own house and see how much no-name stuff you have. I'm sure you'll find some, and you've probably used many of them as well, but they will probably represent the minority of products in your home. Next time you are at the store and you're deciding between two brands that appear equivalent, pay attention to how you internally feel about the one with a familiar name and logo versus the one you haven't seen in advertisements. Real, powerful psychology is at play here.

This also works against all of our health because doctors themselves succumb to this psychology, and in a big way. Over and over again, drugs are chosen just because the name is out there and the pharmaceutical reps have been pounding the pavement telling doctors how great their meds are, handing out pens and other trinkets with the new drug name on them. It works so well that, even in recent years, many drugs have still been prescribed at high levels despite being found to be poorly effective or downright dangerous. A good example at the time of this writing is the diabetes drug, Avandia™

This has become such a problem that a growing number of physician residency programs and medical student groups across the country have now forbidden pharmaceutical reps from visiting or sponsoring any lectures. I don't let them in my office either, nor do I accept any drug samples. I suggest you ask your medical providers to do the same. This would be a step in the right direction. Now we just need to get their ads off the TV and out of magazines and journals. Only the U.S. and New Zealand currently allow television advertising of pharmaceuticals; every other country has apparently realized that is a terrible idea.

What the advertisers are counting on is that we won't effectively use those big frontal lobes we have in our cranium. We, more than the lower animals, have the ability to make decisions based on more than our senses and our programmed responses. We can actually think! We can de-program ourselves if we put our mind to it and program in a healthy skepticism and mistrust of anything we see in any advertisement; just like we already disbelieve most used car salesmen and pretty much anything someone from the opposing political party is saying without even really listening to them.

Information overload

The advertising problem is compounded by the sheer tonnage of stuff that is thrown at us. We get propaganda and advertisements on the radio, television, signs, billboards, in print, and electronically. We can't even check our e-mail without seeing half a dozen ads along the way. They are even starting to send out mass advertising text messages to people's cell phones. All of these advertising people know that the name we hear the most often is probably the one we will choose when the time comes. So they flutter at us like a hover of hummingbirds with little banners trying to gain our attention. How are we supposed to get away from it all?

Another problem with medical information overload comes when we legitimately try to research something on our own. This is a big problem for are a layperson as well as for a medical professional. I hear people complain all the time that they've tried to research their symptoms or diagnosis on the internet and found conflicting information from many different sources. Frustrated and discouraged, at times, they can develop a sense of helplessness and despair. Unfortunately this isn't really an avoidable problem because there will always be gaps in knowledge and diversity in theories. Because of this, I don't think a computer will ever replace a good medical practitioner. There are just too many variables and individual factors to consider when making medical decisions. When patients come in and tell me how they went through this frustration, I simply say, "welcome to medicine".

The fact is that medicine is not an exact science. In truth, much of it today is not science at all. The most important information for me to acquire is that which I can get directly from the patient. But many don't know what information is important. When researching their issues, many people will pick one symptom perhaps, and find that way too many possibilities show up. They may accept a diagnosis that they were given by a provider, or one that they think is appropriate from their own study, and research that only to discover that they don't meet all, or even most, of the criteria. It's very frustrating.

What do we do when there is too much information out there and the stuff we do find doesn't seem to give us the answers? Eventually, we go to a doctor. Too often, unfortunately, doctors have the same sorts of problems. Even more unfortunate is the tendency of physicians and other medical providers to believe what they *think*, rather than admit they don't really *know* at all. What you really need is someone who has a systematic way of sorting through the information and possibilities in a safe and efficient manner. Certainly, the general public is not typically equipped to do this and, unfortunately, many of our medical providers are not either.

Medical dogma in society

Although this was mentioned previously in the failings of medical attitudes discussion, I just want to emphasize how this is another barrier to individual success and health. Adherence to the prevailing dogma certainly slows medical progress and knowledge overall, but it can be used inadvertently as a direct assault on the individual as well. I have had many patients tell me they left their other provider because "they just wouldn't listen to me." This often means that the provider would not listen to what the patient was saying because those ideas conflicted with the practitioner's own medical beliefs based on the dogma of our current system.

One example of this may include a patient who is sure that their beta blocker (a blood pressure drug that typically slows the heart and decreases the workload of the heart muscle) makes their heart race and skip around. Many doctors would likely not believe or have trouble believing this because the drug usually works in the opposite way and is even used to treat the symptoms of palpitations. They are likely to suggest that the patient has had too much caffeine intake or was just imagining it. In reality, a person can experience this as an allergic reaction to a drug (even one which is supposed to slow the heart) or it can be a reflexive response to overly decreased blood pressure, or perhaps it is due to the way in which a new drug influences an entirely different drug the patient was already taking. The way to figure things out is to first *believe what the patient is saying* (what a concept) and then try to make sense of it in some way. Why would the patient lie about something like this, anyway?

A common issue I've come across is a patient who seems to gain weight even though they are restricting their diet to only a thousand calories or less per day. Typically, their provider doesn't believe them because of our generally accepted ideas about calorie usage based on body weight. The doctor just may not believe the patient is telling the truth about their calorie intake, so he/she doesn't bother to look for a metabolic explanation. Well, I can assure you that a person with inadequate thyroid metabolism can certainly gain weight even with this low level of food intake. I've proven this phenomenon repeatedly in practice. What makes this common scenario even more of a problem is the fact that many providers are taught to believe a laboratory test over their clinical impression of thyroid adequacy.

Hypothyroidism is one of the most common maladies afflicting our culture these days, and the majority of cases go undiagnosed because of our narrow-minded modern medical dogma.   In a later section on hormones I will further discuss this topic along with the dogmatic issues surrounding proper vitamin D dosing (because it's actually a hormone too, not a "vitamin" – that's just ignorant dogma too), as examples of medical dogma leaving many people without what they really need.

To further complicate the calorie-intake issue, there are a number of other factors that influence metabolism as well. The individual may have issues with other hormones like cortisol, estrogen or testosterone, toxicity issues, yeast overgrowth, food allergies, or some other source of chronic inflammation that affects metabolic and weight-regulating processes. I usually have to sort them all out and address each possibility before the individual will begin to successfully lose weight.

There are many other dogmatic beliefs in health and medicine that our culture falsely holds true. I am constantly confronted with errant cultural mythology regarding ideas on cholesterol, antibiotic prescribing, calcium intake, food and dietary issues, salt, and other issues. I will elaborate on each of these topics in the following sections. Many patients embrace my more scientific and logical viewpoints on these subjects while others simply look at me with open skepticism.

Access to care and services

Again, this is not a new discussion in this book. I mentioned earlier how access to health care and services is a huge failing of our health care system, but it is truly a problem on an individual basis only. I have many patients who have two insurance policies that may completely cover all of their care. I see a similar number of people who end up having to pay out-of-pocket for most or all of my medical care because they either have no medical insurance or they just have "catastrophic" coverage with a high deductible. Whenever possible, most of these individuals without insurance just go without medical care. They may go to the emergency room, but only if they are squirting blood, having crushing chest pains, or have something else they deem serious.

Most of our senior citizens have insurance through Medicare but can't get in to see a doctor because none of their area doctors will accept that program. Some of these patients even have secondary insurance coverage or have lots of money and are willing to pay cash. They often still cannot get care because of the problems providers have with Medicare. The secondary insurance usually refuses to pay or cover much, if anything at all; and yet they charge the same high premiums.

As a result, many Medicare patients frequently end up in hospital emergency rooms or urgent care centers. They don't just show up for real emergencies either. They show up at the ER to get their daily medications refilled, get a flu shot, a obtain a referral to an orthopedist for their arthritis or some other need which should have been fulfilled by a primary care physician. The problem is that they can't get a primary care provider to see them, and the ER can't legally turn them away. Both patient and provider are caught in this quagmire because it is illegal for a participating doctor to accept cash payment from a Medicare patient. In addition, doctors cannot bill "around" Medicare to a person's secondary insurer.

However, there is a way around the Medicare problem. If a provider "opts out" of the Medicare system by signing a contract with Medicare which states that they are not participating providers and will not bill Medicare for medical services (we can do this, but most doctors don't know about it), they may then treat Medicare patients and accept cash payment from them. The patient cannot get any reimbursement from Medicare either, but they can try to bill their secondary insurer if they have one. I can tell you that the odds of that secondary insurance kicking anything in are still quite poor. They tend to just blame the patient for not choosing a Medicare provider, and they refuse to pay anything. I'm not sure why that's legal, but it is the way this typically goes.

It is also possible for a person to decline Medicare coverage on an individual level. People will be automatically be enrolled at age sixty-five, unless Medicare is contacted and the individual files to opt out of coverage. For many, it seems ridiculous to turn down free insurance, especially when taxes are paid to fund the program one's entire working life (meaning it isn't "free" at all). The system is such a mess right now, however, many people may want to decline coverage, especially if they have continuing private insurance from an ongoing job or retirement package. Those who can afford to pay for their care out of pocket may choose to see practitioners on a cash basis as well.

For most people, the biggest barrier to accessing good health care is financial. The very cost of our modern health care services is often out of reach. Often, the insurance policies are unaffordable and many families do not have the out-of-pocket money to get care when they need it. As I mentioned earlier, it doesn't matter how great our medicine is if people can't afford it and don't get to utilize it.

Individual responsibility still comes into play here. People can prioritize their finances in favor of their health a bit better if they wish. I've seen plenty of patients on Medicaid say they can't afford the three-dollar co-pay for their visit, while holding a latte in their hand that cost them more than that, and they often smoke cigarettes as well (an expensive habit indeed!). There have been many of families who have had to make huge financial sacrifices to cover catastrophic medical care and still managed to get by. Most people could afford to spend a bit more on their health if they cut back spending on the things that harm them or things that really aren't necessary. Most of us just don't think that way it seems.

Food availability

I will discuss the issues of food quality and safety repeatedly throughout this book because the availability of truly safe and nourishing food is certainly a barrier to individual health in the United States. It isn't that we don't have enough food for everyone here, because we are clearly getting more than enough. A national news report in June 2012 stated that Americans in total comprise one third of the total human body mass on the planet, even though we only account for five percent of the total world population!

A big part of the problem lies in our processed food because it sucks in terms of nutrition, and it's dangerous! Most of the food consumed in this country is now processed in some way, even if that just means having products with bleached, white flour instead of whole grains. Our "manufactured" food is also laden with dangerous chemicals, especially if it is not organic.

I'll get more into the dangerous aspects of our food again later. Here I want to discuss the scarcity of truly *good* food. Its lack of availability is a factor working against individual health in America. We certainly don't lack in available calories, but we may in fact lack in terms of safe healthy food. Some of the more common complaints I hear involve people not knowing what to eat, where to shop, or how to prepare healthy food. They also complain about the apparent cost of healthy food, which once again is a potential barrier for some individuals or families.

Our food supply has been depleted of nutrients over the generations by repeatedly growing the same few crops on the same large areas of land and by using synthetic fertilizers rather than biological material. Our food animals have become more ill and toxic through inadequate nutrition, polluted inorganic feed, administration of drugs and hormones, crowded living conditions, and inadequate exercise. The hormone-supplementing practices in American meat production led to a ban on the importation of American beef by the European union in 1989 that was later supported by the World Trade Organization because of the concerns regarding increasing human cancers.

These animals are not fit for human consumption, regardless of how their meat is processed and prepared. At best, they are suboptimal nutritionally and, at worst, they are directly toxic to us if we eat them. This is the main reason, in my opinion, that vegetarian diets seem to offer better health benefits than the standard American diet.

Our processed and manufactured foods (I still don't understand why we need to "manufacture" food) offer very little nutritionally and contain numerous harmful chemicals. However, somehow, they are often cheaper than fresh foods. It costs more money to transport fresh, vital foods in a manner that is quick enough and under the right conditions (i.e. refrigerated or frozen) to maintain quality. I guess that if we turn our foodstuffs into things that don't rot, we can store them longer and ship them slower.

It seems paradoxical that fruits and vegetables cost less when they have chemicals sprayed on them. Don't those chemicals cost money? The cost difference is in the possible crop yield and the extra production when those chemicals are used. In terms of cost, nonorganic produce is less expensive at the store, but we will certainly "pay" for it in other ways.

For sure, the availability of healthy foods also varies by region. If you live near a Whole Foods©, Trader Joe's©, or some other organic marketplace, you may find healthy forms of everything you need. In my opinion, if you have your own farm and raise your own animals for meat, milk, butter, and eggs, then you have an ideal situation. If, however, you live in rural Alaska, where there is only one small store that tends to only supply things in cans, bags, and boxes, then you may have a major problem finding many healthy foods to choose from.

Of course, those people could do what people in those regions did for millennia and hunt or gather everything they eat. In truth, that would be their ideal diet but most cannot conceive of doing that these days. The processed foods are so much easier to obtain and consume. Many in rural communities all over the country still hunt and fish for part of their diet. Unfortunately, they still eat a lot of the bad processed foods, often because they don't know they are bad.

Today, I believe the average American lives close enough to a grocery store with an organic produce section and a "natural foods" section (doesn't that imply that the stuff in the rest of the store is "*unnatural* food"?) that they have most of the necessary food items available in a relatively edible form. The bigger problem for most people is that at many stores and restaurants, the overwhelming majority of foods to choose from are not healthy at all. If you were to run blindfolded through a store and randomly acquire food items, you would probably get healthy food less than 10% of the time, and get poisoned in some manner the rest of the time.

Busy lifestyles

A busy lifestyle is somewhat of a cultural expectation for us, but it can manifest problems on an individual level. For too many of us, the American way of life has evolved into some sort of constantly stressful experience and riddled with long periods of physical inactivity. We have jobs that may take up more than half the day, commutes that may take over an hour each way, kids' activities which may require driving to multiple places in the same evening or weekend, and sometimes obligations to clubs or organizations outside of these things. Much of this is unnecessarily self-imposed.

Some of us work, go to school, and raise children all at the same time, while we are young adults and trying to get ahead in life. Too many of us keep working hard well into our senior years as well. When do we have time for ourselves? When do we have time to relax? When do we have time to prepare a healthy meal and actually sit down with our family to enjoy it? When do we have time to exercise? When did we let this happen?

Our energy has become more and more directed away from things that really matter and that promote good health. It is too often directed toward things that are more self-destructive. It doesn't have to be that way, but our culture has come to expect it. We stress ourselves to the max to get the things that we think are important, but we leave little time to enjoy them or notice the world around us.

Individual failures or self-destruction-

Ignorance

Now, I don't see ignorance as a character flaw or an insult to anyone's intelligence. Being intelligent means you can understand something when it is presented to you, solve problems, and make sense of information. Ignorance just means you don't have the necessary information; we are all ignorant of more than we truly know. However, that doesn't mean that we have no responsibility for our ignorance. In this modern information age there is incredible access to information; the problem is sifting through the garbage that's out there passing for "knowledge".

Intelligence is thought to be somewhat fixed, as determined by our genetics and what occurred in the womb or at birth. To some degree, intelligence is also influenced by other factors such as our environment, food and drug habits through our lives, head injuries, education, and intellectual stimulation, and maybe by how much reality TV we watch or how much time we waste on social networking sites when we could be having *real* human interaction.

As I mentioned before, we are so inundated with false information and advertising, that we don't feel we have the time or ability to sort through all the nonsense and try to find the truth about anything. Therefore, we are at the mercy of the producers and purveyors of the nonsense to tell us what they want us to know.

I, for one, don't have a clue about how to fix my car if anything even a little bit complex seems wrong with it. Therefore, I am at the mercy of the mechanic when I take it in. If it is going to cost less than a hundred dollars, I usually don't ask too many questions. But the more expensive the repair, the more I start to ask about what's involved, and I try to investigate the validity of what the mechanic is telling me.

Most people don't take the time to look up their medical problems or symptoms to try and figure out what's wrong on their own. Therefore, these people have to rely on the keepers of medical "knowledge" to tell them what to do. Some patients do come in with a pile of research from the Internet, or they are maybe armed with what their wife's sister's uncle told them because they are a nurse or doctor or maybe even a veterinarian.

That's cool too, because it shows that the patient is trying to take an interest and some control in his or her health care. Eventually, many "researcher" types end up in *my* office because they eventually know more about their problem than their previous doctor. And, usually in part because their last doctor didn't want to listen to them.

I'm not suggesting that everyone should go buy a bunch of medical textbooks, head off for nursing or medical school, or even watch all the past episodes of "E.R." again on DVD. I'm just suggesting that one's health is extremely important, or at least it should be, and if we want to stay healthy, there is a lot to learn about our daily habits and our environment these days.

There is also a lot to learn about medicine in these times and it is best to not always take a doctor's advice at face value. I have had patients figure out, on their own, that there was a potential interaction between something new I prescribed and some other drug that they were already taking or had been prescribed. I have learned tons about natural methods of health and healing from patients, and often the first place I hear about a new drug or treatment is from a patient (since I don't let drug reps in my office).

My own ignorance never ceases to impress me, but I am always looking to make it a little smaller in scope. We can never know *everything,* but I suggest we all try to learn as much as we can about what is important. Reading this book is hopefully a step in the right direction for many of you; and I also hope many readers already know much of what I have to say.

Acceptance of the status quo and observed "normal" state

Previously I mentioned that, as a failing of society, our tendency is to *accept* what we commonly see in our population as being normal. I think the real problem is that we then begin to equate that "normal" to something that is OK for us too. "Society" is really us. It's made of individuals and social attitudes are the product of individual attitudes. Social norms will not change until we, as individuals, change our perspectives.

We need to stop justifying your own behaviors or complaints based on their commonality in those around us. Just because there are six other cars in that drive-thru, it doesn't mean the food sold in that fast food restaurant is good for you. Just because the guy in front of you in the checkout line has a case of soda and five TV dinners in his cart, doesn't mean that stuff is safe for us to consume. Just because some of our friends smoke, drink lots of alcohol, snort cocaine, or huff glue, it doesn't mean it's a good idea. Just because you know seven people who are on antidepressants, it doesn't mean you need one too. Most people drink coffee, but that doesn't make it good for us.

Many cities have fluoridated water, but fluoride is a known poison (it says so right on your tube of toothpaste). We may see hundreds of SUV's on the road with just one person inside, but it doesn't make that behavior socially responsible. Just because everyone around you is overweight and tired all the time, it doesn't mean that is a normal state in which to live. Gaining weight, developing high blood pressure and cholesterol, and having fatigue and back pain are not consequences of normal aging no matter how common those maladies are in people by age fifty. And, an average life expectancy of seventy-five years is actually a failing grade upon realizing the potential human life span exceeds 120 years.

It's time to stop following the herd and pay attention to what is good for us as individuals. We shouldn't need "plus sizes" or a "chair and a half." (You didn't think that was meant for two people did you?) Twenty-five per cent of adults shouldn't have fatty livers, and half our teenagers shouldn't be overweight or obese. There should be no market for cholesterol drugs, asthma inhalers, or antidepressants. We should not need doctors who specialize in fertility treatment. We shouldn't still need to burn fossil fuels for energy, and we shouldn't have to be afraid of our food. The first step toward progress is a rejection of the status quo.

The way I see it is that the psychological problem perpetuating this is acceptance or tolerance of adverse conditions. We readily adapt to our circumstances, whether they be good or bad. Those with millions of dollars often seem to still want more, and those living in squalor can still seem content in their day-to-day lives. In psychology, there is an adaptive response to stress called "learned helplessness" which some of us resort to when in an unhappy relationship or working at a job we hate. I think many people exist in that state of acceptance and helplessness in our society, and it's not benefiting us.

We must wake up from the trance and realize we can achieve much more. It requires a fresh perspective and higher goals. The mindless droning existence that many in our culture have resorted to is holding the whole group back. If enough of us start pushing the masses toward healthy lifestyles, we may begin to make more progress. It seems to me, we are nearing a tipping point in our modern history. We just need a few more people to jump to the other side of the teeter-totter.

Complacency

This is admittedly a continuation of the preceding rant. Our cultural acceptance of the way things are is the definition of complacency. Allowing social norms to continually slide downward is, to some extent, all of our faults. It is a crime of negligence to sit idly by and watch the health of our children, population, planet, and our own selves deteriorate.

Complacency is the easy, default pattern of behavior. It's sitting and watching rather than doing and participating. It's accepting and observing rather than guiding or changing. Of course, it isn't really helpful to just sit and complain about the way things are without offering up any solutions or taking action to help fix them either. Granted, there are plenty of things about the world that we truly cannot change, and those are the proper objects of acceptance.

It seems that complacency is the most common way to be in human society because there are usually only a few leaders while there are lots of followers. There needs to be more leaders out there among us for whom this complacency is no longer acceptable. Those who have strong feelings should voice them and those with strong voices need to make sure the right people hear them. How many people do you know who casually talk about all the problems with the government or society, as if they have all the answers, but do nothing to try and change things? Well, that's not really very helpful.

Social change begins with *individual* change. Environmental responsibility is the compilation of individual responsibilities. Government, in a democratic society, is supposed to represent the will of the people. So it's time for more of us to make those changes, speak our minds, take responsibility, and force change in the right direction, if we are to have a future. Also, it takes informed, knowledgeable people in order to force this change and ensure it is in a better direction. True progress also requires the realization that you may have to change course frequently, based on the assimilation of new information.

If that sounds extreme, that's part of the problem. We have a tendency to sit and watch things gradually deteriorate past the point of no return, and then act surprised when there's nothing we can do to get ourselves out of the situation. How many people knew, even openly predicted, the stock market was going to collapse years before it did? How many people got slowly deeper and deeper into debt and then were shocked when they had to file bankruptcy?

How many of us watch too much TV and eat too much fast food, then wake up one morning surprised to find we don't fit into our pants? How many people smoke for forty years and then act like it's somehow unfair when they have a heart attach or develop lung cancer? How many people only find religion when they are on death row or have a terminal illness?

Perhaps this complacency problem is an unavoidable aspect of human nature, and it is going to gradually flush us all down the toilet, with surprised expressions on our faces as we get sucked into the drain. We all have an opportunity to prove that wrong. We can go forth and cause some trouble – in a positive way. Remember, nobody ever made history by behaving themselves and following the rules all the time. We make the rules after all.

Self doubt

This is possibly a major underlying cause of the complacency problem. Most of us don't see ourselves as capable of creating much change on an individual level, much less a local or global level in society. Well, why the hell not?

Have you ever heard of Ghandi? How about Martin Luther King Jr.? Mother Theresa? Adolf Hitler? Okay, so we don't want to be equated with Hitler, but you have to admit he caused a great deal of social change and awareness around the world, didn't he? Hitler wasn't hampered by thoughts of inadequacy or a feeling that he was just one person and couldn't really change anything. And he *was* just one person, like you, like me.

All of these people, and every president we've ever had, started out as little helpless babies in their parents' arms. Actually, we all start out thinking that we are the center of the universe and then we gradually lose that sense (well, most of us do). We tend to go the other direction, and, at some point, decide we are totally insignificant. It is called "maturity" when we start to realize more and more that the world doesn't revolve around us. Unfortunately, we all know people who clearly haven't gotten there yet; but many of us have also taken it too far and made ourselves too unimportant.

Sometimes it's those egocentric and narcissistic people who get themselves into positions of power because of that very lack of maturity. They don't limit themselves by thinking they can't make something happen. They don't put their ideas or desires beneath everyone else's. The fact is, in general, we all have the same makeup and essence. So, why should anyone else's voice be heard above our own? Why shouldn't our opinions mean as much as others?

I forget who first said, "some are born to greatness, others have it forced upon them;" but that's not the whole story. Perhaps we are all born to greatness, and it's just that most of us never allow ourselves to believe this or see ourselves in that light. Some people succeed because they just can't help themselves, or they don't have those same mental shackles. Others are just such obvious leaders that they are followed, by more and more people, until they find themselves in a position of responsibility by default. Then there are those who feel self-righteous in taking power and control by force or by immoral action. If you don't want to be a leader yourself, make sure you support the right people.

Well, it's time to stop doubting ourselves. Time to stop thinking we can't change our personal habits. Stop thinking you have to stay in our current job or career even though you hate it. It's time to stop thinking you have to stay in an abusive relationship because you can't make it on your own; to stop thinking your opinion isn't important enough to be heard. If you start looking around, you'll find the rut you're in is not deep enough to keep you stuck, and your feet aren't nailed down. Perhaps you just never really looked around before.

Misplaced trust

The above-mentioned self-doubt and resulting inaction, creates a reliance on *others* to provide what we need in life. Most of us don't produce our own goods or food. But if we did, I imagine we would try to make sure it was safe. You would never willingly put something toxic into the food you give your children. We would not knowingly expose ourselves to harmful substances at home or work, which may damage our system and shorten our life span (well, most of us wouldn't anyway). We need to realize that we shouldn't accept these things from outside sources either.

In today's modern world, we don't have direct control over our food or over the safety of all the things in our environment. We have to get those things from other places. We all like to feel that our society, government, "fellow man", or whatever, would not offer or sell us things that are harmful. We put our trust in employers, producers, manufacturers, and regulatory governmental bodies. Well, we have to stop doing this.

The food being produced and manufactured is too often toxic, and of poor quality. Commonly, the goods being sold to us have toxic metals and chemicals in them. The air that we are breathing right now probably contains numerous harmful chemicals, metals, and particulates from the effects of industry.

We cannot trust that everyone producing the things we need and use has our best interests or our health in mind. We need to start reading labels and questioning what those chemicals are and what they might do in our body. We need to know about the effects of plastic chemicals on our hormones, of microwaves destroying the nutrients in our food, and of cell phone radiation penetrating into our children's brains, as well as other modern daily exposures.

The fact is, we just can't trust them, whoever "them" is. We have to wake up and smell the sewage that we are all living in now. We have to stop trusting that we can go to the store and safely consume or use whatever we find there. We have to stop trusting that our neighbors, or our government, are going to ensure there is a world here for our grandchildren to enjoy. If we've lived in a nice neighborhood, where everyone was required to have a lawn, neighbors may have been spraying weed killer and fertilizers on their grass that may easily get into our drinking water. They don't know any better, and there is no clear warning about such practice.

Don't take it personally; it's just business. The people who make money from chemical production will deny that their products are causing problems with human health, or at the very least, they'll say it's up to the consumer to use them safely. The fact is we, and our planet, could do fine or even better without these chemicals. We don't need corn syrup in our foods. We don't need pesticides and herbicides in agriculture. We certainly don't need lead or cadmium in the paint on our babies' toys, as well as so many other toxins placed knowingly in our purchased goods every day.

Skewed priorities

In modern times, many people have lost sight of what is truly important and this distraction is a major barrier to good individual health. I know that, to some extent, what seems important is a personal choice and a matter of opinion. However, I believe that in terms of individual and family health, some things are undeniably more important than others. Whereas many of the things we put ahead of health are obvious luxuries others are only to maintain the current state of our lives and, in my opinion, are not truly that important. But, of course, this is for each person to decide.

The primary goal of every organism, as driven by its DNA, is to reproduce and make sure that its genes go on into the next generation. People may not know this consciously, but this is why adolescents and young adults tend to have strong sex drives and a certain difficulty in thinking straight at times when around an attractive, potential mate. It is also, therefore, why Viagra can sell just fine for $20 per pill.

After having children, there should be a strong, innate desire to keep those offspring safe and give them what they need. This is another important part of successfully forwarding our DNA, seemingly more prominent in women than men. Priorities clearly change at times, but maintaining individual health is paramount in any other endeavor, really. The common saying, "well, at least you've still got your health" seems to suggest that health is a very important thing. This is certainly true because we require a certain level of health in order to reproduce, earn a living, and care for our children.

When did we lose sight of this? Is it when we started having distinctly meaningless jobs? Is it when we created beer and football? Is it when the DVD came out, or maybe the television? It's possibly around the time that we became "civilized", which in real terms means when we stopped looking out just for ourselves, and our families, and became part of a larger community with new perceived responsibilities. When we developed societies and divided the workload we acquired a lot more free time. Perhaps this led to a desire for "entertainment" and a decreased need for attention to self-support.

I like movies, so let's trace this a little through cinema, shall we? If you've seen *"Quest for Fire"*, *"Clan of the Cave Bear"*, or even *"Caveman"*, you can understand the primitive attitudes of self-preservation. People who should have been helping each other out based on modern concepts of community were still clearly looking out for number one; they steal food from others fairly close to themselves, and males take mates by force.

Move on to *"10,000 B.C."* (not a great or realistic movie, I know), and you see some pretty primitive groups still, but they are mixed in with others and result in having a much more developed social structure. The more advanced cultures kidnap the less advanced individuals and use them as slaves or even sacrifices to their gods (definitely a new priority at some point in human development). This sort of thing happened in many early cultures around the world.

Jump forward to *"Little House on the Prairie"* (I know, it's a TV show and not a movie) and you see a more modern culture where neighbors do look out for and help each other at times, but in general, families still had to provide most of what they needed on their own. From the resources around them, they had to build their own homes and structures, grow their own food, raise their own animals, hunt, fish, and basically, independently subsist for the most part. However, there already depicted significant reliance on the skill and production of others even in what was a much harsher time. Pa had to go to the store in town for nails, windows, tools, and such.

People used tools and equipment such as guns, axes, lanterns and other items made by someone else, perhaps even in a factory. That has become far more commonplace in today's industrialized society. When was the last time you made your own computer or cell phone from raw materials? Some of you today may make your own clothing, but I doubt you harvested the textiles from your back yard and spun it into fabric yourself. Many of you probably grow some of your own food and raise your own animals, but I'll bet you purchased your seeds and baby animals from somewhere else, rather than cultivating wild plants and domesticating wild animals.

This is running on and seems a bit ridiculous I know, but I'm trying to show how dramatically we have lost our way from the basic needs of life. The point is that others now do the vast majority of the work needed to sustain our lives. Most of us don't actually make a single thing we use, produce any of our own food, or even really know where our food and other goods come from. Just trying to survive used to be a full-time job, but now all we have to do is buy things, use them and then throw them away. This makes it very difficult to control what is getting into our bodies.

And what the heck do we do with all the resulting new free time? Today, instead of depending on subsistence or barter, we have *money*. Instead of plows and rifles, we have phones and computers. We don't get to have all our stuff for "free" now. Well, we didn't get it for free then either, it was just a much more direct result of our considerable labor, whereas now there are all these contrived intermediate steps. We have to work to earn money (or perhaps collect money from the government in some way, which is even more dependent on the labor of others), which is some attempt at a tangible representation of the stuff we need.

We then have to give other people our money in exchange for things we need, like food and shelter. This progression leads to an "economy," which is a construct of complex human social behavior but not a real thing in its own right (I laugh every time the news talks about problems with the economy as if it were something separate from us). So our new priority becomes: working. Well, our old priority was working too, but now other people do most of that work and, aside from the paycheck, our new job is probably less directly linked to our needs.

In his classic book, *Walden*, Henry David Thoreau describes how he could either choose to work in a manual labor position for a week so that he could earn enough money for a train ticket to where he was going or, in about a week's time, he could just walk there instead. Either way, he gets there in a week. He chose to walk and, if you think about it, most of us have similar choices. We could choose to make certain things for ourselves or spend time hunting and growing our own food, and therefore work less time at a *job* trying to earn money to buy those things.

Many of us now work at some sort of inherently meaningless occupation, meaningless in terms of meeting primary needs. Modern civilization and society creates such jobs to employ and engage people who are not truly producing any of the basic needs (food, energy, shelter). Many of these occupations serve to drive us continually farther and farther away from our prior natural existence (e.g. rocket scientists, computer software designers, television producers, politicians, etc.).

Perhaps, you have an utterly meaningless, "dead-end" job, and thus some subconscious feeling of lower self-worth because you aren't really producing anything you need on your own. I think this may be true for many people today, and I'll bet that if any of you have ever actually made something that you needed with your own two hands or produced something for your family to eat, then you know that feeling of satisfaction which is sadly missing from most modern occupations. Furthermore, if you make more money than what you need for the basics of life, what are you going to spend it on? If you have a spare eight hours after work as well as free time on the weekends, what are you going to fill that time with? This is where we diverge from the skewed priorities of society, as we've changed it, to the skewed priorities of individuals, which is more personal.

If you're somewhat "responsible", you might invest or put money away for the future and look forward to a time when you don't have to work any more. Isn't retirement a nice modern luxury? I strongly suggest that you find something meaningful to do with your time in retirement though, because that's when people really start to fall apart as they lose their sense of productivity and purpose. In reality, we spend an inordinate amount of money on the huge category I call "entertainment". Entertainment could be considered to be anything we do to make our lives more enjoyable in an immediate sense that does not satisfy a basic need.

For some reason, we in our culture seem to be very deficient in the capacity for self-stimulation (not the kind you're thinking of) and self-entertainment. I'm always shocked to hear how much money entertainers such as movie stars, television actors, professional singers, musicians, and professional athletes, make in our society. Why on Earth should an actors or actresses make millions of dollars for repeating some lines and pretending to be something they're not? Don't most guys in a single's bar do that? Why should a professional baseball, basketball, or football player make millions for playing a game that they already love? Wouldn't they probably play for free, like the rest of us, because it's fun? Why should a celebrity's baby pictures be sold for millions of dollars when my kids are every bit as cute and have just as much potential for greatness? I think our cultural priorities are royally screwed up!

While the professional fakers and overgrown schoolboys are making millions of dollars, which they will have to split in their eventual, high-profile divorces (whatever they don't squander on ridiculous luxury items, that is); our teachers and police officers, in relative terms, make far less money than they deserve. If you think about it, don't you agree that the school teacher, who is going to help shape your child's intellect and attitudes about the world, is more important than an anorexic woman who pretends to be passionate on camera, or an extremely tall man who can jump up and stuff a ball through a hoop?

Teachers had to go to school for a minimum of four years, only to get a stressful and largely thankless job that barely enables them to pay off their student loans. I realize these people chose to be teachers in spite of the predictable stress and poor pay; this is possibly because of a passion for teaching and a desire to do something positive for others. I postulate that we would get the best quality of teachers, however, if we paid them more accordingly to what their job is worth.

The huge amounts of money that entertainers make costs us in a number of ways because, ultimately, the money they are paid comes from us via multiple means. An athlete gets millions because corporations will pay millions to advertise during the broadcast. Their advertising expenditure significantly raises the cost of their goods, and then consumers have to pay more for them. This affects our individual household "bottom line" every day. It is a hidden cost of our desire for these kinds of entertainment.

If we paid our teachers more, perhaps our kids would fare better on international testing and aptitude comparisons. If we paid our politicians more, maybe they wouldn't be so tempted to sell the welfare of the country and its citizens for personal gain (though the personality types that go into politics may remain just as corruptible). Instead, teachers can barely make a living while celebrities and professional athletes can make millions. Our misguided priorities definitely affect us adversely in a variety of ways. We just don't usually think about it.

How does this problem of misguided financial priorities directly affect our health, which is the main topic of this book? When we spend our disposable income on videos and cable television instead of a gym membership or exercise equipment, it definitely affects our health. When we buy soda pop and cigarettes, but won't pay a little extra for organic food, it adversely affects us as well. When we spend hours every evening watching TV and movies instead of directly interacting with our kids, it probably changes their future (for the better or the worse perhaps, depending upon our moods and parenting skills).

Drug use is a very poignant example of how altered priorities can destroy lives. When someone first starts to use drugs it is a conscious choice, but probably not a life priority yet. I suspect no child grows up aspiring to be an alcoholic or drug addict. When drug addiction sets in, that substance often becomes the strongest and primary focus of that person's life. Everything else falls by the wayside. It takes extreme will and redirection of the addict's priorities to break free of those addictions. But it can be done. It has to start with a change in focus and direction.

I think that changing priorities in terms of how we buy food, direct our physical energy, and spend our free time, should be much easier than getting off heroin or cocaine. Later on I will explain how making these changes doesn't really have to cost extra money. These changes won't take time away from our entertainment or the things that many of us feel make our lives worth living in our current culture.

Hedonism, laziness and lack of willpower

We're definitely getting more personal now, and this is possibly the most difficult personal failing to overcome. If people really don't want to do something, they probably won't. In the case of many Americans, even when they do consciously want to make a positive change in their lives, they still don't. Why? It's easy to make excuses and give external reasons as to why we don't do what's good for us but, in reality, it often comes down to the fact that we are just plain lazy.

I'm even talking about people who have legitimate fatigue problems due to biomedical causes or illness, which I will discuss in detail later on; those people may need to have their underlying causes addressed before they will be capable of doing any major *exercise*, but they can still make the right choices in terms of nutrition, environmental control and other things.

I'm talking about those who can, but *won't*, get things done; this includes everyone who is not quadriplegic or severely mentally handicapped.

Anyone who can move his/her arms or legs (it doesn't even have to be both) can exercise. Anyone who can read or hear can educate themselves about food and health. Anyone who has money to spend on soda, chips, cookies, fast food, microwave meals, cigarettes, or alcohol, has the ability to buy healthy food. The vast majority of people who say "I can't" probably *can*. They first need to stop saying "I can't."

Successful change comes down to maturity, priorities, and willpower. Hedonism is opting for what gives a person the most pleasure, usually without paying heed to what is best. This is how children think and behave. I think that hedonistic tendency is what keeps most processed American food on the shelves. Nobody really thinks that cookies, chips, soda, and sugar-enriched breakfast cereals are healthy. They buy these foods simply because they taste good. Everyone knows that smoking cigarettes kills people, alcohol consumption can lead to all kinds of problems, and we all know that, at some point, we should turn off the TV and go do something active or more enriching. Many of us tend to opt for the "immediate-gratification, but long-term-suffering" option too often. We know we shouldn't, but we do anyway.

So, why do we do it? Why do we eat and drink so much junk, watch so much TV, exercise so little, and spend so little time enriching our kids or ourselves? I think it's because we are naturally geared toward conserving energy and our minds really gravitate toward passive stimuli. Clearly, some of us are more easily self-motivated or have more willpower than others, and this tends to show in multiple areas of those people's lives. It was mentioned in the *TIME* article, which I repeatedly cite, that only 6% of those with graduate-level degrees in this country smoke cigarettes, while the overall smoking rate is 19.8%. Conversely, about 50% of the U.S. men who smoke cigarettes have only G.E.D. diplomas. This does not mean that smoking causes you to drop out of high school.

Instead it suggests that people who make poor decisions, or have poor aptitude or resilience, tend to behave consistently through all aspects of their lives.

In the natural world, jogging or running for no apparent reason would be considered a foolish waste of energy. That is, unless you were headed toward a watering hole, food source, or to a potential mate. As you may have noticed in nature shows, the majority of animals primarily sit around all day doing nothing, or they graze on food that is easily within reach.

They generally sit and observe, which expends very little energy, and that is also what we are naturally geared to do. Unnecessary activity is a potential waste of energy resources, which would be a problem if calories were hard to find, such as in nature. This is not a problem in modern society.

Unfortunately, our current civilization provides us with readily available calories, requiring extremely little energy to obtain. It also provides methods of transportation that require minimal effort to go a great distance. Just think how hard it would be to gather 1000 calories of food in the wild. Just think how much energy you would use to walk or bike ten miles to work and back every day. It would be extremely difficult to become obese in a more primitive setting. It appears things are far too easy in our society.

In reality, our bodies and our nature are geared toward conserving energy, and it is completely unnatural for us to want to exercise, or to pass up food when it's just laying there. Hedonism and laziness may sound like character flaws, but, for us, they happen to be the natural order of things. In our current environment, and in order to stay healthy, we have to overcome these powerful forces. This requires intellectual awareness and extreme willpower at times. It requires using our big frontal lobes to make the right *choices*, against what our inner animal nature wants us to do. In some ways, arguably, it is far more difficult to maintain good health in this modern society than it was in more primitive times. We ate all wild and organic foods then because there was no alternative. We got plenty of exercise every day out of necessity.

Unlike in nature, it is not just the strong who survive the incredibly easy lives that we have created through modern civilization. Now, instead of infectious diseases, most of us will die of chronic "lifestyle" diseases like heart attacks, strokes, and diabetes, or cancers and autoimmune diseases which, in many cases, are related to environmental toxins. Our young are rarely dying from infectious diseases or famine and, as a result, we are able to survive into adulthood easily on a very poor diet and unhealthy lifestyle. In many ways, as a species, we have "de-volved" rather than improved over the past several hundred years. And it will take a lot to change that course.

Excuse-A-Palooza; a collection of common excuses and why they're bogus-

This is meant to address the reasonable and unreasonable excuses or explanations, that I often hear for why people don't take better care of themselves. Admittedly, some excuses may be legitimate for some people, however, there are usually ways to get around them. I'm sure there are some great excuses that I've not heard, and some I forgot to list. This is just a sampling of several of my favorites that I hear most often.

"I'm too busy" (to cook, eat healthy, exercise or whatever...)

Okay, so you spend twelve hours a day at work, drive your kids around all evening to their various activities, and then barely have time to watch *American Idol* or *The Biggest Loser* or whatever. You may even work two jobs and go to school (I've been there) or be in medical residency working a hundred hours per week (been there too). In actuality, I think most of the people who use this excuse, work forty to sixty hours per week at the most, and spend maybe five to ten hours per week with those extracurricular activities.

That leaves 100-120 hours per week, or forty-four to sixty-four hours per week, if you sleep eight hours per night. I'll spot you four full hours per day for preparing food and eating, getting ready for the day in the morning and getting ready for bed; that leaves sixteen to thirty-six hours per week. Using these figures, you've got time enough to exercise, learn a new language, take some college or enrichment classes, do volunteer work, be politically active, write a book, or sit around and watch a few hours of TV every day (I believe most people just do that last one)!

Even when I was in medical residency and had three kids to spend time with, I still managed to exercise a few hours per week and, most of the time, I still cooked real food. As chief resident, I even had extra administrative duties on top of my resident work load, and I took an extra three hundred hour training course in medical acupuncture. In spite of all that time commitment, I still found time to stay fit. And this is only because I made it a priority. I realize most people don't have my drive and stamina, but come on!

What I'm trying to drive home, is that it comes back to the issue of priorities, time and time again. In reality, which is where I try to spend most of my time, we all get the same twenty-four hours in a day and 168 hours in a week to budget for ourselves. We just have to decide how to spend that time. By resetting your priorities, you may discover that maybe you don't need to have the more expensive car or clothing, and you can work a few less hours. Maybe each of your kids doesn't have to be in two sports and take additional music lessons; then you might spend more quality time together. Maybe you don't have to watch three hours of TV per night, or maybe you can cook or exercise *while* you're watching TV (multitasking!).

You'll have to do some introspective thinking and see where you may be spending time on things unnecessarily. Maybe you could get a job closer to home rather than commute an hour each way. Maybe you can get to work five minutes early and take the stairs rather than the elevator. Maybe you can bike to work. Maybe you can learn an instrument with your kids or play soccer with them at the park. If you think about it, there are so many positive "maybes," they can quickly outnumber your doubts about not having enough time. Just decide what is really important to you and then figure out how to make it happen.

"I don't have time to exercise"

Many people think that in order to exercise, you've got to purchase a gym membership, a home treadmill or other expensive equipment. It's easy to not go to the gym when it may be ten minutes or more away. You feel like you've got to make yourself presentable before you go, and you may not have time for all of that. Somehow, even when people have exercise equipment in their homes, they still don't find time to use it.

Whenever the opportunity presents, you can get more exercise in your everyday life just by making things a little tougher on yourself. Park further away from the door at the store. Take the stairs. Stand instead of sitting when you watch TV, jog in place, or do push-ups and sit-ups during the commercials. Do dumbbell exercises or deep knee bends, or walk on your treadmill while you listen to an audio book or help your kids with their homework. Multitask with your exercise routine.

I've been getting most of my exercise while watching movies or television with my family for years. I have stayed in good shape exercising just a total of two to three hours per week without need of a gym membership or expensive exercise equipment. I have some very encouraging advice about exercise in section three that will help you realize it is quite easy to get the exercise you need in very little time.

In actuality, we all have the same amount of time per week, and we all intentionally allot time in our schedules for things that are important to us. Successful people *make* time for their health. You can't wait to *have* time; it's already there! That *TIME* magazine article from December 2008, reported that 40% of U.S. adults get no exercise at all. There is really no excuse for this. Forty percent of us are not quadriplegic.

"I don't have time to cook"

Honestly, I think that this is one of the lamer excuses I hear. Everyone has to eat and someone cooks it, whether they do it themselves or not. Even just going through a drive-thru takes time out of your day (and, most likely, some time off of your life). One possible answer to this is for me to simply say, "then don't cook, just eat your foods raw most of the time." You can eat vegetables, nuts, fruit, cheese, and olives without cooking anything. I'm just suggesting that you stay away from processed snack foods and fast food meals.

The better answer to this familiar excuse is to acknowledge that preparing healthy food does take time, even if you're just cutting things up and putting them into containers. Cooking takes time also, but actually not that much hands-on time. Making a salad demands far more direct time than making a roast.

By re-evaluating your time, most of you probably get at least one day off each week or have several non-committed hours here and there (if you don't, then you need to work harder on your priorities). Take a few of those hours to make a bunch of food and store it, possibly in meal-sized portions, to eat for meals or snacks all week. Cook a big pot of rice, make a big pot of oatmeal, steam some vegetables, cook some steaks, fish, or chicken breasts, or boil some eggs.

For goodness sake, it doesn't have to be fancy. Just take a little time for your health. Make a big pot of soup with your leftover meat and some vegetables. Anyone who can turn on the oven or boil some water can cook. It takes only ten minutes of labor to make a roast with vegetables and potatoes; you just have to plan ahead. It takes about that long to order a pizza sometimes, and it's much cheaper to eat food prepared at home. This isn't rocket science, people.

"I don't know what to eat"

Sadly, this excuse is somewhat forgivable in today's America. If you make it through this book you will know much more about what to eat, but right now there is prevailing ignorance and misinformation about this. People are being misled by advertising and the inherent trust in our food producers, not to mention the government with their ridiculous and fraudulent food pyramid.

Many of the people who say this are actually trying to figure it out. They may have given up soda pop and the obvious junk foods. They may have started buying microwave meals that claim to be healthy (but unfortunately are not), instead of going to a fast food joint for lunch. They may feed their kids hot dogs only three times a week now, instead of five. It honestly baffles me what many people think is decent food in our culture. I've heard from a number of Europeans that they lose weight when visiting America because they can't stomach most of our food; and they are far thinner than us to begin with.

Knowing what to eat is truly difficult when 90% of the food in the store is unhealthy. In spite of this, people who are truly motivated to improve their health usually do pretty well by simply realizing food in its natural state is likely to be better than processed foods. They eat more fruits and vegetables, lean meats, and maybe switch to whole grains. As much as possible, many of them will try to buy organic foods as well. In my opinion, making these changes should seem obvious to everyone. Those who just give up and keep eating the food that they know darn well is bad for them, while using ignorance as an excuse, are lying to themselves.

"I can't afford to eat healthy"

Not being able to afford healthy food is a very common excuse. I've heard it so often that I once went through my local grocery store and made lists of common healthy foods and junk foods to compare prices based on weight. I found that junk foods frequently cost *more* per pound than healthy foods. For example, chips cost nearly five dollars per pound in many cases, while organic brown rice costs less than two dollars per pound, and that's before adding all the water weight from cooking. The rice is probably less than fifty cents per pound after cooking. Cookies cost three to four dollars per pound, while organic apples can often be found for around $2.50 per pound, even in Alaska.

It is also important to note that when you eat healthy whole foods, full of nutrients, you feel much more satisfied more readily. Junk foods tend to promote blood sugar swings and hypoglycemia, which lead to more gorging on the same type of processed sugary junk. This means that eating the healthier food saves you even more money because you need less food overall.

Admittedly, organic produce and animal products are a bit more expensive to buy. Hopefully, you can try to buy produce from local growers and save some money there. If possible, hunting and fishing to get your own wild meats (admittedly much easier for us up here in Alaska) may help with quality and expense. In reality, spending the extra money on organic or wild *animal* products is the most important (because pesticide levels in animal foods are much higher than in plant foods). In my opinion, there really isn't much that is more important to spend money on than quality food.

Sadly, rather than putting a little more money into their primary source of health, which is food, many people still spend money on junk food, cigarettes, unnecessary cosmetics and, of course, entertainment. They usually own television sets, video players, video game systems, cell phones, recreational toys, and other devices totaling many thousands of dollars that they apparently consider to be more important than what they put in their bodies. I've seen mothers who smoke cigarettes, color their hair, sport expensive manicures, and carry four-hundred-dollar handbags, tell me with a straight face that they can't afford to feed their kids healthy food. Amazing!

"I can't afford a gym membership"

I've already mentioned that you don't need a gym membership to exercise. Actually, I think this is pretty intuitive because we all took P.E. in school and got exercise without going to a health club. We all know how to walk and run outside, do push-ups and sit-ups, jumping jacks and other exercises that require no equipment whatsoever. There are piles of exercise videos out there to help get you in shape at home with little or no equipment. Surely, you can probably afford a pair of dumbbells and some stretchy bands or something. It requires little or no money to get adequate exercise.

"I don't have room for exercise equipment"

So don't buy any. Just jump up and down. As long as your ceiling is at least a couple feet above your head you should be fine. Go outside and jump rope (I'm sure you can afford one of those), do some lunges across the house a few times or run some sprints outside. All you need in order to do push-ups is a floor, two hands at the most, and a little bit of space. If you can't afford a fifty-dollar set of dumbbells or some stretchy exercise bands, then lift rocks, bags of flour, small children, or cans of food. Eventually, most people just use a treadmill for a clothing rack anyway. Make use of the things you already have.

"I don't know how to exercise"

I don't hear this one a lot, as most people in our society do know a certain amount about how to exercise and stay fit. For those who honestly claim not to know, I suggest you try to think of something in the past that you did physically that made you sweaty and out of breath, and do that some more. Exercise is basically an activity that makes your muscles burn, makes your heart beat faster, your breathing deeper and more rapid, and eventually makes you sweat. It's often more fun with a partner, so you can try to find someone else who may know more than you do.

Also, in the modern information age, not knowing how to do something like cooking or exercise is an easy thing to remedy. You can read books, magazines, or seek online information and educate yourself. There is a plethora of exercise videos out there as well; many of these can be sampled for free at your local library. I'll bet that many who use this excuse didn't know how to use their computer, I-Pod, or cell phone at first either, but they were more motivated enough to figure those things out. Information and guidance in terms of exercise is readily available, if you care to look for it.

"I'm just getting old" or "I can't exercise"

NO! For crying out loud, I hear this from people in their forties and fifties! You are not supposed to get fat and tired as you age, and you cannot accept it as normal. You are not supposed to develop debilitating aches and pains and have significant fatigue probably before age ninety or so. You are supposed to be fit enough to plow your own field, shovel your own driveway, kill and carry your own deer, until you are a hundred or more in my opinion. Basically, you are supposed to be able to do whatever feat of manual labor that a caveman would fit into his daily life well into your eighties or beyond.

People seem to think that getting older is a license to dwindle and fade away, and they are allowing it to happen to them at younger and younger ages. People seem to think they are getting old in their thirties! I've seen women in their nineties still going to yoga classes, and men in their nineties still chasing thirty year-old women around. I've also seen obese men and women in their forties and fifties telling me they have no energy, they have pain in their backs or other places, and errantly blame it on their age.

I'm sorry, but if you are falling apart before you're in your eighties, you probably have yourself to blame more than anything else. I'm sure that some of you were injured in an accident, contracted some terrible infection, have a genetic condition, or something else that wasn't your fault. In my experience, those individuals usually don't blame it on their age, so, for the sake of this rant, we are just talking about chronic diseases associated with lifestyle which are, by far, the most significant causes of death and morbidity. I know that the environment has gotten pretty darn bad, our food supply is depleted and poisoned, and our lives are more stressful than they should be. However, the human lifespan potential is over 120 years, and I'm only willing to spot you forty years for those factors beyond your immediate control. The rest is up to you.

"I might die tomorrow, so why bother?"

This is a great one actually, because it makes for a much simpler office visit. People who don't really care about their health and longevity are much easier appointments for me, because I can just prescribe them symptomatic treatments like conventional doctors do. They can take a pain reliever for their back pain, a blood pressure pill for their hypertension, and maybe a little blue pill for their erectile dysfunction. Most will eventually need an antidepressant to cope with how bad their life sucks. With this kind of patient, I don't have to think hard at all. It probably wouldn't surprise you that the vast majority of people I see with this attitude are men.

You may certainly choose to live every day as if it is your last, because you never know when the end is coming. However, maybe you have no concern for your health and longevity, and just focus on how you feel from day to day, hedonism again perhaps. I find this is a common attitude in young adults who still think they are immortal; in middle aged men who really just don't give a damn and hate going to doctors; and in older people who feel that they've lived a long and fulfilling life already and are just looking to enjoy their later years.

The downside to this kind of thinking is that you may actually live a really long time, and toward the end be miserable for a lot of it. I've seen numerous smokers who weren't lucky enough to die of a heart attack or stroke spend their last ten to twenty years trapped inside a body that can't catch its breath, and suffer even doing minor things like combing their hair. I've seen many people who had a stroke but didn't die. They just became unable to care for themselves and now need to have someone else feed them and bathe them. It's the lucky ones who live hard and then have a blissful sudden death.

You may get lucky enough to go out in a blaze of glory while you still have some vitality, or you may not. You may develop diabetes and, due to poor attention to your disease, have progressively shorter feet and then lose your legs, as you have one amputation after another. You may develop dementia and forget who your loved ones are. You may damage your heart just enough to become a cardiac cripple and be unable to go up a flight of stairs but not quite be dead from your series of small heart attacks.

I see many men who have had this sort of cavalier attitude about health their entire lives, change their position when they have their first heart attack, a minor stroke, or especially when their penis stops working. Yes, good old erectile dysfunction should be the big wake-up call for men. It indicates that something is terribly wrong with you. If you can't get an erection you can no longer breed; and if you can no longer breed, perhaps it's because your health is bad enough to exclude you from the gene pool (of course, there is an upper age limit for natural breeding potential, but that shouldn't prohibit sexual functioning at any age).

This is one way of looking at it anyway. The fact remains that reproduction is the primary function of an organism, and that function is very strongly preserved, in spite of all sorts of other problems. If one has erectile dysfunction, low sperm counts, ovarian dysfunction, recurrent miscarriage, or any other type of functional infertility, then something is really wrong. In my opinion, staying in good general health should keep men and women sexually functional, though not necessarily fertile, past one hundred years of age, no matter how distasteful that may sound to some of you.

Many people have the attitude that if you try and take better care of yourself, you will just delay the inevitable: dying. In a pure sense, death is absolutely unavoidable. We are all going to die some day of course; nobody gets out of here alive. The real expected benefit to a healthy lifestyle is something termed "compression of morbidity." Compression of morbidity means that if you live a healthy life, you will have vitality and function well into old age, then quickly deteriorate and pass away, without suffering through a long, drawn-out, chronic disease. These are major benefits of taking good care of yourself, having all of your years be good ones, and having more of them, as well.

Basically, we all have to make decisions about our health, right at the start. We either give a damn, or we don't. If you don't give a damn about how long you live or how easy the road to death is, then that's fine, and I never fault anyone for feeling that way. After all, we've all got our own priorities, right? I still see plenty of patients who want to keep up their self-destructive habits and continue taking prescription drugs for their symptoms with the expectation they will be saved by the medications rather than by their own actions. That is, unfortunately, pure fantasy.

I have learned that the people who are truly motivated to learn and willing to change their personal habits in the interest of their health benefit the most from my care. As a result, honestly, I try to focus most of my energy on them. I refer some of the others, who just want medications to soothe their self-inflicted suffering, to local conventional doctors. Most all I can do, in a very real sense, is educate people. It is then up to individuals to do what they need to do to achieve optimal health for themselves. Even if I prescribe a drug for someone, that doesn't guarantee they will take it. I can suggest all sorts of dietary and exercise advice along with a list of helpful supplements, but I won't go shopping for you or run behind you and yell encouragement.

The fact is people have to be self-motivated and fully engaged in their own health care if they wish to be successful. Health is a personal responsibility. If you want good health you have to be very proactive. You have to seek out the knowledge and expertise you need, prioritize your life and your time accordingly, and *do it*. Being healthy is an active process, not passive; you aren't going to be healthy by default in this world.

Moving on...

I believe I've ranted enough about what I think is wrong, so let's move on to discussing what we can all do about *solving* the problems.

The following sections will be about my general approach to health and medicine, discussing the important aspects of health in terms of lifestyle practices, dietary issues, toxicity, physiology, and mechanisms.

SECTION III

NOURISHING THE BODY AND MIND

Introduction

The goal of this section is to provide information about the food, water, and other nutrients your body and those of your children need. I also discuss concepts of physical, mental, and spiritual "nourishment" because they contribute significantly to total health. This is the section in which I explain what you need to do for yourself in order to be healthy; your own efforts are often much more important than most of what a doctor can do for you.

This topic is enormous, so I do not attempt to present a comprehensive description of all the ways nutrition affects your health or all the specific conditions related to deficiency of specific nutrients. It would require an encyclopedia of texts just to describe the examples we know about today, and there are sure to be an even greater number we know nothing about yet.

The goals of this section are to convey why nutrition is important and how categories of nutrients influence your health, to provide an overview of how nutritional factors relate to disease, to discuss the benefits of different types of exercise to meet different goals, and to open your mind to the idea of mental, energetic, and spiritual enrichment as necessary in promoting total health.

If you want to read more about nutrition, I suggest starting with *Clinical Nutrition: A Functional Approach* from the Institute for Functional Medicine (Liska et al. 2004), *Nourishing Traditions* (Fallon, 2001), and possibly *Nutrition and Physical Degeneration* (Price, 2006) and *Healing with Whole Foods* (Pitchford, 2002). I also suggest getting the newsletter from the Price-Pottenger Nutrition Foundation.

Chapter 1 – Some Generalizations Regarding Food

You are what you eat

"You are what you eat" is one of those statements that just sounds true when you hear it. It is so plainly obvious that I find it particularly egregious when medical schools neglect proper training in nutrition and how it relates to our health. What could be more important than what you choose to eat? What you drink and what you breathe are more important than what you eat because we die faster without air or water—although we can't last much longer without food. I'll discuss air and water in this section as well.

We can solve many health problems through nutrition, but we need to know what it is we need from food, when we need it, and how much of it we need. We also need to know what should *not* be in our food, and in a very practical sense, we need to know how to get the food we need.

What may be even more important than what you eat is what your *mother* ate when you were growing in her womb. Her particular intake of nutrients and toxins set the stage for your future health in many ways. Some of those mechanisms involve the epigenetic issues I discussed at length earlier. Some of it dictates how well you developed physically and mentally in utero and how close you may get to your genetic potential later on. It may start with your DNA, but how your mother nourished you as a fetus has a great deal to do with whether you will succeed in the world and who you become.

Of course, this information doesn't help you now as an individual, but it certainly can help future generations if these concepts and principles are put into play prior to conception. These concepts are important not only for women; men need proper nutrition (and detoxification in many cases) in order to produce high-quality sperm and do our small but important part to create a healthy and fully functional child. To those of you still planning to have children, who would like to improve the overall quality of our human product, I say this: pay attention.

What does food do for us?

Most everyone realizes that food provides energy; we know from an early age that, if we don't eat, we start to feel weak and to function poorly in a variety of ways. Unfortunately, many people today seem to think that energy is just about all food is good for. They think managing body weight, for example, is a simple matter of counting calories eaten versus calories burned. This is a huge miscalculation, evidenced by the nearly universal failure of calorie-restrictive diet programs.

Food is just a solid mass of many individual chemicals. Some of them, such as sugars, starches and certain fats, are useful only for energy production. We need some of them, including essential fats, cholesterol, and the amino acids from protein, to make our tissues and chemicals. Some, primarily vitamins and minerals, are needed as chemical cofactors for our physiological reactions. Others include plant-derived chemicals that can augment our healthy body processes in a variety of ways.

Food is vital to our existence and function. It provides our structure and body mass. It provides what we use for energy. It provides the substrate from which we make the chemicals that make things happen in our bodies, such as hormones, enzymes, and neurotransmitters. It provides nutrients that influence how well all our physiological reactions and processes work—the myriad factors that directly influence our health.

Pretty much everything that goes right or wrong with your body and your health is influenced in some way by your diet and the foods you did or didn't eat. This is an undeniable truth, yet somehow it has escaped our conventional medical training and most of its practitioners. I could give you many examples of people who corrected their metabolic problems using dietary changes and nutritional supplements in place of the prescription drugs they were using when they came to see me.

For some reason, when I try to explain this to most of my conventional colleagues, they either disbelieve what I am saying or they think the examples are anecdotal, so they do not change their practice of prescribing drugs. This issue goes back to philosophical problems with our training and to the personality issues in doctors I discussed earlier.

It makes sense that if food is the basis of how everything works in our bodies, it may also be part of the cause of dysfunction and part of the solution. I have seen many people with high blood pressure because of too little salt in their diets, even though that sounds completely backward based on our current cultural thinking on the subject. I have seen depression and anxiety treated effectively using solely nutritional therapies because, as I like to say, depression is not a (insert antidepressant of choice) deficiency.

Food is the basis for how we look, how we feel, how we grow, and how we age. It is the basis for our success and our failure in many ways. It can explain how well we cope with environmental change and how well we heal from injury or recuperate from illness. If you include air and water in the huge category of what we call "food" or nourishment, you could make the argument that food is the basis for everything that goes right or wrong for you. Of course, it isn't that simple, and the issues discussed in the next section should elucidate this idea of nourishment further.

What food is supposed to provide

For the sake of this discussion, let's divide the topic of food into broad categories of macronutrients, micronutrients, phytonutrients, enzymes, and other food constituents (One should always have an "other" category in mind when making lists to remind us that we don't know everything and probably never will.)

Each of these separate topics is so extensive they are organized into chapters of their own.

CHAPTER 2 – MACRONUTRIENTS: FATS/LIPIDS

Most people have some understanding of the concepts of the big three macronutrients: fats, proteins, and carbohydrates (sugars), so I use those subcategories here.

Defining fats

The words "fat" and "lipid" are largely interchangeable in biology, so I use them both here to mean the same thing. These nutrients are big molecules—hence, the prefix "macro"—and they include fats, oils, cholesterol, phospholipids, sphingolipids, myelin, and other cellular components in your body. Cholesterol, fat, and oil tend to get a bad rap these days, but that is a big misunderstanding for the most part.

There has been a huge campaign against the consumption of fat in most any form in our food advertising, as well as in the propaganda from the American Medical Association (AMA) and the American Heart Association (AHA). This anti-fat campaign is very misguided in my opinion since, at the same time that we have reduced our fat consumption as a population, we have seen our health problems increase. What's more, we have found examples of human cultures that consume the majority of their calories in the form of fat who have excellent health (the Masai of Africa and the Inuit of Alaska, to name two).

The term "fat" describes molecules made primarily of carbon and hydrogen (which makes it a "hydrocarbon" like gasoline, something our cars use for fuel, right?) that will not mix with water in a stable fashion. If fat is liquid at room temperature, we tend to call it "oil," but some tropical oils, such as coconut oil, are solid at room temperature, so sometimes the boxes we try to put things into just don't fit well.

Fat functions

Fats may be used as energy, which is what we are all familiar with, but they are also extremely important structural components for every cell in your body. Every one of your cells is defined by a membrane made primarily of fats called phospholipids. Phospholipids have a long, fatty tail with a water-soluble head at one end that contains phosphorus. In a water-based setting, such as the human body, they spontaneously arrange themselves into a double layer with water-soluble heads oriented away from each other and long, fatty tails touching each other, creating a continuous layer of fat molecules inside the resulting membrane.

Interspersed in this membrane is cholesterol to add rigidity, stability and integrity; there are also protein channels, signaling molecules or receptors, and enzymes that perform various functions. The membrane is the most metabolically active area of the cell and the most important place for communication between that cell and the rest of your body.

Most hormones, neurotransmitters, and other signal molecules have to transmit their messages to the cells via its membrane in some way. Nutrients must get into your cells through the membrane in order to nourish you and provide what your cells need for all their functions. If you don't have the right makeup of lipids in the membrane, these processes will not work properly.

Do you know what organ in your body contains more fat than any other? It's your brain. *Now* do you think fat is important? This is one reason why lipid-lowering drugs like the statins cause impenetrable brain fog in many people and why some vegetarians (especially vegans) may have issues with memory, sleep, anxiety, and other brain-related functions.

Low-fat diets and fat-reducing drugs have even been associated with depression and suicide (Fallon, 1999), not to mention certain cancers and degenerative conditions. Have you ever noticed how your dog's coat improves when you feed him or her more animal fat like meat scraps or bacon grease? Your skin and hair will improve greatly with the right fats in your diet as well.

It's staggering to think how much more is known about nutrition in conventional veterinary medicine than in human medicine. Veterinarians know how to solve all sorts of problems with food. I've seen a number of experienced animal owners who admitted they feed their animals much better than they feed themselves and who still did not realize the role their own diets played in their health. I see a lot of dry skin and hair, fatigue, depression, anxiety, and other problems in the general population because our diets are often poor in the right fats.

So what are the right fats? We can make some fats inside our own bodies to store energy. (That's the fat with which we are all too familiar that fits too snugly into our jeans.) The saturated fats from foods like meats and butter are examples of this type of fat, though those fats do other beneficial things for you as well. In our culture most of the undesirable stored fat was converted from excess sugar we ate. Other fats provide mostly structural or functional support to the important cell membrane I was discussing earlier.

Fat forms (and more about functions)

"Essential fats" are the fats we need for normal health, structure and function that we cannot synthesize internally, so we must get them from our diet. These include the omega-3 fats we hear a lot about these days from sources like fish and flax oils. Omega-3 fats have been shown to be important in preventing inflammation in the body, improving brain and cellular function, generating regulatory chemicals in the body, and influencing liver function, among other benefits. In fact, it is safe to say the drastic decrease in our intake of omega-3 fats, coupled with the huge increase in our sugar consumption, is one of the strongest nutritional factors behind the dramatic rise in some of our most common chronic diseases and killers.

An important and lesser-known essential fat is conjugated linoleic acid (CLA), which is almost exclusively found in the meat and milk products of wild or grass-fed hoofed animals. Notice I said "grass-fed" animals, which means it is *not* present in our modern livestock, which is fed corn and the other garbage we make our animals eat for cheap meat production. I have to wonder if a cow made from corn is a cow at all, since cows are supposed to be made from grass.

CLA has been shown to decrease cancer and cardiovascular risk to an extent that would thrill pharmaceutical manufacturers, if there were a chance one of their drugs could ever achieve the same thing. Do you think many Americans are getting any CLA in their diet of corn chips, fast-food burgers, pizza, fries, macaroni and cheese, and soda? Are you getting any on a vegetarian or vegan diet? Do the cows your milk comes from eat grass? No! Well, "no" for the vast majority of you; I'm sure some of you know this already and are milking your own grass-fed cow or goats to get your dairy products and eating primarily wild or grass-fed meat.

This is a good example of the principle of animal-based food being what it itself eats, and it is only good food if it was fed well itself. This is a concept I will bring up repeatedly, and if it starts to sound like a broken record, that's good; maybe it will stick. It is one of the most important concepts to glean from this book.

Cholesterol confusion

Cholesterol is another very important lipid, especially since there is an enormous smear campaign going on against it in this country and most other industrialized nations. Cholesterol is a complex lipid molecule comprised of several rings of carbon atoms with their attendant hydrogen and maybe an oxygen atom here and there. (I don't imagine you really want to see organic chemistry symbols and drawings, so I'm glossing over the details.) Most other lipids or fatty acids are long, linear molecules that are sort of floppy and flexible. A round, reinforced molecule, cholesterol is used largely to provide rigidity and strength to cell membranes, so it influences cell membrane structure and how things pass through or move within the membrane.

Therefore, cholesterol is important for the integrity and function of your cell membranes. (Again, the membranes are the most important part of the cells you are made of, sort of like the walls of your house.) When you don't have enough cholesterol in your cells, the membranes may be weak and fragile, which is part of why liver and muscle cells can burst and die when people take statin drugs like Lipitor™, Zocor™, and Crestor™. The other big problem with those drugs is that they prevent normal energy production within cells, which is why cells with higher energy needs are the major targets for dysfunctional side effects. Nerve cells also suffer when you lack cholesterol because nerve cells are supposed to have thick lipid sheaths around them like the insulation on an electrical wire.

So why do we make cholesterol in our livers? On average, only about 20 percent of the cholesterol measured in your blood comes from what you eat; you produce the rest yourself because it's important. Why would we intentionally produce this terrible substance in our livers if we didn't need it? Does it make any sense to spend billions of dollars per year on drugs to stop this production?

Studies have shown a loose association between elevated cholesterol and cardiovascular disease, but the association is weak, and it does not prove or even imply cause-and-effect at all. Further, the abject failure of cholesterol-lowering drugs to prevent cardiovascular death should have convinced us we are off track.

Another vital note about cholesterol is that it is the substance from which you make many important hormones. Specifically, the "steroid" hormones are all derived from chole-"sterol." The steroid hormones include testosterone, cortisol, estrogen, and progesterone. Do you think statin drugs could therefore affect your ability to make these hormones? I'm not sure there is a clinically relevant effect of statins on hormone production, but these drugs certainly can't improve it.

Vitamin D is also made from cholesterol. It behaves much more like a hormone than a typical vitamin, with far-reaching benefits I discuss later in the "hormone" chapter. Some statin drugs surprisingly cause vitamin D synthesis to increase, rather than decrease (Ertugrul, 2010). Statins in general have been shown to have metabolic activity mimicking vitamin D in various ways, which likely explains all of the benefits they seem to offer (Grimes, 2006). So, why don't we just give people vitamin D and avoid the potential toxicity of statin drugs?

I should explain the "cholesterol" measurements in your blood tests. When a lab tests your cholesterol it is actually called a "lipid panel". The report lists LDL and HDL numbers, triglycerides, and a figure called "total cholesterol," which doesn't make sense since most of your cholesterol and fats are in your cells, rather than circulating in your blood. You see, the L at the end of HDL and LDL stands for "lipoprotein," and a lipoprotein, as you may derive from the word, is a substance comprised of both lipids (fats, including cholesterol, but also triglycerides and other fatty acids) and protein molecules. Picture a basketball full of butter with the outer shell comprised mostly of protein so the whole thing is soluble in water (blood).

These particles are manufactured by your liver as a means of delivering the fats every cell in your body needs to your body in a form that can travel through the blood. They are little care packages of energy and raw materials for your hard-working cells. Your liver wouldn't make them if you didn't need them. If you don't have enough or if you suppress their production too far, such as with a drug or extreme dietary restrictions, you will probably get sick.

Since fat is less dense than water or protein, the "low density lipoproteins" (LDLs) contain relatively more fat than the "high density lipoproteins" (HDLs). This is why we refer to "good cholesterol" for HDL and "bad cholesterol" for LDL. However, the cholesterol molecule itself is only a minor constituent of LDL or HDL since most of the fat in LDL is fatty acids like triglycerides, which are mainly an energy form of fat. The amount of cholesterol itself could be exactly the same between HDL and LDL particles. Triglycerides measured in your blood are there primarily for energy, and when we don't use that energy, those LDL particles end up delivering the energy to our fat cells for storage, rather than being used immediately by more metabolically active cells.

Sometimes those unused lipids end up accumulating in a fatty plaque that forms on the inside of a blood vessel because of some inflammatory injury (which is the *real* cause of cardiovascular disease, not high blood lipids) and cause that plaque to accumulate. Therefore, high blood triglycerides have been associated with a greater risk of heart attack and stroke, independent of the LDL or total cholesterol readings. The fats end up in those plaques by accident; if you have a large amount of fat in your blood, you may well build up the plaques faster, but that does not mean those fats are the cause of the plaque in the first place.

The more important factors regarding lipoprotein particles now appear to be particle size, rather than density, and the presence of "oxidized" LDL. Some labs can perform "VAP" or "NMR" testing, which shows the average size of your LDL and HDL particles, when they run your cholesterol readings. The smaller the particles, the worse it is for you because those little particles can infiltrate your vessel linings and settle into atherosclerotic plaques more readily when they are small. Small particle size has been associated with metabolic syndrome, diabetes, and obesity syndromes, and it is likely a key element of the cardiovascular disease risk seen in people with those conditions.

Therefore, you can have high cardiovascular risk because of small particle sizes even if your LDL and HDL parameters appear to be in the proper range. Cholesterol drugs like the statins *do not* improve this particle size issue, which is probably why they don't have any positive effect on cardiovascular death. All you can do to improve particle size is to eat healthfully, exercise regularly, maintain a healthy weight, and improve your overall health. If you are concerned about your cardiovascular risk, the next time you have your cholesterol checked, make sure they run a VAP or NMR type of panel.

Oxidized LDL (LDL-ox) particles exist in the blood of people with inflammatory processes going on in their bodies causing oxidative stress. The oxidized lipid particles are the ones that accumulate most readily in blood vessel walls and pose the greatest health risk. Statin drugs do seem to effectively decrease LDL-ox, so these people are the ones likely to truly benefit from one of these drugs. The problem is, we don't have mainstream tests available for LDL-ox yet. The real solution lies in improving overall health and addressing whatever is going on in the person to cause the oxidative stress in the first place (e.g. smoking, heavy metals, psychological stress, fast food, etc.).

It is reasonable to believe that an increase in your LDL or total blood cholesterol readings means one of two things: you are eating too much sugar or you have some type of inflammation or cellular injury going on in your body and are trying to heal yourself by synthesizing more tissue components. The first example should be corrected by lowering your sugar and simple carbohydrate intake; the second should be addressed by figuring out the real cause of your inflammation or injury. Neither of these should only be treated with a drug that blocks the production of cholesterol molecules (statins like Lipitor™, Zocor™, Crestor™), prevents absorption of fats from your diet (Zetia™, Orlistat™ or Cholestyramine™), or shoves your triglycerides into your blood vessel walls (Lopid™, Tricor™ and Trilipix™, which have been shown to increase death rates, rather than decrease them).

Some plants and other organisms produce "sterol" substances, which look something like cholesterol. Some of these come from soy and can have major beneficial effects on your liver and lipid profiles; others seem to modulate the effects of estrogen or other hormones in your body in either positive or negative ways. Fungi produce sterol substances in their cell walls, but I don't believe it is clear yet whether they are good or bad for us nutritionally.

The lipid physiology lesson aside, how this relates to food is the crux of this discussion. What you need to know is that excess sugar consumed in your diet ends up being turned into triglycerides and the "bad" fat in those particles from the liver. We eat much too much sugar in our society, and when you can't use it all right away, your liver turns it into fat and sends it out to be stored in the fat cells all around your body. The dramatically increased sugar consumption in our society over the past hundred years is the most likely dietary contributor our rise in cardiovascular disease; it is not the unfairly vilified fats and cholesterol from natural food sources, especially since our fat consumption as a culture has significantly decreased during the same time.

That last part is critical to understand. The source of fat and the type of fat you consume is extremely important. You can eat all the butter you want as long as that butter comes from the milk of cows raised organically on grass, in which case the butter is rich in CLA, vitamin A, and other nutrients that are essential to your health. There is no reason to think it will harm you, and if you read Weston Price's work, you will find repeated examples of people enjoying excellent health while consuming large amounts of pure, wholesome dairy products.

Unfortunately, if you buy butter, milk, or other conventional dairy products from your grocery store today, you are not getting the same product at all, so when I tell my patients "butter is good for you," I have to qualify emphatically what butter is supposed to be and where real butter comes from.

Fat digestion

The process of digesting and assimilating fat is complicated. Fat in food often comes in the form of large, complex molecules like triglycerides (three fatty acid chains attached to a glycerol molecule), which must first be broken down into individual fatty acids before they may be absorbed. Acid in the stomach helps break up fat a little but not as effectively as it does other types of food compounds (which may be why fatty foods tend to cause more heartburn in some people). Enzymes called "lipases" perform this function; some lipase is produced in the mouth from glands on the tongue, but most is produced by the pancreas and mixes with your food after leaving the stomach.

You may recall that fat and water don't mix, and this is where bile comes in. Your liver produces a continuous trickle of bile, which is normally stored in the gall bladder between meals. When you eat something fatty, your gall bladder dumps a load of bile into your small intestine alongside your pancreatic juice and its digestive enzymes. The bile creates soluble particles, called micelles, which are comprised of bile salts and fatty acids that may then be absorbed by the intestine.

If you lose your gall bladder, you may still digest and absorb small amounts of fat at one time just fine, but you may have trouble handling a large load of fat until the common bile duct enlarges to act like a surrogate gall bladder. This is not a lasting problem for most, but some people develop bowel irregularity issues after their gall bladders are removed, and it is theoretically more likely that they will have trouble absorbing adequate amounts of fats and fat-soluble vitamins. You can purchase digestive enzyme supplements containing bile salts for use with meals, which should correct this problem.

When something like cystic fibrosis, chronic alcohol use, toxins, or certain medications damages the pancreas, fats cannot be digested normally, and the individual can become nutritionally deficient. Certain drugs are designed to block fat absorption, which I feel is a horrible idea. Some children are born with genetic conditions that affect their fat digestion or absorption mechanisms. In this instance, it is vital to know that certain types of fatty acids can absorb directly, without the normal mechanisms of fat digestion.

Fatty acids come in short, medium, or long lengths, based on the number of carbon atoms in the chain. Medium-chain fatty acids have six to twelve carbons, can be absorbed directly, and do not require energy for absorption, utilization, or storage. They are critical sources of nutrition for those with fat-malabsorption syndromes or conditions. The best food sources of medium-chain triglycerides (MCTs) are coconut and palm kernel oils. People whose gall bladders have been removed may do well to use these oils preferentially.

Scary fake fats

Margarine and other butter substitutes artificially produced from liquid vegetable oils are not good for you at all and cannot be metabolized correctly. Some cause inflammation and certain kinds of physiologic dysfunction and have been associated with higher rates of death. Apparently, margarine was originally made as a lubricant for machinery, and that's where they should have kept it. Some health problems from margarine are the result of "trans fats," which you have probably heard about on television and in product marketing.

The word "trans" refers to the direction of bond angling between carbon atoms in a long fat molecule. When fats are made biologically in an organism, the bonds are all in the "cis" configuration (meaning the molecule bends in the same direction on both sides of a double bond), which is the opposite of trans. When a polyunsaturated fatty acid from a plant like corn or soy (omega-6 oil) is artificially altered, as it is in "hydrogenated oils" or "partially hydrogenated oils," they add hydrogen atoms into the chain and eliminate the double bonds, and some of the new bonds end up in the trans formation.

So what? Who cares if the bonds are cis or trans or something else? What does that mean to me?

In biological systems, everything is three-dimensional, and biochemical reactions often take place with one large molecule needing to fit into another just right, like a protein into a digestive enzyme or a fatty acid into a cell membrane. Our enzymes and cellular structures are designed to work with natural substances, not unnatural manufactured ones. Sometimes the artificial molecules fit differently or don't fit at all into our enzymes, because their physical structure is altered from the norm. This lack of fit may have no biological effect at all, it may cause a beneficial effect (as is the intention with pharmaceutical drugs), or it may result in negative physiological effects ranging from inconsequential to severe (as is the case with many).

The problem is that the trans configuration in a fatty acid does not mesh with our enzymes and cell membranes so the fatty acids don't fit into the enzymes that are needed to break them down for use as energy, and they don't arrange correctly within our cell membranes.

So what do these molecules do when they get in our bodies? Fatty acids in cell membranes play a vital role in controlling the inflammatory process, and abnormal fats promote or exacerbate inflammation, rather than helping to control or modify it like omega-3 fats do. Abnormal fats can't be used for energy the same way a normal saturated fat is, so they persist and accumulate in places they don't belong, promoting higher rates of cardiovascular disease, brain and neurological problems, inflammatory problems like arthritis and other pain conditions, cancers, and other maladies.

If we can't use these abnormal fats or break them down right because they don't fit into our enzymes, what do our bodies do with them? That is the last part of the problem. Our bodies have systems in place to break down, detoxify, and excrete normal biological molecules, but we can't always do a good job with abnormal molecules (like acetaminophen from Tylenol™, which causes rapid liver destruction in cases of overdose). Therefore, the trans fats may just linger in your body, promoting inflammation for long periods until they are eventually metabolized or excreted. In other words, a little may go a long way, and no amount is truly safe.

You should not eat margarine or any product with trans fats or any type of hydrogenated oils. The key to avoiding them is to look for the listing of hydrogenated or partially hydrogenated oils in the ingredients list and not to believe the listing of "zero grams of trans fat" in the nutrition information because, by current regulations, the product can contain more than half a gram of trans fat and still say "zero" on the label. (That's your government *not* protecting you from the food industry.)

All the food manufacturer has to do is to alter the "serving size" until they have less than the reportable amount of trans fat in a serving, and they can report "zero trans fat". Unfortunately, products containing trans fats are everywhere in our stores, and every time you see this stuff on the shelves, you should shake your head in disgust as I do. It is nothing more than the food industry trying to sell you an agricultural waste product with a false promise of better health. Don't buy it!

Of course, even I eat trans fats on rare occasions. I confess this sin so I won't be called a hypocrite. (Our culture loves to call people hypocrites at any opportunity, thereby somehow discrediting everything the person ever said, right?). I also want to show my understanding of how difficult it is to follow a truly pure diet. I like some pie on Thanksgiving and Christmas just like the rest of you do. I also like some kind of whipped topping on my pie, and I am allergic to milk, so I have to decide between the stomachache and stupor I may get from the dairy-based topping or the small amount of time off my life I might suffer from the non-dairy stuff, which is made mostly of corn syrup and hydrogenated oils. (I suppose I could eat pie without the topping, but what would be the point?)

I do not mean to condone the consumption of these toxic foodstuffs, but we all have to live in the world and to decide how well and how long we want to live. I eat the stuff without guilt on those rare occasions when I choose to because I am fully informed about the danger, and I avoid them the vast majority of the time. Don't use this confession as license to pollute your body daily; just try to do better for yourself. I see patients at the grocery store all the time, and they are always curious to see what I have in my cart. I suspect this is in hopes of catching me eating something bad so they can justify it themselves. Humans are fascinating creatures.

Good fats and oils

Healthy types of fat in the diet come from both plant and animal sources. I've already discussed CLA and the healthy natural saturated fats from butter and tropical oils (coconut and palm oils, which appear to be healthier than our northern oils discussed below). These are good sources of energy, and they promote the normal function of your cells, which discourages disease. The large-scale "Kanwu" study suggested that increased dietary intake of saturated fat improves insulin sensitivity, so it should help to improve metabolic syndrome and blood sugar levels in those with type 2 diabetes.

There are also "unsaturated" oils, which have double bonds between some carbon atoms so they can hold more hydrogen atoms if they are so inclined. The "hydrogenation" process takes an unsaturated oil and fills in those spots with more hydrogen atoms. (I know I'm repeating myself, but understanding a little biochemistry will arm you against those pretty tubs of butter-substitute on the shelves.) Unsaturated oils come in two general categories: "polyunsaturated" (PUFA, which have more than one double bond in the chain) and "monounsaturated" (MUFA, which have just one double bond).

Monounsaturated oils appear to be very good for us in terms of cardiovascular health. Studies involving the Mediterranean diet (high in MUFAs) have shown significant reductions in cardiovascular events and vascular death (Gardener, 2011), which trumps anything that big pharma has put out. Increasing MUFA intake has been shown to promote healthier blood lipid and cholesterol profiles, to decrease breast cancer risk, and to decrease a number of inflammatory markers and disease conditions.

Good sources of MUFAs like oleic acid include olive oil (the most promising in practical terms because of its ease of use and availability), avocados, almonds, macadamia nuts, hazelnuts, and their oils. There is also a high amount of MUFA in sunflower and safflower oils, but their content of omega-6 fatty acids is also high, possibly outweighing the benefit. Some MUFA is created in the production of artificially hydrogenated soy, canola, and other oils as well; but that also means trans fats are produced along the way, so definitely don't go there.

One extremely important category of polyunsaturated oils comes largely from fish in the form of the anti-inflammatory and brain-strengthening omega-3 fatty acids (the "EPA" and "DHA" on the label of fish oil). These healthy fats should be a priority in your eating habits because a higher intake of omega-3s has been associated with decreased risk of cardiovascular diseases, improvements in brain and neurological function, decreases in arthritis pain and autoimmune disease symptoms like those of in rheumatoid arthritis or Crohn's disease, and improvements in anxiety, ADHD, and insomnia.

Other food sources of omega-3 include nuts, flax, and canola oils, but fish is the best source. (Sorry, vegans.) Some other sea foods also have notable omega-3 content. Algae are being farmed as a nutritional source of EPA and DHA, and you can also find them in grass-fed beef and wild red meat—but not in the grain-fed stuff you typically get at grocery stores and restaurants. All of the plant sources of omega-3 fats also contain omega-6 fatty acids, which have pro-inflammatory properties and may cause problems like increased inflammatory symptoms and cardiovascular risk. You really need animal sources of omega-3 fats to truly improve your overall inflammatory profile.

Increased intake of isolated omega-6 oils has been linked to higher rates of breast and prostate cancer as well as higher rates of heart attack, stroke, cardiac arrhythmia, arthritis, osteoporosis, and even mood disorders like depression. (You can find this information with primary literature citations on Wikipedia.) This is one area where balance is extremely important; you need some omega-6 fats along with all the other types of fats, but it's a matter of ratio. Studies have suggested that one of the biggest negative differences between our modern diet and indigenous diets is the 3:6 ratio in these PUFAs, referring to the overall amount of omega-3 fats in the diet relative to omega-6 fat intake.

It appears that diets like the indigenous Eskimo diets and the traditional Japanese diet contain these PUFAs at a ratio of about 1:3 or 1:4. (They still get more omega-6 than omega-3 because the omega-6s are more abundant.) This level is recommended as a target in your diet for excellent health, as achieving this ratio has been suggested to drop your risk of cardiovascular disease dramatically. The diet in Greece is even lower at 1:2, which is probably an even better target because it seems to be associated with a significant decrease in cancer incidence, along with the drop in cardiovascular disease. Certain labs now offer tests that show the ratio of these fats in your red blood cells.

Of course, there are other differences in the diets of various cultures, so estimates like these, which come from epidemiologic data, are not definitive; it is possible some foods commonly eaten in Greece have phytonutrients with anti-cancer effects separate from the fatty acid ratio. We can't be sure of the effects of the 3:6 ratio by itself, but it has been a consistent factor in repeated studies across numerous cultures and is certain to be significant in its own right. Japan and Greece both represent modernized cultures but seem to maintain a healthier dietary fat balance through high consumption of sea foods.

Our food-fat tragedy
The typical modern American diet is so full of soy, corn, and badly raised meat and dairy products (not to mention the vegetable oils used in

our commercial baked goods) that our 3:6 PUFA ratios are now commonly 1:20 or worse! That is a huge difference from the healthy ratios described above, and it may explain a good portion of the increases seen in many of our chronic diseases. Many authorities and authors have postulated that the 3:6 ratio is one of the most important dietary factors affecting our health today.

Grass-fed beef and wild red meats (moose, elk, probably bison) have a 3:6 ratio of about 1:1 and high amounts of CLA, which makes them extremely good for you. Beef raised on corn and grain (pretty much all the beef in a typical grocery store; even if it says "organic," you need to find the words "grass-fed" also) has no appreciable CLA and a 3:6 ratio of about 1:20—not even considering all the toxic chemicals, antibiotics and hormones; this means the meat should not be eaten.

Remember that this warning also applies to dairy products, such as butter, milk, yogurt, sour cream, and cheese. If the cows ate grass, they made the right types of fat; if the cows ate corn, they made corn-milk or something (whatever you want to call it, it isn't good for you). These same principles apply to pregnant and nursing humans.

Vegetable oils in general contain much too much omega-6 and should not be major sources of fat in your diet. Vegetable oils includes oils like flax and canola, which do have some omega-3 fats and are often promoted by vegetarian/vegan types as being the best oils to consume. Unfortunately, the presence of all the omega-6 fats can counteract those omega-3 benefits, especially if one consumes a diet high in carbohydrates. Most vegetarians have higher carbohydrate diets than non-vegetarians do because vegetarians don't eat the common high-protein foods as often.

Other common plant-source oils that contain primarily omega-6 oils include sunflower, safflower, rapeseed, grapeseed, cottonseed, soy, and corn oils. Those last two make up a huge amount of the "vegetable oil" in our manufactured food products because they are cheap and can be easily mass-produced. The vast majority of salad dressings, for example, are made of these types, of oils, and it's difficult to find alternatives. (Look for dressings that contain olive oil.) If you want to, you can put down this book right now, go to your kitchen, and chuck all the products in your refrigerator and cupboards that contain trans fats or omega-6 oils. I'll wait.

Okay, good.

Many Americans are too busy trying to avoid fat to notice what fat does for them and how important it is to their overall health. This is not their fault; it is the result of erroneous beliefs propagated by people who make money by selling you agricultural waste like soy and corn constituents or maybe even by people who make money from human illness (like pharmaceutical companies or the AMA and American Heart Association, who continue to make dietary recommendations that conflict with the prevailing science). We need to dispense with some of our cultural myths about food, and our current mainstream idea about fat is a great place to start.

Fatty acid supplements

Although there is proven benefit to consuming higher amounts of omega-3 fatty acids, some would argue that the recommendation may refer only to eating more high-omega-3 foods, not to taking fatty acid supplements. Although many studies have been done now showing the clinical benefits of taking fish oil supplements for a variety of medical conditions, it is true that you must pay attention to the dietary aspect of your oil intake. It is all about the balance of oils within your total intake. When you eat more of the healthful foods, you will likely eat correspondingly less unhealthful food, thereby improving your health in two ways: eating less of the wrong foods that can hurt you and eating more whole foods with healthy fats that can provide you with other beneficial nutrients present in those foods.

Conversely, if you keep eating doughnuts for breakfast, burgers for lunch, and pizzas for dinner, but you start taking a fish oil capsule every day, you aren't likely to live any longer. That's like trying to put out a house fire with a squirt gun; you're kidding yourself. You would have to take a lot of fish oil capsules every day to generate a 1:4 ratio of PUFAs while still eating the standard American diet (termed "SAD" for short, which I think is very appropriate).

This follows the "tack hypothesis," which states that it takes a lot of aspirin to make if feel good if you are sitting on a tack. It's better to get the tacks out of your diet! I frequently have folks ask me how much fish oil they need, and I can't answer them correctly without knowing what they eat. The other point I want to make here is that you need a whole-food fatty acid source rather than a product containing extracted EPA and DHA or other PUFAs.

There are about ten different types of fat in typical fish oil, and EPA and DHA are just two of them. I mentioned earlier the advantages of a whole food source over a supplement with extracted nutrients, and this issue is no different. Taking a supplement of whole fish oil (processed to remove mercury and other contaminants) is better than taking a concentrated EPA/DHA product without the other oils present in natural balance.

Many products have omega-6 fats added to the omega-3 because the manufacturer suggests you need them all "in balance." I don't think this is a good idea. We get too many omega-6 fats in our diet as it is, so taking a supplement of omega-3 fats without any omega-6 fats is a better way of trying to get back in real balance. Find a good-quality fish oil supplement, and take at least the equivalent of 800mg EPA per day. Along with a healthier diet overall, this should make a huge difference for you.

You can find vegan-friendly types of omega-3 supplements made from plant sources like flax or hemp (hemp has about the highest EPA content), but I don't think they are as good as fish oil. The studies that showed health improvements were looking at a diet that acquired omega-3s primarily from fish and sea foods rather than from hemp and flax seeds (because we don't do that naturally; it takes some convincing to get us to grind up or eat a bunch of hard little seeds). The studies were not based on people eating krill or algae either, because that just doesn't happen normally.

It is possible that increased fish consumption, with all the other nutrients fish possess mixed in with higher intakes of omega-3 fats and correspondingly lower intake of omega-6 fats, is the true savior here. Until studies are done that show that the use of non-fish oil supplements to raise your omega-3 levels is beneficial, we won't know. A number of studies have proven fish oil supplements can help various conditions and lower your blood lipids, but those studies generally didn't pay attention to the diet the subjects were otherwise consuming. The doses of fish oil required to show improvements were often quite high, and we can't put that into perspective without knowing other dietary factors.

I know I keep harping on the need to eat foods rather than taking supplements, but fish oil—along with vitamin D, iodine, magnesium, and often zinc—is one of those I routinely do recommend because it is difficult to get them in sufficient amounts in the diet. It isn't that difficult to get fish, but there are problems with fish that I discuss in the chapters on environmental toxicity. The issues we have with heavy metals and chemical pollutants in fish these days mean it may be safer to take purified (look for the words "molecularly distilled") fish oil rather than to consume a lot of fish.

Chapter 3 – Macronutrients: Proteins

Proteins are large, complex molecules comprised of long chains of individual amino acids folded into various shapes. Proteins are used for structure in the body, such as the collagen fibers found in muscles, tendons, and bones. Proteins may also become functional components of cell membranes, such as ion channels and signaling complexes, enzymes that perform all the chemical reactions necessary for life, large carrier molecules in the blood like albumin or hemoglobin, hormone-binding proteins in the blood, clotting factors that keep you from bleeding to death when you cut yourself . Well, you get the point. The body uses proteins for lots of purposes.

Protein structure and amino acids

Most of the dry weight of your body should be made up of proteins. (I say "should" because some people have extremely high body fat percentages, and their fat may outweigh their muscles and bones) Each type of protein is comprised of different combinations of amino acids (as is also the case for your food sources). It is important that you get all twenty-two of the standard amino acids in your diet, but eight of them are considered essential because we can't synthesize them ourselves from other amino acids so we must consume them in our diet or die.

The twenty-two standard amino acids are termed such because all our myriad proteins are made up of variable combinations and amounts of just these twenty-two acids, like thousands of words are comprised of just twenty-six different letters. In addition, there are a much larger number of non-standard amino acids that our bodies normally produce for us through various chemical processes but are not incorporated into our proteins. Some of these non-standard amino acids are extremely important as signaling molecules, in chemical reactions, or as neurotransmitters.

The eight essential amino acids everyone must get in their diets are leucine, isoleucine, lysine, methionine, phenylalanine, threonine, tryptophan, and valine. Others are also essential for young children because children's chemically immature bodies lack the capacity to make enough of them; these include tyrosine, histidine, arginine, cysteine, and taurine. It is important to get all of these and more in the diet for optimal health.

It is particularly important to mention taurine because standard baby formula is sorely lacking in this amino acid. Taurine is extremely important in heart function and detoxification of the body; it also acts like a neurotransmitter to calm down unnecessary aberrant electrical activity in the brain. I use it therapeutically to treat insomnia, anxiety, hyperactivity, and even seizures with notable success.

Many amino acids can become "conditionally essential" in an adult because of illness, environmental toxins or stressors, or other circumstances that cause faster nutrient depletion. Deficiency may also occur because of disease and dysfunction in those tissues that produce it for you. Emotional stress increases your need for the amino acids used in making neurotransmitters, and heavy metals or chemical toxins increase your need for the sulfur-containing amino acids used in detoxification.

Arginine, which is made in the kidneys, is needed to produce nitric oxide, the small molecule that dilates your blood vessels when needed. (This is how Viagra works—by increasing production of nitric oxide from arginine.) If your kidneys are damaged or if one has been removed, you may be deficient in arginine. Tyrosine is the precursor for some of the stress-related neurotransmitters like epinephrine and norepinephrine. If you are under stress (anyone you know meet that criterion?) you will burn through your tyrosine faster than otherwise, and you may suffer depression, anxiety, and insomnia, among other problems. You may also have hypothyroidism because the thyroid hormone is made from tyrosine.

Food sources of protein

It is important to know where the essential amino acids come from so you know what kind of protein you need to eat in order to get them. Animal proteins are "complete proteins," which means they have all the amino acids you need in appropriate amounts and ratios (because we are animals too, right?). You can get all the right amino acids from the proteins in meat, poultry, fish, eggs, milk, and cheese.

It should make sense that milk has all we need in it because, as mammals, we are grown on milk exclusively for the first and fastest-growing part of our lives. Of course, the nutritional value of human milk depends upon what the mother is eating. I often wonder how vegans feel about breast-feeding; after all, human milk is an animal product.

Some vegetarians may still consume fish, eggs, and/or milk. As long as they eat one or more of these at least a few times each week, they are likely to be okay. But what about my friends, the vegans? However are they to stay alive and functional without any animal products?

Next to animal products, the next most complete proteins (considered "near-complete") are found in foods like quinoa (pronounced "keen-wa"), buckwheat (which is not at all related to wheat), hempseed (put that in your pipe and smoke it!), and amaranth. Quinoa is touted as the most complete plant protein. If early humans had groped around the forest for a while, they may have accidentally eaten these things, but they were probably never staples in the diet. These days they are pretty obscure and uncommon constituents of our diet.

People who don't eat meat like to point out that soy has a near-complete protein, but it is a legume, so it is too low in sulfur-containing amino acids like cysteine and methionine. These aminos are very important for detoxification, fighting infection, and running the methylation cycle, which helps control gene expression and other vital processes. Other problems with soy I should mention here include that it contains problematic substances like trypsin inhibitor and phytic acid.

Trypsin is a digestive enzyme produced by your pancreas to break down and digest proteins in your food, and if it is inhibited, you may have problems getting the amino acids you need from your food. Phytic acids, which are found in many types of plants, bind up minerals (zinc in particular) in your food, preventing absorption. Soy in its usual form could theoretically cause problems with digestion and absorption to some degree, but if it is fermented, these offending chemicals are broken down and it may offer better nutrition. This conflicts with research suggesting that *non*-fermented soy has cancer-prevention properties and fermented soy may actually increase certain cancers, as I will discuss in the chapter on "super foods" later in this section.

Fermented soy products include soy sauce, tempeh (not tofu), miso, and natto. There are other benefits of soy, such as the sterols discussed previously and other compounds that may favorably influence hormonal issues for some. I don't want to discourage you from eating soy; I just want you to know that the benefits of eating soy foods in various forms are still unclear. Also recall that soy oil is high in omega-6 fatty acids so they should not be a major component of your diet.

You can get proteins with most of the necessary amino acids from grain products as well. Wheat, corn, rice, and other common grains have some protein, but they tend to lack lysine, tryptophan, and some other amino acids to some degree. The relative strengths and deficiencies of legumes (soy, beans) and grains complement one another so they are traditionally eaten together in some cultures. This is true of beans and rice in American cultures, soy and rice in the Asian cultures, and corn and beans in many Hispanic dishes (often rice as well in modern times).

If you try to follow a vegetarian or vegan diet, it is important to pay attention to the balance of amino acids in your food. Many of vegetarians tend to eat far too much grain, which is low in protein, especially when it is processed and refined. Grain at that point is primarily starch and chemicals and much too high in carbohydrates, relatively speaking. This is not at all a good strategy in your diet. You should be sure to eat significant amounts of protein from beans, soy, nuts, and the near-complete plant proteins, such as quinoa, buckwheat, and amaranth.

Alternatively, you could eat free-range organic eggs for breakfast every morning, fish for lunch or dinner here and there, and a juicy wild or grass-fed organic steak once in a while as well. If you needed three ingredients for a recipe, would you rather go to three different stores to get them or make one stop? Animal protein may be considered one-stop shopping for your required amino acids.

Functional proteins

The body uses much of your protein for structural purposes, such as the collagen in bone, cartilage, and ligaments; the large protein fibers in muscle cells; and even disposable tissues like hair, nails, and the outer layers of skin. The more "exciting" types of proteins are those that perform chemical functions in the body. These are your enzymes, the little molecular machines that keep everything humming along on a cellular level. Without enzymes, nothing works in your body; it would be like having a mansion with no power or no people in it. When your enzymes stop working, you're dead, and death may result from the lack of only one enzyme. For example, you can be completely paralyzed for surgery using a drug that blocks a single enzyme (acetylcholine esterase).

Enzymes are three-dimensional structures made of long chains of individual amino acids folded up in just the right way. Their production requires the presence of the right amino acids from protein in your diet, just like the protein in your muscles and bones does. I imagine making enzymes takes priority over larger tissue synthesis, so restricting protein intake is not likely to cause metabolic dysfunction that is due to a resulting enzyme deficiency unless it is a severe or prolonged restriction.

Amino acids and neurotransmitters

I want to cast my vote for tryptophan as the most often clinically important essential amino acid. Tryptophan is the precursor to the neurotransmitter serotonin, which—thanks to drugs like Prozac and its relatives—many now know is very important in conditions like depression and anxiety. Tryptophan converts downstream to melatonin, which helps regulate sleep. Turkey is high in tryptophan, which may explain some of the sleepiness we feel after eating on Thanksgiving. Other poultry and dairy products are the best additional sources, while soy and other vegetarian foods are relatively poor sources.

If your diet does not include animal products, you are likely to run low on tryptophan and to be at risk for some of these neuropsychiatric issues and other problems. If you are under a lot of external stress, you may use up your serotonin much faster and run out of tryptophan even if you are consuming it in decent quantities. Therefore, during times of stress, it is important to increase your intake of proteins that contain tryptophan; this need may explain why many people are "stress eaters." It is possible to purchase tryptophan as a supplement or to use whey protein as a whole-food supplement, provided you aren't allergic to milk.

5-HTP is a modified version of tryptophan, moved an important step closer to becoming serotonin itself, and it works much better than plain tryptophan as a therapy in these circumstances. If you are using an antidepressant drug that boosts serotonin signaling, you may have an adverse reaction between the two. This doesn't mean you should avoid 5-HTP if you are on an anti-depressant. Anti-depressants cause you to burn through your serotonin faster without providing more, leaving you even more serotonin-deficient than you were before. This is why patients often need to increase the dose of their anti-depressants or to add another drug over time.

Taking supplemental 5-HTP along with an antidepressant will help the drug work better for you, or it can even replace the drug (my preference) in some cases. Supplemental 5-HTP also makes it easier to get off the antidepressant without the withdrawal symptoms, which drug companies call "discontinuation effects." (They use that term because they don't want withdrawal to sound as miserable as it usually is when the time comes to stop the drug; and just so you know, the training in my medical school was to treat depression with drugs for only up to a year before trying to wean off them—but the drug company influence over medical education seems to have overridden that teaching.) If you try supplemental 5-HTP, be sure to start at a low dose if you are on a serotonin-related drug, and take supplemental magnesium and a good B complex with extra folic acid.

Tyrosine can also be a helpful amino acid in depression and anxiety because it is the precursor to some other neurotransmitters involved in those symptoms. Again. the best food sources are animal products; chicken, cheese and beans are particularly good options. Drugs like Effexor® and Cymbalta® affect norepinephrine, and the drug Wellbutrin® affect dopamine transmission, in addition to serotonin. The older tricyclic antidepressants like amitriptyline and imipramine work primarily on norepinephrine. Norepinephrine and dopamine are made from tyrosine originally, so I often prescribe tyrosine for people who are taking or withdrawing from these medications.

Tyrosine in foods can turn into tyramine during pickling, fermentation, or aging. Tyramine mimics or triggers the release of norepinephrine and dopamine closely enough to cause some physiological effects, such as blood vessel constriction, leading to migraine or increased blood pressure. Those prescribed an old class of antidepressant called a monoamine oxidase inhibitor are instructed to avoid all these foods or risk developing life-threatening reactions that include extremely high surges in blood pressure. Patients prone to migraine would also do well to avoid tyramine-containing foods, lists of which are readily available on the internet.

More reasons to eat meat

Two more specific amino acids I want to mention here are carnitine and taurine. Both are non-essential because they can be synthesized in the body to some extent, but both are frequently needed in greater amounts, making them "conditionally essential." Carnitine is used to help create energy from fatty acids (yes, it helps you burn fat off, in case any of you have extra fat to lose), and it is vital for nerve health and brain function.

I frequently prescribe it therapeutically for people with fatigue, nerve or brain problems, high blood triglycerides, or obesity. Genetic problems with carnitine production often lead to seizure disorders and poor muscle tone or function.

Taurine is useful in neurological and psychiatric conditions and is essential for cardiovascular health and cellular detoxification in the liver and other tissues. Infants cannot produce it well, so any formula you feed your baby should be adequately fortified. You can even add a little taurine to a bottle every day. I prescribe taurine frequently for various nervous and neurological issues, and it seems to have no adverse effects. Deficiency can manifest as nervousness, insomnia, hyperactivity, tremors, seizures, increased muscle tension, or high blood pressure.

I bring up taurine and carnitine now because of their importance in your health and so I can pick on vegetarians a little more. There are no adequate plant sources of these particular amino acids. "Taur"-ine is called such because it was initially found in ox bile, and it is present in most red meat and poultry as food sources. Carnitine is obtained adequately only from red meat (eaten by "carni"-vores). Your body can make both taurine and carnitine internally, but infants and small children, who really need them, cannot. However, even adult bodies can't always keep up with the demand in some circumstances.

If you want to have good physical muscular stamina and neurological health in the face of life's stresses, you would do well to find a healthy red meat source once in a while. I try to encourage my vegan-oriented patients to eat some wild game, organic grass-fed beef, or bison at least once a month. In my opinion, the healthy fat content, complete protein, and the extra beneficial amino acids make a strong and compelling argument against pure veganism. For more science in support of this idea, I suggest reading Loren Cordain's book, *The Paleo Diet*, on the nutritional aspects of a prehistoric human diet (Cordain, 2002).

Protein quantity

The last point I want to make about protein is how much you should consume. You hear recommendations like "one gram of protein per kilogram of bodyweight per day" (that's 100 grams if you weigh 220 pounds, 50 grams if you weigh 110 pounds), but how much protein you need is based on your age, size, body composition, growth rate, exercise level, stress level, reproductive stage and state, medical problems, healing requirements, and other factors.

There is also a common belief that too much protein can be harmful to you, but don't tell the Masai or Inuit. Excessive protein may be a problem if you have kidney or liver disease of some significance, but otherwise your body can handle very large amounts of protein just fine. We can use excess protein as an energy source, which is why you lose muscle mass just as quickly as fat (even faster for most people) when you starve yourself.

If you are trying to lose weight, you should have a higher relative intake of protein and fat than sugar. If you are actively trying to build muscle or to get in better shape, you had better be getting adequate protein in the right forms. You also need more protein if you are trying to heal an injury or wound. If you are a developing child, an adolescent, or a pregnant female, you need to take in more protein than if you are not. Remember that you are what you eat, and most of your body, outside of the water content, is supposed to be made of protein.

CHAPTER 4 – MACRONUTRIENTS: SUGAR AND CARBOHYDRATES

Sugar and carbohydrates are a category with which we Americans have far too much experience. We need a certain amount of carbohydrate and starch in our diets, but our culture has taken this requirement to an extreme for the last century or so. We don't need that much sugar in our diets, and we don't need any processed or refined sugar at all. If you want to see the consequences of excessive carbohydrate intake, look around you next time you're in public, or tune in to an episode of *The Biggest Loser*. We are fatter than ever before, and we owe it in large part (pun intended) to our intake of sugar.

Before I go too far over the edge with that tirade (and it's a doozey, so don't get me started), let's discuss the good things about sugar. Sugar is an essential class of nutrients because it is the preferred energy source for our body, especially the brain. Natural sugar can be burned rapidly and efficiently and with little to no waste. If we don't have any sugar (glucose) in our blood, we will die straight away.

Simplest sugars or monosaccharides
The form of sugar that circulates in our blood is primarily glucose or dextrose, and that is the form our cells are geared to utilize for the most part. Glucose is what is termed a "monosaccharide" because it is a single, simple six-carbon sugar and it stands alone as a complete, discrete molecule. Monosaccharides can be absorbed from the gut directly, without needing to be digested or broken down first. We may also use a couple of other important monosaccharides, namely fructose from fruit and galactose found in milk from humans and other mammals, for energy.

There are other types of simple sugars we can't use for energy metabolism, such as mannose. Mannose absorbs into our bloodstreams, but we can't effectively break it down or metabolize it, so over 90 percent of the mannose absorbed ends up flushing right into our urine. It turns out that the common bacterium E. coli absolutely loves the stuff. E. coli causes about 80 percent of urinary tract infections, and bladder infections clear completely just by taking mannose, which is often available at health food stores for this very purpose. That's integrative medicine using basic biochemistry at its best!

Disaccharides and sugar digestion

It is also common to get "disaccharides," sugars that are slightly more complex because they are a combination of two simple sugar molecules, in our diets. Common examples include sucrose (a combination of fructose and glucose), our common table sugar (usually derived from sugar cane), and lactose (a combination of glucose and galactose found in milk). Maltose is a disaccharide that is comprised of two glucose molecules commonly found in malt, barley, and related grains.

If you are going to digest a complex sugar, you must have the proper enzyme to break it down. You may have noticed that sugar names all end with "-ose," and it is easy to identify their corresponding enzyme because it is much like the same word, but it ends with "-ase." Therefore, we use sucrase to break down sucrose, lactase to break down lactose, maltase for maltose and so on.

Failures of sugar digestion

There are many other mildly complex sugars in our foods, some of which we don't break down so well. One called stachyose is a sugar commonly found in beans. Stachyose is a "tetrasaccharide" that is comprised of two galactose molecules, a single glucose, and a fructose in series. This is important because we don't have the right enzyme to break this stuff down ourselves, leaving the job for bacteria living in our intestines that do have the ability to break it down through the process of fermentation. Fermentation produces gas as a byproduct, and this is why beans make you fart. (Isn't science fun?) If you want to fart less, you can soak your beans for at least twenty-four hours before you cook them so the sugar will dissolve and break down somewhat.

You may have noticed that you also get terrible gas when you consume milk products, which is probably due to the condition we call "lactose intolerance." Lactose intolerance is technically the normal state for humans after the age of two or so. In fact, lactose intolerance is present in 75-80 percent of humans on the planet, making it the normal state; the ability to digest lactose as adults is a genetic mutation.

The lactase enzyme is not produced by the pancreas as most of our other digestive enzymes are. Instead, it is found in the cells that line our intestines just at the tips of the little finger-like projections called villi. In most humans, these cells stop expressing the lactase enzyme at some point, perhaps after lactose stops being around for a while. In humans with the right mutation, the cells continue to produce lactase until something happens to damage those intestinal cells.

Why is this? Maybe it was a way to encourage weaning naturally after a couple of years so the mother could get ready for the next baby, or maybe it was just a passive occurrence because primitive humans did not have access to milk. Some cultures apparently broke this rule out of necessity; people who migrated a long way from the equator to where it was cold in the winter turned to consuming high-fat dairy products like milk, yogurt, and cheese as a way to survive.

Following evolutionary or adaptive theory, one could imagine that those individuals who could still digest lactose would fare much better than their lactose-intolerant cohorts. Way before toilet paper or indoor plumbing, running out in the freezing cold to have explosive diarrhea after every meal could have had adverse health and social consequences. Many cultures have individuals here and there with the ability to tolerate milk, but it is the light-skinned northern European and Russian groups, along with those in some other isolated cultures like the Masai and Mongolians, who consume dairy most commonly.

Sugar and diarrhea

What is also interesting about this is that people can develop lactose intolerance at any age. Perhaps sometimes this is due to eating a poor diet that does not adequately nourish those intestinal cells correctly or that contains too many chemicals or harsh ingredients like alcohol, caffeine, or spices. One important instance I see often is the development of lactose intolerance following infection with the giardia parasite. This parasite appears to munch away those cells at the tips of your intestinal villi, leaving you without lactase forever because the cells that express the lactase enzyme never regenerate and are replaced by non-lactase-producing cells. This is a common way to acquire lactose intolerance in adulthood.

It seems highly likely to me that other parasites or intestinal inflammatory problems may also cause this effect over time; we haven't figured that out yet. My advice is that, if at any time in your life you begin to have chronic or frequent diarrhea and gas, you try going off dairy products for a while to see if that's the problem before you spend a bunch of money seeing doctors. Most gastroenterologists are just as likely to stick a scope up your butt, for a thousand dollars, as they are to shake your hand in my experience. A colonoscopy is usually a waste of money when it comes to diarrhea issues; most cases of chronic diarrhea are caused by relatively benign "functional" problems, and the colon will usually look normal. Save the colonoscopy until these more common issues have been ruled out.

If you can't absorb something properly, it will stay in your intestinal tract. Basic chemistry principles require that dissolved substances retain a certain amount of water around them in varying amounts for each substance. If there is a significant amount of non-digested stuff and its attendant fluid in your intestines, it flows out more quickly and with greater water content, and you have diarrhea. We use this aspect of osmosis to our advantage in medicine to treat constipation or to clear your gut for procedures like colonoscopies. Many laxatives are either fiber-based or magnesium-based because those substances retain lots of water in the bowels. The most powerful agents are sugar-like substances, which do not absorb at all but instead pull lots of water into the intestine with them (i.e., Go-Lytely, Fleet's Phosphosoda, and others).

More on sugar digestion and absorption

Digestion in general is a very complex and extremely important function in the body. Most of our food is not presented in a way that could be injected right into the blood stream and assimilated by our cells properly. We have to break down complex sugars into monosaccharides before they can be absorbed, and we need to break down protein into amino acids before they can be properly absorbed and used. Some fats (the medium-chain fatty acids) can be absorbed straight away, but most require some level of digestion and complex processing in the gut before they can be absorbed. If you don't have a working pancreas to make the necessary digestive enzymes, it doesn't matter what you eat; you'll starve to death without digestive enzyme replacement.

If you don't have enough acid from your stomach because of surgery, antacid drugs, or possibly the normal effects of aging, you won't digest things right and won't absorb certain minerals well. If you are missing large stretches of your small intestine, which is where you absorb most of your nutrients, you will end up horribly malnourished. In my experience, this is the eventual outcome of most gastric bypass surgery patients; even though they may lose a ton of weight and feel great for the first few years, the patients think it's a big success, and the surgeons think they are the greatest heroes on Earth, I'm here to tell you that the gastric bypass is a slow death sentence for most. In my opinion, it should not be performed unless the plan is to reverse it right after the weight is lost.

Post-gastric-bypass patients may experience what is called "dumping syndrome," when they eat large amounts of sugar or carbohydrates. This is because the digestive enzymes from their pancreas no longer mix with their food immediately after leaving the stomach, but they encounter each other fifteen to twenty feet downstream. Since sugars pull a lot of water with them, these patients can experience florid diarrhea if they eat a large amount of sugar in excess of what they can absorb.

Carbohydrate metabolism

Starches, large carbohydrate molecules found in many of our common foods, are metabolized as quickly as pure sugar. The technical name for digestible starch carbohydrate is "amylose," so the corresponding digestive enzyme is "amylase." You have some amylase enzyme in your saliva—presumably to help get the sugar ready for absorption right away and to make sure you taste the sugar even when you are eating starch rather than simple sugar—and in larger quantities from your pancreas. As a result, starches are rapidly broken down, and the sugars are absorbed just as fast as if you had drunk a cup of glucose solution. This fast absorption is very important for diabetics, pre-diabetics, and those struggling with obesity.

The concept of the "glycemic index" (the prefixes "glyc" or "glyco," they refer to sugar like glucose) is an important one. The glycemic index refers to how rapidly the sugars from a given food are absorbed compared to consuming an equal quantity of straight sugar. Something with a high glycemic index causes a rapid rise of sugar levels in your blood. This is desirable if you are running a marathon or are about to be active in some way because you can get the sugar to your muscles quickly. However, if you are sedentary at the time (which most of us are while we eat and for a time afterward), something with a high glycemic index will spike your blood sugar, and insulin from your pancreas will then rise as well (unless you're a type 1 diabetic) to prevent your blood sugar from going too high, which causes problems metabolically. The result is that excess sugar is quickly converted to fat and then sent to the storage cells we Americans tend to accumulate in our love handles, saddlebags, man-boobs, muffin tops, beer bellies, cankles, thunder thighs, trunk-junk, or whatever you want to call it.

We don't need very much sugar at one time to be active because it is such an efficient fuel source. We eat so much more sugar now than we used to—up to fifty times more than we did a hundred years ago, by some reports. This rise in sugar consumption is clearly one of the greatest causes of our obesity problem, so let's talk about where sugars come from and which ones are better to consume than others.

First, I want to say something about fiber, which is comprised of long chains of sugar molecules. If you link long chains of glucose molecules together in a particular way, you get starch or amylase, which is a viable energy source. However, if you link the glucose molecules together in a different way, you get cellulose (see how it still ends in "-ose"?), which is the tough fibrous stuff in plants we call fiber or "roughage" because it is too rough for us to digest.

We don't have the enzymes needed to break down cellulose and get the energy out; if we did, we could eat grass like cows do or wood like termites do. It is the bacteria those animals keep in their stomachs that technically break down cellulose, so no animal has these enzymes.

You can see the sheer amount of energy contained within sugar when you burn wood. All that hard fiber in wood is a whole lot of sugar molecules put together in a way we cannot digest. (If we could, I might just nibble off a bit of my desk if I ever forget my lunch.) What we see when we burn wood or paper is the raw energy being released from the sugar molecules, and what is left is black ash made mostly of the leftover carbon, other minerals, and noncombustible stuff that was trapped in the wood. When we burn carbohydrates for energy, we generate carbon dioxide ("carbo") and water ("hydrate") internally.

Animals exhale carbon dioxide because carbon dioxide is the byproduct of producing energy from sugars and fats. In the intensive care unit, we can tell when we are feeding a mechanically ventilated patient too much sugar because their carbon dioxide levels may rise too high and cause problems. As for the water that is produced, sometimes it settles in your ankles and lower legs by the end of the day. If you have problems with water retention, try avoiding sugar for a few days rather than avoiding salt, which often helps improve water management.

More on fiber and the glycemic index

The fiber content of foods is very important for several reasons. One is that it provides some roughage to increase the bulk and water content of our stool, helping to ease our bowel movements and promote normal elimination and detoxification through that route; we know this has some effect on reducing colon cancer risk and some other problems. A second reason is that it helps bind up some of the toxic substances our liver puts out in our bile so they leave the body without being reabsorbed. Fiber also binds up sugar and fat from our food somewhat, which slows its absorption, spreading it out over a much longer time. This is why eating whole oats lowers your cholesterol and blood fats (Cheerios™ don't count).

Fiber content is a major factor in the glycemic index of foods because the energy content of the fiber itself is counted in the total calories of a given food; they figure out calorie content by burning a sample of the food and measuring the heat energy released. I often tell my patients counting calories is a waste of time because, offering the analogy that my desk holds many calories worth of energy (if you burn it a lot of heat will come out right?), but none of them are bio-available to me. The same thing is true of the fiber in vegetables and whole grains.

Therefore, if you juice a carrot, there will be a large pile of orange fiber left behind; the caloric energy contained within that fiber is included in the total calories of that carrot, but you don't absorb the energy from that fiber, so a hundred calories' worth of carrot may only yield two-thirds that amount or so in usable calories. This same thing holds true with grains, making it particularly important to eat "whole" grains (meaning they still have the outer fiber layer on them). I tell people not all calories are created equal; it is the type of food you are eating that is important.

The glycemic index of a food is partly determined by how much protein, fiber, and fat is in it alongside the sugar. The more fiber, protein, and fat the better, unless you need rapid energy. Juice is an excellent example of this. If you eat a hundred calories of a whole apple, a good portion of it is fiber that will both bind up the sugar in the apple for you and reduce the portion of available total calories from that food. If you drink apple juice, which has much less fiber, you absorb virtually all the sugar rapidly. If you eat real oatmeal, the sugar does not absorb as readily as it does from "instant" oatmeal, which has had most of the fiber stripped away. Whole grain breads have a much lower glycemic index than white bread and so on.

Sugar becoming fat

With a rapid rise in the amount of glucose in our blood from eating starches in breads, pasta, crackers, baked goods, rice, or potatoes, we get more sugar in our blood than we can use for energy in the short term, so that sugar will have to be stored in some way. Some ends up as glycogen in our muscles and liver. Glycogen is our animal version of starch, a chain of glucose molecules linked together. It can be rapidly broken down into glucose molecules for immediate use in your muscles or released from the liver into the bloodstream when your blood sugar levels drop.

If you exceed the amount of glucose that can be stored as glycogen, which is easy to do, especially if you don't have much muscle mass, the excess sugar is converted to fat and transported to your fat cells for later use (hopefully). This conversion occurs primarily in the liver, so high sugar intake can lead to fatty liver disease. Fatty liver disease, which is now present to some extent in about 25 percent of American adults, can even progress to cirrhosis and liver failure if not properly addressed. There is no effective drug for this problem, and there never will be; you have to fix your diet.

Most Americans already have a fatty butt, fatty hips, and a fatty belly. Most of that visible fat is also a testament to the excess sugar eaten by the individual. Many nutritionists (and the American Medical and Heart Associations) still propagate the erroneous idea that dietary fat causes obesity, but obesity is clearly more often due to dietary sugar, especially that obtained from processed grain products and processed sugar or sweeteners like corn syrup.

Let's talk about corn syrup for a minute because this one really irks me. True "corn syrup" is just a sweet liquid extracted from corn. Primarily glucose in composition, it has been around for many decades as a natural sweetener. Although it's largely pure sugar, your body can process and deal with naturally. "High fructose corn syrup" (HFCS), on the other hand, has been chemically processed and is a mixture of glucose, fructose, and other crap, including chemical and heavy metal toxins.

Mercury has been found in a significant percentage of HFCS samples with one 2008 study showing over 80 percent contamination rate among the sources sampled (Wallinga, 2009). Various other studies in the past several years have found measurable levels of mercury in 30–50 percent of processed foods containing HFCS. Given the extreme toxicity of mercury and the fact that Americans consume gallons of corn syrup annually, this is bad news indeed.

In addition, we do not appear to process HFCS correctly in our bodies. HFCS is an artificial substance, so our cells do not possess the enzymes designed to break the stuff down correctly; this results in an inflammatory response within the body, increasing various disease symptoms and cardiovascular risk significantly. Our inability to break it down also results in a more rapid accumulation of fat in the liver and elsewhere because the stuff ends up being stored rather than utilized. The type of fat created from HFCS doesn't seem to be readily usable either because I see people having one heck of a time losing it.

I have been shocked and disgusted by recent TV commercials that attempt (and, no doubt, often succeed) to convince the public that HFCS is just a natural sugar derived from corn that poses no health risk. The rates of obesity in this country have clearly increased sharply since we banned importation of cane sugar several decades ago and switched to this domestically mass-produced sweetener. A number of food companies have acknowledged this problem and switched to natural sugar sweeteners again in an effort to attract the informed consumer.

Carbohydrates in food

It is obvious that foods with a sweet taste, including the berries and fruits or junk food sweets we all love so much, contain sugar. Other very important sources of sugar are grains, root vegetables, and starches. Breads and cereals are largely sugar in the way they are typically presented at the grocery store. In addition to the fact that many breakfast cereals are up to 50 percent sugar in the form of added sucrose or corn syrup, the grains themselves have been so heavily processed they no longer offer any nutritional value other than the energy from the carbohydrates.

Breakfast cereal is one of the worst damn things you can eat, in my opinion, but it has, unfortunately, become a staple of the American diet, with an entire huge aisle devoted to it at the store. Most of the stuff comprising many breakfast cereals today is pure sugar and food coloring, along with a list of other toxic chemicals. It's not part of anyone's "balanced breakfast"; in fact, it will throw your kids so far out of balance that they can't sit still or focus during school, so stop buying it!

Wheat and corn are the most popular grains in this country, and they and the other cereals occupy the biggest tier on that idiotic food pyramid promoted by our government, which was created with heavy input from the grain growers and other factions of our agricultural industry (the food pyramid was finally replaced in 2011, but the new diagram still overdoses us on grains and carbohydrates). I have already stated that we don't need that much sugar in our diet, so we do not need much grain either. Grain is not something indigenous hunter-gatherer humans would have encountered, so it is a relatively new introduction to our diet. In reality, we don't need to eat any of the stuff at all, yet grain now comprises the largest portion of our modern diet.

In truth, most grains hold an abundance of nutrients when produced on rich soil and not processed to death. Wheat bran and wheat germ, for example, are excellent sources of B vitamins, Vitamin E, and many minerals. The problem is we don't get that in our commercially made bread; what we do get is lots of sugar and gluten. You have to buy the healthy part of wheat separately in the "natural food" section of the store—the wheat bran and wheat germ are sold separately, sort of like the batteries and action figures that go with your kids' toys—while the carbohydrate energy-source portion is within our bread products in abundance.

You need fiber with your food to slow the absorption of sugar, but it's not there in most flour products. You need vitamins like the B complex in order to process your food and derive the energy from the carbohydrates properly, but those have been largely stripped away in grain processing as well. So what do we do with our processed grain flour products? We get fatter.

Natural sugars, such as fructose from fruit and sucrose from sugar cane and other sources, are high-energy as well and also induce fat deposition when eaten in greater amounts than necessary. The important difference between natural sugars and unnatural items such as HFCS or artificial sweeteners is that they are processed by the body in a safer manner and are more readily utilized without causing inflammation or other biochemical problems. Natural sugars don't automatically come with any chemical or heavy metal toxins if obtained from a clean organic source.

Sugars in fruit are more abundant than sugars from vegetables to be sure, which is why fruit tastes sweet and vegetables typically do not. Therefore, if you are trying to lose fat, you may do well to limit your fruit intake a bit, especially those fruits high in sugar like grapes and melon, to eat relatively more vegetables, and to strictly avoid grains. There are many vital nutrients in fruits, which we discussed in greater detail later, so you should not exclude them from your diet. In fact, natural fruits and vegetables contain extremely high amounts of essential, healthful nutrients that help you metabolize sugars and promote health overall, which makes them a superior food choice over processed grains and starches.

Carbohydrate caveats

Corn is not a vegetable! Corn is a grain, as it is technically a grass seed. Anyone who has raised livestock knows you can use corn to fatten up the animals and "marble" their meat. This works on humans too, as it turns out, and that is terrible for your health. Marbled meat is muscle riddled with fat, where it doesn't belong, and animals (including humans) who have fat-marbled muscle are likely also to develop fatty livers and other health problems. In his book, *The Omnivore's Dilemma*, Michael Pollan describes how cows forced to eat corn instead of eat grass, their natural food, must be given large amounts of antibiotics to prevent the bloating in their stomachs that occurs when their natural stomach bacteria ferment all that sugar.

Potatoes are not vegetables either; they are root tubers with an astounding amount of rapidly absorbed starch and a high glycemic index. However, potatoes are more healthful sugar sources than corn and other grains. Studies of weight gain and markers of inflammation have found that people are less likely to put on fat or to have increased systemic inflammation if they eat potatoes than if they eat grains. This is because foods provide information signals to your body, not just calories. Make no mistake though: excessive intake of potatoes will fatten you up.

Carbs and kids

American children eat very little fruits and vegetables. The government and major medical associations have suggested our kids get at least five servings (a half cup is a serving size) of fruits and vegetables per day for optimal health, but national nutrition surveys like NHANES (National Health and Nutrition Examination Survey) have shown that fewer than half our kids get this much, and that's only if you count corn and potatoes as vegetables (which they are not). If you remove those grain and starch products, the percentage of our kids who get adequate healthful produce drops below 20 percent. One of the most commonly reported "vegetables" eaten was French fries! Come on, people!

The problem is not just what our kids aren't getting; it's also that those healthful foods that are absent from their diets are replaced by processed grains and added sweeteners. It's no wonder our kids are developing obesity and type 2 diabetes at alarming rates. The American Academy of Pediatrics (which I no longer trust at all because of this) is now even advocating the use of cholesterol-lowering drugs (the statins) in kids as young as eight years old if their lipids are high. If we would simply feed our kids like humans rather than like livestock or chemical waste dumps, they would be much better off.

Sugar-loving genetics

Why are we doing this to ourselves? Why do we eat dense sugar sources in such mass quantities and then go back for more? Are we trying to commit slow, sweet suicide? Are we just stupid? Is the food industry putting addictive chemicals in our processed foods? (Yes, and HFCS and artificial sweeteners are among them.) There is a logical explanation for this. We aren't as much in control as we think we are.

Carbohydrates are a rich source of readily available energy. Many foods that are naturally sweet (e.g., fruits and berries) are excellent sources of important nutrients, such as vitamins and antioxidants. If you were living a prehistoric or hunter-gatherer lifestyle (no supermarkets or agriculture to speak of), you would eat every berry and piece of fruit you could stuff in your gullet when you happened upon a bush or tree bearing such dietary treasure. Such natural sugar sources are uncommon in the wild, so they are precious. Other omnivores like bears will sit in a berry patch for days, tediously eating the tiny morsels until they're all gone, even though it seems ridiculous for an animal that weighs hundreds of pounds to toil over such tiny bits of food.

Our primitive brains have regions that are triggered by sugar intake or a sweet taste, and this trigger suddenly increases our appetite and relaxes our stomach so we can stuff it with goodies. If you happen upon a berry bush or fruit tree, your brain and body will help make sure you attempt to eat as much as possible because they're so good for you. Unfortunately, if you instead come upon a box of doughnuts or a plate of brownies (which are *not* our natural foods and which have no essential or beneficial nutrients to offer with their sugar), your brain will still tell you to eat them all if possible, and your stomach will relax to accommodate much more than usual.

Our primitive brains don't distinguish between what is a healthy natural sugar source and what is an artificial, toxic food source. We also can't seem to tell an artificial sweetener from a real one; studies have shown that people who consume diet soft drinks in an attempt to lose weight apparently gain just as much weight and fat as if they had been consuming the HFCS-containing versions. The cravings kick in for them too, so many will go find some real sugar sources to satisfy those cravings.

The other problem is that, in modern society, where our modern foraging habitat includes fast-food restaurants, soda fountains, and vending machines, not to mention the vast majority of foods at most grocery stores, sugar is not at all rare. In fact, it is so abundant that we have to exert great effort to avoid sweets in our environment. Just about every processed food has some kind of added sugar or sweetener (check the label of any loaf of bread), probably in an effort to ensure we enjoy their food product and buy more.

Therefore, you can no longer rely on your primitive brain areas to guide your food choices. You have to lean on those big, fatty frontal lobes of yours, the part of your brain that solves problems, helps you figure your way through social interactions, and keeps you from ramming the car in front of you that just cut you off on the highway. This part of your brain enables you to read labels and avoid those foods with the tasty, tempting toxicators. This is critical because, as you know, if you eat the first bite, you're in trouble.

You can't just decide that you have the willpower to control your portion intake because that caveman brain will kick in and grunt urgently at you to stuff your face. You may have noticed that the strategy of eating lots of dinner so you don't have room for dessert goes out the window once you have that first single bite of dessert. It seems that, no matter how stuffed I am after eating my healthful dinner, I suddenly have all kinds of room in there if I eat a bite of brownie or cookie or a piece of dark chocolate with almond butter on it. (That last one is my guilt-free healthful dessert.) My advice is this: when you start looking at the dessert tray, go brush your teeth instead; that usually extinguishes the sugar cravings.

Non-energy sugar uses

I have a couple of miscellaneous things to discuss about sugars; one is the non-energy-source aspect of sugars, and the other is in regard to alcohol. Some sugars—not the glucose, fructose, and galactose types of sugars we use for energy—play structural and regulatory roles in our cells. They are more rare sugars that are, in most cases, obtained from natural plant sources.

One common structural sugar is ribose. Ribose is most often made from glucose in your own body and is used as the structural backbone in DNA or RNA. (It's the "ribo" in deoxyribonucleic or ribonucleic acids.) Ribose is also an excellent fuel source for your mitochondria, the little power generators in all of your cells. It is sold as a supplement for treating fatigue syndromes like fibromyalgia and cardiac problems like heart failure.

A new field, termed "glycobiology," is elaborating some of the important signaling processes involving certain types of sugars. The importance of this is only beginning to be realized; products like "Ambrotose" are coming out in the nutraceutical market with some very interesting positive results (including in a few of my own patients). Stay tuned on this one.

Another common use of sugar in the body is the production of mucous. This is a structural use, I suppose, although the purpose is not to support any body tissue. Mucous is produced as a barrier to invading organisms or irritant substances in your "mucous membranes," such as the nasal and airway linings, gastrointestinal lining—in the stomach, mucous protects us from our own acids—and other places. You may have thought mucous was made primarily of fat or some other substance because it's icky and doesn't taste sweet, but think of how sticky it is; that's from the sugar. The fats and oils we use as protection on our skin feel oily and slippery rather than sticky.

Alcohol

Alcohol is metabolized very much like sugar, which should not come as a surprise since alcohol is just modified sugar. We make our edible alcohol, ethanol, by exposing natural sugar sources to brewer's yeast and letting the fungi ferment it into alcohol. This is how we make beer from grain, vodka from potatoes, whiskey from corn, sake from rice, wine from grapes, and so on. It is the sugar in each of these plants that is converted to alcohol. You can't do the same thing with proteins or fats because they get rotten or rancid, producing unpleasant odors and toxic substances.

Alcohol is technically a toxic substance also, which is why consuming too much of it is called being in-"toxic"-ated. Most of us are fully aware of the toxic effects of alcohol and that you can kill yourself in short order with a massive sudden overdose (e.g., frat parties on college campuses). It seems like a dumb idea to produce alcohol from our grains and other plants, so why do we do it?

Alcohol may have been developed as a way of preserving nutrition sources throughout the year because they are seasonal items and arrive in mass quantities too great to consume before they spoil. If you try to store your excess wheat or corn all winter, much of it will get moldy or rotten, or the mice and weevils will eat it.

If you enlist the help of brewer's yeast, you can turn it into something that will not grow mold and that the varmints won't eat. It makes you feel warm inside too, an effect that may have appealed to many. It is also somewhat addictive, as most of us know, a fact that I'm sure played no small part in the spreading popularity of brewing practices.

Could alcohol be good for you at all? The health properties of red wine and sake, which have been fairly well established, exist in part because they contain antioxidants and the nutrient resveratrol, which has been shown to extend life expectancy significantly in laboratory animals, to help reduce some chronic disease markers in people, and even to inhibit cancer growth in cell cultures. Traditionally brewed, dark, rich beers and some other alcoholic beverages still contain a good amount of nutrients, including B vitamins and antioxidants, which can promote health.

Alcohol is also a source of pure energy. If you don't believe it, try lighting some hard alcohol, greater than 150-proof, on fire and watch it burn. You can even run cars on the stuff. It is energy for your body as well, and it is burned very much like sugar in your cells. In addition, like sugar, if you consume more than you need for energy at the time, it will be converted to fat and stored—hence the resulting "beer belly."

I once saw a nutritionist on TV (whom I determined had been put on TV because she was pretty rather than smart, as too often happens) adamantly state that "there is no such thing as a beer belly because there is no fat in beer." I have repeatedly run into areas where our modern nutrition education, even for our supposed experts, is extremely lacking. If you consume too much alcohol, you will convert it to fat, just as if you were consuming too much sugar. Similarly, people can have corn-bellies, potato-bellies, and pasta-bellies.

Your problems are worse with alcohol, however, largely because the alcohol itself is a potent toxin in its own right. Alcohol is directly toxic to your liver, nerve tissue (like your brain and the nerves to your feet), bone marrow, heart, stomach, joints, and generally every other tissue in your body. We have probably all known someone who damaged himself or herself through chronic excessive alcohol use. There may be healthy nutrients in some alcohol sources, but they should still be taken only in small amounts for optimal health.

Okay, enough about sugar for now, and that does it for our macronutrient discussion.

CHAPTER 5 – MICRONUTRIENTS: VITAMINS

Definitions

The word *vitamin* is short for "vital amine," which indicates that the earliest discovered vitamins were of the "amine" category in organic chemistry and that they were found to be vital for life and health. Most vitamins are comparatively small molecules that assist our enzymes (a role termed "cofactor") in vital metabolic processes. Vitamins come in somewhat arbitrary categories like "B complex" and "fat soluble," but each is a distinctly important substance with its unique job and source.

The usual working definition of vitamins includes the characteristic that they are not be produced by the human body, so it is vital that we get them in our diet. This is not the case with a couple of notable "vitamins," niacin and vitamin D, as we can produce them in our bodies. They are typically considered vitamins because we frequently need more than what our bodies provide and because there are deficiency diseases ascribed to them ("pellagra" in the case of niacin, "rickets" in the case of vitamin D). Vitamin D is much more like a hormone than a vitamin, so I will discuss it in that section.

B vitamins

The B vitamins are essential for physiological processes such as energy production, detoxification and neurotransmitter creation. Folic acid, which is often grouped with the B vitamins, is vital in neurotransmitter production and an important metabolic pathway called "methylation," which I discussed in the section on epigenetics. (Methylation is an important way to turn genes on or off.) Folic acid has been added to all bread and cereal products in the U.S. for some time now because a dietary deficiency in pregnant women could lead to neural tube defects, such as spina bifida.

In my opinion, it would make more sense to encourage pregnant women or those seeking to become pregnant to consume more foods naturally rich in folate, such as green leafy vegetables, fruit, mushrooms, and moderate amounts of whole grains. Folate is one essential nutrient the vegans can hold over the carnivores' heads because you don't get it from meat sources in significant quantities. I've even read that folate comes from plant sources exclusively, but I have to believe there is some form of folate to be obtained from animal sources since otherwise those populations that consume extremely little plant material would not have enjoyed such excellent health.

The substance in meat representing folate could be something called "biopterin," an enzyme cofactor created in animals in part through the help of folic acid, which they get in abundance from plant-based diets. Isolated deficiency of biopterin, which is usually due to a genetic mutation that causes an inability to produce it, causes very similar problems to those caused by folate deficiency, such as neurotransmitter deficiencies, brain damage, and higher rates of gene mutation or inappropriate activation. I suspect it's possible to get all the benefits of folate through animal consumption in the form of biopterin.

Folic acid can be deficient because of poor dietary intake or excessive physiologic demand resulting from such conditions as pregnancy or chronic stress, and some medications. The drug methotrexate inhibits folic acid metabolism, which is how it works against cancer and your own immune system, so patients who take it must supplement with folic acid. Most all anti-seizure drugs cause folate depletion to some degree, a fact not generally appreciated by conventional doctors, so anyone taking a drug in this class should supplement with folic acid. Anyone with depression, anxiety, or cardiovascular disease likely needs extra folate as well. The ideal forms of folic acid to use as a supplement are thought to be "5-methyl"-folate or "5-formyl"-folate because they are the activated forms.

Other B vitamins, such as riboflavin (B2), thiamin (B1), niacin (B3), and pantothene (B5) are clearly involved in cellular energy production from sugar and other sources. These B vitamins can be found in both plant and animal foods. Riboflavin is found primarily in animal products and tissues and may be the cause of another subtle deficiency in some vegans.

Riboflavin is most commonly used in my practice to treat fatigue and migraine headaches, problems that may result from insufficient intake of B-2. Vitamin B-2 may be best taken in its activated form, riboflavin-5-phosphate, if you can find it.

Another B-vitamin, called biotin, can be found in foods as well. For most of us, biotin is largely provided by the friendly bacteria inhabiting our intestines; this is why antibiotic use can lead to relative biotin deficiency. Biotin is helpful in sugar utilization and energy production, hair and fingernail growth, and some other physiologic processes. Diabetics can see improved blood sugar levels with mega-dose biotin supplementation (15,000mcg or more daily), and there is no known toxicity. Research has recently suggested that babies born with cleft lips or palates may, in some cases, have suffered from biotin deficiency during gestation.

Pyridoxine (B-6) deserves special consideration because of its use as a cofactor in more metabolic processes or enzyme reactions than any other vitamin. It is particularly necessary for brain and nerve function, detoxification, muscle function, and many other vital areas of physiology. Vitamin B-6 is found in many foods—brewer's yeast is the highest source—but it is commonly used up too fast because of excessive emotional stress and ingestion of environmental toxins. The medication isoniazid (INH), which is used to treat tuberculosis, is also notorious for causing vitamin B-6 deficiency. Many other drugs may do this as well simply because they have to be detoxified.

Here is an interesting bit of clinical nutrition knowledge: if you have a dominant second toe, meaning it's longer than the neighboring big toe, you may have trouble "activating" vitamin B-6 to its functional form, pyridoxal-5-phosphate (P-5-P), so you will suffer more readily from B-6 deficiency problems because of a mutation in the enzyme that performs the vitamin activation process for B-6. It is important to note that excessive intake of vitamin B-6 can cause peripheral nerve damage; this toxic effect is seen most commonly at doses greater than 1000mg per day. There may also be a potential for B-6 toxicity and neuropathy with chronic daily intakes that exceed just 200mg per day, because occasional case reports of toxicity have been associated with those lower doses (Katan, 2005).

Those with functional B-6 deficiency may display symptoms like anxiety, insomnia, muscle tension problems, and other neurological or muscular issues. B-6 deficiency doesn't usually cause debilitating or life-threatening problems unless it's severe; however, it often results in chronically nervous and uptight people who have trouble sleeping and get a lot of tension headaches, constipation, and muscle cramps. Those with the genetic activation problem can be helped by taking P-5-P as a supplement to get around their enzyme problem (orthomolecular medicine and functional medicine at their best). Magnesium should always be taken in addition because the two nutrients work together.

Vitamin B-12 is heavily involved in nerve health, methylation, detoxification, and blood cell production, among other functions. B-12 deficiency is known to cause fatigue, nerve damage or dysfunction (numbness and weakness at the extremities), psychosis, depression, and anemia. Many people are familiar with using B-12 shots to treat generalized fatigue, which does help many people. We are also using B-12 shots for the treatment of autism with impressive results.

Vitamin B-12 is special because you have to get this essential nutrient from animal sources; there are no acceptable plant-based sources of vitamin B-12. The best source is red meat, preferably from an animal that ate grass or its natural diet. Vegans and vegetarians will tell you there is some B-12 in flax oil, but it is not the same form of B-12 as that found in animals and may not work the same. I don't know the specific biochemistry of this issue, but I've read it in several places. It's possible what I read was just malicious anti-vegan propaganda.

There is a staunchly vegan population of east Indians called the Jains who are forbidden to harm any living thing. Consequently, they don't eat any animal flesh at all, they don't eat root vegetables or other plant parts that would require killing the plant, and the devout followers are said to sweep the ground before them as they walk so as not to step on any tiny insects in their way. I'm sure they don't have a military or a football team. Some of the Jains get small amounts of B-12 from dairy products and eggs, but these devout vegans must struggle to get an adequate intake.

It has been proposed that the strict Jains in India survive on B-12 from trace amounts of insect parts eaten accidentally on their wild or cultivated vegetation. (Don't tell them because it probably means going straight to hell or something.) This is suspected because, although they enjoy survival and adequate health in India, where their food is mostly wild and unprocessed, when they have moved to Britain, where the food is clean and processed, some individuals develop signs and symptoms of B-12 deficiency. I think that this deficiency could also be explained by the increased toxic exposure upon moving to industrialized Britain, which causes them to consuming their available B-12 more rapidly.

There are a number of other B-vitamins I didn't discuss in detail; I will hit a couple highlights of some for you now before moving on:

B-1 (thiamin) is needed for nerve health and energy production; it can be depleted in alcoholics, leading to psychosis and cranial nerve paralysis. It has no known toxicity or potential for overdose.

B-3 (niacin) is most often used to raise your "good" HDL cholesterol and decrease triglycerides; it has also been clearly shown to decrease cardiovascular events such as heart attacks and strokes, and may even reduce death from heart disease (Duggal, 2010). It has also been shown to be useful in schizophrenia at high doses, as an orthomolecular therapy (See the work of Dr. Abram Hoffer.) It does appear to have the potential for liver toxicity in doses exceeding 500mg per day and may certainly cause intensely uncomfortable and disturbing flushing reactions (red, hot skin all over) if you take too much too fast.

B-5 (pantothenic acid) is mostly for energy production, both via its action as a chemical cofactor in the Krebs cycle (becoming Coenzyme A), deriving energy from glucose, and because of its use in the adrenal gland. There is no known toxicity or overdose potential. B-5, like biotin, is made for us to some extent by the bacteria in our intestines. The best food source is royal jelly from bees (the stuff that turns common workers into queens). I use it in a lot of nutritional IVs in the office.

That pretty much covers it for the B vitamins. I suggest to most people that they take a good B complex vitamin daily to help ensure they get enough of all these. Most of them have no known toxicity, but watch your total daily intakes of B-3 and B-6. You may have noted there are a lot of numbers missing in the B vitamins (no B-4, B-7, B-8, and so on); That is because some of these nutrients were renamed, and others were thought to be vitamins at one point but were later reclassified. Inositol falls into the latter category; it was later reclassified because it was found to be derived from glucose within the body and is therefore not an essential nutrient.

Some of these reclassified B vitamins go by their own names now, such as folic acid, formerly B-9. Biotin used to be called "vitamin H", but is included with the B group now as vitamin B-7. The B vitamins are all water-soluble and tend to act as cofactors in biochemical reactions. Initially it was thought there was just one "vitamin B", first placed between vitamin A and vitamin C, until some of the individual substances were elucidated. That's why they still have the "B" designation, in addition to their specific chemical names. It's all somewhat confusing, I realize; and as

261

I said, some of these classifications are largely arbitrary or their significance has become obscure over time.

Other water-soluble vitamins

Other water-soluble vitamins include Vitamin C, which we all know helps fight infection and prevents scurvy, and beta carotene, which could be considered a water-soluble vitamin but is just a precursor to the fat-soluble vitamin A. I'll discuss the benefits of beta carotene and vitamin A later.

Vitamin C can be found in quantity in both plant and animal foods, (The highest concentration in an animal is in the adrenal gland, which we don't usually eat.) Vitamin C is a vitamin for us because we primates and can't make it ourselves. The vast majority of other mammals will produce their own internally and can increase production as needed to fight off infection, cancer, and other problems.

Vitamin C is not just an antioxidant; it is also an essential cofactor in the formation of collagen, the main structural protein for most of our tissues. This is why vitamin C deficiency leads to scurvy; structures such your skin, gums and the ligaments that hold your teeth in lose their integrity and fall apart. (They technically "melt" at body temperature without the chemical modification catalyzed by vitamin C.) It has also been observed that people with vitamin C deficiency have heart attacks at a high rate. (On long ocean voyages some sailors would suddenly fall down dead before even showing the typical signs of scurvy, presumably from sudden cardiac death.). Vitamin C has been shown in numerous studies over the years to help prevent heart attacks and atherosclerosis (Frikke-Schmidt, 2009).

Fat-soluble vitamins

The fat-soluble vitamins may be involved with physiologic processes around the cell membranes, which are largely comprised of fat. They are also involved with complex cellular signaling processes.

Vitamin E, which is vital to the integrity of the cell membrane, helps protect your cells from the effects of free radicals on the lining of your blood vessels and other tissue surfaces. It is also important for neurological health because nerve cells are extremely long and have correspondingly large membranes.

The term "vitamin E" describes a diverse group of compounds in two distinct groups called "tocopherols" and "tocotrienols." Tocopherols are the compounds with which we are more familiar and are the found in most vitamin supplements. They come in various forms and have Greek letter designations like alpha, beta, and gamma.

It was thought for a long time that the alpha form was the most important, so a synthetic form of the alpha type of vitamin E is what is in most supplements, including all the cheap ones (dl-alpha tocopherol). It has since been determined that gamma tocopherol is probably the most important of the group, so you should look for a supplement with "mixed tocopherols," about half of them in the gamma form.

Studies have been done in which vitamin E supplements were used over a long period of time, resulting in an unexpected increase in mortality from various causes. These studies almost certainly involved the use of primarily dl-alpha tocopherol supplements. As a result of these studies, conventional medicine would have you believe that all vitamin E is bad for you, which doesn't make sense when it has been established that it is essential to life. It is more likely that you need a mixed form of tocopherols and that taking large amounts of just one may throw things out of balance.

Vitamin E supplements are usually in gel caps made of soybean or other plant oils. These pills can become rancid over time, and those rancid oils may generate more free radicals and cellular injury than the vitamin E within them is capable of extinguishing. Therefore, I suggest buying only high-quality vitamin E supplements in small bottles so you can rotate stock quickly.

I discussed a similar study previously in which researchers found that giving smokers a high amount of beta carotene without the other antioxidant vitamins C, E, and others appeared to increase their risk of developing lung cancer over time. One would think that these nutrients should be only health-promoting, but the problem is that we are very complex biological systems, and sometimes one chemical reaction alone produces conditions that are more toxic than their precursors were. Everything has to be in balance.

For this reason, it is important to get most vitamins and other nutrients from food sources, where the proper mixtures of various forms should be present in biologically appropriate ratios. It is also likely that some vitamins or forms of vitamins haven't been discovered yet. Vitamin E can be found in various animal and plant sources, with the tocopherols somewhat richer in animal products like milk, eggs, butter, and meat. The tocotrienols are not well understood, but they appear to be important for nerve health, while the tocopherols are more associated with the antioxidant functions. The tocotrienols are very high in some plant sources like spinach, other leafy greens, and avocados and in oils like wheat germ oil, palm oil, and others.

There are no good supplements available for the tocotrienol forms of vitamin E, so you need to get these essential nutrients from eating whole foods. A recent study of American children found that fewer than half of our children get the recommended daily intake of vitamin E, probably because they eat mostly processed food. It's no wonder that learning disabilities, attention deficit problems, hyperactivity, and mood disorders are on the rise among our children.

The form of a vitamin when it is taken is often very important, as is the case with vitamins E, folate, B-2, and B-6, for example. This is a complicated issue that is specific to each vitamin and the condition for which it is being used. A full discussion of this issue would require too much detail to include in this text, as is a complete discussion of every nutrient, its action, dosing, and therapeutic applications. For more information on vitamins, minerals and macronutrients, I direct you to *Clinical Nutrition: A Functional Approach*, published by the Institute for Functional Medicine (available at www.functionalmedicine.org). This book is easy to read, contains useful and concise information, and will tell you what foods contain the most of each known vitamin and mineral. I refer to it frequently.

Vitamin A, also a fat-soluble vitamin, comes in different forms as well. Many consider beta carotene to be vitamin A, but the carotenoids—there are a bunch of them, not just the "beta" form—likely have some of their own important health properties. No toxicity has ever been described with excessive intake of naturally occurring beta carotene, although toxicity from overdose of vitamin A itself is widely reported (such as from eating polar bear liver). Vitamin A toxicity is thought by many integrative and nutritional practitioners to have been exaggerated, and some believe there is no real toxicity at all.

It's the carotene content that provide the yellow and orange colors for many natural plant foods like carrots and red and yellow peppers; they are also highly represented in most green plant foods, though the green chlorophyll overpowers them in terms of color. The carotenes are found strictly in plants, while pre-formed vitamin A can be obtained from animal tissue or dairy products. Herbivores and omnivores presumably derive some from the carotenes in their diets, and carnivores get vitamin A by eating other animals.

You may have noticed that if a child eats a lot of carrots or sweet potatoes, his or her skin will turn somewhat orange. This is just from accumulated carotenes in the skin; you can differentiate it from jaundice (which is due to accumulated bilirubin) because the whites of the eyes do not turn yellow from hypercarotenemia, but they are the first area to become yellow in jaundice. This is because bilirubin has an affinity for elastic tissue, while carotenes do not. The hypercarotenemia reaction may indicate iodine deficiency because you need iodine to convert carotenes to vitamin A. The richest sources of real vitamin A are butter and liver, including the cod liver oil your mother or grandmother may have forced upon you.

It is hard to tease out the specific benefits of the carotenes, but vitamin A is clearly very helpful for eye problems and vision. The chemical name is of vitamin A is "retinol" because it is present in the retina of the eye, and vitamin A deficiency classically causes night blindness. Other symptoms include skin problems like eczema and acne and respiratory and cardiovascular issues. Vitamin A is also important for the manufacture and metabolism of steroid hormones in the body, and it is an antioxidant, along with vitamins C and E. I use it most often in high doses for acute respiratory infections or skin conditions like acne.

You require iodine to produce vitamin A from beta carotene. I will discuss iodine more at length in the next section of this chapter, but note that a person who looks deficient in vitamin A may instead be primarily deficient in iodine. This condition is most prevalent in those who eat little or no animal products and who depend upon conversion of beta carotene for most or all of their vitamin A. They may have impaired night vision, dry, bumpy skin, dry eyes or mouth, and yellowing at the bottoms of their feet (because of early carotene accumulation).

Because of complicated issues like these, it is important to find a physician or other practitioner who knows something about nutrition and biochemistry to help solve your health problems. Every chemical process in the body is linked to various others, and it is often extremely difficult to sort it all out.

The last fat-soluble vitamin to discuss here is vitamin K. Vitamin K comes in several forms. The two naturally occurring forms are vitamin K1 (phylloquinone) and vitamin K2 (menaquinone). To make things even more complicated, vitamin K2 comes in various other forms based the number of a certain added chemical group that is attached. The most common ones are menaquinone-4 and menaquinone-7, the latter version being the most potent and important.

To make things even more complex, as the pharmaceutical industry often does, there are three synthetic versions of vitamin K, termed K3, K4, and K5. These were developed so they could be patented and sold for use in pharmaceuticals and OTC vitamins for nutritional replacement. Of course, they don't work the same as natural vitamin K, and K3 was even banned by the FDA because of serious toxicity problems. This is another example of how a tiny change in a molecule can have extreme consequences and why we shouldn't mess around with nature.

Vitamin K1, the first version discovered, is found primarily in green plants like parsley, spinach, chard, broccoli, kale, avocado, and kiwi. It has been primarily associated with improving blood clotting, thereby preventing excessive bruising and bleeding problems. This is why patients are often cautioned to avoid high intakes of these foods when they are on the anticoagulant (blood-thinning) drugs Warfarin or Coumadin. This important action is also why these nutrients are termed "vitamin K" in the first place; the K stands for "koagulation" in German.

Vitamin K2 is found primarily in animal foods like meat, eggs, and milk; but especially in fermented dairy products because it is largely produced by the bacteria used to culture them. It is also found in significant amounts in natto, a fermented soy product, again because it is produced by the bacterial cultures, and not because it is contained in soy. A considerable amount of your daily vitamin K in all forms comes from your intestinal bacteria, which is one reason patients on Warfarin have to be cautious about taking any antibiotics, as they will lose a lot of vitamin K suddenly and risk serious bleeding.

Vitamin K2 (especially menaquinone-7) is so important for proper bone development that it is thought to be Dr. Weston Price's "X-factor." Dr. Price postulated that there must be something in the natural foods indigenous people were eating that caused the dramatic difference in the formation of their facial bones, jaw, and teeth as well as their overall health. Many of these populations were consuming raw dairy and fermented raw dairy in great amounts, while others ate green plants from the land and sea. (There is a large amount of vitamin K in seaweed.)

That vitamin K2 is essential to bone development may be one of the reasons that cooking the milk or meat fed to Dr. Pottenger's cats led to such disastrous health. The heat likely degraded this fragile chemical and contributed to the rapid generational changes in bone structure he witnessed. In addition, those with liver disease usually become vitamin

K-deficient because they can't store it properly, and drugs like aspirin and barbiturates have been shown to induce deficiency.

Vitamin toxicity

It seems to be very difficult to induce the vitamin A toxicity that is so widely feared. The stories about eating bear livers may be true, but how much vitamin A that entails has not been determined. Nutritionally minded practitioners, myself included, sometimes prescribe as much as 400,000iu of vitamin A daily—the RDA is 5,000iu for adults—for as long as a few weeks to clear severe acne, maintaining patients on 50,000iu daily for long periods without seeing any sign of toxicity. High quantities of vitamin A are supposedly toxic to the liver, but I have never seen a specific amount published. The most important caution is for pregnant women because vitamin A in daily intakes greater than 10,000iu per day is thought to cause birth defects. This warning may be based on questionable data but why take the chance?

It is widely believed that the fat-soluble vitamins may cause toxicity because they can accumulate in your tissues, while the water-soluble vitamins won't cause toxicity because they just flush out in the urine. However, that is not true since it is theoretically possible to overdose on anything. Still, I've not heard of a case of overdosing on vitamin K, one of only four fat-soluble vitamins, provided you count vitamin D as one. There is some neurological toxicity reported with high amounts of vitamin E supplementation.

Most of the water-soluble vitamins have no toxicity at all, even at extremely high intakes. This includes vitamin C; though you'll get wicked diarrhea with high oral intake, I have given 100,000mg at a time intravenously to cancer patients with no adverse effects. I have mentioned the lack of toxicity for some B vitamins, such as thiamin, B-12, folate, B-5, and biotin. However, niacin has well-described toxicity, which can cause serious liver damage at doses exceeding 2,000-3,000mg daily. Of course niacin is produced internally, so technically it isn't even a vitamin.

Vitamin B-6 may allegedly "antagonize itself", by overloading its own binding sites and enzymatic conversion process. Neurological problems, primarily damage to sensory nerves, are the main asserted symptoms of toxicity. Toxicity was thought for many years to occur (in adults) only at doses of 500mg per day or greater (Cohen, 1986), but has since been shown to occur at much lower doses in some cases. The widely accepted safety limit in adults is currently 200mg per day. There have been cases of suspected toxicity reported at doses lower than that taken over extended periods of time, but there could be genetics or numerous other factors involved.

It is important to revisit the concept of biochemical individuality because one person may experience toxicity from a nutrient at a fraction of the dose that would be required to harm another person. There are factors involving genetics, nutrition, and toxicity status that play a role in an individual's tolerance for a given substance. You don't usually know who you are in this regard, so it is important to proceed with caution and work with a knowledgeable professional if you want to practice orthomolecular medicine with therapeutic doses of nutrients. Functional tests, such as urine organic acid panels, work best for this purpose.

Vitamin supplements and the RDA

I've discussed most of the known vitamins, but there are likely many more we have not yet identified. For this reason and many others, it is important to eat natural, whole foods, many in their "raw" form, so as not to break down any important chemicals. (I eat raw red meat from bison, moose, and other wild or naturally raised animals, but I can't recommend this practice for you.) It is vital you try to get vitamins in their proper form from foods rather than relying strictly on supplements, even if they are carefully produced from natural sources.

I don't mean to discourage the use of vitamin supplements, as they can be extremely helpful for ensuring adequate intakes and treating specific conditions therapeutically. In some cases, it may be very important to supplement your diet with particular vitamins. This includes taking significant amounts of vitamin D if you live far from the equator or high amounts of vitamin C if you are regularly exposed to environmental toxins or germs.

The pitiful handful of vitamins and minerals put back into "enriched flour" after all the nutrients have first been stripped from the grain through processing is a cruel joke, and most processed food has nothing of value to you any more except as an energy source. Since most Americans are carrying around enough stored energy to last for weeks, this is a very poor foraging strategy. Eating a highly processed diet will also lead to multiple nutrient deficiencies in most people. On that note, I want to close the vitamin discussion with a tirade about the "recommended daily allowance" (RDA) and the concept of deficiency.

The RDA for individual nutrients was originally based on the amount found necessary to prevent severe deficiency diseases, taking no account of how much might be optimal for human health. It's not that the RDA isn't useful information; it's just that it's a ridiculous basis on which to base nutrient supplementation. In most cases, there is a huge difference between the amount of a vitamin or mineral that barely keeps you from death or terrible suffering and the amount that enables you to function at your best. As a healer and a parent, I want to know how much is good or optimal to take, not how much I need to survive.

A good example most can relate to involves intake of vitamin C. The RDA for vitamin C in adults is about 60mg. That's right, just 60mg. Can you find me a vitamin C supplement anywhere that contains just 60mg? It may be found at that level in some cheap multivitamins because it is a bulky nutrient and they are just covering the RDA for everything, but everyone knows that if you feel you are getting ill, you take vitamin C on the order of thousands of milligrams per day. Sixty milligrams is just "pissing in the wind" when you're sick, but at least you won't get scurvy, right?

The RDA for most B vitamins is in the single digits in terms of milligrams per day, and in the cases of B-12, folate, and biotin, it is mere micrograms. It may take only 2mg per day of thiamin to prevent beriberi, but we give a standard 100mg to alcoholics when they hit the emergency room. It may only take 20mg of niacin per day to prevent pellagra, but 2,000mg per day might make a huge difference in schizophrenia or significantly lower your cholesterol. The list goes on for the B vitamins, most of which have no documented toxicity.

Similar issues exist with many minerals, which are the topic of the next portion of this chapter. Many minerals have the potential to cause toxicity in excessive doses, but most have health benefits when taken at levels far above their respective RDAs. What makes this whole concept even more ridiculous is the recent proposition by the FDA to limit all OTC nutritional products to no greater than the RDA for any individual nutrient per serving. I wonder who's behind that nonsense. Could it be the drug companies, which benefit financially when people are sick?

CHAPTER 6 – MICRONUTRIENTS: MINERALS

I have less to say on minerals than I did on vitamins since this book needs to be light enough to carry around. For an excellent account of the major minerals, their purpose in the body, their food sources, and potential toxicity, I refer interested readers to the text on clinical nutrition published by the IFM. I mention here some important concepts about minerals in general and discuss individually some of the more important minerals in medical practice.

Definitions

Minerals, as they are discussed in medicine, are the pure individual elements that are found in the periodic table of elements you may recall from chemistry class. Some minerals, such as calcium, magnesium, and iron, play an important role in our health, and some, such as mercury, arsenic, and lead, cause terrible toxicity. Others have no role in the human body, but have no inherent toxicity either. Remember, just because something is "natural" doesn't mean it is good for you!

Many other "mineral" substances are in rocks, dirt, and the earth's crust, including compounds like granite and quartz. For the sake of this discussion, I refer here only to those elemental minerals important to health and normal function. I also discuss some individual solid elements that aren't usually called minerals but that play important roles in your health.

Examples in this last category include iodine, which is in the elemental category termed "halides," and the minerals sodium and potassium, which are typically referred to as "electrolytes," rather than minerals. Chloride is usually grouped with the electrolytes, although it is technically a halide like iodine. I discuss sodium, potassium, and chloride in the section on salt because they serve mainly electrical or membrane transport functions. The discussion focuses on those elements most typically referred to as beneficial minerals.

Functions of minerals in the body

The nutritionally vital minerals have been identified as such because of noted symptoms of illness resulting from their deficiency in the diet. Some minerals are needed for structural support (e.g., calcium in bones), but most are needed because they are cofactors for enzymatic functions in the body or because they perform other necessary biochemical purposes (e.g., iron in the hemoglobin complex). Recall that enzymes are large protein molecules that perform biochemical jobs like the transformation of other molecules, digestion, detoxification, neurotransmitter formation, and many other processes needed to support life and health.

A cofactor helps a given metabolic reaction run faster and more efficiently. Many enzymes use minerals bound in certain places on the enzyme to make the enzymatic reactions move many times faster, with little or no enzyme function if the necessary mineral is absent. This binding of minerals can frequently be the difference between health and illness or even life and death. For example, you need zinc and copper in order for vital immune system and antioxidant enzymes to work and for the normal formation of collagen important for skin health and wound healing.

Minerals other than sodium, potassium, and chloride can also perform important electrically relevant functions on nerve and muscle cells, including those in the heart and brain. Magnesium and calcium are the two most important minerals in this area; significant deviations in their levels in the blood can rapidly lead to death from electrical disturbances in the heart. Magnesium is the primary treatment indicated for a cardiac rhythm emergency called "torsades de pointes," which is likely to be fatal without the rapid administration of intravenous magnesium. Drugs won't fix it.

You can have too much of a good thing, however, because hypercalcemia (too much calcium in the blood) or hyperkalemia (too much potassium) can lead to fatal heart arrhythmia as well, and excessive administration of intravenous magnesium can lead to respiratory suppression, heart failure, and coma in short order. However, it takes a lot of calcium or magnesium to cause these negative effects.

Mineral balance and toxicity

Mineral utilization in the body is complex; some minerals need to be in proper balance with other particular minerals or nutrients for proper absorption and function. For example, you absorb calcium better if it is taken with magnesium, but that is at the relative expense of the magnesium itself, and it also depends greatly on your level of vitamin D. You need sufficient stomach acid and the co-ingestion of vitamin C to absorb iron properly; magnesium assists the performance of more than three hundred biochemical reactions in the body but generally also requires the presence of adequate vitamin B-6 to do so.

Most minerals have well-described deficiency symptoms, and most have some degree of toxicity at certain levels intakes as well, with the ranges of deficiency and toxicity varying widely among the individual nutrients. An adult man needs about 10mg per day of zinc minimum, probably 50mg per day optimally when supplementing, while 100mg per day may well be too much for some people over time; this results in about a 90mg difference and ten-fold range between too little and too much. Zinc doesn't seem to have much toxicity of its own at these levels, but it causes a copper imbalance problem, resulting in copper-deficiency anemia and neurological issues. Therefore, about 1mg of copper for every 50mg of zinc is recommended to prevent this imbalance.

Similarly, adults need a minimum of about 50mcg of selenium per day, and about 200mcg per day optimally for most people. (These are my suggested levels, not the RDAs). Selenium can become toxic with chronic daily supplementation above 400mcg per day, so there are only a few hundred micrograms (a thousand times less than a milligram) difference and an eight-fold range between "adequate" and "potentially harmful."

In contrast, calcium has to be taken at extremely high doses to create toxicity from supplementation alone; calcium toxicity is more typically caused by some metabolic derangement, such as cancer, hyperparathyroidism, or sarcoidosis, conditions that can metabolically cause hypercalcemia.

Chromium is a mineral needed at only about 200mcg per day. It has no documented toxicity, even up to daily supplemental doses of 70,000mcg, which gives it a much wider margin of safety and therapeutic range than our previous examples have.

Different minerals are required by our bodies in very different amounts, and they have highly specific dosing and safety considerations. You need ten thousand times more magnesium than selenium daily, and only two hundred times more magnesium than manganese daily. (Magnesium and manganese are similar words but entirely different minerals.) These days you will never likely find a product on the shelf with a toxic dose of a nutrient in one serving, and you will usually be completely safe if you follow the directions on a product bottle. However, you may run into trouble when you ingest multiple products with some of the same ingredients in substantial doses.

I want to share with you a case of a ten-year-old boy I saw who had a rare autoimmune condition that attacked his kidneys and caused him to swell up all over unless he took high doses of suppressive steroids. His mother had taken him anywhere she could think of to find help for his condition. One place they had been was the office of a chiropractor who used certain herbal/nutritional products prescribed based on the manufacturer's suggested protocols in particular disease conditions or symptom complexes.

The well-meaning practitioner had prescribed ten to twelve different supplements from this catalog, following the company's standard recommendations based on the boy's apparent problems. The boy and his mother showed up at my office with a large shoebox full of these products, and when I reviewed the ingredients I found a number of duplications of some herbs and nutrients. Most of these did not amount to anything worrisome, but one mineral was greatly overdosed: he was getting a daily dose of 40mg of manganese.

Manganese is usually therapeutically in doses of 4–10mg daily, and the RDA is 2mg (not that you should care too much about that, as discussed above). One of the main issues with manganese overdose is toxicity to the kidneys, which was the boy's initial problem to begin with. If his kidney function had worsened, the condition may have been attributed to his autoimmune disease. Why would anyone look for a cause like manganese toxicity?

You must do careful research before trying to correct your own problems with nutrient supplementation, and seek out a trained professional if safety is not clear. Obviously, you should also be careful about who you choose as a provider. The well-intentioned chiropractor in the example above was just following protocols from the supplement system guidelines. (I'm not mentioning the particular company here even though I don't particularly like their products for the most part and don't like their promoting habits.)

Like medical doctors, chiropractors get no formal training in nutrition or the use of nutrition as medicine. Even a chiropractor who calls himself or herself a "natural chiropractor" may have no nutrition training. He or she may do muscle strength testing for allergies or prescribe these same supplements, but the only doctors you can feel certain have had some formal nutrition training are naturopaths. Make sure you quiz your practitioners about their specific training in nutrition and research their background yourself if possible. I encourage my patients to research everything I suggest and to bring their questions and concerns to me.

Mineral forms and supplements

Another important issue related to mineral supplementation is the form in which they are presented. In general, minerals don't absorb well in their pure form. Minerals usually have to be bound to other elements, such as oxygen or sodium, or to organic molecules, such as amino acids, in order to be absorbed well. In addition, the "chelated" forms, minerals that are bound to amino acids, absorb the best by far. Therefore "selenomethionine," which is the mineral selenium bound to the amino acid methionine, absorbs and works better than "sodium selenate," which is selenium bound to sodium, and "magnesium glycinate," magnesium bound to the amino acid glycine, absorbs better than "magnesium oxide," magnesium bound to oxygen. Magnesium oxide is the cheapest form of magnesium, and it also causes the most diarrhea because of poor absorption.

I should mention there is another use of the term "chelated" in nutraceutical manufacturing. You will see some products listing simply "chelated" minerals on the label, without naming the chemical form itself (such as selenomethionine). This can refer to a process by which raw mineral substrates are sprayed with a protein substance such as hydrolyzed whey protein. The expectation is that the minerals will end up stuck to amino acids within the protein applied, but that is not a safe assumption at all. You really want to use products that have specific amino-chelated forms of minerals named on the label. If you do, you will get something worthwhile for your hard-earned money, rather than something that may largely end up in the toilet.

You should also notice whether the amount of a mineral listed on a supplement label is related to the mineral itself or to the bulk form it is coming in. For example, 1000mg of magnesium oxide yields only about 400mg of actual magnesium; therefore, if the label says "magnesium oxide – 400mg" you are getting 160mg of actual magnesium, and if it says "magnesium (from magnesium oxide) – 400mg," you are getting 400mg of magnesium in 1000mg of magnesium oxide.

This distinction is especially important when you're trying to get a certain dose of a mineral, and it's one way the supplement manufacturers can trick you. The other way they trick you is with the "serving size" on the label, which they hope most people don't read. I frequently see patients who take one capsule of a supplement daily thinking they are getting the doses listed on the label. However, the serving size required to achieve the listed dose may be two, three, or even more capsules. In my opinion, all labeling should be consistent and should list only what is in one capsule, one packet, or one dose in order to avoid confusion and errant dosing.

Some minerals may occur in slightly different forms in nature, based on their electric charges or other factors. A good example is iron, which comes in either "ferrous" or "ferric" forms. The ferrous form is the kind your body can use, and the ferric is the form from which metal tools are made. In my college chemistry course, the professor once placed a magnet in a beaker of water with some bran flakes that advertised that they were "iron fortified.". When he stirred the solution, a bunch of iron filings emerged from the bran flakes and stuck to the magnet, showing that it was the ferric form of iron they had added, not the form the body can use for health. Did they lie on the box? Not technically. Is it a dishonest, despicable, deceitful trick? Yes.

Mineral sources

How are we supposed to get minerals naturally, without having to mess around with these confusing supplements? We are supposed to get them from food, and this, after all, is still the "food" section of the book. Minerals are certainly best absorbed from natural food sources, and you can get them from both plant and animal sources to varying degrees depending on the mineral.

Of course, iron is most easily obtained from red meat, although you can get some from lentils, spinach, and some other plant sources. It's difficult to get enough iron from plant sources, and many of those poor vegetarian/vegan types I keep picking on, especially menstruating females, will be iron-deficient to some degree. Magnesium is found in any green plant because it is the mineral in the center of the porphoryn rings of the chlorophyll that makes plants green, similar to the iron in the rings of hemoglobin that creates the red color in our blood. Magnesium is also present in decent amounts in nuts, seafood, and meats.

The best source of zinc is oysters, but it is also present in the outer layer of most whole grains, so you get it only if you don't "process" the stuff first. Selenium is best obtained from Brazil nuts, but it's also present in alfalfa, garlic, and meat. I can't think of a mineral other than iodine that you won't get from meat, but iodine is a special case, as it is, without doubt, the most commonly deficient mineral in our culture. It is mainly found in kelp, which we rarely eat (and therein lies the problem), but it is also present in animal sea foods, although to a far lesser degree.

Two of the key points about obtaining minerals from your diet relate to how we grow and process food. If you want zinc, copper, manganese, and magnesium to be present in your meats, vegetables, and grains, it has to be present in the soil. We have tended to produce a great deal of our food from the same areas of land over and over again, depleting the soil of minerals. Complaints of this sort have abounded in agricultural and nutritional literature for more than half a century.

The creation of nitrogen-based fertilizers enabled farmers to grow more food than ever before, but these fertilizers did not help to replace valuable nutrients. Certainly the plants grow better in nutrient-rich soil, but you can keep producing a lot of nutritionally poor food by driving growth artificially with fertilizers; you can churn out tons of corn, wheat, and soy on depleted soils using chemical fertilizers and pesticides. You need even more pesticide to protect plants grown without proper nutrients because they are lacking things they would normally use to protect themselves. Minerals don't just end up in plants by accident; the plants use them to promote their own health and protection just as we do.

It follows that animals fed mainly mass-produced nutritionally poor grain and waste foods may not have the mineral content in their tissues to promote normal health for themselves or those who eat them. When cattle graze in a region that is low in soil selenium content, they develop a condition called "white muscle disease," where their muscles are so weak they can barely stand on their own. Consequently, their survival is not good unless their food is supplemented with selenium. The Matanuska-Susitna Valley, where I grew up, is known for growing freakishly large vegetables, such as eighty-pound cabbages and other colossal crucifers, but it is also known to produce cattle with white muscle disease if they are not given supplemental selenium.

How do the minerals get in the soil in the first place? They must all exist in the earth's crust initially, of course, and then the movement of water redistributes them. The ocean has every mineral we need dissolved in solution. They end up there in runoff from rainwater that leaches minerals from the soil on its way to the sea. Iodine can be found in crops grown near the ocean, but not those grown far inland. Plants tend to grow very well and to be nutrient-rich near deltas where rivers flow into the oceans. Soils, provided they have not been depleted through repeated farming, are also rich where there has been flooding from rivers and where the land was once beneath an ocean.

Volcanic activity also puts minerals into the soil. Eruptions and ash fallout sprinkle the landscape with all sorts of trace minerals, but also some toxic ones, such as mercury. We had a lot of volcanic activity in south central Alaska near the end of the winter in 2009, and the region produced multiple heads of cabbage at the fair that fall that exceeded the old weight records. In fact, this valley benefits from both glacial run-off with minerals from the mountains and from fairly frequent regional volcanic fallout. It seems odd that we don't have enough selenium.

It is clear there are regional differences in the mineral content of soils. My area has low levels of selenium but high levels of arsenic in the well water at many local houses and community water supplies. Fluoride is naturally high in the ground water in some regions of China, and the people in those areas are prone to crippling arthritis problems and skeletal fusions because of it. (Look up "skeletal fluorosis" to learn more about that particular toxic effect of fluoride.)

Iodine is so closely linked to the oceans that some people in the central regions of every inhabited continent suffer from endemic goiters (enlarged thyroid glands) because they had virtually no iodine intake from their diet. If you want to raise animals or subsist off your own farming, find information about the mineral content in the soil in your area.

Macrominerals

Now let's talk about some specific minerals because I often find them useful or because there is considerable general misinformation about them. Again, we could spend an entire textbook discussing just minerals and their role in human health, so consider this a scratch on the surface of what you could learn from other sources.

Calcium is the first mineral I'll address individually, both because of its importance in the body and because of the widely held myths regarding the need for supplementation. Calcium is probably the most abundant mineral in the body by weight since it makes up a significant proportion of your bone mass. It is very important as an electrically active mineral in blood and is a frequently utilized signaling molecule within and between cells. Because of all these functions, we focus an appropriately large amount of attention on getting adequate calcium intake in our diets, and our culture pushes dairy products as a vital part of the diet.

Here's the problem though: we get calcium from many different types of foods—most everything we eat has calcium in it to some extent. Calcium absorption is somewhat dependent on other factors, the most important being the presence of vitamin D. In my opinion, if you have a decent vitamin D level, you will absorb adequate calcium from most any diet, including one completely devoid of dairy products. Calcium supplementation is generally unnecessary for most people, and too much can cause harm.

How dare I say such blasphemy? Will the dairy industry have my head on a platter?

Think for a moment about who tends to get osteoporosis (which is alleged to be due to calcium insufficiency, although that's not correct either). It's the northern-living, pale-skinned, milk-drinking, cheese-eating folks. Recall the earlier discussion about lactose intolerance being the norm for most humans; it's mainly the northerners who evolved to tolerate milk into adulthood. Why is it that folks who eat more dairy products seem to more often get a disease thought to be related to calcium deficiency? The fact is that osteoporosis is now understood to be the result of other factors, such as chronic inflammation (Tilg, 2008) and hormonal deficiencies (including vitamin D), resulting in poor bone formation and maintenance.

Calcium resides in bones as a storage place, not to make bone strong and resistant to breaking; this is why bone density scans do not correlate well at all with risk of fracture. If you don't have enough vitamin D, your cells and body will not handle calcium well. Recall that calcium is a common signaling molecule in cells, and some of those signals trigger reactions that can cause harm. Biochemical research has clearly shown that there is widespread intracellular calcium dysregulation and abnormal accumulation in those with vitamin D deficiency (there are a myriad of articles published on this topic, too many to list).

This poor regulation can lead to chemical reactions that cause cellular dysfunction and disease. Poor regulation of calcium from vitamin D deficiency can lead to calcium's being deposited in places it does not belong, forming what we call "calcifications" in soft tissue like the breast and the blood vessels. Breast calcifications are common mammogram findings in breast cancers, and we know vitamin D helps prevent breast cancer. You can see coronary artery calcifications on a CT scan, and we now know that vitamin D helps prevent heart attacks too. Bone spurs are comprised of calcium deposited at the edges of joints, where it doesn't belong, and some people get calcium crystals inside joints in a condition that mimics gout. Both of these conditions can be helped tremendously by – you guessed it - vitamin D.

So most of you should top stuffing yourself with calcium supplements, it's likely that you get plenty in your diet. Just make sure you have adequate vitamin D. In addition, since calcium can be dangerous in high amounts, make sure you don't go crazy with the antacids. Toxic calcium overdose can result from high intake of antacids and milk, which used to be the prescribed treatment for stomach ulcers; the resulting toxicity was called "milk-alkali syndrome."

Magnesium is my favorite mineral. It is the third most common supplement I suggest, after vitamin D and iodine. Magnesium is the third most abundant major mineral in the body based on my definition, after calcium and phosphorous, and it is involved in so many biochemical processes in the body that it would take volumes to enumerate them all. Our bones should be full of stored magnesium along with calcium, but it is much harder to get adequate magnesium in the diet. Good dietary sources include green vegetables (since the green color comes from chlorophyll, which contains a magnesium atom in each molecule), nuts, seeds, legumes, cocoa, avocados, wheat germ, bananas and fish.

There are many reasons why magnesium deficiency is so common. We don't store magnesium as efficiently as we do calcium, it is harder to get in the diet, and it is involved in many body processes that effectively consume it. It is excreted into the urine in excessive amounts if one consumes any caffeine or alcohol, takes a diuretic drug for blood pressure or swelling, or is under any degree of mental or emotional stress. (Do any of these conditions apply to you?). Some sources, including the NHANES studies, have suggested as much as 85 percent of the U.S. population is relatively magnesium deficient, which means that most of us have some physiologic processes that aren't working as well as they should because of decreased availability of this mineral.

Rather than supplement with calcium, which I think is not necessary except for individuals with rare hormonal deficiencies and perhaps those with bone density loss, you should supplement with magnesium. I say this with confidence because deficiency is so common that taking a little extra usually improves something for everyone, and it is essentially impossible to overdose with oral magnesium. There is one important caution, however.

If you have kidney disease, you may accumulate much more magnesium than normal, which can cause some of the problems typically seen only with intravenous magnesium administration. Protection from oral overdose lies in the fact that too much magnesium intake will cause diarrhea, flushing the excess right through your body without harm. Magnesium is the active agent in many common laxatives because, if you push the dose up far enough, it will cause runny stools in nearly everyone. A bottle of magnesium citrate laxative solution at the pharmacy contains over 17,000mg of magnesium; almost anyone (those without serious kidney disease) can drink the whole bottle at once without risk of harm other than an increase in toilet paper usage and a sore anus.

I most commonly recommend magnesium for problems like high blood pressure; heart palpitations or arrhythmia; muscle cramps; spasms or tension headaches; smooth muscle tension problems like constipation; migraines or high blood pressure; neurological excitatory problems like ADHD, anxiety, or insomnia; neurotransmitter production problems; detoxification issues; blood sugar problems; obesity or weight problems; and any chronic fatigue condition like fibromyalgia. I suggest it to just about everybody.

Most physicians and conventional practitioners who can order labs will make the mistake—and, yes, it's a mistake—of checking a *serum* magnesium level in blood to determine whether you are magnesium deficient. This is a mistake because a serum level checks only the amount dissolved in the liquid portion of your blood. Since this portion is electrically important, your body goes to great lengths to keep the concentration within a narrow range, no matter how much or how little you have in your body as a whole. Therefore, the amount in your blood does not directly reflect the amount in your body. If your serum level is low, the rest of your body is probably nearly completely depleted, and it will require a long period of supplementation to get back to normal.

Consider the analogy of your wallet versus your bank account. You may keep twenty bucks in your wallet as a rule, whether you have a million dollars in the bank or are down to your last hundred. The money in your wallet is the amount you choose to have readily on hand, but it does not reflect your total net worth. Checking a serum magnesium level is like looking in your wallet; just because your serum level is normal doesn't mean that you have plenty of magnesium in your body. Your doctor may be certain that checking the serum level is adequate, but certainty never makes someone correct.

The better test is an RBC (red blood cell) magnesium test, which involves dumping off the liquid portion of your blood sample and testing what is inside the blood cells themselves. This test measures an actual tissue level of magnesium and is more appropriate for assessing your body level of the mineral. You can measure RBC levels of many different minerals, and it is generally a much better way to assess nutritional status than testing the blood serum level.

Another problem is that nobody knows what a "good" level of magnesium is for any individual. We know what a toxic level may be in serum magnesium, so it is worth checking this if you are someone who is at risk of toxicity, such as a dialysis patient, others with impaired kidney function, or a pregnant woman with preeclampsia who is receiving large amounts of magnesium intravenously (up to 2000 mg per hour). Magnesium is the only treatment shown to be life saving in this last condition, so hooray for orthomolecular medicine once again! The RBC magnesium ranges posted on labs are not based on any kind of clinical science or experience I am aware of, and they go way too low; just make sure your level is at least above 6.0 (micrograms per gram of hemoglobin).

Because of the variability of the laxative effect, I suggest that people start at between 300mg and 600mg of magnesium per day and gradually increase their dose until they feel the desired effects or they get soft stools. If you push it up to the point of loose, frequent stools, it will also interfere with your absorption of other minerals and nutrients. If you get diarrhea with even low doses or can't tolerate enough to make a therapeutic difference, you should take magnesium glycinate, a more absorbable form.

Intermediate minerals

For the sake of organization, I created this category for minerals that are typically required at levels between 10mg and 100mg per day. These minerals aren't as abundant in the body as the macrominerals calcium and magnesium, but they are more abundant and prominent than the "trace" minerals required in even smaller amounts. Of course, it is important not to lack in any mineral, no matter how small the amount the body requires.

I address iron first because of its clinical importance and the fact it can be toxic, so one has to be careful with it. Most of us know that iron is used to make blood, which is its best-known role and certainly an important one; many patients tell me they "had their iron checked" when all they had was a CBC (complete blood count) to look for anemia. The truth is you can be anemic for many reasons other than low iron, and you can have many problems related to low iron without being anemic. If you want to know your "iron" status, you have to test it specifically in the blood. I recommend you have this test done if there is any question that you may need iron, rather than supplementing iron based on assumptions from a CBC.

Most people who eat meat do not need to supplement with iron. Some groups, such as pregnant women and young children, typically have iron added to the multivitamins that target them in order to support higher levels of growth and development. Dosing of iron is based on body weight, age, and circumstances like pregnancy and degree of deficiency. The form of iron in a supplement is very important; a chelated form, such as iron picolinate, gluconate or citrate, is much better than the common "ferrous sulfate" form, but the most effective form of supplement I have seen is an "iron water" product from a health food store. It absorbs remarkably well even though the actual iron content per serving is comparatively low.

If you have your blood tested for iron, ask for an "iron panel," which looks at the iron concentration itself and the level of iron-binding proteins to calculate the "iron saturation" (ideally 40-55%). You should also request a blood "ferritin" level, which is thought to reflect the amount of your stored iron in a form bound to protein. If you have taken or eaten iron recently, you may have brought your iron saturation quickly up to normal, while your ferritin may still be low. The problem with the ferritin test is that it may erroneously report elevated levels if you have an inflammatory condition like an infection or autoimmune disease, giving you a false sense of sufficiency or suggestion of excess. It is best to check both a ferritin level and iron panel.

If you are moderately low in iron you can have problems with fatigue even though you are not depleted enough to be anemic (which is why a CBC is not adequate), because iron is used as a biochemical cofactor in the enzyme reactions that create energy in your cells (the Krebs cycle). Therefore, you get iron-deficiency fatigue before you get iron-deficiency anemia. Iron is also required to make neurotransmitters like dopamine, so iron deficiency can cause tremors, muscle twitches or spasms, ADHD and other concentration problems, depression or anxiety, teeth grinding, insomnia, and restless legs syndrome.

If someone loses a lot of blood either acutely (as in hemorrhage from injury, childbirth, or surgery) or chronically (as in women with long and heavy menstrual bleeding and people with undiagnosed gastrointestinal cancers or other bleeding sources) or if someone eats a severely iron-poor diet for a long period of time (vegetarians/vegans usually, especially the menstruating females), he or she may end up with some or many of the problems related to iron deficiency. This will also happen over time to almost everyone who has had gastric bypass surgery, partial or total stomach removal for ulcers, and some on strong antacid medications like omeprazole (Prilosec™) and the others in that class; you need strong stomach acid to absorb iron.

If the loss of iron is severe and sufficiently prolonged, you may lose substantial amounts of iron from the brain stores and develop the psychological issues, tremors, and the restless legs problems mentioned above. These issues are sometimes difficult to correct with oral iron supplements alone and may require a series of intravenous iron infusions. I've seen a number of people resolve their restless legs issues after replacing their iron quickly with a few infusions, and they usually feel better in many other ways as well. Many people with this degree of iron deficiency will crave ice to the point of ruining their teeth by chewing through multiple bags of ice per day. I think this craving may be related to the fact that ice in nature is often full of minerals (e.g., glaciers).

I mentioned that iron has some potential for toxicity so I should elaborate on that. Iron has both acute and chronic toxicity potential, which means it can kill you quickly if taken rapidly in excess (acute), or it can kill you slowly if accumulated gradually in excess (chronic). You may have noticed that vitamin products that contain iron in any amount, including prenatal vitamins and kids' chewable multivitamins, have childproof caps. That cap is there because small children can overdose easily on iron, and deaths have occurred as a result.

Iron is important for life, but it reacts very strongly with oxygen. While we're all familiar with the rusting of ferrous metals from exposure to oxygen, iron can also trigger the formation of free radicals called "reactive oxygen species" (ROS) from oxygen within the body. Our bodies have systems in place to deal with oxidative free radicals, which is what "antioxidants" are for, but one can overwhelm the system with a large dose of iron. Symptoms may include vomiting, hemorrhage from the stomach region, neurological symptoms, even leading to death in severe cases.

It would be difficult or most people to experience chronic accumulation of iron, but it is a special consideration for certain groups. Some people who take many nutritional supplements could overdose on iron over the long-term, especially if they're not menstruating women. Some people of certain Asian or African ethnicities have genetic blood conditions called thalassemias, which involve genetic changes in hemoglobin structure that look like chronic anemia because of small red blood cells that are similar to those seen in iron deficiency. Here in the US, where thalassemia is uncommon (it doesn't tend to occur in Caucasians), these patients are often prescribed iron supplements by unsuspecting health care providers. If their actual iron levels aren't checked toxic iron accumulation can result over time.

The adverse effects of gradual iron accumulation may be best demonstrated by the genetic disease called "hereditary hemochromatosis," which is sometimes reported to be the most common genetic disease condition in Caucasians. Hemochromatosis is the word for long-term iron overload from any cause, and the hereditary component relates to certain genetic mutations in iron-carrier proteins that cause affected people to absorb iron at excessive rates.

The body typically regulates iron absorption tightly because of its risk for toxicity, but those with hemochromatosis readily absorb iron even when the tank is already full. Over time, the iron accumulates in the body tissues and can cause organ dysfunction. The most common clinically relevant organs affected are the liver, potentially leading to cirrhosis; the pancreas, leading to type 1 diabetes and malabsorption; and the heart, leading to potential heart failure. Treatment for these folks is surprisingly simple: donating blood regularly.

Zinc is important because of its physiologic impact and the high rate of relative deficiency in our population. Zinc is used as a cofactor in many vital processes involving immune system function, detoxification, antioxidant function, hormonal functions, tissue formation, and wound healing. Because of the increased levels of toxins in our modern world and what we have done with our food production and processing, our need for zinc is much greater than it was in the past. Because of these two changes, we now see zinc deficiency as a very common problem.

Signs of zinc deficiency can include poor wound healing, easy bruising, frequent infection, a poor sense of taste or smell, hair loss, fatigue, widespread hormonal deficiency symptoms, and other problems. An important physical examination finding for zinc deficiency is white spots under your fingernails.

Go ahead and look at your nails now.

If you have smashed a nail in the last year or so, there may be an isolated white spot from that, or if you have had a major stress sometime within the past few months, it may show up as white lines from side to side on multiple nails the same distance from the nail base. However, if you have multiple white spots that are randomly placed, then you are likely to have zinc deficiency. However, the lack of white spots does not mean you have plenty of zinc.

The zinc taste test is arguably the best clinical test for zinc adequacy. The test is performed by swishing a solution of zinc sulfate around in your mouth for 20–30 seconds. If it tastes like water to you, then you are zinc-deficient to some degree. If it tastes like metal, an unpleasant taste for most, then you have sufficient zinc. An RBC zinc level in blood, not a serum zinc level, which has the same problem that was discussed with magnesium—is the next best test.

Zinc is often deficient in those with chronic immune system problems like frequent infections, men with hormonal deficiency or prostate problems, any kid on the autism spectrum, anyone with heavy metal toxicity problems, people with eating disorders such as anorexia nervosa, and many others. I have already mentioned typical dosing ranges and that copper should be given as well if high doses are to be taken, although this may not be indicated for autistic kids because many of them retain too much copper. Oysters are by far the best food source of zinc, which is probably why they are considered a male aphrodisiac.

Trace minerals

Trace minerals are those with recommended allowances ranging from about 50mcg to 5mg daily. "Ultra-trace" minerals are with no established RDA or those needed at only extremely small amounts, such as less than 50mcg per day.

Selenium is the first mineral on my list here, not because it is needed in a greater amount than other trace minerals but because I think it is particularly important to be aware of and that probably everyone should supplement with it. Selenium has the lowest therapeutic dosing of all the minerals I often recommend clinically, but it is extremely important.

Selenium is important for the body in several ways. Like most minerals, it is used as an enzyme cofactor; some of the important enzymes with which it is involved include those important for detoxification, proper conversion of thyroid hormone, and combating oxidative stress. A series of separate reactions is required to extinguish a given free radical molecule, in which the intermediary compounds created may get more toxic along the way before the whole thing is resolved. Therefore, an imbalanced complement of antioxidants can potentially lead to more damage than if all were deficient; this is because some of the toxic intermediate compounds will be generated at higher amounts by early reactions in the chain, but one may not be able to clear those effectively due to lack of the antioxidants required further down the chain of reactions.

I realize this is confusing, so imagine a process of clearing snow off your roof (remember, I'm an Alaskan) by rolling it into a ball and then pushing it off the edge. The snowball you are creating in the process gets heavier and heavier, and risks caving in your roof more and more as you go through the process, until you finally push it off the roof and get rid of it in the final step of snow clearing. Things get more dangerous through the process of elimination, until the very end when things are resolved definitively. Selenium is a key component of the antioxidant complex at the end of the series, it finally pushes the snowball off the roof, so it could be considered most important.

Peroxides, such as hydrogen peroxide, are produced in the body to help kill invading organisms and also produced incidentally in the process of metabolizing free radicals. The worst of these free radicals is peroxynitrite (NOO-), an extremely toxic molecule that is neutralized by peroxidase enzymes utilizing selenium as a key cofactor. We know oxidative stress is a key component in the development of cancer through DNA damage. Epidemiological studies have shown higher rates of certain cancers, such as gastrointestinal, lung, skin and prostate, in selenium-deficient regions such as China and Russia. Well-controlled supplementation trials in the 1990's showed significant reductions in the rates of all these cancers, except skin cancers, in US populations (Fleet, 1997).

I should point out there is significant debate about this however, with numerous conflicting studies, so the selenium supplementation question is still unclear in terms of cancer prevention. For example, the "SU.VI.MAX" study suggested a 50% decrease in prostate cancers for men supplementing with 100mcg per day of selenium, while the more recent "SELECT" trial found no change in prostate cancer risk for men taking 200mcg per day. Many integrative practitioners and organizations feel the SELECT trial was intentionally designed (and its statistics skewed) to refute numerous earlier studies suggesting benefits of selenium.

People with who have issues with heavy metals and those with thyroid problems usually need increased selenium since selenium plays a key role in the detoxification and clearance of heavy metals and binds directly to mercury, inactivating it directly. For this reason, people with high heavy metals exposure or burden become depleted in selenium, which may partly explain why some toxic metals increase cancer rates.

Thyroid function relies in part on selenium because normal gland activity produces free radicals as a byproduct of metabolism, and the selenium-dependent "thyroid peroxidase" is the major enzyme responsible for combating this oxidative stress in the thyroid. Selenium is also required by the enzymes that process thyroid hormone, converting T4 to T3. People without adequate selenium run an increased risk of autoimmune thyroid disease and functional hypothyroidism. A certain type of cretinism, or congenital hypothyrodism, occurs in selenium-deficient regions such as China.

In my opinion, most people today should supplement with selenium, especially if they have breasts, a colon, or a prostate (and chances are you have two out of three). Supplementation may consist of eating a handful of Brazil nuts every day, eating lots of garlic or alfalfa, or taking 100-200mcg per day in a supplemental form for most, although it may be taken in doses up to 400mcg for those with relevant medical problems. Recall that the chelated form selenomethionine is probably the best supplement. Many manufacturers make good multi-mineral products that combine decent amounts of selenium, zinc, copper, manganese, and others, and these products are usually a convenient and economical way to go.

Analysis of data from the SELECT trial suggested that selenium may be associated with an increased rate of type 2 diabetes, but there are serious scientific problems with that conclusion. The primary problem with this conclusion is that the SELECT trial looked at rates of prostate cancer, not diabetes, and therefore they did not control for other factors predisposing people to diabetes (e.g. obesity, family history of diabetes). Given that type 2 diabetes appears related to the accumulation of chemical and metal toxins and that selenium aids in detoxification, it seems ludicrous to believe that study's outcome without more specific investigation.

I must caution the reader that selenium isn't totally safe either; it has a fairly narrow therapeutic range, and overdose can occur with chronic supplementation exceeding 400mcg per day for adults (less for kids of course, depending on their size). Symptoms of overdose may include neurological problems like tremors, numbness or tingling; brittle hair and nails; and a garlic odor from the body.

Copper is a common trace mineral used in supplements to improve your hair, skin, and nails. Copper is needed to make collagen, which supports those and other tissues, but it is also needed for blood cell production, wound healing, and immune function, among other purposes. I usually suggest 0.5–1mg daily, and it is important to get about 1mg for every 50mg of zinc taken. Copper can accumulate in the body and cause neurological toxicity, so staying within recommended amounts is important.

Molybdenum is a trace mineral needed for the detoxification of certain chemicals, such as sulfites. It also has other uses in the body, but I'm just hitting some highlights here, and sulfite sensitivity is the condition for which I usually prescribe it. Those with sulfite sensitivity should try taking a couple milligrams of molybdenum daily. General supplementation should range 200-500mcg daily for adults; check your multimineral/multivitamin to be sure it provides the required amount of molybdenum.

Chromium, which is fairly well known for improving blood sugar regulation, is a key part of a large physiologic molecule called the "glucose tolerance factor." Chromium is in many supplements geared toward weight loss or diabetes management. It is usually in the chelated form chromium picolinate, which is ideal; however, it is hard to find in doses greater than 200mcg, and you may need at least ten times that much per day if you want it to help. I suggest people take at least 500–1000mcg with each meal if they want a therapeutic effect. The RDA is only 120mcg, but to my knowledge there is no described toxicity under 70,000mcg per day. It is important to note there are very toxic forms of chromium, such as "hexavalent chromium", which is a waste product of certain industry and was the subject of the community lawsuits depicted in the movie *Erin Brockovich*.

Manganese is an important cofactor in many metabolic processes, including energy production, collagen formation, bone development, blood clotting, and protein digestion, and it is also an antioxidant. Deficient adults may experience loss of hair color, skin rashes, and low HDL cholesterol (that's the "good" one). The best food sources by far are nuts and grains; very little is found in animal sources. (Score one for the vegetarians!) You should try to get 2–5mg per day, which takes only a few ounces of pecans or Brazil nuts.

Ultra-Trace Elements

The names of trace minerals may be more recognizable, but some of the lesser-known ultra-trace elements have been found to be extremely useful for some health conditions. I will go through a few of the major ones here—the ones I recommend for specific health conditions. There are dozens of these rare elements found in health supplement products like clays, glacier-derived minerals, coral calcium, and other products. It isn't yet clear what all of them do in the body or how much of them are needed.

Silica seems to be useful in the formation of healthy collagen and subcutaneous tissue. I recommend patients drink water high in silica, such as certain spring waters and commercial bottled water products, if they are having fat-reducing injection therapies or liposuction.

Boron seems helpful for bone density. We often recommend supplementing at 1–3mg daily for those with osteoporosis, though daily needs are much lower than that.

Strontium also seems helpful for osteoporosis; it has also been shown to increase the tensile strength of bone significantly, thereby reducing risk of fracture. 150-250mcg per day appears to be enough for this effect.

Vanadium is often recommended for diabetics to aid in blood sugar regulation and insulin function. 1–2mg daily is a typical suggestion in this case.

I'm sure there are many other minerals we need in very small amounts but don't get from our depleted, highly processed modern diets. The ultra-trace elements are often not well understood and are absent from most nutritional supplements. I think the key is to eat a broad whole-food diet, perhaps including plenty of seafood, in hopes of getting all everything you need from your diet. It may also be helpful to supplement with sea salt, coral calcium, clay, or some other trace mineral product. Just be sure the supplement you find is derived from a clean source.

Iodine

Iodine is a "halide," And our need for iodine ties us inescapably to the ocean. The only truly rich sources of iodine are seaweed and other foods from the sea. Goiters, caused by a lack of iodine, have been historically prevalent on every continent where people live a long way from the coast. Those of us who study nutritional medicine affectionately refer to the middle of the U.S. as the "goiter belt." Significant iodine deficiency based on World Health Organization (WHO) criteria has been thought to be relatively low in America due to consumption of iodized salt, but still estimated present in ten percent of American school children based on data collected from 1993-2003 (De Benoist, 2003). Iodized salt intake has been known to decline further in our culture since then.

Who cares about a lump in the front of your neck? If that were the only problem you had from iodine deficiency, you could just wear a scarf, and life would go on. However, iodine is needed for thyroid *function* as well, so iodine deficiency leads to a whole mess of problems. I will review the symptoms of thyroid dysfunction in greater detail later on, but suffice it to say that thyroid hormone affects just about every process in the body. Because iodine deficiency is so common, thyroid problems are also extremely common.

Iodine is also used in every estrogen-sensitive tissue in the body, including the breasts, ovaries, uterus, and the prostate gland. In women the tissue that comprises a man's prostate gland instead grows into a uterus; they are analogous structures. Prostate tissue therefore still has estrogen receptors on it, which affect growth and differentiation (processes relevant to cancer formation) of that tissue in response to estrogen levels. Women low in iodine will be prone to fibrocystic breast disease, which usually goes away with iodine supplementation, as well as ovarian cysts, menstrual problems, and infertility. Iodine-deficient women are more prone to the development of breast cancer; in fact, some studies have shown up to 50 percent reduction in breast cancer risk when hypothyroid women supplement with iodine (Derry, 2001).

Another important feature of iodine is its role in brain development before birth and in early childhood. This effect may be related mainly to thyroid function in the fetus and infant, but iodine could have its own independent activity in regards to brain development as well. It is well known that hypothyroid women who do not receive proper thyroid replacement during pregnancy are more prone to miscarriage and more likely to have babies with cognitive problems. The World Health Organization has estimated that iodine deficiency affects up to 2 billion people worldwide, and is the most common preventable cause of mental retardation (WHO report 2007). Children may be mentally retarded if their mothers are significantly iodine deficient during pregnancy.

This iodine deficiency problem isn't just a problem in far-inland underdeveloped countries and our interior states. NHANES data has shown a significant portion of the US population gets less then the RDA for iodine. Speaking of the RDA once more, our suggested intake guidelines for iodine are based on the amount needed to prevent big goiters from showing up in children; they have nothing to do with promoting optimal thyroid function or preventing cancer or cardiovascular disease. The RDA is currently just 150mcg, with 200mcg suggested for pregnant women.

This is likely not nearly enough for optimal health of the mother and fetus during pregnancy.

An endemic iodine deficiency problem was discovered here in North America in 1811, so this is not a news flash. It took until 1924 for the government to iodize salt for the public and to put iodine into flour for commercial baked goods. While these measures provided a tiny amount for the average person, they were at least a step in the right direction. Unfortunately, in the 1970s the iodine was removed from flour products because of some misguided research that suggested iodine may actually bad for you. Iodine deficiency again became a significant problem for our population, and to make things far worse, they chose bromine to replace iodine in those food products. Bromine is a poison that works directly against iodine and all it should be doing for the body. For more information and references on this discussion, see Dr. David Brownstein's book *Iodine: Why You Need It, Why You Can't Live Without It* (Brownstein, 2004).

Other modern factors contributing to iodine deficiency are exposure to substances that block the uptake or utilization of iodine. Perchlorate is a chemical substance found in rocket fuel, explosives, road flares, fireworks, car airbags and some fertilizers. It can now be found in our food and water with some regularity. It has been shown to interfere with the uptake of iodine into the thyroid gland, potentially resulting in thyroid dysfunction. US Food and Drug Administration studies (Total Diet Study) conducted since 1961 have shown significant intake of perchlorate by our population. Infants and children have the highest relative exposure because they take in more food and water relative to their body weight. Those deemed at greatest risk were the fetuses of pregnant women who may have hypothyroidism or iodine deficiency. This same study found average iodine intakes in our population to be only 138 to 353mcg per day. (Murray, 2008)

Fluoride will be discussed again later in the toxicity section, but I will here briefly mention it's relevance to iodine deficiency. Fluoride is a "halide", similar to iodine, meaning it carries a single negative charge when in ionized form and has certain chemical behaviors similar to the other halides. The halides we need nutritionally are chlorine and iodine, the ones we don't utilize physiologically are fluorine and bromine. Bromine and fluorine are both smaller in size than iodine, and can displace iodine atoms from their positions in thyroid and other tissues in the body, thereby effectively contributing to a functional iodine deficiency problem. (Brownstein, 2004)

Perchlorate can displace or obstruct iodine because of the chlorine within it, another halide. We now have fluoride exposure from toothpaste, water systems and manufactured beverages, as well as other sources. Bromine, as mentioned above, is now present in most flour and also some manufactured beverages and other products. One way to combat all these adverse substances in our world today is to supplement with greater amounts of iodine, making sure there are far more iodine atoms to outcompete these other substances and saturate the thyroid gland. For this reason, I suggest iodine supplementation to pretty much everyone, particularly hypothyroid patients, pregnant women or women hoping to become pregnant.

Aside from the prevention of thyroid, cancer, and retardation problems, repeated studies have also shown that iodine supplementation prevents cardiovascular disease and heart attacks. Feeding rabbits dried egg yolk powder can induce the formation of cholesterol plaques in their arteries, but if the rabbits are fed iodine before and during the experiment, those plaques do not form. This study was first done in the early 1930s and has been repeated at least three times since (Brownstein, 2004), yet this knowledge is left out of our medical education in this country. Why wouldn't they teach me that when cardiovascular disease is our number-one killer?

The rabbit studies may not be enough for some people, especially since rabbits are vegans biologically and don't naturally eat eggs, but there is also a convincing study from human populations that confirms the protective effect of iodine against cardiovascular disease and death. Japan has notably lower rates of cardiovascular disease than we do, although its population's smoking and drinking rates are about twice ours. There are two main differences in their diet: one is fish consumption, and the other is their rate of iodine consumption, derived mainly from the seaweed in their diet. The average daily intake of iodine in the Japanese diet is about 12,000mcg, which is eighty times greater than our RDA (Hoption-Cann, 2007).

But wait, there's more: Finland had extremely high rates of heart attack and cardiac death as a nation but noted that the rates were significantly lower among those near the coast versus than they were among those inland. The government performed a country-wide diet survey and determined that the greatest difference in intake between the coastal and inland populations was the amount of iodine, with those at the coast getting significantly more from seafood consumption (Roine, 1958). Finland added significant amounts of iodine to their bread products, salt, agricultural fertilizers, and animal feeds and saw the national rate of heart attacks fall about 50 percent after this intervention. This information was all presented at an IFM conference in 2007 by Dr. Stephen Hoption-Cann, who conducted extensive original research regarding iodine intake and disease epidemiology.

Why wasn't I taught anything about iodine in medical school? It only costs about five dollars per month to take iodine supplements in the same amount the Japanese get per day, and studies suggest it could cut breast cancer rates in half, cut heart attacks by as much as half, cure fibrocystic breast disease, and promote normal thyroid function. It costs $125 or so per month to take a statin drug to lower your cholesterol, which doesn't fix a damn thing, doesn't extend your life one bit, but does have loads of side effects! Tell me the drug companies don't run our medical education system.

Iodine has not been shown to have any inherent toxicity to humans at all. There is a condition called "iodism" that can occur at variable doses, even low doses, in some people; this generally includes red eyes, nasal congestion and a red bumpy rash. It is also possible to have an allergic reaction to iodine, but true allergic reactions are extremely rare. It is common for patients to have bad reactions to the injected contrast used for CT scans and then be told they have an "iodine allergy"; but those injected substances contain a large synthetic organic molecule *bound to* iodine, and it is the artificial molecule to which they are actually allergic.

It is also common for people with shellfish allergy to be told they are reacting to iodine in the shellfish. This is not correct, as it is really a muscle protein from the animal triggering the allergic response, not iodine. If someone were truly allergic to iodine they would react much more strongly to seaweed than to any shellfish because the iodine content of seaweed is far greater.

The issue that has caused the most trouble regarding concern over iodine supplementation is a physiological phenomenon termed the Wolff-Chaikoff effect. These two researchers (Wolff and Chaikoff) observed a transient suppression of thyroid function when the "iodide" form of iodine was administered. This effect is thought to last 7-10 days and then is overcome by the body, with resumption of normal function in spite of the iodine supplementation. That hardly constitutes *toxicity* in my opinion, and in my experience it is not a clinically relevant effect. We have prescribed what would be considered extremely high doses of iodine to at least one thousand patients through my clinic and never seen anyone become clinically hypothyroid as a result, not even for a few days. We have seen the opposite however, rapid improvement of hypothyroid symptoms, in a small proportion of cases.

Because of the dogma surrounding the Wolff-Chaikoff effect conventional practitioners are inclined to interpret iodine research in a negative light. For example, one recent study found a strong correlation between elevated urinary iodine levels and subclinical hypothyroidism (defined by a mildly elevated thyroid stimulating hormone, or TSH, level) in pregnant women. The researchers interpreted this to mean that the women taking higher amounts of iodine were adversely affecting their thyroid function; this was thought to agree with the dogma that iodine "overdose" suppresses thyroid function (Sang, 2012).

The problems are that they didn't actually assess iodine *intake*, just looked at urinary iodine and *assumed* it reflected intake. That is a huge error, and leads to the exactly wrong conclusion. Many individuals need vitamin C supplementation in order to take up iodine into tissues such as the thyroid. If they do not get adequate vitamin C with their iodine, the iodine will just spill out into the urine. We have observed this phenomenon repeatedly in our practice when doing iodine loading tests over time in women we are supplementing with iodine. It is my interpretation of this study that the women with higher urinary iodine likely had a sodium/iodine symporter defect and could not assimilate their iodine, which is precisely why they also had relative hypothyroidism.

Appropriate products to use for supplementation include the *iodide* (usually potassium iodide) and *iodine* (I-I, two iodine atoms bound to each other) forms together in a roughly 3:2 ratio. Lugol's iodine is a concentrated liquid product that can be found in this ratio with approximately 6,250mcg per drop. We typically suggest one drop daily for children, two drops daily for teens and adults for general supplementation purposes. Note that two drops provides just a little more than the average daily adult Japanese individual gets in their diet, as discussed above. There is a liquid iodine solution available with a super-saturated solution of potassium iodide alone (termed "SSKI") but that is not ideal because it lacks the iod*ine* form, which is assimilated better by the thyroid gland.

There are a number of companies now offering dry capsules of iodine with the same ratio as Lugol's solution, usually containing 12,500mcg total iodine per capsule. One of these capsules daily would be appropriate for general daily use in adults. This is an attractive option for many because liquid iodine taste quite bad to most people. If one does try to use liquid iodine I suggest putting the drops into a strong-flavored drink such as coffee, tea, dark juice like grape or pomegranate, or possibly milk.

If we have patients with iodine-deficiency conditions such as hypothyroidism, fibrocystic breast disease, cardiovascular disease, breast cancer, prostate cancer, or cancers of any type for that matter, we often suggest they start out supplementing with 50,000mcg iodine per day for the first three to six months. As discussed, iodine is found in very small amounts in the typical American diet. It is therefore something with which I suggest everyone supplement using iodine solutions, capsules or even kelp capsules if a whole food source is desired. In any case, I advised taking about 2,000mg vitamin C with any iodine supplement, to help ensure absorption and assimilation into tissue.

If you want to test for iodine status the best test is an "iodine loading test". This test involves taking 50,000mcg (4 capsules of an appropriate product, or 8 drops of Lugol's solution) oral iodine, then collecting twenty-four hours of urine afterward. The total amount of iodine excreted can be calculated from that sample, then divided by 50,000mcg to get the percent excreted. Someone who is saturated with iodine should excrete more than ninety percent of the iodine load (>45,000mcg) in twenty-four hours. If the sample contains less than fifty percent (25,000mcg) it indicates significant deficiency.

If you want more information on iodine, I suggest you read the excellent, well written, easy read by Dr. David Brownstein mentioned above.

Bad Minerals

There are also well-known toxic minerals out there. Arsenic, lead, mercury, cadmium, antimony, and others are naturally present in the earth's crust and have clearly described health consequences that I discuss later in the toxicity chapter. Theoretically, we could have evolved or adapted to utilize mercury or lead as essential nutrients, and selenium and zinc may have been toxic to us instead, but that's not how it worked out in this universe. Remember, just because something is "natural" doesn't mean it is good for you.

Along those same lines, I should mention something regarding the safety of nutritional supplements. Many essential minerals may coexist in nature with toxic minerals, and many nutritional products are incidentally contaminated with heavy metals through environmental contamination of their natural source (e.g., fish oil), irrigation of commercially cultivated herbs with contaminated water coming through lead pipes (herbs from China and India most commonly), or during processing with certain solvents or chemicals. (Recall most samples of high fructose corn syrup contain mercury because of processing.)

There have been many case reports of patients who accumulate toxic amounts of lead from herbal supplements or other products. You should get your nutritional supplement products from a reputable manufacturer who can prove that every batch of raw materials is tested for toxic substances. These may cost a bit more, but they may cost a lot less in terms of your health. One of the websites you can use to find out about the quality and safety of specific nutritional products is www.consumerlab.com.

CHAPTER 7 – OTHER ESSENTIAL NUTRIENTS FROM FOOD

We are supposed to get much more from foods besides protein, fat, carbohydrates, vitamins and minerals as discussed above. The "vitamin" classification can be a dubious distinction for some molecules. Some nutrient chemicals that we need in significant quantities for optimal function are synthesized by our bodies to some extent, so they are not categorized as vitamins (though niacin and vitamin D are–I don't know who makes these rules), but we often require more than we can produce on our own and they are therefore considered essential nutrients by most authorities. I also discuss some other healthy chemicals and enzymes from plants in this chapter; these are molecules we cannot produce ourselves that provide significant health benefits for us, but we can live without them so they are not technically vitamins or essential nutrients.

"Almost" Vitamins

Choline is a small "amine" molecule the body uses in all cell membranes and as a signaling chemical. In membranes it is usually bound to a lipid, as in the case of phosphatidylcholine (PPC), a supplement I often recommend for problems with liver inflammation or brain function. Acetylcholine contains choline and is a very important neurotransmitter in the brain and the part of the peripheral nervous system involved in memory functions, pupil dilation, sweating, intestinal movement, and many other processes.

We can synthesize a little choline on our own, but not enough to function optimally without added dietary intake. Most types of foods have some choline in them, but a person who does not eat eggs or meat may have trouble getting adequate amounts, especially if he or she has a neurological or liver condition that would benefit from more choline. Soy and wheat germ are the richest sources for of choline for vegans. You can supplement with PPC, which is usually derived from soy, and many processed foods have lecithin from soy or eggs added to them. Lecithin contains PPC, is readily available at the grocery store, and is a more cost-effective way to supplement than purchasing PPC capsules.

One caution is that choline in excess amounts may be converted to a chemical called trimethylamine, which has a strong fishy odor. Some people genetically don't break down their trimethylamine very well so they exude a strong fishy odor if they consume too much choline. This condition is appropriately called "fish body odor syndrome," although it has nothing to do with fish. You can help these folks out by suggesting they avoid foods high in choline.

Inositol was considered a vitamin for a time after its discovery and was initially labeled "vitamin B-8." It was later discovered that our bodies can synthesize it from glucose, so it was de-classified as being a vitamin. Inositol assists the chemical signaling between and within cells and helps modulate hormonal (e.g., insulin) and neurotransmitter (e.g., serotonin) activity. It has been shown to be extremely important for neurological and brain function. The best food sources of inositol are plant foods like fruits, beans, grains, and nuts. (Score another one for the vegans!)

Some clinical studies have suggested a therapeutic role for inositol in the treatment of obsessive-compulsive disorder and benefit that is equal to or better than that of drugs like fluvoxamine (Palatnik, 2001). That may sound exciting but the doses of inositol used for therapeutic effect were extremely high, up to 18,000mg per day, and would be hard to achieve in reality. Even at those high doses, reported side effects were still less than those seen with fluvoxamine (Palatnik, 2001).

Inositol also appears to be potentially helpful in treating psychiatric conditions depression, anxiety, panic, and bipolar disorders. It has shown some promise in reducing blood cholesterol levels and great success in treating polycystic ovary syndrome (PCOS). Suggested dosing for PCOS typically starts at 1000–1200mg, but most clinical research studies seem to use 4,000mg per day. Inositol has been shown to improve ovulation, menstruation, fertility, pregnancy rate, and also the insulin-resistance problem seen in PCOS. One study showed sixty-five percent of patients resuming normal ovulation with 4g/day inositol plus 400mcg folic acid daily, while only fifty percent had similar success with 1500mg daily of metformin, a diabetes drug prescribed as first-line treatment for PCOS.

The successful pregnancy rate was correspondingly higher in the inositol group as well (Raffone, 2010).

I'm sure there are many other essential nutrients from foods that are known and many more not yet discovered. I am just bringing to your attention the incredibly wide array of nutrients in food that we need to sustain life and optimal functioning. You must to eat diverse, natural, whole foods in order to get adequate amounts of what you need. Processed food has had the vast majority of what's nutritional stripped out or destroyed, and you cannot live well by consuming those foods in place of what will promote life and health.

Phytonutrients

Phytonutrient is a new designation for nutrients in plants that promote health in some significant way but are not "essential" for life. Of course, some of the vitamins I have discussed, such as beta carotene and tocotrienols, which come from plants almost exclusively, could themselves be considered phytonutrients. There are many different chemicals found in plants that play well-defined roles in our body chemistry, as if we were meant to consume them for our health, or our bodies adapted over time to use them in beneficial ways.

Some of these other plant-derived nutrients also have positive effects on our health and life span, to the point where, in my view, you could almost consider them vitamins. After all, what else would you call a chemical compound that you have to obtain from foods because you can't produce it and without which you would suffer some health problem and not live as long? The issue also raises the question: What's the difference between a plant-based "nutrient" and a plant-based "medicine"? I think the difference is that a phytonutrient promotes normal physiological functions in a beneficial way, and a plant-based medicinal chemical alters normal physiology in some way that creates a clinical effect like that of a drug (e.g., caffeine, aspirin, digitalis, and ephedrine). These lines are crossed frequently by some of the compounds I discuss below, but I won't go into that philosophical conundrum any further here.

Chlorophyll is the primary green pigment in plants that, as you may recall from high school biology, enables the plants to perform the process of photosynthesis, creating sugar for us to eat and oxygen for us to breathe. Therefore, without chlorophyll in the world, we would all die—and we haven't even eaten it yet! Chlorophyll is a large, complex molecule very similar to our hemoglobin so it contributes nutritionally to our ability to make hemoglobin for our red blood cells. There is a magnesium atom in the center of each molecule so it is a source of this vital mineral as well. Chlorophyll is often purported to have health benefits by factions of the complementary and natural medicine community, but none of these suggested benefits seem to have been proven. My search of PubMed, a biomedical research database including thousands of publications and more than 21 million citations, yielded precisely zero studies on the health benefits of chlorophyll in humans.

Proanthocyanidins are long polyphenol compounds in the category of nutrients called bioflavonoids. They are potent antioxidants, are noted to improve cardiovascular disease risk factors and outcomes (Schroeter, 2010). These are the compounds found in red wine that are thought to be responsible for the cardiovascular risk reduction seen with regular moderate wine consumption. These compounds are present in red wine to a significant degree, as well as in pine bark and grape seeds at fairly high concentrations. People pay lots of money to buy pills containing pine bark and grape seed extracts and to drink red wine for the benefits of these molecules.

In reality, grape juice has levels of bioflavonoids that are nearly as high as those of red wine. Dark berries also often have good amounts of bioflavonoids. Most dark fruits and berries have extremely high ORAC (oxygen radical absorbance capacity, a measure of antioxidant potency) because of these and other compounds. The real kicker here is that apples have eight times the level of these beneficial compounds as red wine ounce for ounce, so the old expression "an apple a day" has a physiological basis. Save your money on pine bark extract—people don't naturally eat bark—and put down that second glass of wine. Have an apple instead. (Make sure it's organic, of course.)

EGCG is the common abbreviation for "epigallocatechin gallate," which is an extremely important phytonutrient chemical that is obtained primarily from green tea. It has been shown to reduce cancer risk and potentially helps to treat many cancers to some extent (Rouzer, 2011). These benefits are related to antioxidant activity of EGCG and also various complex molecular effects suppressing tumor cell formation and division.

EGCG can be found in many health and nutritional supplements, but you are better off getting it from green tea with the other compounds found there. Green tea, white tea and black tea are made from the same plant, but the leaves are fermented in the making of black tea and the

EGCG is destroyed. The unfermented varieties, white and green tea, still contain EGCG and other beneficial compounds. It is important not to brew green tea longer than two or three minutes, or you may lose most of the beneficial compounds.

Curcumin is an important plant chemical from the spice turmeric, which is found in foods like curry and mustard. Turmeric is used in East Indian ayurvedic medicine for treating infection and inflammation. Curcumin acts biochemically to reduce inflammation, using mechanisms similar to those of drugs like corticosteroids (e.g., prednisone) and nonsteroidal anti-inflammatories (e.g., ibuprofen) (Bland, 2004). These two types of prescription drugs act on the inflammatory cascade in different ways, but curcumin covers both functions without any of the toxic side effects.

Curcumin also performs other biochemical functions, offering additional benefits in preventing cardiovascular disease and degenerative conditions like dementia and cancer (Basnet, 2011). It is now also being used increasingly in the treatment of autism because of its ability to decrease brain inflammation. Extensive study has been done on the benefits of curcumin and many of the cellular and physiological mechanisms have now been worked out. My PubMed search for articles involving "anti-inflammatory effects of curcumin", conducted in November of 2011, yielded 2,523 articles. There are likely more added every month.

You can find the extracted curcumin chemical in many nutritional supplements now, but it is usually far better to get these compounds from their whole food sources to maximize proper absorption and effect. It's best to use the whole turmeric herb rather than extracted curcumin, since nutrients generally absorb better from whole food sources. Supplements often contain piperine or bioperine, from black pepper extract, which are purported to greatly increase the absorption of curcumin. Some nutraceutical companies are producing "liposomal" curcumin formulations, packaging the molecules into fat-soluble complexes, which also appears to improve absorption (Bisht, 2009).

Cruciferous vegetables like broccoli, cauliflower, cabbage, and Brussels sprouts have been shown to decrease the risk of cancers that are estrogen-sensitive, such as breast cancer (Boggs, 2010). Uterine cancer and prostate cancer also fall into the estrogen-sensitive category, but the bulk of the research has involved breast cancer. There are a number of active agents within cruciferous vegetables that have been proven to help fight cancer development.

Two important active chemicals in crucifers are indole-3-carbinol

(I3C) and diindolylmethane (DIM). When you eat cruciferous vegetables, you get I3C; after your stomach acid has worked on the food, the I3C is converted to DIM, which appears to be the more the effective compound, although there is some controversy about that. There are other compounds created from I3C as well, of unclear significance for health. Antacid drugs used by many Americans today may well impair the conversion of I3C to DIM.

Indoles such as I3C help fight cancer through multiple concurrent cellular processes (Marconett, 2011). They also facilitate the detoxification of estrogen in the body. I know it seems odd to suggest you need to "detoxify" your own hormones, but as I discuss in greater detail in the hormone chapter, detoxification is of particular importance in the case of estrogen. As your estrogen is detoxified and chemically converted through the liver, it can become a variety of intermediate compounds, some of which are more cancer-promoting than others.

You can find supplements that contain I3C, DIM or both on the shelves of health food stores, but as usual I suggest you obtain these nutrients from foods if you can. However, some people dislike cruciferous vegetables and will not eat them regularly, so a supplement is better than nothing. The best food source by far is broccoli sprouts, which are more palatable to many people than the adult crucifers.

Another category of healthy nutrient derived from crucifers are the sulforaphanes. These compounds have been found to suppress many different types of cancer cells, through a variety of cellular mechanisms (Kim, 2011). Supplements are not readily available with these compounds in isolation, but extracts of broccoli seeds (the highest content by weight) and cruciferous vegetables are available in capsule form for those who don't like to eat these types of vegetables (and there are many such folks out there).

Lastly, it is very important not to overcook or microwave your cruciferous vegetables because prolonged cooking destroys the beneficial nutrients fairly quickly. Just steam or boil these vegetables for about a minute, leaving them still a bit crisp.

Resveratrol is a phytonutrient that has had considerable press in recent years. Animal studies have shown benefits in the areas of diabetes control, cancer prevention and treatment, cardiovascular disease, dementia, and life span. Resveratrol has been shown to extend the life of fruit flies, a worm species, and a fish species in the lab, but has not yet done so in mammals. (The only intervention shown to do that for mammals is general calorie restriction.) However, dosing at 22mg/kg daily did decrease cardiovascular mortality in the mice (Baur, 2006). High dosing (3-5g daily) in a human study showed improved blood sugar levels (Elliott, 2008), but it takes a long time to study life extension in humans because we live so long.

The resveratrol content of red wine typically ranges from only 0.3-2.1mg/L, with levels in white wine of only 0.1-0.2mg/L (Mozzon, 1996). In most studies, the doses of resveratrol proposed to achieve adequate benefit in humans are higher than what is practical since the supplements are expensive, and one would need to drink thousands of glasses of red wine per day to achieve the levels that showed efficacy in these studies (not recommended). For this reason, many researchers have concluded that the benefits seen in laboratory studies of small animals are not relevant to human health at all, and the supplements I've seen are too expensive for most of us to consume in doses adequate to improve our health significantly.

However, in the process of digging up some of these details on Wikipedia—it's not primary literature, but the references are there and it's easy—I learned something interesting about resveratrol: it absorbs much better from the inside of the mouth than from the digestive tract. One study showed 250 times better absorption from holding a solution containing resveratrol in the mouth for a minute than from swallowing it (Asensi, 2002). The problem with absorption in the digestive tract appears to be that the chemical is rapidly changed into other (still beneficial, but not the same) compounds in the cells of the human intestine.

Resveratrol can be found in grapes, blueberries, bilberries, and mulberries, but it is found in much higher amounts in Japanese knotweed, so this weed is the most common commercial source for supplemental forms of resveratrol now. Japanese knotweed grows well all over Europe and North America—so well that it is considered an invasive weed and a biological pest of the worst sort. In Chinese it is called Hu Zhang, and its root has been used as a traditional remedy for various conditions there for millennia. You can grow a huge patch of this weed in most parts of the U.S. (not Alaska), but be careful because it spreads rapidly and could tick off your neighbors.

Before you go making knotweed salad for dinner, consider that the plant contains other compounds, as all plants do, some of which can act as a potent laxative or can aggravate gout, arthritis, or kidney stones. I have to wonder, though, if you could achieve all the benefits and none of the negative effects by chewing on the root for a while and then spitting it out. We know that you will absorb the resveratrol much better from the inside of the mouth than if you swallow it, and this way you may avoid exposing your stomach and intestines to the irritating components. Just a thought. According to Wikipedia, some companies are now attempting to produce chewing gum with resveratrol, to take advantage of the oral surface absorption.

Lycopene, a carotenoid phytonutrient that is present in high amounts in tomatoes, has shown promise in reducing cancers of the prostate, breast and colon. Suggested molecular mechanisms behind this effect are antoxidant function, improved cellular communication, decreased lipid peroxidation and DNA damage (Kelkel, 2011). It is important to note that there is dramatically superior absorption of lycopene from tomatoes when the tomato product is cooked with olive oil, as in cuisine typical of the Mediterranean diet (Fielding, 2005).

Lutein and zeaxanthin are antioxidant carotenoids found in dark, leafy, green plants, such as kalye. They have been shown to both prevent (Ma, 2011), and cause significant improvement in, age-related macular degeneration (ARMD) and associated vision loss (Weigert, 2011). This should make increased kale and spinach consumption a standard recommendation to those with ARMD or at risk for the condition.

Pycnogenol is a powerful antioxidant compound that has purported benefits for cardiovascular problems and other chronic degenerative diseases via various mechanisms (Iravani, 2011). Pycnogenol and other potent polyphenolic compounds are primarily obtained from pine bark and grape seeds. Since we don't eat pine bark and since grape seeds are quite small, this phytonutrient is difficult to get from your diet in quantities sufficient to make a difference. The supplements tend to be expensive, so this is not a very practical intervention for most people.

There are many more beneficial nutrients discovered in plant foods, and there are likely hundreds more we know nothing about yet. Most of the time you are much better off getting these nutrient chemicals from whole foods, although you may need to be careful how you cook or process them to ensure that the chemicals are not changed or destroyed.

Research has shown that isolated curcumin supplements do not absorb well at all so they provide no real clinical effect. However, their lack of effect does not stop manufacturers from trying to sell them. Taking a supplement of the whole herb (turmeric) plus the substance bioperine from black pepper increases the absorption of curcumin incredibly. You can get curcumin into the blood and the brain by eating curry as a turmeric-containing food, and human studies from Singapore have shown a relationship between curry consumption and reduced rates of dementia (Ng, 2006).

Cooking some foods seems to improve the availability and absorption of other compounds, such as lycopene, from tomatoes. Cooking tomatoes in the presence of an oil like olive oil increases the availability and absorption of lycopene. Nutrients such as the indoles in cruciferous vegetables are rapidly destroyed by cooking; therefore, those foods should be eaten raw or just lightly cooked. There is so much to learn about all this! The Price-Pottenger Nutrition Foundation is a great place to look for ongoing research into nutrition and how food relates to health; I encourage you to get their newsletter and other publications they offer.

Enzymes

Enzymes are large proteins that cause a chemical change in another substance. Some may build tissue up, while others tear it down. Some fruit enzymes, such as bromelain from pineapple and bananas, perform important anti-inflammatory activities, while others, such as papain from papaya, aid in protein digestion. It is believed that most whole foods also contain the enzymes necessary for you to obtain the food's nutrients most efficiently.

One benefit of eating a raw, whole food is that the enzymes you need to digest and assimilate the nutrients in that particular food will be present, whereas if you cook it or process away much of the substance, you may remove or destroy these enzymes and will no longer be able to glean all the nutrients from the food. This is because enzymes are generally somewhat fragile proteins and are fairly heat-labile. This is one of the key points behind the "raw food" movement.

You can find a multitude of commercial digestive enzyme products containing plant-derived enzymes to aid in digestion. There are also combination enzyme products marketed to help break down scar tissue, fibrous tissue in your gut and elsewhere, and plaque from your arteries or to combat inflammation in joints and elsewhere. Wobenzyme™ is a prominent example; designed in Germany, it has been shown to significantly decrease inflammatory mediators and prevent postoperative adhesions and intestinal obstruction problems following abdominal surgery (Minaev, 2006)

Digestive enzymes are typically intended to be taken with food, but in the treatment of systemic disease problems these products are meant to be taken on an empty stomach so the enzymes will absorb into your bloodstream rather than getting caught up digesting food. These types of enzyme products are also popular for the treatment of arthritis and other types of chronic inflammation. I did find one German study showing Wobenzym™ to be as effective as diclofenac (a prescription non-steroidal anti-inflammatory drug) for osteoarthritis of the knee. The enzyme treatment used required taking seven pills four times per day, rather than two pills twice daily for the diclofenac, and Wobenzym™ caused more adverse gastrointestinal symptoms during the course of the study than the diclofenac (Singer, 1996). Therefore, the enzyme product may be a good option for those who cannot tolerate the pharmaceutical medication, but may not be that appealing to people in general.

Serrapeptase and nattokinase are proteolytic (which means they break down proteins) enzymes derived from a bacterial species common in the gut of the silkworm and fermented soy, respectively. They are both frequently suggested by alternative and integrative practitioners to help dissolve atherosclerotic plaque in blood vessels and to prevent heart attacks or strokes. Oral nattokinase has been shown to actively dissolve intravascular blood clots in animal models (Sumi, 1990). A similar enzyme, pinokinase, was shown to completely prevent blood clots and swelling in the legs of humans after long (7-8 hour) airplane rides, while there were clots found in 7.6% of the control group (Cesarone, 2003).

Serrapeptase has been shown to have excellent anti-inflammatory activity in vivo (meaning in a living animal, not just a laboratory experiment), even better than aspirin (Viswanatha, 2008). However, my search of Pubmed yielded no studies involving serrapeptase and blood clots. I also found no articles at all involving these enzymes and atherosclerosis. The suggestion that these enzymes may help reduce vascular plaque in those with cardiovascular disease is therefore still just anecdotal.

Some of the most beneficial substances in foods are enzymes, which are easily destroyed or depleted by food processing and cooking, so it is important to eat food in its whole, natural state whenever possible. This goes for animal products as well as plants, since important enzymes in milk are destroyed by pasteurization and homogenization. Weston Price, DDS, author of *Nutrition and Physical Degeneration*, noted that certain groups never seemed to get tuberculosis until they were told to boil their milk (yet another dumb idea brought to the people by their government). Other aspects of their health deteriorated notably as well, apparently because of the devitalization of enzymes and nutrients in a dietary staple (Mudrak, 2008-9). Many other types of food processing began around the same time, so the changes in health may not have been related exclusively to changes in milk.

It is nutritionally ideal to consume only unprocessed and unpasteurized dairy products if possible and to cook red meat and fish as little as you can tolerate. The problem in our modern society is contamination by bad bacteria and parasites. If you buy poultry from the store, you should cook the heck out of it because it may have salmonella bacteria, and beef and pork may contain tapeworm eggs. Many species of fish have tapeworms or other parasites as well, which is why it is traditional practice to eat wasabe (that spicy-hot green paste) when you have sushi with raw fish: it kills the parasites.

Remember the lessons learned from the work of Dr. Francis Pottenger and his cats. They began to deteriorate rapidly when their milk was heated and their meat was cooked, at least in part because of the destruction of enzymes. Think about what you are putting in your mouth and what it is supposed to be providing you in terms of your health.

Chapter 8 – Water

I know water isn't food, but our bodies certainly need it. Without water you will die far faster than you will die without food. Water is second only to oxygen in terms of intake your body needs to survive.

Why water is important

Our bodies are comprised mostly of water, with estimates ranging from 60 percent to 70 percent of our total body weight. That alone should be enough to convince people to drink more water, but many people have trouble doing so. You need to consume water in its pure form some of the time, because if there is always sugar or other stuff in it, you may not achieve proper balance. You need some pure water to flush the toxins and waste products out.

People often tell me they get enough water because their coffee, beer, or soda is mostly water; they drink these concoctions because they hate the taste of water. If you don't like the taste of water, you should inspect where you are getting it; if it's good water, then your system may be extremely screwed up!

Coffee, tea, and alcohol have diuretic properties, meaning they leech water from your system and make you pee a lot more than you would otherwise. If you drink these liquids, you'll have to drink even more plain water to replace what you're losing. On top of that, these diuretic substances make you waste important electrolytes and minerals like potassium, magnesium, and calcium.

You need water in every one of your cells as the base for the solution where all the body's chemical and metabolic reactions take place. If you get dehydrated, your body becomes like a pond that's drying up with all the fish thrashing in small puddles separately rather than swimming around freely and interacting. Your cellular functions will not work as well: you will not be able to detoxify substances or eliminate waste well, and you will not be able to synthesize proteins and other molecules or generate energy in your cells as well.

Of course, you also need enough water in your blood to carry oxygen and nutrients around to your various tissues and take toxic waste products to your kidneys and other organs of elimination to be excreted. If your blood volume is low because you're dehydrated, your vascular system will constrict, shutting off blood flow to many capillary beds that serve less-vital tissues like the skin and mucous membranes. That is partly why you will feel sluggish and fatigued when you are dehydrated even though your blood pressure is still maintained. Your body will maintain the water inside your blood vessels at the expense of some water from your tissues in order to maintain circulation to vital organs.

Without adequate water intake, your stool will be drier and will not pass easily, causing you to retain more toxins and develop bacterial and fungal overgrowth in your gut. Your kidneys will have to work harder, and your urine will be more concentrated. Your cells will not be able to excrete their individual toxic byproducts into circulation as well, and the lymphatic drainage from your tissues will stagnate.

Where water is in the body

Since water makes up the bulk of your body mass, when you get dehydrated, you will feel wilted, like a plant that has not been watered. You've seen the floppy, rubbery carrot that sat in the refrigerator too long? That's because most of its structure and rigidity is due to the cells' being full of water, and when it loses water from sitting out in the air too long, it loses that rigidity.

Normally, only about a third of your total water is outside your cells, while roughly two-thirds of it is intracellular. Of the third that resides outside the cells, about a third is circulating inside your vessels as the fluid portion of blood and the rest is in your tissues, occupying the intercellular space. That means a 150-pound person, who has about a hundred pounds of water in his or her body, will have sixty-six pounds of it inside the cells and about eleven pounds (eleven pints) in the blood stream, with the remaining amount between the cells in the tissues and outside the vascular circulation. The water between the cells in the tissues is the most variable and flexible portion of your body water.

If you receive intravenous fluids for some reason, such as during surgery or labor or because you're extremely dehydrated, you may notice that your socks and shoes don't fit the same for a while or that your feet and lower legs swell to the point at which you can press a finger into your flesh and make a dent that disappears only slowly after you remove your finger. You may also note this effect after flying in an airplane or driving in a car for a while or even after being on your feet all day. We call that swelling "edema," and it represents excess water in the intercellular space (outside your cells) of your tissues.

When we run fluid into people intravenously, typically only about a third of it stays in their blood vessels, while two-thirds goes to that interstitial space between their cells. We call that "third-spacing," with the blood vessels and insides of cells being the first two "spaces" for water. Accumulation of water between the cells also occurs with pressure changes, such as from the weight of your water pushing down toward your feet all day and when it is prevented from easily returning back to your heart if you sit with your knees and hips bent for a long period of time.

Did you ever wonder why you sometimes have to pee so badly in the middle of the night, even though you haven't had anything to drink for many hours? It's partly because the pooled water in your legs from being vertical all day returns to your circulation when you lay flat through the night and finally has a chance to filter through your kidneys. The swelling in your feet and ankles goes down when you put your feet up for a while because of the effect of gravity. In the end, we are just bags of water walking around.

If you get a chance, look closely at the skin of someone over the age of seventy or so and note how it looks crinkly like crepe paper at the surface. You can usually pull it up away from the flesh on the back of his or her hand, and it will stay that way for a little while even after you let it go, rather than snapping back flat onto the hand like a young person's skin will. That is what chronic tissue dehydration looks like; it occurs as we age because we tend to lose our normal sense of thirst as our brains age and gradually lose normal function. Elderly people with dementia will lose their sense of thirst even more dramatically, contributing to an even more rapid physical decline.

How much to drink

So how much water do we need to drink? Our bodies are designed to function well enough for life over an extremely broad range of water intake, but we will die at either extreme. (Yes, you can overdose on water.) Every time you urinate, you lose water; whenever you sweat, you lose water; and every time you exhale, you lose water. You constantly lose water through your skin, depending on your metabolic rate and temperature, and you cannot reabsorb it through your skin. All of this water has to be replaced to maintain a reasonably constant amount in your body.

A long-held standard has been that adults drink eight eight-ounce glasses of water daily for a total of sixty-four ounces, or half a gallon of water daily. I agree that is a good target for most normal-sized adults. A study out of Loma Linda Medical School (The Adventist Health Study, started in 1976) showed a nearly 64% percent relative risk reduction in heart attack rates when patients drank five glasses of water daily compared to those drinking two or fewer glasses daily, so there is some science to back up the recommendation (Chan, 2002). It is important to understand, as with everything else in your body, there is a big difference between "sufficient" and "optimal" water.

Your brain is supposed to tell you when you need more water; your thirst is there to prevent dehydration. You would think all you have to do is drink a little water when you feel thirsty and you'll be fine, but you definitely do better on more than the bare minimum of water intake. In addition, there are instances where that regulatory thirst mechanism malfunctions. As we age our thirst sensors become less sensitive, and at the opposite extreme are certain psychiatric conditions (schizophrenia and other psychotic syndromes) that cause people to have excessive thirst and feel compelled to keep drinking water. These latter individuals can kill themselves by drinking in excess of four gallons of water or so daily. That level of water consumption can drastically dilute blood sodium levels, which causes their brains to swell within their skulls, triggering intractable seizures.

One problem with the eight glasses of water suggestion these days is that it's a one-size-fits-all recommendation, and we people come in vastly different sizes. Does a hundred-pound woman need the same amount of water as a two-hundred-pound man? One would think the heavier person needs more water, but I'm not sure need is based on body weight. Oil and water don't mix, as we all know, and having a tremendous amount of body fat, for example, may not entail the need for correspondingly greater water intake. That fat tissue does have blood vessels running through it that need water to fill them, and there will be increases in water-containing tissues like skin and intercellular space, so there is going to be some degree of increased need in obesity—but how much?

Most old recommendations were based on a prototypical adult weight of 110–150 pounds, but this range is clearly not the average adult weight range these days. That's roughly one glass of water for every 15-20 pounds of body weight, which may be a better recommendation—up to a maximum of one gallon—for most people. The suggestion should be based on parameters like "lean body mass" and "total body surface area" because those are the factors that determine, for the most part, water content and water loss. Activity plays a major role as well; if you sweat a lot, you must put that water back in.

Signs that you need more water may include headache, constipation, indigestion, fatigue, poor concentration, irritability, and muscle tension or cramps. You are also likely to have back pain and stiffness that is due to loss of water from your intervertebral disks. The color of your urine is often a good indicator; it should be a pale yellow color unless you take a lot of B vitamins, which make it a darker yellow. It should not look like apple juice or amber beer, nor should it look like straight water itself all the time because that may suggest one is drinking too much water.

That being said, there is a great deal of flexibility in our systems; our kidneys and cardiovascular systems adapt to promote proper body functioning over a wide range of water intakes. Just make sure you drink lots of water a few times each day and extra when you feel any sign of thirst, and you will probably be fine.

We have had a tendency to suggest restricted salt and large amounts of water in this culture, but people who try to follow those recommendations to the extreme will progressively dilute the essential salt and minerals out of their bodies. You cannot urinate pure water, so every time you pee, you lose salt, minerals, vitamins, and other beneficial elements along with your waste products.

We also consume water and mineral-wasting diuretic drinks like coffee and alcohol, which means even more water and nutrients need to be replaced. Some would suggest you replace all the coffee, caffeinated sodas, tea, and alcohol you drink with equal amounts of water in addition to your eight glasses or so per day. For many Americans, that would entail consuming two gallons or more of total fluid per day, and is therefore totally unrealistic. The answer there is to stop drinking the bad stuff, of course.

Types and forms of water

Talking about the kind of water you should drink may sound strange because, in a pure sense, there is only one kind of water, which is made up of one oxygen atom and two hydrogen atoms. The source of your water is probably the bigger issue. Most authorities agree that drinking only distilled water, which is the purest water, is a bad idea because it has no minerals in it. PubMed has numerous articles suggesting cardiovascular and other disease processes are to some degree influenced by the mineral content of water in different regions. You always lose some important minerals in your urine, so you have to get somewhere, and it turns out the trace minerals and salts from ground water is a good source.

You could conceivably drink distilled water and take a trace mineral supplement, but we don't necessarily know everything you need. We can't assume that all ground water is good either; residential wells may have excessive arsenic, iron, fluoride, or other potentially toxic substances, and treated water from city supplies in the U.S. is typically contaminated with things such as chlorine, fluoride, prescription drugs, solvents, benzene, trihalomethanes, and other chemicals.

If you have a well, you should have the water tested, and if you use a city water system, you may want to filter your water—even the water you use for bathing, because many chemical toxins found in water can absorb through the skin. You should also avoid water bottled in plastic, which severely limits the options for people in some regions. I discuss these issues more in the section on environmental toxicity.

One last thing I wish to discuss about types of water is ionized alkaline water. There are a number of systems available for generating this water, such as LIFE™, Enagic™, Jupiter™, Tyent™, KYK™, Alkalux™ and others. This technology uses a machine that passes water by electrified titanium plates. This ionizing process alters the way in which water molecules dissociate, move about and aggregate with each other so the water may become transiently more alkaline (higher pH) and forms much smaller water molecule clusters in solution. My view is that the changed pH has little to do with the perceived health benefits, because your stomach acid will immediately make neutralize that pH and "alkaline" water is not really adding any truly basic (meaning the opposite of acidic) chemical substance to the system.

The real potential for benefit of this water probably lies in the smaller water molecule clusters. Smaller aggregates may allow water to circulate throughout the body—in and out of cells—much more readily. This would improve the nourishing and detoxifying properties of the water significantly because nutrients, cellular signaling molecules and toxins would all be able to pass membranes and move about the body much more efficiently. This type of water should therefore be able to improve the efficiency of all the body's processes, thereby improving overall health.

Small animal studies have shown major improvement in metabolic acidosis conditions (caused by experimentally causing kidney failure in test animals) using alkaline ionized water, both orally and through dialysis (Abol-Enein, 2009). Japanese research in the mid-1990's, by Watanabe and colleagues, found very interesting results giving ionized alkaline water to pregnant rats, then through their two-week nursing period, and subsequently to the infant rats themselves out to fifteen weeks. Positive results included significantly faster growth and physical development in the test subjects given the ionized water throughout the study period (Watanabe, 1995). This seems like a clearly beneficial effect, but in-depth tissue and biochemical study of the rats yielded some surprising negative results.

Giving ionized alkaline water to mother rats, and subsequently to a subset of the offspring, was shown to increase the calcium and electrolyte content of breast milk and significantly increase the growth rate in offspring; however, those baby rats had unusual foci of necrosis (tissue deterioration) in their heart muscle (Watanabe, 2000). Biochemical analysis suggested that increases of certain enzymes' activities caused increased metabolic demand and resulted in damage to the heart muscle of these infant rats because their cells could not compensate for the change in energy usage and metabolic stress (Watanbe, 1998). Further biochemical study of these rats found increased red blood cell hexokinase enzyme activity, another marker of overall increased metabolism, and elevated potassium levels (which may indicate increased availability of potassium in the mothers' milk, or widespread cell damage and death in the infant rats themselves) in the rats whose mothers were given ionized water through gestation and nursing, then given ionized water themselves to fifteen weeks of age (Watanabe, 1997).

So, as is so often the case with medical and biomedical research, there are some conflicting and confusing results. Ionized alkaline water seems beneficial on the surface because it accelerates growth and development in test animals, also improves metabolic acidosis conditions in animals with experimentally induced kidney failure. On the other hand, it appears to cause heart muscle damage and metabolic imbalance in growing young rats as well. It may be that whatever causes more rapid growth and development also causes more rapid aging and tissue death; after all, growing and aging are inseparable processes. The biochemical studies do show increased nutrient delivery and suggest improved nutrient delivery around the body and increased overall metabolism, which may be enough to outweigh the potential negatives as long as there are ample nutrients in the diet and a favorable balance of toxicity and metabolic stressors (all of which are extremely unlikely in the modern human).

My search for articles regarding ionized water on PubMed yielded only these few animal studies discussed, and no human studies at all. We really don't know what the real overall benefits of ionized water are or may be in humans. It is reasonable to conclude from the available research here that ionized water should improve nutrient delivery and detoxification, improve acid-base balance and increase overall metabolic rate. The real question is whether or not that will be truly good for someone overall in the long run. The delicate balance of homeostasis may be disturbed in unfavorable ways here, potentially increasing metabolic stress, tissue death and the inevitable aging process that will eventually take us all.

A number of my patients claim their health issues improved notably when they began drinking ionized alkaline water, and this may be a "real" effect. The problem is this could be short-term reward in exchange for long-term harm. I don't know what the truth is here, but for now I would suggest those with ongoing chronic health problems or a need for short-term healing consider trying ionized alkaline water; but, those looking for something to just improve overall health and vitality and possibly slow the process of aging may want to look elsewhere. If you are sick or need accelerated healing, the probable benefits of using ionized water may certainly outweigh any potential long-term risks. I cannot, however, at this time suggest that ionized water is a good thing to use for preventive medicine and long-term health promotion or "anti-aging"; it may in fact be just the opposite.

CHAPTER 9 – SALT AND ELECTROLYTES

Salt is one of the most misunderstood nutritional items in our culture. Our cultural mythology surrounding salt is one of the common beliefs I have to try to dispel—along with the whole cholesterol thing. My goal here is to get you to start thinking about salt differently and realize its importance to your overall health.

Salt misconceptions

Like cholesterol, salt gets an unfairly bad rap in our society. What we know as "salt" is sodium chloride. The conventional medical belief is that salt is bad for you and that you should eat as little of it as possible—as little as two grams per day or some such nonsense. The main concern medically is high blood pressure and its consequences, and the rationale is that eating too much salt may cause you to retain water, thereby increasing your blood volume and ultimately your blood pressure. This makes me wonder why they don't tell you to avoid water, when blood is predominantly water. Does this sound odd to anyone else? The research into this question, as with much of medical research, is conflicting.

The U.S. National Health and Nutrition Examination Surveys (NHANES), which present extensive data with careful scientific analysis, are good examples of the benefits of salt in this regard. Data from the NHANES I (conducted 1971–74) demonstrated a 14 percent *reduction* in cardiovascular death and a 31 percent reduction in mortality from all causes with *higher* levels of sodium intake (Alderman, 1998). Data from the NHANES II (1976-80) showed roughly 30 percent *increased* cardiovascular and all-cause mortality for those who consumed *less* than

2.3 grams of sodium daily compared to those who had higher salt intakes (Cohen, 2006).

These results run contrary to the prevailing medical community dogma that suggests that higher salt consumption leads to cardiovascular death. The best modern evidence cited in favor of reduced sodium intakes is derived from the DASH diet study (Dietary Approaches to Stop Hypertension) conducted from 1993 to 1997 on over 5,500 patients. Patients who followed the lower sodium diet (strictly kept to <2g per day total sodium) demonstrated significant reductions in blood pressure and in rates of death from stroke (possibly near 90%) and all-cause mortality (roughly 30%), but there was no demonstrated reduction in cardiac death (Parikh, 2009).

That sounds convincing, but those results cannot be attributed to sodium restriction alone. The DASH study diet also involved reducing processed foods, sugar and sweets, and dramatically increasing the intake of fresh fruits, vegetables and whole grains. The study group had a highly increased intake of potassium, which could have had just as much to do with the beneficial outcomes as the reduced sodium did, if not more (Parikh, 2009). Therefore the DASH study showed that a healthier diet helps reduce blood pressure and mortality, but it did not prove that lower salt intake is the beneficial intervention. The NHANES data argues against salt reduction's being an important factor because the analysis teases out the salt intake as a single variable. The problem is it is an epidemiological study, and therefore does not clearly indicate cause and effect.

What the establishment has gotten right is that you need salt to retain water in your body. Since you are comprised of 60–70 percent water, and water is pretty darn important, what's the problem? Furthermore, only one-ninth of your body water is in your blood vessels, and water is free to flow back and forth between the vessels and your tissues. With too much water and salt, you could also just urinate more and eliminate the excess, so the whole thing never made much sense to me, and neither did the practice of prescribing diuretics ("water pills" as many people call them) to reduce blood pressure; after all, if you dehydrate someone with a diuretic, what's to stop him or her from just drinking more water? And, don't we believe that drinking more water is good for you?

Salt is a precious commodity here on land. In fact, people used to kill each other over salt and control of salt resources. (Do you remember the scene in *Ghandi*, where the Indian men were all lined up to take a beating from the guards at the salt mine so the people could regain control of it?

Did they all have a death wish or something, trying to eat all that salt so they could stroke-out in the streets?). We give soldiers and athletes salt pills or replacement drinks when they are sweating out in the heat, and farmers put out salt licks for their animals because they need it. The water inside every one of our cells and in our blood stream has roughly the same salinity as seawater. The message here is this: without salt and regular salt intake, you will dry up and die in fairly short order.

I think it is safe to say (because I say it all the time and nothing bad has happened to me) that salt is vital in supporting your life, following only oxygen and water in importance. Every time you urinate or sweat, you lose significant quantities of salt, and it must all be replaced in order to maintain the right concentration of saline in your blood. Sweating is a bigger problem than urinating because sweat always contains a high concentration of salt, and your urine concentration varies based on your salt intake. The kidneys and adrenals help regulate salt retention in the body, as well as water.

You can't keep water in your body without salt; therefore, the water-forcing, salt-restricting people in our society risk are becoming gradually salt-deficient. Shouldn't that be good, considering how horrible salt is for us? No, it's not good at all. Sodium and chloride, along with potassium, are extremely important for electrical balance in the body. In my opinion, magnesium and calcium are electrolytes as well because they affect the membrane potential and electrical balance of your muscle and nerve cells.

Salt definitions and biological functions

Here I digress briefly into a little complex biochemistry in order to explain the importance of salt. The term "salt" describes a simple chemical compound that readily separates into its two ionic constituents when dissolved in water. Sodium chloride is the most common form of salt in our diet; when you mix it in water, positively charged sodium ions and negatively charged chloride ions in equal amounts result. They readily bond and dissociate, and since there are equal numbers of positives and negatives, the overall total charge is electrically neutral. Potassium chloride is a salt in the same way, as are magnesium chloride and calcium chloride; you can also have potassium iodide salt, which uses iodine as the negative ion instead of chloride, and so on.

The most complicated part involves "membrane potential." For our nerve cells to be able to send electrical signals, an electrical charge must be created. (The same is true in muscle cells like those of the heart.) We measure these electrical activities and patterns with devices like the EKG (electrocardiogram, measuring electrical activity of the heart) and the EEG (electroencephalogram, measuring electrical activity of the brain). In a sense, we are living batteries, and if our electrical activity stops, we are dead—flat-lined on the EKG and EEG. That would be true "equilibrium," which is not a good thing in this case.

In order to create an electrical charge across the cell membrane in every cell of our bodies, which is how we get all sorts of routine things done chemically in our cells, we expend energy to pump sodium and potassium ions across the membrane in opposite directions, generating dramatic gradients. At equilibrium, half of our sodium ions would be outside our cells and half inside, right? Instead of maintaining equilibrium, we constantly expend great amounts of cellular energy keep 96–97 percent of our sodium outside our cells and 96-97 percent of our potassium inside, with chloride remaining fairly balanced to keep the total charges inside and outside neutral.

These steep gradients (96% on one side and 4% on the other) create great electrical potential because, if you were suddenly to open a gate and allow free movement of sodium across the membrane, there would be a dramatic rush of positively charged sodium ions into the cell in an attempt to achieve equilibrium for sodium. If you don't allow free movement of potassium as well, a major difference in electrical charge between the inside and outside of your cells will result. Your cells then harness that power to send nerve transmissions, transport substances in or out of the cell, or perform other important activities.

When the signal needs to stop—just a tiny fraction of a second later—the gates are opened to allow potassium to move across the membrane as well, and the positive potassium ions rush out of the cell, reestablishing overall electrical balance. Energy is then expended to pump the ions back against their gradients to their previous imbalanced concentrations so it can all happen again. This occurs over and over again every second in an activated cell.

This dance of dissolved salt ions goes on all the time in every cell of your body, consuming massive quantities of energy in the metabolically active tissues like your brain—which consumes 20 percent of your calories even though it is only 2 percent of your body weight, so if you want to lose weight, just think more—muscles, intestines, liver, heart, bone marrow, skin, and other organs with ongoing metabolic function. What doesn't consume much energy is fat tissue; it just sits there. That's why people who have lots of fat seem to be able to eat less than their leaner counterparts and still gain weight; that fat tissue does not really use energy, it *is* energy.

Now perhaps you have a better understanding of why sodium and potassium are important: you need them to generate all these vital cellular processes that keep you going. What is also important to understand from this discussion is that you are supposed to have more potassium than sodium in your body, which is why you shouldn't eat processed food crammed full of excess sodium, which tends to have no potassium in it at all. Let me explain this more clearly.

More salt chemistry – sodium and potassium

I described how you have pumped most of your potassium inside your cells and most of your sodium outside. Potassium and sodium are dissolved in your water mass, and, as I discussed earlier, two-thirds of your body's water is inside your cells and only a third is outside. This means that twice as much water mass has an extremely high potassium concentration relative to your sodium, so you probably need to have about half again as much potassium as sodium in your body in order to maintain proper balance and function. Your blood volume is important too, of course, so your kidneys and adrenal glands work constantly to maintain your sodium content, and they have great influence over your blood pressure.

If you have ever looked at your lab report from routine metabolic lab tests, none of this will make sense to you. In fact, I didn't figure it out until I had been in medicine for about seven years. The normal sodium range reported in your lab work is 140–145, while the potassium range is only 3–5, which would seem to suggest that you need much more sodium than potassium. However, as I just discussed, the concentrations are reversed when you look at the intracellular fluid, which holds twice as much of your water volume as that outside your cells (such as the liquid portion of your blood that was measured for your test). In addition, we know clinically that the range of potassium is far more critical than that of sodium; if your potassium level drops to 2.0, you may stop breathing, and if it goes up to 7.0, you may die of a cardiac arrhythmia in short order. In contrast, sodium levels can range down to 120 or up to 150 without a major emergency for most people.

This is the real reason why eating processed food full of imbalanced sodium or consuming lots of table salt comprised of purified sodium chloride is such a problem: it creates an imbalance between your sodium and potassium that is difficult to overcome. You can find potassium salts in "salt substitutes" (which, of course, is a misnomer because they are still technically salt), and these would be a good option for many. It is best to get potassium from foods; it can be found in high quantities in many fruits and vegetables, including oranges and whole potatoes. If you ate an all-natural diet, you would certainly get more potassium than sodium.

Salt forms in the diet

So what type of salt should you have in your diet? Salt from natural whole foods is always fine; the issue is what type of salt to add to food in cooking or at the table. "Table salt" is processed salt comprised of almost entirely sodium chloride and it is not good for you. Raw, unrefined sea salt, which you can find at almost any grocery store, is what you want. Raw sea salt has color to it—it almost looks like sand—because it contains numerous other minerals including potassium, magnesium, calcium, and a multitude of trace elements. If you get a white granulated or clear crystal form of "sea salt", it has probably been purified to be just sodium chloride.

Some processed foods such as canned soups and other prepared food items are now using what they list as "sea salt", but that could mean anything. The labels on most processed foods report "sodium" content, which is pure sodium without any potassium or other minerals to balance it out. Limiting sodium intake from labeled food to less than one gram (one thousand milligrams) per day is a good idea. You should be able to add liberal amounts of raw, unrefined sea salt in addition to that however.

Raw sea salt is balanced physiologically and has trace minerals you aren't likely to get in your diet otherwise. For most of us, it should be seen as a vital part of our diets and not feared. Dr. David Brownstein's book, *Salt Your Way To Health* (Brownstein, 2006), is a quick easy read that clearly explains all this in much greater detail. I recommend it to everyone.

Therapeutic uses of salt

I suggest that my patients supplement with sea salt for several reasons. In my experience, most people's blood pressure decreases if they consume moderate amounts of real sea salt while avoiding table salt and processed foods with unopposed sodium. After I read Dr. Brownstein's book, I tried taking ½–1 teaspoon of sea salt (I use *Redmond* salt) dissolved in the quart of water I use to take my vitamins every morning. I had positive and surprising results.

For years, when I stood up quickly, I would get light-headed and see black for several seconds, often having a few heart palpitations as well while my cardiovascular system tried to adjust to the rapid change in position. Those events totally disappeared within a few weeks of my starting this daily sea salt routine. I also had less muscle tension, and the typical uncomfortable dryness of my nose and lips from our extremely dry Alaskan winter disappeared.

I had never had high blood pressure; it was usually 115–125 over 65–75. After I had been consuming this salt for about a month—because, of course, I was afraid of the high blood pressure we all "know" you get from consuming too much salt, and I was getting 2.8-5.6 grams of salt in just that one dose every morning—I was amazed to find my blood pressure had dropped to around 90/50.

It was hard for me to fathom how my dizzy spells had gone away. My body was clearly better hydrated, but my blood pressure was even lower then before—and I was taking in heretical amounts of salt! The explanation lies in our need for the electrolytes from real sea salt and the potassium and other minerals from a whole-food diet (which I was already following in general for years) in order for your physiology to work correctly. If you give your body everything it needs, it will function properly, and most people's bodies will dispense of any extra sodium just fine.

For most of us, if we restrict our salt intake and drink lots of water, we will just dilute the salt and electrolyte levels in our bodies, with the result that important functions work less well. This salt depletion increases hormone signals from your kidneys (renin) and then your adrenals (aldosterone, which can easily be measured in your blood). Higher levels of aldosterone cause retention of sodium in the body, while dumping more potassium into the urine; this is bad because we need potassium more than sodium if you recall. If you take a diuretic drug on top of that, you will further deplete your potassium, magnesium and also sodium, potentially screwing yourself up even more.

I now routinely stop diuretics on my hypertensive patients to see if they will do okay without them, and the vast majority do. I cautiously recommend to my mildly or moderately hypertensive patients that they try phasing quantities of real sea salt into their diets or even taking the half teaspoon every day while watching their blood pressure closely. I can report anecdotally (which is not valid evidence by the tenets of conventional medicine) that most people's blood pressure falls as a result, especially if they get rid of the high-sodium processed food like sodas, soups, crackers, chips, pickles, and lots of other items.

Anyone who gets dizzy when he or she stands quickly should have a salt trial or at least proper laboratory evaluation to assess salt management, including blood and urine measurements of sodium and creatinine to calculate their "fractional excretion of sodium." Leg or foot swelling and apparent water retention problems will often resolve with real sea salt taken in this therapeutic manner as well. It seems amazing at first, but now I see it as common sense.

Risks of salt supplementation

Ten to fifteen percent of the population is truly "salt-sensitive" based on genetic factors and will often have unexplained high blood pressure. Those with these genetic mutations have difficulty managing salt through the kidneys, and their blood pressure will rise if taking in greater amounts of sodium in any form, including sea salt. These folks are the target group for which diuretics are the drugs of choice for managing high blood pressure. Many drugs have their place in certain subsets of the population, the key is to use the right drug in the right person.

This physiologic salt-retaining type may be more common in people whose origins are in hot climates, such as Africa, Central America, South America, or the Middle East, probably because there was a tendency to lose excessive amounts of salt through sweating. Studies that reviewed the DASH diet results have commented that greater benefits from sodium reduction were seen in African Americans than in Caucasians (Parikh, 2009), further reinforcing this idea.

My advice to anyone who has borderline or mildly high blood pressure is that you try taking sea salt only in gradual amounts and that you monitor your blood pressure closely. If it goes up just a little the first week, that may be an adjustment period, but an increase of ten points means you are likely to be salt-sensitive. In that event, you should eliminate all processed sodium from your diet, use only potassium salts at home, and take as much magnesium as you can tolerate. Diuretics may be the drugs of choice for hypertension in these individuals, but most everyone should concurrently take magnesium and potassium supplements when on diuretics.

In review, you need salt to survive but excessive, unbalanced sodium is not natural salt and is the real problem in our diet. Everyone should switch to real, raw unprocessed sea salt for cooking and food seasoning at home, dispense with processed foods and beverages that contain loads of sodium, and consume greater amounts of natural plant foods to get adequate potassium.

More about potassium

Potassium may be the most important "mineral" or electrolyte in your diet. It is the primary electrolyte in your body, even though the lab reports suggest that should be sodium. Potassium maintains cell volume and structure because of its pull on water into the cells, so it is important for the structural support and function of every cell in the body. It is vital for processes like detoxification and cellular communication, but it is commonly deficient in the American diet because we don't eat enough fruits or vegetables and we tend to consume far too much processed sodium, which throws everything out of balance.

Most who are taking a typical diuretic drug should take supplemental potassium because diuretics deplete potassium through your kidneys. Patients who are prescribed blood pressure medications designed to "spare" potassium (spironolactone, triamterene, ACE inhibitors, angiotensin-receptor blockers, and a few others) may not need to supplement. Prescription potassium pills given to patients on diuretics are usually large and difficult to swallow and assimilate. They are also typically very high-dose; anyone on these sorts of medications or potassium replacements should have their blood levels checked regularly because of the risks that can occur when potassium levels in the blood are out of range. The people most likely to have problems with potassium toxicity or overdose are those with severe kidney dysfunction; patients with acute kidney failure and those on dialysis may quickly develop critically high levels of potassium, which suggests that the kidneys normally excrete quite a bit of potassium per day.

The foods with by far the greatest potassium content are dulse and kelp. Foods like sunflower seeds, wheat germ, nuts, raisins, dates, and figs are also high in potassium based on weight. We don't tend to eat large quantities of any of those foods, so the most important common foods seem to be potatoes, bananas, broccoli, and oranges (especially the little mandarin oranges). Another great source of daily potassium is apple cider vinegar; mix about a tablespoon with honey daily, and dilute in water to taste.

Because of the fermentation involved in making it, apple cider vinegar contains potassium citrate, a compound that aids in detoxification and tissue growth. If you get added potassium citrate, all your cells will function better, your water balance and movement will improve, you will detoxify your body more efficiently, and many chronic symptoms may improve. The book *Folk Medicine* by D.C. Jarvis, MD gives repeated accounts of the benefits of daily apple cider vinegar. My wife and I started taking it after I read Jarvis' book, and we both notice within a couple of weeks that our hair and fingernails grew about twice as fast as they had been and that they became thicker, healthier, and stronger.

Chloride

Chloride is the most common negatively charged ion found in salts. It is measured on your lab reports, but it is rarely out of range. In general, people do not need to pay any attention to the amount of chloride in their diets.

Chloride is most relevant in the stomach, where it is a key component of the hydrochloric acid used to break down your food. Some people need to supplement with acid, usually in the form of betaine HCL, to improve digestion or treat acid reflux problems. (Yes, adding more acid to the stomach decreases reflux and improves digestion.)

The other area where chloride may be relevant is in those with cystic fibrosis. These patients have genetic mutations that impair their ability to move chloride across cell membranes properly, resulting in excessive amounts of salt being lost through the skin. In fact, diagnosis is often made via a chloride sweat test. People with cystic fibrosis may benefit from supplementing with sea salt as well.

Chapter 10 – What Food Is Not Supposed to Provide

You truly are what you eat, so what happens if you eat something that you are *not* supposed to be made of? People naively assume their bodies are smart enough to get rid of anything harmful that happens to get in. Wrong!

We will discuss what is bad for your body more in the chapter on environmental toxicity, but here I want to discuss some of the content in today's foods that are not good for you. Some of these toxins occur naturally, but most are added by food manufacturers. The naturally occurring toxins are the focus here because manufactured toxins are discussed in a chapter of section four.

"Natural" does not mean "safe"

Not all the dangerous substances in food are put there by man. Many plants, such as hemlock and poison ivy, produce harmful substances naturally. We have even turned some of these substances into drugs. Digitalis, for example, is a chemical made from the foxglove plant to treat heart failure, but even in mild excess it can kill you. Aspirin was originally derived from the willow tree, and although we use it commonly to treat pain and fever and to prevent death from heart attack, it can cause stomach ulcers or bleeding into the brain. These examples aren't relevant to food because you probably don't eat willow bark or foxglove.

However, there are many milder substances in foods that are harmful; some are commonly consumed, and just as with anything else, it is possible that certain individuals are more sensitive to them than others are. It is important to know that the word "natural" means nothing in terms of food advertising; it has no formal, legal definition like the "organic" has. Don't be fooled by food advertisers who use the terms "natural" or "all-natural" on their products, since their products can contain preservatives, pesticides, antibiotics, high fructose corn syrup, trans fats, added sugar, hormones, and much more—all the while being "natural" because they are all derived from naturally occurring substances originally.

Many naturally occurring plant chemicals are toxic to some degree. Herbivorous animals contend with them, and some adapt to become the only animal that can eat them. The happy little koala, for example, is about the only critter that can safely consume the leaves of the eucalyptus tree. I say they are "happy" because they apparently exist in a constant state of mild intoxication from the plant chemicals they ingest from the eucalyptus, which would be lethal to other animals. If you watched the Discovery Channel's production *Planet Earth*, you may have seen the elephants that walk a hundred miles to eat clay from the bottom of a particular water hole, presumably to get what they need to absorb and excrete the toxins from plants they regularly consume for food. Humans sometimes use clay to detoxify as well.

Common toxic beverages

Coffee

Coffee and alcohol are two very popular beverages, and my vote is that both are more bad than good for your health. One has a stimulant chemical and the other is a depressant and cellular toxin. Both get tossed around as health foods from time to time, and perhaps in moderation there are some benefits, but Americans are no good at moderation for the most part.

Coffee and many alcoholic drinks do have some antioxidant substances that cause some sources to suggest they are good for you, but I think, considering the loss of nutrients they cause and the adverse effects they have on your adrenal function and your sleep, the bad outweighs the good. A large population study could find no association in either direction between coffee intake and breast cancer risk (Glerach, 2011). Similarly, data from one of the largest nutritional studies ever done in women, the Nurses' Health Study, found no clear association between caffeine consumption and cardiovascular death or all-cause mortality in either direction, though there was a non-significant trend toward increased death rates in the group with the highest caffeine intake (Lopez-Garcia, 2011).

Both alcohol and caffeine may be considered "anti-nutrients" in that they cause more depletion of nutrients than they offer. Coffee not only leeches water and minerals from your body, it causes your adrenal glands to be abnormally stimulated, which is partly where that false sense of energy comes from. Caffeine contributes substantially to the adrenal burnout we see in our society today; it simulates the fight-or-flight response in your body, which is not a state you are supposed to be in very often.

Drinking caffeine also interferes with your sleep, which is common knowledge. What most folks don't realize is that the caffeine you drink in the morning will still disturb your sleep even hours later, when you try to go to sleep at night. People who like coffee seldom believe me when I tell them this, so I ask them when it is that they get their caffeine-withdrawal headache if they stop drinking coffee. The headache typically sets in by the afternoon of the following day, about thirty hours after their last intake, which means they had sufficient caffeine in their systems for well over 24 hours.

We use caffeine to prevent apnea (that's where you forget to breathe) in premature babies, and it is dosed only once per day because the chemical lasts more than a day in the body and brain. The half-life in adults is listed as being from three to seven hours; this means it takes somewhere between fifteen and thirty-five hours (five half-lives) to get it out of the system, depending upon your detoxification capacity. That means the cup of coffee you drink at 7:00 a.m. may interfere with your sleep rhythms all night long, even if you think you're sleeping soundly.

I hope I've made my point here and that, if you have trouble sleeping, you will try eliminating all caffeine from your diet before you try a sleeping pill. If you want those healthy antioxidants found in coffee, you can switch to a little dark chocolate instead; anything 75 percent cocoa or higher is fair game because it wont have as much added sugar or milk.

Tea also contains caffeine, of course, but if you choose green tea you get very little caffeine—about 20mg per cup rather than the 110mg in coffee. Green tea is also valuable for the anti-cancer properties of the compounds it contains, such as EGCG. Again, you need to make sure your tea is organic in order to reduce your burden of fluoride rather than increase it.

Alcohol

Alcohol is a natural byproduct in many fermented foods and drinks; its concentration levels depend on the beverage. Just like coffee, there are beneficial nutrients in many alcoholic beverages, particularly red wine. However, in my view, those helpful chemicals are not enough to make an alcoholic beverage a healthy food because the toxic effects of alcohol quickly overpower the benefits if you consume more "moderate amounts" of alcohol, usually defined as more than two drinks per day. Numerous epidemiologic studies truly have shown a significant *decrease* in death rates for those who drink *moderate* amounts of alcohol compared to those who don't drink at all; but those differences also involve significant confounding variables, such as the potential reasons (i.e. chronic health problems) why people may abstain completely from alcohol (Holohan, 2012 and Holohan, 2010).

Alcohol has been shown to increase estrogen levels to some degree. This effect, combined with the inherent toxicity of alcohol, is likely responsible for the observed increase in breast cancers seen in women who consume alcohol. Having just one drink per day appears to increase a woman's risk of breast cancer by 4%. Having three or more drinks per day increases risk by 40% or greater. Because of this, has been suggested that approximately 50,000 cases of breast cancer worldwide may be attributable to alcohol consumption (Seitz, 2012). I think it is safe to take away from this body of evidence that drinking mild to moderate amounts is likely not detrimental to most of us, but it is probably *not* something that should be considered "healthy".

Alcohol is a toxin, which is why having too much makes you in-*toxic*-ated. It is directly harmful to every tissue in your body, including your nerves, heart, bones, liver, bone marrow—everything. Having one or two glasses of organic red wine daily may benefit most people more than it harms them, but you are likely far better off with a glass of organic dark grape juice, pomegranate juice, or something similar. Beer has less alcohol per volume than wine, and a rich, dark beer has a lot of nutritional value (the watered-down beers consumed by most of our society do not count however). The problem here again is moderation; just one or two beers should be a stopping point for anyone.

Alcohol has a diuretic effect similar to that of caffeine (as most who have had much experience with it know), and like caffeine, it causes large amounts of magnesium to be wasted in the urine. This leeching of magnesium may have something to do with the "holiday heart" phenomenon, where some people who drink more alcohol than usual for a few days may suffer from a new rapid heart arrhythmia and some degree of reversible heart failure. In addition, the diuretic effect that causes dehydration and the waste of magnesium is likely responsible for the headache and other symptoms associated with a hangover.

Alcohol, like caffeine, also interferes with sleep, causing disturbed sleep rhythms and tending to make people wake in the middle of the night. People who try to self-medicate their insomnia with alcohol may get worse sleep than before without realizing it. "Passing out" and being *unconscious* is not the same thing as *sleeping*.

Oxalic acid

Oxalates or oxalic acids are common in many foods, including coffee (one of my favorite foods to pick on), tea (darn, I like tea), chocolate (double darn!), spinach, and peanuts. Oxalate combines with calcium to form crystals that can accumulate in your body's tissues or urine. If they build up in the brain, you can get psychiatric manifestations (some autistic kids have major problems with oxalate accumulation) or headaches; in other organs you will get chronic pain or see specific physiological consequences related to those organs; and in the urine you will get kidney stones.

Kidney stones are common, and the most common form of stone by far is calcium oxalate. One suggested solution is counter-intuitive: to eat more food that contains calcium or take calcium supplements because the calcium will bind up the oxalates in your food and keep them from absorbing into your body in the first place. Drinking lots of water to dilute your urine also helps. I think one of the best plans is to take a good dose of vitamin D, which helps regulate calcium activity in every way. If you are prone to kidney stones, especially if they run in the family, you may have inherent trouble managing oxalates and may want to eliminate high-oxalate foods from your diet. Thiazide diuretics, which keep calcium out of the urine, are helpful as well.

One other important thing to note about oxalates is they are also produced by organisms in your gastrointestinal tract; particularly yeasts like Candida. If someone has very high oxalate levels in urine it is very likely they have an overabundance of yeast in the gut. Restricting oxalates in the diet may be helpful to some extent in this case as well, but clearing the yeast load is the more effective intervention for sure. Consider this issue if you are prone to calcium oxalate kidney stones as well.

Cyanide

Cyanide is a known poison, right? Cyanide is a simple molecule with a negatively charged carbon-nitrogen (CN-) group that is highly reactive. The major toxicity of cyanide is in its binding to certain molecules we need to produce energy in our cells, causing widespread system failure and death. Cyanide occurs naturally in foods like walnuts, almonds, and cassava root, and in the seeds of fruits like apples, mangos, and peaches.

It would be difficult to eat enough walnuts and almonds to cause significant harm from the cyanide, but there is a wide range of sensitivity and susceptibility to cyanide poisoning. Cassava root is a staple in the diet of some tropical cultures, and it can cause poisoning in those who consume it in very large amounts. Tapioca flour is derived from cassava; those of us on gluten-free diets may consume significant amounts of tapioca flour, but it is unlikely to be enough to cause harm.

One medically relevant issue here is that the most common form of vitamin B-12 is a synthetic form called "*cyano*-cobalamin," which has a cyanide group attached. You are not likely to get quantities sufficient to cause harm because doses of B-12 rarely exceed a few milligrams daily. Other forms of vitamin B-12 work much better than the synthetic cyanide-containing forms, so you should seek out *methyl*-cobalamin or *hydroxo*-cobalamin, which are the forms I use in my office. Unfortunately, your local pharmacy will almost certainly have only the *cyano*- type available by prescription.

Toxins from processing or cooking

Some harmful substances are created when natural substances are modified in processing or cooking. These dangers may or may not be labeled explicitly on food items, and they will not be listed anywhere if they appear from your own cooking or processing at home. Trans fats are one such toxic byproduct of plant oil processing. They are labeled to some extent, so remember to look for any type of "hydrogenated oil" on the label and not to believe the label when it reports "zero" grams of trans fat because manufacturers are allowed to have more than half a gram per serving and still report zero trans fats (totally condoned by the FDA).

Advanced glycation end products, or "AGEs," are created when food is cooked with sugars in the presence of fats or proteins. The best example I can give you is grilled or overcooked meats. When meat is cooked at high heat, the sugars in the meat bind abnormally to fats and proteins—what cooks call caramelization—turning some of the meat brown or black.

It may make the food taste good, but those AGEs increase the body's inflammatory responses and seem to be associated with cardiovascular disease risk, particularly in diabetics (Yamagashi, 2007).

There are also carcinogenic (cancer-causing) chemicals produced by grilling meats over fossil fuels (propane, charcoal, natural gas) or smoking meats. Smoked foods have been found to increase the risk of cancers such as those of the stomach (Compare, 2010) and nasopharynx (Chelleng, 2000). The carcinogens come from the smoke or fumes from the burned fuels or wood that bind with the food substance. The safest ways to cook meat are in water (boiled, steamed, stewed), baked or roasted over long periods at low heat, or grilled as briefly as possible to adequately kill germs or parasites ("well done" is not so good). The traditional Alaskan Native method of drying salmon was likely very safe, but smoked salmon contains toxic substances.

Man-made toxins in food

A whole host of man-made substances are put into your food while growing plants or raising animals, and during processing, packaging, preparing, and cooking. I discuss many of these in a chapter on environmental toxicity, but a few categories should be addressed here because they aren't as directly toxic as many environmental toxins, but they frequently cause health complaints.

Sulfites, such as sodium sulfite, metabisulfite, and bisulfite, are simple sulfur-containing molecules that are commonly added to certain foods in the U.S. to preserve freshness. Sulfites are added to wine to kill the residual yeast and stop the "aging" process. Some people who are sensitive to these chemicals have asthmatic symptoms, headaches, heartburn, or flushing when they eat them. I personally get flushing through my face and chest and feel like I have to clear my throat frequently for a while after eating sulfites, and one of my eyes usually turns red.

Sulfites are added to most dried fruits (e.g., raisins, prunes, apricots) and wine and juices, such as grape, lemon, and lime. Unless you specifically seek out "sulfite-free" wine in the U.S., you can expect the wine to contain sulfites. Italian wines and other wines from foreign countries may not contain sulfite until the wine gets to this country, where we then add it as a preservative. Sulfites are also very commonly sprayed onto the lettuce and other foods in a salad bar to prevent wilting while it sits out in the open. Sulfites are often on prepared fruit such as pre-cut apple wedges for the same reason.

Artificial colors are put into foods to entice you to eat them by preying on your natural attraction to colors in food, which in nature would indicate the presence of beneficial nutrients. Chemical coloring agents like yellow dye #5 (tartrazine) and red #40, which can cause health problems in sensitive individuals, are present in a staggering array of foods. These chemicals do not seem to have significant direct toxicity, but it is somewhat common for people to report allergic or immune-based reactions to them, particularly kids on the autism or ADHD spectrum. I am somewhat sensitive to both of these additives, and I routinely find them in foods I would not have expected because the foods aren't yellow or red! (So why do they need to put yellow or red dye in them?)

In my experience with allergic and chemically sensitive patients yellow #5 is a common trigger for asthma and upper respiratory irritant symptoms like runny noses and scratchy throats. Red #40 tends to cause neurological symptoms like headaches and mental fogginess, but you can see allergic-type reactions to any of the artificial coloring agents. Kids often manifest these reactions as behavioral changes, becoming agitated, irritable, and inattentive. (ADHD, anyone?) Blue dyes seem to have particularly effects in many sensitive kids, manifesting as temper flares and serious behavior problems. The effects a small ingestion can last for several days.

Many people self-report suspected reactions to artificial dyes in foods, but scientific confirmation is lacking. Most attempts to look at this question find no clear association and conclude that the incidence of true allergy to these chemicals is grossly over-reported and exaggerated (Elhkim, 2007). I often suggest people take these chemicals out of the diet if they suspect sensitivity, then "challenge" with them to see if there is notable reaction. It is very relevant for certain individuals.

Monosodium glutamate—most people know it as "MSG"—is both a food additive and a naturally occurring byproduct of preparation or cooking. Examples include whey protein and other dairy-based products that are high in the precursor amino acid "glutamine" and fermented foods like soy sauce, steak sauces and Worcestershire sauce. MSG is often added to food in restaurants to enhance the flavor because of its salty taste and stimulant effect. Glutamate, a simple amino acid, is the most important and abundant excitement neurotransmitter in the brain. MSG is thought to cause widespread and unregulated excitation in the brain, potentially triggering headaches and leading to the death of nerve cells. These concerns have not to my knowledge been confirmed by scientific research.

MSG may also be found on labels as "glutamic acid," "hydrolyzed vegetable protein," "hydrolyzed gluten or wheat," "hydrolyzed yeast," "yeast extract," "soy extract," or "protein isolate"; you can also infer the presence of MSG if you find "disodium inosinate" or "disodium guanylate" on food labels. These ingredients are on the labels of many commonly consumed foods, including sauces, salad dressings, soup stock, bullion, seasoning mixtures, meat jerky, chips, other snack foods (especially if they have a salty taste), and prepared foods like frozen dinners and other quick-meal products. You can ask for food without MSG in restaurants, but you may limit your choices; also, they may not know it is there, as it may have been added before it reached their establishment. In any case, your server may have no idea whether it is in the food or not.

I have encountered many people who feel they are sensitive to MSG in some negative way, but the FDA has concluded after what they feel is extensive study that MSG is completely safe for most people, even in extremely large amounts. Your job is to figure out whether you are included in "most people" or not. The FDA does acknowledge that some people anecdotally report symptoms like asthma or headaches, but it feels that these adverse effects are not satisfactorily reproducible or supported by research. A significant minority of the population's experiencing minor harm from a completely unnecessary food additive is not enough for the FDA to ban its use, which I find reprehensible. There is absolutely no good reason for a non-nutritive food additive to be allowed if it could harm even one person in ten thousand.

CHAPTER 11 – DEVITALIZED FOODS

I mentioned earlier that many vitamins and minerals are often stripped away from plant-based foods when they are initially processed, through the removal of outer husks, smashing, pressing, or grinding. Additional problems with nutrient destruction occur when foods are heated during processing. Nonorganic, or "conventional" farming methods also serve to decrease the nutrient content of foods.

The vitamins in any type of grain product that has been cooked to high heat have been destroyed, along with most phytonutrients it may have had. The sugars and proteins may also have been modified into something potentially harmful, such as AGEs. Common examples of these sorts of foods include almost all breakfast cereals ("part of your balanced breakfast"–if you want to die young), fried tortilla or potato chips, crackers, and anything that has been "puffed." Rice cakes are widely seen as some sort of health food, but all the nutritional content has likely been destroyed by intense heat and the cake is nothing more than refined carbohydrates with chemical byproducts.

Pasteurized dairy products are another large group of foods that were once healthful and now pose far more harm than good nutritionally. The heating process destroys important enzymes in raw milk that help digestion and assimilation of food. Heating also alters the proteins and fats so they are far less healthful. Dr. Francis Pottenger observed a wide array of health problems in his experimental cats when he cooked their milk, and Dr. Weston Price described how tuberculosis ran rampant through a rural Swiss community after their government's health department urged everyone to boil milk prior to consumption (Mudrak, 2008).

Other beverages, such as fruit and vegetable juices, are also pasteurized.

Pasteurization was developed because certain bacterial infections, such as E. coli from certain combination juices and Listeria from apple juices and soft Mexican cheeses, have been linked to unpasteurized foods. A bacterium found in dairy products, *Mycobacterium avium paratuberculosis,* is thought to be linked to inflammatory bowel disease such as Crohn's disease. It is mostly killed by pasteurization, yet it can be isolated live from up to 5 percent of the pasteurized milk on grocery store shelves. (This claim is based on a personal account from a gastroenterologist who is researching the subject.) Therefore, foods aren't completely safe even when they are pasteurized.

Homogenization also causes problems by liberating more of the enzyme called xanthine oxidase, which promotes inflammatory processes in your body and changes the way fats are absorbed (Hyman, 2008). Safety in dairy products and juices and other animal products or produce is mainly an issue of growing or raising conditions, animal feeding, crowding, clean processing, and harvesting. If the apples didn't come into contact with animal poop, they wouldn't have high quantities of bacteria on them. If a cow is fed only grass, it will not develop abnormal bacterial overgrowth. Most of our problems come from the unhealthful practices inherent in mass production, and the nutritional value of the foods is further decreased by the measures required to ensure safety.

Let me rant a bit more about breakfast cereal for a moment. Breakfast cereals are terrible, even if they claim to be low in sugar or to have five vitamins added. Go throw it all away right now. Breakfast cereal may be slightly better than eating doughnuts, Pop Tarts, toaster waffles, or instant pancakes for breakfast, but not much better. Even taking away the fact that many breakfast cereals are half added sugar by weight, they were almost all carbohydrate to begin with. I used to try to find the cereal with the most fiber content on the shelf, thinking I was providing a healthful breakfast for my kids (who would inevitably complain about wanting a sweeter cereal), so I understand the resistance to this idea.

However, the fact is that almost all breakfast cereals consist of grain products, which are inherently allergenic to begin with, stripped of their nutrient-rich outer layers, further ground up and stripped of more nutrients, heat processed, and probably puffed or mashed into some unnatural shape like a flake or a shamrock. To make matters worse, these cereals are typically bathed in some non-organic, pasteurized, and homogenized cow's milk. Loren Cordain's book on the Paleolithic diet provides a clear picture as to why humans would probably be better off without eating grain products at all, and T. Colin Campbell's book, *The China Study*, clearly depicts the potential harm in consuming dairy products. Eating breakfast cereal involves consuming both of these foods.

Eating instant oatmeal is akin to having processed, sugary cereal without the milk (unless you like milk in your oatmeal; then it's the same thing). Instant oatmeal is "instant" because the fiber has been stripped away by processing so you don't have to cook it for twenty minutes or longer. Eating unprocessed, steel-cut, oats may be a relatively healthy breakfast option, even if oats are still a form of grain. However, if you have instant oatmeal with flavors and sugars added, you may as well have toaster waffles or Pop Tarts™.

Similar severe devitalization occurs in most other "instant" food products, such as minute rice, instant mashed potatoes, and ramen noodles. Those are foods that have been processed and treated to such an extent that they no longer have anything to offer you as real food. Try to keep in mind that the reason you eat is to nourish your body, generate healthy tissues, and support normal immune function and brain processing. You don't eat just to fill your belly, store energy, or to satisfy hunger or specific cravings.

I've mentioned that organically produced foods contain far greater amounts of vitamins and other important nutrients; I think this warrants some more specific examples. A study comparing organic versus nonorganic spinach found roughly 60% higher levels of vitamin C and 25% greater flavonoid content in the organic produce, while levels of nitrate (which are not good for you) were far higher in the spinach produced through conventional methods using synthetic fertilizers (Koh, 2012). Recent studies have shown similar differences in the content of vitamin C, flavonoids and beneficial phenolic compounds in organic versus nonorganic tomatoes (Hallmann, 2012). Modern conventional agricultural methods have also been shown to decrease the overall mineral content of cultivated plant foods (Reeves, 2011).

If you start eating natural, nutrient-rich foods, your hunger will likely decrease and your bodily functions should all improve. This is because you will be getting more adequate amounts of the things you really need from your food, rather than just excessive calorie content. You will also probably find that your tastes change; you may start to enjoy nutritious, whole foods more and will likely feel sick if you eat processed food and junk foods.

CHAPTER 12 – WHAT WE
ARE SUPPOSED TO EAT

One of the most common questions I get from patients is "what *should* I eat?" This question often comes with some angst behind it after I have told them many of the things they should *not* eat, such as processed foods in general, cereal, bread products, pasteurized dairy, and all the other "food" they may have lived on most of the time. People are full of excuses for why they don't have time to prepare or can't afford healthful food.

This is a huge topic, and there have been myriad books published suggesting the perfect diet for this or that reason. Successful human civilizations have eaten a wide range of diets from primarily vegetarian to nearly purely carnivorous. We are fortunate to be omnivores, which allows us to subsist on many different foods, but the issue here isn't survival; it is a search for the ideal diet.

The reality is that the ideal diet may be different for everyone. The factors that determine your perfect personal menu include your genetic and geographical heritage; environmental stressors like temperature, water availability, and pollution; individual genetics (e.g., single nucleotide polymorphisms, epigenetics); stress and activity levels; reproductive status (e.g., pregnancy or preparing for pregnancy); age; and allergenic profile. Many people try to convince you they know your ideal diet, but they can't all be right—and probably none of them are. There are so many individual factors that it is impossible to know what is best for anyone else to eat.

The best I can offer may be some important guiding principles and some advice about how to go about your own investigation into your ideal diet. I have already touched upon many of the important principles in previous sections, but I will try to collect them for you here. If you want a diet to follow, I'd suggest the Mediterranean diet or the Paleolithic diet (the "caveman" diet), both of which include natural, nutrient-dense foods.

The Paleolithic diet is my favorite because it doesn't include any of the grain products that are so prevalent in the modern American diet and that are, in my opinion and the opinions of many people more prominent than I am, responsible for a great many health problems. The Mediterranean diet does include wheat and other grains, and if you were to move to the Mediterranean you could probably eat those foods as they produce them there; however, wheat and other grains here in the U.S. are bioengineered to have greater gluten content and polluted with chemicals, making them highly allergenic and pro-inflammatory. Organically grown wheat has been shown to have significantly easier digestible protein (Nitika, 2008), so one may do somewhat better on organic wheat products.

As I've said repeatedly, it is ideal to eat pure, natural foods without chemical pollutants, meaning only wild or certified organic foods. It is also important to avoid foods with added chemicals that are put in during processing or manufacturing and that have nothing to do with the organic designation, so they may be present even in foods labeled "organic." I have not reviewed all the toxins put into our foods yet, but I hope that the information presented in later sections will help convince you of the importance of eating "clean" food.

I previously reviewed some of the problems with food processing, including mechanical grinding, stripping of outer layers, cooking, and homogenization. If you want to be healthy, it is important to eat foods that still have their nutrients. I can't stress enough the importance of eating whole foods. Eating foods like fruits, vegetables, and nuts raw is a good idea; you may get into trouble eating animal products raw, but milk products should be raw, if they are from healthy animals raised only on grass, to get the best nutrition. Cooking many plant and animal foods to some extent can make them less allergenic and more digestible, so don't go too crazy with the "raw diet" thing either.

Diet composition is the big question here. I've spent a fair amount of time criticizing vegetarian and vegan practices to stress the importance of having some meat and other animal products in your diet. Some may cite a number of studies in the modern literature suggesting improved health from eating a strongly plant-based diet or even a vegan diet in the U.S., where we arguably consume more meat than we need, but I believe the real problem with our meat is how poorly raised our animals are. The fats, nutrient content, and toxin contents of meats depend wholly on how the animal was fed and raised.

Campbell's book, *The China Study*, makes a compelling argument for strict avoidance of animal foods, specifically milk products, to reduce cancers, cardiovascular disease, and some other common chronic medical problems. In my opinion, the studies mentioned in Campbell's book are all confounded by the fact that they were done in modern times with the modern problems of mass-produced animal foods. You cannot equate the consumption of lunchmeat and processed feed-lot-raised fast-food burgers with eating wild Alaskan salmon and moose meat. You can't equate mass-produced milk with grass-fed, organic raw milk.

Campbell points almost exclusively to studies that used casein (from cows' milk) as the protein source, resulting in poor outcomes, and then extrapolates those results to include all "animal protein" conceptually. It is widely known that there is something uniquely bad about the way our bodies respond to casein; it is far more inflammatory and harmful than any other type of animal-derived protein (Cordain, 2002). The book is also clearly biased because of its long discussion of how immune reactions to cows' milk can trigger autoimmune disease, while the fact that wheat and gluten (plant-based food) are also responsible for a great scope of problems, including autoimmunity, is ignored.

The book does help to reaffirm my previous conviction that we must move away from modern, mass-produced animal products as much as possible. Those foods are killing people every day. Because of the limited availability of high-quality, healthful animal products in the modern marketplace, moving toward a vegetarian diet is practical and is likely to result in health improvements for Americans. That does not mean, however, that we should go vegan.

If you are eating feedlot-raised meats from animals fed corn and soy and riddled with hormones and pesticides, then you're probably going to feel better, lose weight, and have a better chance of beating cancer or heart disease if you go vegan, but that doesn't make it the ideal. Natives of Alaska and Greenland are good examples of people who experience robust health on a diet comprised largely of animal products (up to 99%). Since their diets have become filled with modern convenience foods, these populations have rapidly deteriorated (Price, 2006). In my experience, Alaskan native children now often have terrible dental problems and recurrent ear and other infections, and adults get cancer and heart disease at fairly young ages compared to the white population. There is a (unfortunately small) movement among Alaskan natives to move back to a more traditional diet. They have even produced a cookbook designed for people with cancer that describes how to find and prepare native foods.

The most important factor with animal products is how they are raised and produced. If you have access to Alaskan salmon, moose, elk, venison (from deer way out in the woods, not the ones grazing at human farms), organic natural free-range eggs, pasture-fed beef and dairy products, wildebeest, zebra, ostrich, or other natural animal foods, then you should eat those animal products to your heart's content. If you don't have access to those types of healthy animal products or you can't afford them, don't replace them with commercially produced beef, chicken, pork, pasteurized milk, or non-organic corn-fed butter and cheese. You may die much younger if you eat these foods.

Yes, I said "die." Sometimes that's the only word that catches a person's attention. Food has a major impact on your life expectancy, and when you're really sick is way too late to make much difference. If modern, toxic products are the only animal foods available to you, you truly are better off eating an organic vegetarian diet.

Again, don't think you can eat whatever you want and then go to the doctor for a magical solution when you develop medical problems. We have extremely poor success treating obesity, diabetes, cardiovascular disease, and cancer, so odds are you will end up on a bunch of expensive drugs that make you feel sicker in a variety of ways and that prolong your life just a little longer, accelerate your decline, or even kill you outright. Medical care has been shown to be responsible for over two hundred thousand deaths in America every year and has become roughly our third leading cause of death overall, depending upon how you calculate things (Starfield, 2000).

Modern, mass-produced animal products in the U.S. and many other developed nations may cause you to die prematurely from diseases like cardiovascular disease, cancer, neurodegenerative diseases, and autoimmunity. Therefore, although I advocate eating meat and animal products, I am clearly *not* saying, "Eat all the meat you want." You must know where your food is coming from, how it was grown or raised, how it was produced and processed, what was added to it, and how it was packaged.

As far as what you should drink, drink water! To be more precise, drink only water you know is clean and safe: filtered water in a glass or metal container or water from a well or spring that has been tested and found free of toxic metals and other substances and bacteria, and don't drink bottled water from plastic!

Other beverages you may drink in moderation are organic green tea, yerba mate and herbal teas, organic fruit and vegetable juices (in glass jars), and perhaps the occasional healthful alcoholic beverage but only one or two drinks per day. Don't partake of soft drinks, whether diet or regular, don't drink excessive coffee or espresso, and stay away from energy drinks (too much caffeine and sugar) and sports drinks (too much sugar and always in plastic).

Regarding milk, you should not be drinking milk as a beverage if you're older than three unless you need to gain weight. Milk is a growth formula! Haven't you seen how fast baby cows grow on a steady diet of milk? Even if you are getting only natural, grass-fed, raw milk, don't drink it as a beverage unless you are a growing, developing child or you have some sort of medical problem with gut absorption issues or increased nutritional needs. Perhaps make yourself some natural kefir, yogurt, butter, and cheese out of it, but don't just drink it. It isn't that the milk is bad for you in this case; it's just a lot of calories you may not need. I've seen extremely obese people who just needed to stop drinking milk—some were drinking up to a gallon per day—to start readily dropping weight. Of course, if the milk is the mass-produced grocery store stuff, you are poisoning yourself and your family on top of all that.

Plant foods may constitute as much as 85 percent of your daily diet, but you should also include modest amounts of healthy animal products like natural eggs, fish, and butter and have a naturally raised or wild red meat at least a couple times per month. It's worth the money to buy grass-fed meat. To avoid gaining weight, have more protein-dense plant and animal products and very few grain products. In addition, be careful about what you put on your plant foods, as many salad dressings will torpedo your calorie-control plans if you aren't paying attention.

One issue with grains like wheat, rye, barley, corn (not a vegetable, remember), and other grass seeds is that they tend to be highly allergenic and to cause inflammatory responses in the body. They are also just pure carbohydrate energy; grain is what ranchers feed livestock to fatten them up for slaughter after all. Also, excessive grain consumption often leads to intestinal yeast overgrowth. I've seen many obese vegetarians who consume too many bread products and grains, so don't do that if you want to eat a mainly plant-based diet. Junk foods like potato chips or corn chips, breakfast cereals, crackers, pretzels, popcorn, cookies, brownies and other high-calorie goodies can all be part of a vegetarian diet as well, and are clearly not healthy.

Eat fruits, vegetables, beans, tubers, nuts, and seeds, and use moderate portions of potatoes and rice as your starches. Don't go crazy with soy, and make sure your soy products are fermented varieties only (tempeh, miso, natto). Buy produce locally in season as much as possible, make sure it is all organic if at all possible, and go for frozen products if you can't get it fresh because the nutrients in canned foods have been destroyed by heat, and the food is typically polluted with plastic or metal and may contain added sodium or sugar.

When we are young or very active—teenage athletes or people with physically demanding jobs like lumberjacks, laborers, iron-workers, and people who carry lots of heavy stuff around all day, not people who are fifty pounds overweight and try to convince me they don't need to exercise because they walk three miles at work every day in a retail store—then you may eat more starches and carbohydrates for energy and get away with it. If you ever start to pack on extra fat, cut the sugar and starches down first.

People tend to want meal plans and specific lists of what to eat, but everyone's needs are so different and their allergies are so specific that you are much better off starting with this list of guiding principles and paying attention to how your own body responds to foods. I would love to write more about weight management and obesity, but that will have to be the subject of its own book some day. If you want good resources to learn more about food and how to eat it, read books such as Pual Pitchford's *Healing With Whole Foods,* Mark Hyman's *Ultrametabolism,* Barry Sears' *The Inflammation Zone,* and the natural cookbook and nutrition resource *Nourishing Traditions* (Fallon, 2001).

It is vitally important to learn to pay attention to your body. If you don't feel bright and energetic or if you are progressively gaining weight, then change your diet as I've described and see if you feel different. Learn which foods make you sleepy, irritable, bloated, nauseous, or itchy and stop eating them. Investigate the chemical additives in foods and how they affect you, because there is no good allergy test for that. I will discuss this more in the chapter on allergy.

Keeping a food diary is cumbersome, but it is invaluable in the task of figuring out what is good for you as an individual. Track what you eat and drink every day, along with your body weight and a scoring system regarding how you feel from day to day. For example, rate yourself from one to ten every day in terms of energy, mental clarity, mood, quality of sleep, and chronic pain or medical symptoms you may have. Your food may affect you within minutes or hours or even the next day. This exercise is invaluable in determining what you should and should not eat.

I realize this advice will not seem helpful to many of you, and some of you will be irritated at my failure to provide you with a straightforward diet plan that allows you to remain blissfully ignorant about food. I want to teach you to fish, rather than just giving you a fish, as the saying goes. You need to understand food and why you are eating it. If you want to learn to read, you start with the alphabet, not phrases or sentences; I'm trying to give you the dietary alphabet here, the basic principles. You need to know what foods are safe and nourishing and what foods to avoid. You need to pay attention to yourself and learn what's best for you.

It is also important to note that healthful food doesn't have to require a lot of preparation time or fancy ingredients. Many people use their time crunch as an excuse, but I can usually make dinner faster than I can get take-out; the time you spend preparing food is therapeutic for you as well. It takes me two minutes to get my lunch together in the morning, while my office staff often uses much more time than that to pick something up for lunch or they're left impatiently awaiting delivery. I challenge those who say they don't have time to prepare healthful food to find households much busier than mine. It's a matter of making your health and the health of your family a real priority, rather than just claiming that it is.

A brief rant about the Food Pyramid, or "Plate"

Before leaving this discussion on what one should eat, I want to express my contempt for the food pyramid, which was designed by our country's agricultural producers and is, in my opinion, nothing more than capitalist propaganda promoted by our government. The pyramid diagram was replaced by the image of a plate in 2011 but the new diagram suggests roughly the same dietary proportions as the pyramid, just in a more relevant visual format. The bottom tier of the pyramid, or largest portion of the plate, is grain products or "cereals," suggesting that those foods should be the largest component of your diet. I'm reasonably certain that these foods are in the largest portion because they are the foods our country mass-produces with the greatest ease and largest profits, not because they are the best foods for you.

Many of the groupings represented seem arbitrary and contrived. Do beans and nuts belong with meats because they are high in protein or with vegetables because they are plant foods? Do seeds belong with oils because they are high in fats or do they go with vegetables as well? Potatoes and corn are not vegetables, but they were grouped there; the best thing about the new "plate" diagram is they moved potatoes and corn to the starch and cereals group where they belong. Fungi like mushrooms don't seem to belong in these food diagrams anywhere because they aren't animals or plants, and they have some unique nutritional qualities.

Finally, why is there a little triangle space for junk foods at the top of the pyramid and small wedge at the bottom of the plate at all? Why don't they make a little compartment for plastic, artificial sweeteners, preservatives, and pesticides while they're at it? Everyone would probably acknowledge those foods don't belong in a healthy diet anywhere, yet they are represented in the government's depiction of what we should be eating.

In my view, these diet diagrams exemplify our government's support of capitalism over human health. I suggest you ignore them and learn about food in more depth than the simplistic and misleading graphics offer. The food pyramid is just another example of our faulty cultural mythology about food, which is driven by industry. Don't believe the hype!

CHAPTER 13 – "SUPER FOODS"

I think it is important to know what foods to seek out for optimal health—foods that offer the most nutritional bang for your buck. Some are diet staples and others are foods you should not pass up an opportunity to consume.

Protein/Meats/Animals

It isn't just that we need some animal protein in our diet; some animal products are very healthful and do much more than just feed your energy and macronutrient needs.

Wild Pacific salmon is, in my opinion, the best animal to eat; if it's ever on the menu in a restaurant, choose it over other meat options. Wild Pacific salmon differs in important ways from Atlantic salmon, which live for many years and acquire more toxins, and farm-raised salmon, which are fed an unnatural diet full of toxins. Of course, you should avoid many other types of fish, including large fish like tuna, shark, swordfish, mackerel, and halibut, because of mercury content.

Other animal seafoods are very high in omega-3 fatty acids and offer good sources of clean animal protein, provided they are wild and not farmed. Squid is a good option and is always wild so far. Scallops, mussels, octopus, and clams are other tasty mollusks, and crab, shrimp, and lobster are good crustacean options. I suggest you avoid farm-raised shellfish; look for only wild options. Stay away from imitation crab because it usually has gluten, red dye, titanium, and other additives.

Wild red meats like moose, elk, and venison (from the forest, not farm country) are great sources of nutrition. Grass-fed bison (buffalo) and beef are a distant second to wild meat, but they are great sources of nutrition as well.

Wild fowl, such as pheasant, duck, and grouse, is a good choice. Free-range organic chicken is possibly safe to eat, but it is not a super food because the chickens are usually just fed grain. Anyone who has raised chickens will tell you their natural diet consists of wild vegetation, bugs, worms, frogs, mice and anything else they can forage; they are not vegetarians! Any bird that has pale or white muscle tissue (meat) is not truly healthful food because that means the muscle tissue had no exercise.

Organic free-range eggs are an excellent source of nutrition, though again only if the hens weren't fed just grain. If you get eggs from hens eating a natural omnivorous diet the yolks are a deep orange color and have an incredible rich flavor, not like the pale tasteless yolks you get in eggs from the store. I don't recommend eating the regular eggs from a grocery store; it's best to find eggs from a private local producer whose feeding and raising practices are as clean and natural as possible.

Dairy products can be a good source of nutrition for those who are not allergic or intolerant to dairy, but they have to be derived from organic, grass-fed animals that have been given no hormones, antibiotics, or other chemicals, and the products must not be pasteurized or homogenized. Good dairy products include only raw milk, yogurt, cheese, and butter—sorry, but I cannot recommend ice cream. All milk found in American grocery stores is bad, in my opinion—even the organic milk, unless you live where raw milk can be sold. You can find organic, pasture-fed butter and cheese in some stores or perhaps find local producers and co-ops for raw milk products.

Cultured dairy, such as kefir and yogurt that uses the right cultures is a super food. These foods contain nutrients and enzymes produced by the bacteria themselves, which are of great value to us. These include certain forms of vitamin K, biotin and other vitamins, and enzymes such as nattokinase. Other benefits of the probiotic bacteria themselves are discussed later on.

Bone broths are an important source of nutrition that most people in our modern culture never consume. There are nutrients in cartilage, bone, and bone marrow that are highly healthful and aren't represented well in other foods or animal tissues. Cartilage is a unique tissue that is difficult to maintain; consider how common arthritis is at early ages these days.

I have found that taking MSM (methylsulfonylmethane) as a supplement dramatically improves arthritis and even seems to help cartilage to heal.

My mother has a genetic disease that causes osteoarthritis, and some of her hand joints and her ankles have shrunk back to normal size since she began taking MSM 2,000mg daily. I see it as a basic nutritional building block that is very limited in most foods but may be obtained naturally by consuming bone broths or cartilage. Gelatin is also a source for some of the substances needed to make cartilage. It is processed purified collagen from animal tissues such as skin and bone. Perhaps you need to eat the components of cartilage in order to make better cartilage.

I don't have many plant-based proteins in this list because no plants have nutritionally complete protein. That said, black beans are on the list because of their high antioxidant content and beneficial fiber; other dark-colored beans are likely very good as well. Nuts are good sources of nutrition for their healthful oils and minerals and their protein and fiber content, so I suggest eating small amounts of raw, organic nuts regularly. Walnuts may top the list because of their high magnesium content, or possibly Brazil nuts due to their high selenium content. Many people are allergic to nuts, so be cautious.

Fermented soy products like tempeh, miso, and natto may make the list because of the increased nutrient content from the bacteria, particularly vitamin K (menaquinone-7 to be precise). There is research suggesting consumption of fermented soy foods increases bone density and strength and should decrease fracture risk (Ikeda, 2006).

A potential problem and point of confusion with soy foods involves cancer risk. More recent studies implicate fermented soy products as a potential risk factor for developing gastric cancer. A meta-analysis done by the Japanese Cancer Society in 2010 suggested a 22% increased risk of stomach cancers with higher intakes of fermented soy products, and 36% *decreased* risk from consuming *non*-fermented soy products such as tofu and edamame (Kim, 2011). Other large epidemiological studies have suggested a significant decrease in prostate cancer risk for men consuming *non*-fermented soy foods (30% decrease overall, but mainly noted for Asian populations), with no noted effect of fermented soy foods on prostate cancer risk (Yan, 2009). The effects of soy on breast cancer risk have been unclear, with different epidemiological studies yielding diverse conclusions. A recent meta-analysis suggested a roughly 25% decreased risk of breast cancer from higher consumption of soy isoflavones (which are largely destroyed by fermentation, and would require consumption of *non*-fermented soy foods), but only in Asian populations; no such effect was seen in Western populations (Dong, 2011).

Basically, the soy question is a confusing one without a clear answer. Eating fermented soy foods may be better nutritionally because of higher vitamin content, decreased phytic acid and trypsin inhibitor presence (discussed in an earlier chapter of this section), and may be better for your bones. Fermented soy may, however, increase the risk of gastric cancers and fail to reduce the risk of hormone-sensitive cancers such as those of the breast and prostate as may be accomplished by non-fermented soy foods. Non-fermented soy foods may qualify as super-foods because of possible decreases in certain cancers. Welcome to the world of medical research and decision-making. There seldom are clear answers.

Fats and Oils

All the foods mentioned anywhere on these lists must be, without exception, organic or wild varieties to be considered super foods.

Butter is an excellent source of nutrition in its natural form. Ghee or clarified butter is usually safe even for those with severe milk allergies and can be used at much higher heats than regular butter can.

Coconut oil and milk are also excellent sources of healthy fats and may be used with high heat cooking or frying. Kefir from coconut milk is a super food, and cultures for making kefir can be obtained through the Body Ecology™ organization.

Extra-virgin olive oil is part of the heart-healthy Mediterranean diet. All the other olive oils are relatively depleted versions generated by various forms of processing.

Eating whole olives is better than consuming olive oil because of all the additional antioxidants in whole olives; I recommend eating olives of every kind, except perhaps those canned black ones. Black olives have been turned that color via the addition of artificial chemicals; this is often just iron sulfate, which would not be toxic, but you cannot be certain.

Flax oil is an excellent source of omega-3 and other essential polyunsaturated fatty acids. Flax oil is best derived from the seeds and ground just before use, though that is labor-intensive. Alternatively, find a bottle of organic flax oil with high lignans and use that. Remember to keep it refrigerated and never heat it at all. Use it in smoothies, on salads, and in other cold dishes. Putting flax seeds in baked products kills the oil, but at least you get the fiber and lignans.

Lignans are polyphenolic compounds that have some hormone-regulating properties and purported health benefits. Recent studies have suggested as much as a 50% decrease in breast cancer risk for women consuming the highest amounts of lignans versus the lowest, with two lignans in particular (matairesinol and lariciresinol) having the biggest impact (McCann, 2011). Flax is by far the best source of lignans overall, having ten times the total lignan content of the next contender, sesame seeds; however, sesame has much higher content of the two specific lignans that were shown to have the greatest impact on breast cancer risk (Smeds, 2007).

Fish oil is probably the best food source of omega-3 fatty acids, and is best obtained from eating wild salmon, but if you don't eat fish, find a supplement that is molecularly distilled and free of mercury and PCBs. Krill oil is catching on as a supplement, but it is notably more expensive than fish oil and has the same potential problem of environmental pollution. In addition, I am not convinced that krill are among our "natural prey" as humans.

Nuts and seeds are good sources of healthy oils. Try to find organic, unroasted tree nuts like almonds, walnuts, cashews, Brazil nuts, and pecans. Remember that peanuts are not true nuts; they are highly allergenic, and I do not recommend their oil as a healthy food either. Sunflower, flax and sesame are popular seeds to consume and easy to include into your diet. Hemp seed is very high in omega-3, and its oil is now commercially available.

Chia seeds are hot items from South America that have purportedly excellent health value. Chia is high in omega-3 fat such as alpha-linolenic acid, also complex carbohydrates. Chia intake was found to have health benefits such as reduced fatty liver, improved insulin sensitivity, reduced internal belly fat and reduced cardiac and liver inflammation in obese rats (Poudyal, 2011)

Avocado, technically a fruit, is a great source of monounsaturated fat as well, and I am a big fan. Go for the guacamole over the sour cream any day.

Vegetables

Broccoli tops the list for me here; broccoli sprouts in particular have health benefits because they boost glutathione levels better than most any other food. In addition, the compounds in broccoli sprouts have been shown to reduce the incidence and growth of multiple cancers, to prevent cardiovascular disease, to kill H. pylori (the bacterium associated with ulcers and stomach cancer), and to help with conditions that include rheumatoid arthritis, macular degeneration, and some neurological problems (Sulforaphane Glucosinolate Monograph, 2010).

All the crucifers contain healthy compounds that improve the detoxification of estrogen and other toxins. Try to find locally produced Brussels sprouts, red cabbage, cauliflower, and other crucifers. Alternatively, you can buy frozen or even take the ideal route of growing your own.

Kelp is probably second on my list here. It's not a vegetable because it's not a true plant, but it's close enough. Kelp is the only rich food source of iodine, and it contains many other nutrients and trace elements as well. Kelp contains an important form of vitamin K and numerous carotenoids. One particular marine carotenoid, fucoxanthin, is found in brown algae and seaweeds; it has been shown to have properties that may reduce inflammation, cardiovascular disease, obesity, diabetes and cancer. It is being investigated as a possible "drug" (Peng, 2011). Who knows what other treasures lie within seaweed?

Kale, spinach and other dark, leafy greens are extremely healthy. They contain high amounts of carotenes and other phytonutrients like lutein and other carotenoids important for eye health and other things. Just remember the caution about oxalates, which are found in high amounts in dark leafy vegetables. You may want to limit these foods if you are prone to kidney stones or related problems.

Tomatoes are technically a fruit, but I list them here because most people think of them as a vegetable. Slow cooking tomatoes with olive oil liberates lots of lycopene and other healthy nutrients, a key aspect of the Mediterranean diet.

Red onion contains lots of sulfur and compounds that aid detoxification, so eat as much, preferably raw, as your loved ones and coworkers can stand. This goes for garlic as well, which has even more health benefits than its cousin, the onion. Again, garlic should be consumed raw for the best health effects.

Watercress, which is in the same family as broccoli and cabbage, contains similar anti-cancer compounds and is high in iodine, iron, folic acid, and other beneficial nutrients. If it is cultivated with animal waste, it can harbor the larvae of liver flukes, so be cautious about the source.

Many other vegetables are good for you as well, and this food group should comprise a large portion of your diet.

Fruits and berries

Dark berries top the list here, as they contain high amounts of phytonutrients and antioxidants. Eat wild or organic blueberries, blackberries, boysenberries, and acai berries, as well as other dark, sweet things like prunes, every day. I believe these foods are the biggest reason we have a natural craving for sweet flavors. A wild animal that comes across a berry bush wants to eat them all.

Make sure you buy them frozen if you can't pick your own; the fresh ones are often moldy by the time you get them home and, as with all other fruits and vegetables, they start to lose nutrients like vitamin C as soon as they are picked. Frozen organic blueberries are a favorite dessert for most of my children, and I am happy to give them large amounts.

Apples are a must nutritionally. As I discussed earlier, they are even higher in the polyphenol antioxidants (proanthocyanadins) than red wine is. They have other beneficial nutrients as well, and they contain a great deal of soluble fiber, which helps to bind up the toxins from your liver bile and improve bowel clearance. Eating an apple has apparently been shown to improve energy and alertness better than drinking a cup of coffee (my fourteen-year-old daughter learned that in science class, so it must be true). An apple or two daily may indeed keep the doctors away. Make sure you eat the peel and, no, applesauce and apple juice do not work the same way!

Apple cider vinegar is a super food if ever there was one. It improves digestion and nutrient assimilation, promotes weight loss for many, kills some abnormal organisms in the gastrointestinal tract, cures acid reflux for many people, improves resistance to infectious illness, and provides an excellent source of potassium citrate, which dramatically improves liver detoxification and promotes cellular growth and tissue regeneration. Since I've started taking half a tablespoon mixed with an equal amount of honey and diluted with water to taste every day, and my hair and fingernails grow twice as fast and thick as they did before. A great book by D.C. Jarvis, MD, *Folk Medicine*, catalogs the benefits of apple cider vinegar (along with honey and kelp).

Red grapes contain antioxidants and polyphenols similar to those in dark berries, and we all know the purported benefits of red wine. My concerns about grapes are that they contain relatively high amounts of sugar, and they usually get moldy soon after you get them home from the grocery store. You don't generally find frozen grapes at the store, and it is rare for folks to grow their own. The healthiest and most practical way to get your grapes may be in the form of red wine, and many cultures that start this practice at early ages enjoy excellent health.

Grape juice may be a useful alternative, without the toxicity risk of alcohol. Seek out organic varieties with no added sulfites or sugars and hope the grower used grapes with seeds. It is also good for your health to have any sort of dark fruit or berry juice (pomegranate, blueberry, cherry, grape, acai, and others). They should be organic, of course, have no added sugar, and be in glass jars rather than plastic.

Prunes deserve a second mention because they improve bowel transit and are full of antioxidants. Prune skin seems to contain certain compounds that significantly improve detoxification, so that a large nutraceutical company, Metagenics, has made a medical food product with prune skin extract they sell for detoxification. Prunes are a good dessert to have every night.

A couple other fruits are not really "super" but bear mentioning here because they can dramatically improve the health of you and your kids if you use them to replace junk foods in the diet. Oranges are high in vitamin C and potassium. The peel has some healthful substances as well, so you can eat some of the white pith, but the orange part of the peel contains a stimulant chemical similar to ephedra, so don't try to eat the whole thing like an apple. Oranges also come with their own wrapper and are very portable!

Bananas also have some healthful nutrients and come in their own wrapper so they don't require washing. Washing is very important for all fresh produce whose outer layer is consumed, even if it is organic. Fruit is often transported with non-organic items, and you never know who was handling it or what was on their hands. Organic bananas cost only 99 cents per pound even in Alaska, which is only 20 cents more per pound than non-organic bananas and a quarter to half the cost of most junk snack foods like chips, crackers, and cookies.

Herbs

Many herbs have excellent nutritional value in terms of the phytochemicals they have to offer. You should try to incorporate many of these herbs into your foods as much as possible, but I list a few of the key ones here.

Turmeric tops the list for me; it contains curcumin, which I discussed at length in the section on pytonutrients. Consuming turmeric in the form of curry with coconut milk, which is also a super food, has been shown to reduce the risk of dementia, cardiovascular disease, and cancer as discussed earlier (Basnet, 2011). It has been suspected to exert its widely beneficial effects through some epigenetic mechanisms (Fu, 2010). Turmeric is also used in Ayurvedic medicine to treat infections and other problems. I encourage you to eat curry on a regular basis or to find some other way to use turmeric in your cooking.

Cilantro contains compounds that help bind and remove mercury and other heavy metals. Garlic and onions also have sulfur-containing compounds that aid in detoxification. Basil contains antibiotic and antiparasitic compounds, and oregano is helpful in killing yeast and some other pathogenic intestinal organisms. Cinnamon and fenugreek both help control blood sugar. Cinnamon is also helpful in reducing gas, and fenugreek is commonly thought to promote breast milk production.

I have already discussed some of the benefits of green tea. Just be sure your tea is organic and that you brew green tea covered for just a few minutes to get the highest concentrations of healthful compounds.

There are many other herbs we use regularly or have easy access to, and I encourage you to learn the possible health benefits of others.

Miscellaneous

I had to find a place to put chocolate. It's not typically considered a fruit, vegetable, bean, seed, or animal product, so I'm not sure where to put it. Chocolate in its pure form has a high antioxidant load, polyphenols, and healthy oils and does not have much sugar. It also stimulates the pleasure centers of the brain! The catch is that it is almost always mixed with sugar and milk to varying degrees, it may be somewhat addicting (though there are far worse things to be addicted to).

There is an urban legend that chocolate always contains cockroach parts because wild roaches of a certain species lay eggs inside the chocolate beans/berries as part of their life cycle, or because roaches invariably get into the large vats of chocolate during manufacturing. I searched PubMed and the general web for a definitive answer to this question and was met with just widespread speculation. Of course, I feel this just adds to chocolate's charm and nutritional value. In any case, if you are allergic to cockroaches you are unlikely to have trouble with chocolate.

Fermented foods, discussed somewhat previously, deserve special mention in the super food category. Fermented foods include fermented dairy products like yogurt and kefir, coconut milk kefir, fermented tofu products, and cabbage products like kimchi and sauerkraut. Some of these traditional dishes have been around for thousands of years and have persisted because of their clear health benefits. The word *kefir* is derived from the Turkish language and means something akin to "good health."

What separates these fermented foods from their "mother" food items, which are generally healthful in their own right, is the bacteria used to produce them. These organisms produce enzymes we do not have that can derive nutrients from foods we cannot, so they produce new chemicals we cannot create ourselves. They also produce vitamins for us and help attune our immune systems. Using the right organisms and starting with healthful ingredients seem to be the keys to making a truly healthful fermented food. Of course, keep in mind the confusion about fermented soy foods and cancer risk I mentioned previously.

Certain strains of bacteria have traditionally been used for each kind of food, and the bacteria wonderful things for our own health after we ingest them, in addition to the healthful changes they produce in fermented foods. Yeasts, which are also often used for fermentation, are a source of nutrition, but many of us have become sensitive to yeast organisms, so I do not put yeast-fermented foods in the same class as those fermented with probiotic cultures.

Yeast-fermented products have been used for millennia; some of the healthy ones include apple cider vinegar, beers and ales from various roots and grains, wine, and perhaps sake. (I don't think Coors, Budweiser or other mainstream beers are healthful beverages, but old-fashioned, thick, dark, rich beers have a lot of nutrition to offer.) Some yeasts, such as brewer's yeast, which is particularly rich in B-vitamins, is also consumed as food. However, many people become chronically ill from yeast and may be sensitive to beneficial yeasts as well.

For more information and to learn how to make your own fermented foods, look online for the Body Ecology™ organization (http://bodyecology.com) or find recipes in Fallon's *Nourishing Traditions* and other sources.

I am sure there are many other foods deserving of mention as super foods, but this is a good initial list. Try to incorporate these types of foods into your diet every day, replacing less healthful foods. You can make gradual transitions or just jump in with both feet. Start by going through your pantry and refrigerator and throwing away everything that is bad for you. I know you paid for it all, but there's no reason you and your family's health should have to pay for it again by consuming it. "Now" is always a great time to start, because "tomorrow" never comes.

Where to find healthful food

It's always annoying when someone complains about problems without offering real practical solutions, so I'm going to try not to do that. Two of the more common excuses I hear from people is they don't know where to get healthful food and that healthful food is expensive. I've already mentioned how healthful food does not have to be more expensive than junk food; apples cost less per pound than pop tarts, cookies, or potato chips, and brown rice costs less than Hamburger Helper™, for example. Producing your own food is usually cheaper than buying it.

I suggest you look for a whole-food market or natural food store somewhere nearby or find the natural foods section in your local grocery store. Ask your grocers to carry more organic produce and health food items; they will usually be happy to oblige if it means you'll buy it from them. Industries operate based on consumer demand, and food is no different. I have seen the natural foods and organic produce sections at my local grocery store expand dramatically in recent years, possibly in part because I myself have influenced thousands of local residents to change their food choices.

Consumer behavior is one important way we can all change the face of food production. If nobody buys mass-produced eggs, milk, or meat, the suppliers will be forced to stop producing it in the same way and turn to more healthful practices in order to stay in business. In the process, the healthful options will become cheaper.

If there is no suitable local store, look online for buying clubs and whole-food suppliers of dry goods, organic cheeses, butter, meats, and produce. I have access to a number of cooperative organic produce suppliers even in Alaska, and we have local buying clubs that reduce individual costs through bulk purchasing of more healthful foods.

Grow or produce as much food as you can yourself. You can grow herbs and sprouts with minimal space in your house, and if you have space for a garden or greenhouse, there is no better use of your time than producing healthful food for your family. You'll find the labor rewarding in terms of mental and spiritual balance, and you can get the whole family involved.

Hunting and fishing are still practiced in many parts of the country, and you may be able to share the yield with other families. You can also seek out local producers of foods like raw, grass-fed dairy, natural free-range eggs, and other animal foods and produce. Supporting local producers provides you with better food and decreases pollution from long-distance transportation of food. The more we lean toward regionalized food production, the better it is for the planet and future generations.

These are just some ideas to get you started. If you start seeking out healthful food products, you will be surprised how easy it becomes to maximize their use in your diet. I have some patients who live in very rural environments where there is little or no regional food production and the local stores have only highly processed foods to offer. Some of these people hunt, fish, and grow much of their own foods, but others eat the processed foods and complain to me that healthful food is not available. My response is that perhaps they should move somewhere else. You can't sit in a veritable wasteland and complain that you have limited resources.

Eating for health is extremely important, so stop making excuses and figure it out!

CHAPTER 14 – WHEN WE SHOULD EAT

A discussion of how you structure your food intake through the day has mostly to do with weight management. There are a couple of general principles to follow: First, eat when you are hungry. Second, try to consume most of your food in the first half of the day, prior to being active, when you are going to use up the energy. Avoid eating a lot at night prior to being sedentary and going to bed. I doubt that this is news to you. The first recommendation is to keep your metabolism going so it doesn't shift into "starvation" mode. The second recommendation is to distribute your energy intake to when you need it most.

There is that old saying that you should have "breakfast like a king, lunch like a prince, and dinner like a pauper." Breakfast is, as has often been said, the most important meal of the day, and people are much more satisfied in terms of nutrition and hunger if they start the day with foods rich in healthful proteins and fat than if they eat starches and grains for breakfast. Studies have noted people ate 80 percent fewer calories throughout the rest of the day when they had an omelet for breakfast, rather than cold cereal or instant oatmeal (Hyman, 2008). Studies that have reviewed successful diet plans for weight loss have found that eating a good breakfast is one of the few consistently helpful habits.

Probably the best depiction of why you should eat in the morning and not at night is the sumo wrestler lifestyle. You may have never considered how difficult it is to grow a 400-pound Japanese man without steroids or gamma rays, but sumo wrestlers have been doing it with diet for many generations. As described in Dr. Mark Hyman's *Ultrametabolism*, the sumo wrestler's diet and activity program consist of doing several hours of intense exercise in the morning without eating anything, then having a huge lunch and a nap. They meditate or pray in the evening, eat a large dinner, and go to bed shortly afterward. This meal and activity structure appears to stimulate massive weight gain.

How many of you follow the sumo lifestyle inadvertently? How many Americans skip breakfast and run out the door, work through lunch (or eat high-calorie, low-nutrient fast food), then have their largest meal at dinner, after which they sit around watching TV until going to bed?

How many health-conscious people exercise in the morning because that's when they feel they have time, then skip breakfast or eat very little before running off to work? Sometimes all you have to do is restructure your food and activity timing through the day to lose weight and achieve improved health. I've seen it work repeatedly.

Of course, like any generality, this routine isn't applicable to everyone. Many slender, fit people say they skip breakfast because they aren't hungry in the morning or it makes them feel nauseous if they eat before 10:00 a.m. Many people stay fit while exercising in the morning. These aren't the people who should rearrange their days and change their habits; it's those who are not succeeding who should try a different schedule.

A more consistently helpful dietary tenet is that of avoiding periods of "starvation". Eating small, frequent snacks and regular meals seems to be helpful for almost everyone, and trying to starve yourself to lose weight may really shut down your metabolism. Choosing foods with high protein and fat content will allow you to go longer between hunger feelings and to consume fewer total calories for the day. If you eat eggs and meat or possibly nuts and whole grains for breakfast, you will be much more likely to make it through to lunch without feeling hungry or needing a snack than if you have processed bread or cereal products.

If you starve yourself, your body will shift to energy storage mode when you do eat, and everything you put in your mouth will seem to stick to your butt, thighs, and belly. A lot of this depends on other factors, such as hormones and toxicity load, it applies to some extent to almost everyone.

CHAPTER 15 – HOW MUCH WE SHOULD EAT

When we were young, we could get away with eating way more than we could after we hit age twenty or thirty because our metabolic rate slows considerably when we no longer need to grow to flesh out our lean body and bone mass. When we are young, there is often a lot of leeway in how much we may overeat and still not gain excessive weight, but after we reach maturity it is a different story entirely.

Once you hit maturity, you should eat only the amount needed to sustain your basic metabolic needs plus your individual activity level. Before the discovery of resveratrol, calorie restriction to meet minimum energy requirements was the only intervention shown to increase life expectancy in animals, and it is still the only realistic one. Eating anything more than you need stresses your organs, depletes factors needed for digestion and metabolism of food energy and toxins, increases the oxidative stress from burning carbohydrates and fats, and sticks more sugar molecules onto your proteins, overall accelerating the aging process.

Calories vs. activity

You can probably maintain a healthy weight by exercising to burn off extra calories, but exercise also produces increased free radicals and oxidative stress, itself potentially accelerating the aging process. If you want to live as long as possible, you should have moderate physical activity and eat only what you need.

However, many of us don't consider that prescription to describe a great quality of life, so we should all find our own happy medium between indulgence and restriction in terms of food intake and activity. I love both food and exercise, so I'm sure I will not live as long as I might have otherwise, but have come to accept that so I can enjoy the journey.

There are various opinions about how many calories we should consume, but there is no way to get it exactly right. Typical estimates are 25-30 calories per kilogram of body weight per day for adults. Thus, 50kg woman (110 pounds) would need 1250-1500 calories per day to maintain the same weight at a typical activity level. Of course, there are so many variables involved in weight regulation that this rule of thumb really may not apply to a given individual. After all, people who weigh 220 pounds can restrict their food intake to 1500 calories per day and still gradually gain weight.

I don't know how many obese women I have seen who restrict their calories to 1000 per day and exercise five hours or more per week but still do not lose weight because their metabolism is dramatically altered by toxins, hormonal abnormalities, allergies, and inflammation. Then there are 100-pound women who eat like lumberjacks and never seem to gain a pound. Unfair as this may seem, it is related to differences in metabolism. In regard to weight regulation, we are mostly at the mercy of our underlying metabolic rate, not by how much we exercise.

Metabolic rate and calorie needs

Metabolic rate is much more influenced by lean muscle mass than by fat. Muscle consumes energy with every movement, while fat tissue just sits there and traps heat, thereby possibly even conserving energy. You don't need to "feed" the fat tissue—it should be feeding you—just the muscle and metabolically active organs. The amount of lean muscle mass in proportion to fat is partly why leaner people have higher metabolisms, and fatter people continue to gain weight even though they eat the same or less than their thinner counterparts.

Since energy consumption is depends more on the amount of lean body mass and muscle tissue you have than your total body weight, you can't calculate daily calorie needs based on your body weight if you are overweight or obese. Weight training is typically a much better way to successfully lose weight and keep it off than aerobic exercise because you increase the amount of muscle mass that consumes energy and burns more fat that produces energy over time. The ongoing "housekeeping" energy consumed to maintain cellular functions is responsible for 80 percent or more of your daily energy expenditure, while you influence only 15 percent or so of the energy you consume through your daily activity and exercise.

This is why doing light or moderate aerobic exercise rarely helps people lose much weight.

Pharmacists have been trained to calculate daily calorie needs based on "lean body mass" rather than total weight. Lean body mass is calculated based on your gender and height, the first of which changes only gradually in adult and the second of which rarely changes by much in an adult. Measuring lean body mass is a much better estimate of calorie needs for most people who want to achieve a normal weight for their height. Of course, your muscle mass may be greater than average for your height and your activity level may be significantly higher, both of which will require more calories to maintain muscle tissue.

Professional athletes have to eat several thousand calories more per day than the typical person because of their activity level and greater proportion of lean body mass. The Olympic swimmer Michael Phelps is a good example; he reported eating ten thousand calories per day intake when he was training hard, with no weight gain. I myself did some bodybuilding as a teenager and had to eat insane amounts of food in order to gain muscle mass. The point of all this is to show there are many variables affecting caloric needs for any given individual, and it is virtually impossible to calculate what you need precisely.

Counting calories vs. nutrient content

Because of all of these metabolic factors and variables, I almost never recommend that anyone count calories strictly. That doesn't mean it isn't helpful to know the calorie load of different foods and have a sense of what you are actually consuming, but what bothers me about calorie content is that people will limit certain healthful foods like butter and fruit because of their caloric density or sugar load. In my opinion, the calorie content is not as important as the macronutrient makeup and nutrient content of food.

"Empty calories" refer to foods that have no healthy amino acids, fats, fiber, vitamins, minerals, or phytonutrients. Empty calories are rampant in foods high in processed carbohydrates, including junk foods like cookies, chips, and French fries and foods like pasta, white bread, "instant" potatoes, rice, and oatmeal. Some fats and oils like margarine and vegetable oil also have empty calories. No amount of these foods is really good for you, even if you keep your calorie intake down where you want it, because these foods offer none of the nutrients you need to run your metabolism and break them down or burn them off. Therefore, those calories are "empty" and may just become extra fat.

Conversely, eating pasture-fed butter or an organic apple provides you with fat or sugar, but in conjunction with high amounts of beneficial nutrients that improve your overall health. In my opinion, all most people have to do to reach a healthy weight is to focus on eating only nourishing foods, avoiding those that contain poisons, and eating only until they are satisfied. Most of us have mechanisms in place to tell us we have eaten enough, but many of us ignore those signals and continue eating until we have stuffed ourselves, and this is the part to work on.

Some people's bodies contain environmental toxins, yeast, hormonal or neurotransmitter imbalances, and other factors that affect their normal appetite-sensing mechanisms, so they can no longer rely on their innate sense of satiety. Those people may in fact need to count calories to some extent rather than relying on their innate signals. However, most of us can do fine if we just learn to eat more slowly and to stop when we feel satisfied. Overeating can quickly become a habit because of stomach stretching and the resulting ramp-up of your digestive metabolism from high intakes of food, but all that excess processing creates harmful byproducts and free radicals and may contribute to shortening your life span.

To me, one of the biggest scandals in food manufacturing is the ready-made meals marketed to help people lose weight. They are full of highly processed foods with added chemicals and are usually not organic. They have typically been cooked once, and then you microwave them again, which destroys more of the residual nutrients that may have survived the original processing. To top it off, these ridiculous meals are in plastic dishes, the evils of which I discuss later. They may be lower in calories than other meals, but they have nothing of value to offer.

Age and growth needs

Age is another major factor related to caloric and energy needs. Younger people require more calories per pound than older people because their basal metabolism is much higher when they are still growing, and they need more food substance to build new body mass. The faster your rate of growth, the greater your relative energy needs. The fastest rate of growth and development occurs in the newborn period, when your calorie needs per pound (or kilogram) are the highest they will be in your lifetime. In contrast to the 25–30 calories per kilogram of body weight for adults, newborns need about 120 calories per kilogram! If I (weighing a little over 90kg) ate that much for my body weight, it would be over 10,000 calories per day!

Breast milk and typical baby formula have about twenty calories per ounce, so an eleven-pound baby needs about thirty ounces per day—close to four eight-ounce bottles. These numbers are far more consistent than figuring out what an adult should eat because the metabolic rate and activity level of infants is much more uniform. As kids grow, their calorie needs drop off steadily even though their physical activity level picks up.

Babies need that much to ensure normal growth and organ development, and they need the best nutrient-rich food in order to do it. Breast milk fits this bill better than any formula ever will, but the quality of breast milk depends on what the mother is eating and how well she has taken care of herself nutritionally and environmentally. A thorough discussion of prenatal and neonatal health may be the subject of a future book because it is a topic critical to our future as a species.

We should not let our kids eat just anything they want because they may develop weight-related health problems. We are seeing huge rises in childhood obesity, type 2 diabetes, high blood pressure, high cholesterol, joint and back pain, and other complaints related to excess weight. I believe that this problem is caused by the types of food they eat, not by how much they eat; kids on a natural whole-food diet are extremely unlikely to develop any of these issues, and they will likely eat less overall because the food will be more nourishing. Their activity level will likely increase as well because natural foods promote energy rather than sluggishness.

Natural appetite mechanisms

Overeating is a natural tendency. We have a strong natural drive to eat for survival purposes, a drive that evolved in a setting where food was all wild and healthy but far more difficult to come by. In the natural world, animals, including humans, have to expend a lot of energy to get a thousand calories of food, while in modern America you need only to hunt down a couple doughnuts or a drive-through. There are high-calorie, low-nutrient foods everywhere that you can consume in massive quantities with little or no effort. It's no wonder so many people gain weight so easily!

This is why it is so important to focus on the *type* of food you eat, so you eat food that nourishes and satisfies rather than foods that clog your system and keep you hungry for more. The consumption of sugar and processed food generally leads to increased hunger for those things, while eating nutrient-dense whole foods generally leads to a deeper sense of satisfaction and decreased hunger in general.

If you think you can eat just one of those cookies or brownies, you are fooling yourself. If you think that tub of ice cream or bag of chips is going to last you a week because you're just going to eat a little at a time as a treat, you may be surprised when you eat them all in a day or two.

We have to use the advanced part of our brain to outsmart the primitive areas. You have to look at those foods in the store or on the break room table at work and make the smart choice with your frontal lobes. Don't get close enough to smell them if you can help it, and be sure not to try "just one bite" because then your primitive brain takes over and you're likely to keep sneaking back for little bites all day. If not, you may go to the store later, buy yourself a whole box of treats, and find yourself in a sugar coma.

Do you think the food manufacturers don't understand how our innate appetite mechanisms work? Do you think they don't put things into processed foods to make you crave them more and more, like the tobacco industry did with cigarettes? I'll bet they do, and some of those additives include corn syrup (especially HFCS), artificial sweeteners, and MSG. There are also naturally addictive proteins in wheat and other gluten-containing grains (gluten itself), as well as in milk and dairy products (casein) that cause you to crave them and eat more of them than you need.

Of course, our sense of hunger usually diminishes at some point as we age. If you have cared for an aging parent, family member, patient, or client, you may have noted that they don't want to eat or drink much and that they need to be encouraged to do so. This situation occurs because, as the brain ages, the innate mechanisms that signal life-preserving hunger and thirst begin to deteriorate. This problem is most prominent in dementia patients, such as those with Alzheimer's disease. These patients often refuse to eat or drink at some point, accelerating their demise. After all, most behavior is driven at least to some extent by chemical reactions in the brain, which is why they can make drugs with chemicals that suppress or stimulate your appetite.

Calorie confusion

One last point about calories is they are not all created equal. A calorie is just a unit of energy, and it does not necessarily equate to energy your body can use. Foods with high amounts of fiber have significant calorie content that you cannot metabolize. Wood actually contains loads of caloric energy, released as heat when you burn it, but you can't digest it and obtain that energy if you try to eat wood.

In residency I saw an infant who had been hospitalized due to "failure to thrive" simply because his parents did not realize that he could not metabolize high-fiber foods. The infant was around seven months old, and his mother was still trying to breastfeed him, but had become pregnant again so the calories she had to offer were being stretched too thin. The parents were some of the most health-conscious people I've ever met, and they were trying to supplement the baby's intake with only organic foods they had grown themselves.

This sounds great, but the problem was that they were calculating what his calorie needs should have been and were feeding him just that much. He was not growing at all on this regimen, but when we put him in the hospital and fed him formula whenever he was hungry, he grew normally on about the same number of total calories. So what happened here?

When I talked to them later and found out what they were feeding him, I realized that you can't count the total "calories" in a carrot as all useable calories for growth and metabolism because a lot of it is fiber that you cannot use for energy. All they had to do was feed him the same foods but increase the calorie count, and he did fine. The mother also had to make the same logical adjustment to her own diet and stop counting all the vegetable calories as real energy for herself so she could provide both for the baby in utero and the one she was breastfeeding.

The short answer to the question, "How much should I eat?" is "I have no idea." My advice is eat the minimum lean body mass (you can find calculations online based on your height and gender), and to seek the help of a knowledgeable practitioner if that doesn't work. Use a naturopath or integrative physician, not a conventional nutritionist or dietician because their training in this area is lacking. If you are trying to lose weight and failing or if you are having trouble maintaining normal weight, naturopaths and integrative physicians can also help you find the causes of your metabolic dysfunction.

Some useful calorie-and-nutrient-tracking diet programs available on the internet can reveal whether you may have a metabolic problem if your calorie intake and expenditure don't seem to jive with what your weight is doing. There are also devices you can wear, such as the Body Bug™, that calculate how many calories you are burning with activity, and these can be very helpful as well.

CHAPTER 16 – EXERCISE

Exercise is one way of "nourishing" the body, or giving it something it needs for optimal function. For my purposes here, the term "exercise" includes mental activity and engagement in addition to physical activity. How you use your body and your mind is extremely important in maintaining the health of every organ.

If you don't use your muscles, they will shrink; if you don't bear weight on your bones they will thin and weaken; if you don't use your mind, it will fade away. Your brain typically burns about 20 percent of the total calories you burn in a day, even though it usually accounts for less than 2 percent of total body weight.

The need for physical activity

Our bodies need physical activity or "exercise" for normal health and function. Astronauts in zero-gravity environments have demonstrated how fast we can lose muscle mass and bone strength without proper stimulation. I broke my right arm in December 2009, and I was disturbed by how quickly the muscle mass shrank when I couldn't exercise or use it for only a few weeks. Our bodies require physical activity and stimulation in order to form and maintain function properly; it is a "use it or lose it" situation.

Other reasons we need physical exercise include that, when we are sedentary, we tend to become tired and unmotivated. You would think just the opposite, that a person with a sedentary job would be itching to get to the gym or go out and jog afterwards, but inactivity seems to promote more inactivity. Nothing is more draining to me than a long drive in the car, even though it did absolutely nothing to wear me out physically. A body at rest tends to stay at rest (Isaac Newton's first law of motion).

The flip side to this is that, when you do force yourself to get active or exercise, you will generally feel much better, more energetic, more clear-headed, and have more motivation to be active again the next day. If it doesn't work that way for you, see an integrative practitioner to have your adrenals checked. When you put more energy demands on your body, it starts producing more energy. A body in motion tends to stay in motion (also concordant with Newton's first law).

So what are you going to do about this? You're going to get your butt moving, that's what. When you feel totally drained from a long day of sitting, you should eat an apple to perk yourself up and do some jumping jacks to get moving. Once you wake your body up, continue with whatever exercise regimen you have chosen based on the results you are looking for.

Mental exercise

The same concepts apply to mental exercise, which is just as important for brain function and longevity as physical exercise is for physical health and weight regulation. A long-term study of a group of nuns ("The Nun Study") found that those who did crossword puzzles or other mental activities regularly preserved their mental function and avoided problems with dementia at a better rate than did their counterparts who did no such mental exercise. This could have just been a behavior pattern of more intelligent nuns at baseline however. Analysis of the nuns' writing samples through the decades showed that those with poor language and grammatical skill, whose writings lacked intellectual quality, later on developed dementia at a rate of 80%, while those with the best writings in those regards developed dementia only 10% of the time (Riley, 2005).

This may just mean that those with better brains to begin with end up with better brains toward the end; it could also suggest that using your brain more helps it work better longer. Reading books and playing complex games (even video games perhaps) may work if you don't like crossword puzzles or Sudoku, but watching TV and managing your online social network account probably don't count.

Another effect of sedentary mental behavior seems to be depression and a general lack of pleasure. Many people who retire from their jobs quickly become quite pitiful, shuffling aimlessly around the house all day, gaining weight, and shutting down mentally and physically. Others remain very active in retirement; they write, travel, tend a garden, do volunteer work, and help raise their grandchildren, and my experience is that they usually remain happy and active, maintain a better weight and state of health, and live longer. However, I've seen no research on this phenomenon.

The people who become sedentary and mentally and physically inactive after retirement tend to deteriorate not only physically but also in terms of their emotional and mental state. They are much more prone to weight gain and depression, and I suspect they are more likely to develop dementia and die earlier as well. We should maintain goals and interests throughout life, but especially as we age—enjoy hobbies, travel, do a physical sport or activity, learn a new language, play an instrument, volunteer somewhere, or even go back to school or work.

If you find the initial motivation to get going in terms of both mental and physical activity, then it becomes much easier to maintain that momentum. This is very important for both your quality and quantity of life. You also owe it to your loved ones because people who become sedentary also become irritable, depressive, and no fun to be around. They become the grumpy old neighbors you never liked when you were a kid.

Exercise for cardiovascular and neurological health

There are many reasons to do physical exercise. Some people are trying to lose weight, some are training for athletic competition of some sort, some are looking for better overall fitness, some just don't want to die, and others are trying to recover from a near-death event or injury. I try to suggest appropriate activities for folks based on what they are looking to achieve and with what they are most likely to comply.

The best exercise choices for cardiovascular and neurological health include those with sustained alternating movements like walking, which involves repeatedly alternating bilateral arm and leg swinging. This type of activity, sustained for half an hour or more, does a lot to get your nervous system into proper balance and gets your heart and cardiovascular system going faster, depending on your level of intensity.

There are two sides of your brain, each of which controls motor function for the opposite side of the body. The two sides communicate through a conduit in the middle of the brain called the corpus callosum and other areas of crossover for returning stimuli from the body to the brain in the brain stem. Increasing sustained alternating activity, such as walking, jogging, and swimming, improves the integration and overall function of your nervous system, which may lead to increased physical and mental energy, a better mood and sense of wellbeing, and improved physical coordination and balance. This last improvement is especially important for the elderly, where even a little physical exercise has been proven to help prevent falls and resulting hip fractures or other devastating injuries.

These same types of exercise are also good for cardiovascular health, but you must do them at a higher intensity to get cardiovascular benefits. Your cardiovascular system will improve its ability to deliver blood and oxygen efficiently when you regularly put greater demand on it. The amount of intensity you need is based on your level of fitness; since your fitness should improve over time, your exercise tolerance rises and the intensity of exercise you need should increase so you can make gains over time.

If you are very overweight and out of shape or if you are recovering from a heart attack or other cardiac event, you should start out slowly, perhaps after undergoing a stress test on your heart arranged by your doctor.

If you try to go too fast with an exercise routine of any type you are likely to get injured or discouraged, and that will just move you backward. Be patient, ease into your exercise program, and you will likely find your exercise capacity improves steadily. It usually takes years to achieve poor health, and it takes time to get back to a good state of health as well.

The best forms of exercise for your nervous system are activities like yoga and tai chi, which are meditative types of exercise that involve lots of balance and symmetrical neuromuscular integration. I recommend these types of exercise (especially yoga, which you can do in your own home with very little space or equipment) to everyone, whatever their fitness and health goals. Practicing yoga improves general functioning, balance and coordination, sports performance, and resistance to injury and enhances the mind and spirit. Yoga is also frequently therapeutic for back pain and other musculoskeletal problems.

Target heart rates and exercise intensity

For cardiovascular fitness, it is appropriate to exercise at an intensity based on a "target heart rate," that is, you try to get your heart rate up to a certain level, but not much higher. When your heart rate increases during exercise, it's because you are putting a greater metabolic demand on your muscles and your heart has to beat faster in order to increase circulation through the tissues, delivering needed oxygen to the muscles and other areas of the body, including the brain. The increased circulation also aids in clearing the increased toxins and byproducts of metabolism away from the body.

The more demand you put on the system, the faster your heart beats to compensate. Your blood vessels will also dilate in the appropriate muscles, your brain, and other areas in order to deliver more blood where it is needed. Your blood vessels will change in response to exercise in order to improve circulation, as though you were building bigger and better roads in the high-traffic areas of your city; it's good for overall efficiency. You may have noted that people who exercise have larger visible veins in their arms and legs, which is a sign of cardiovascular fitness and a greater circulatory capacity. This should not be confused with varicose veins in the legs, which may look like spider webs or may dilate to very large sizes and look like big blue worms curving back and forth under the skin.

Your target heart rate is typically based on your age because, as we age, our heart muscle tends to stiffen and lose its resilience, making it harder for the heart to fill with blood between beats and to deliver a enough blood with each heart beat. Your total output of blood per minute will drop off quickly if your heart beats too fast and doesn't allow sufficient time to fill with blood between beats. This is why people with rapid cardiac arrhythmias of around 200 beats per minute may get very dizzy or pass out

There comes a point at which your heart delivers less blood, not more, with an increase in heart rate so, your "maximal predicted heart rate" is calculated as roughly 220 minus your age. That means, if you are fifty years old, you aren't expected to stay conscious for long if your heart rate exceeds 170 beats per minute (bpm), but if you are twenty years old, you can probably tolerate a sustained heart rate of 200 bpm for a while. Of course there is significant variability here based on your level of fitness, vascular disease, and other factors; I've seen some people in their seventies and eighties remain completely conscious and lucid with heart rates at 150 or higher from cardiac arrhythmias.

As a general practice, you should not try to sustain your maximal predicted heart rate during exercise. You may get there if you are running from a bear or something, but those are special circumstances. Most trainers will suggest you go for a target heart rate of 80–85 percent of your maximal predicted level instead, where we assume your body is stressed to the point at which it will be forced to adapt and improve your physical fitness and cardiovascular capacity for next time, without nearly killing you in the process.

In most cases a fifty-year-old should aim for a target heart rate of around 136–145 or so, a thirty-year-old for 152–162, and so on. You can usually tell when you have hit the right range because you should feel a bit more mentally alert or even "high," and you will usually break out in an intense sweat because of the adrenaline release that occurs at this level of exercise. If you are very out of shape and/or obese, you may hit your target range with minimal activity, but as your fitness improves, you will have to go harder, faster, and longer to get your heart rate up. One important point is you don't have to exercise for very long to get good benefits, and it is fairly easy to *over*-exercise. Twelve to fifteen minutes is really plenty of time, as will be discussed further below.

Heart rate is a key to your cardiovascular fitness, but if you are just looking for nervous system balance, you don't need to get your heart rate up; time in the activity is a more important factor than intensity for improved brain and nervous system integration. Going for a long slow walk on the beach with that special someone won't increase your physical or cardiovascular fitness much, but it will do wonders for your brain and nervous system. You don't have to break a sweat to make your brain happy, but you should get sweaty and winded if you want to lose weight or decrease your risk of cardiovascular problems.

External influences on heart rate and exercise capacity

Some substances can artificially interfere with your heart rate. A common one is caffeine, one of my favorite whipping posts. Caffeine makes your heart beat faster, as many of us have experienced, but it does not improve your cardiovascular fitness because this increase in heart rate does not represent a physiological response to increased muscular demand. Similarly, fear, pain, and anxiety increase your heart rate and blood pressure but do not represent physical exercise.

Many people consume caffeine daily, and some have it prior to exercise because there is some evidence it increases fat-burning metabolism. If you have caffeine, and it raises your heart rate 10–20 bpm, you may not be able to exercise as intensely before reaching your target heart rate, but part of your elevated heart rate will be artificial, so using caffeine prior to exercise may not be of much benefit if you are doing aerobic exercise. If you are doing resistance exercise like weightlifting, it may be another story.

Other common sources of interference with heart rate are medications and illicit drugs. Stimulant medications, such as the amphetamine derivatives used for ADHD, elevate the heart rate much as or more than caffeine does, so the combination may be deadly: don't drink coffee or energy drinks if you are on these medications! There are black box warnings in the Physicians' Drug Reference (PDR) about these stimulants' potential for causing heart attacks even in children and young adults. Illegal amphetamines and cocaine may stimulate the heart to dangerous degrees as well.

Some medications commonly prescribed to patients with heart problems are designed to slow the heart down. They decrease the demand on your heart by slowing the heart rate and decreasing the strength of the heart contraction, usually lowering blood pressure as well. While these medications decrease strain on the heart and may decrease the risk of future heart attack, they certainly don't help in terms of exercise capacity. The most common side effect from these drugs is impaired exercise tolerance; when you increase demand on your muscles, the heart can't speed up in response with the result that you cannot go as hard or as long. If you are on these medications, your fitness will still improve over time if you keep at your exercise routine. If you find that you are unable to exercise at all because of the medication, ask your doctor if the dose can be decreased, as being able to exercise may be more important than maintaining a high dose of the medication.

Exercise for weight loss and physical fitness
Weight loss is a common reason people seek advice from a doctor. Many believe there is a big difference between exercising for cardiovascular fitness and exercising to lose weight, but there isn't. The best way to exercise for weight loss is the same as for overall improvement of fitness. However, the milder forms of exercise, such as walking, light cycling, or jogging, are frequently not successful for weight loss because of the way people usually do them.

The problem is often that people exercise at a low intensity for a long time. Studies have shown most people must do more than five hours per week of moderate, sustained aerobic exercise to lose weight in this fashion (Hyman, 2008). That is a lot of time, which many of you don't have. Interval training, doing high intensity exercise in brief spurts, is much more effective in far less time.

Of course, if you start running an hour a day, you are probably going to lose weight—marathon runners are awfully skinny, after all. If you push aerobic exercise hard enough, you will lose weight, but most people are not going to carry it that far and will likely not be successful. I see many very heavy people casually or "briskly" walking, and walking, and walking, without ever losing a pound. They aren't sending the right message to their bodies, so they aren't getting the right results.

Walking at a moderate pace tells your body "I'm going somewhere," not "I'm trying to change you." Walking and jogging are *transportation*, not exercise. When we perform sustained activities such as these we tend to make every movement as easy and efficient as possible so we can keep going for a long time. This doesn't really force change in the body; therefore I don't consider it true exercise. Try doing a series of deep lunges across the room and back or down your driveway, and see if you think it has a different impact on your legs than walking the same distance in the same amount of time. The difference is when you do lunges you are making each movement more difficult and demanding more performance from your muscles.

Think of exercise as giving your body a list of demands or requests for future capability. If you run hard for thirty seconds, you tell your body "I need to be able to run faster," and your body will respond by making your muscles faster and stronger. These changes cause metabolic changes that increase your calorie burning and lean body mass and changes in your lungs and cardiovascular system to improve oxygen delivery. If you run at a more moderate pace for miles and miles, you are telling your body you need to be able to sustain activity for a long time; this gives your body very different instructions.

Just look at the difference in physique between a marathon runner and a sprinter. Which one looks fitter? Which one looks healthier? Sprinters have excellent cardio-pulmonary (heart and lung) fitness, performing only short-term exercise at high intensity. Distance runners have elevated heart muscle enzymes in their blood, after running a long distance, which indicate damage to their hearts, and adversely altered heart-pumping activity (Sahlen, 2010). Long, sustained exercise tears your body down and makes it weaker rather than healthier; your heart and lung functions decrease rather than improve (Sears, 2010).

The other bad thing about sustained endurance exercise is that it shifts your body into fat-burning mode because you usually use up your available sugar and muscle glycogen within the first fifteen minutes or less. This sounds great on the surface because you may want to burn off your fat, but the problem is the message to your body says "store more fat for me because I'm going to use it a lot." Endurance athletes may stay lean as long as they continue exercising, but if they stop, they will likely pack on fat more quickly than a more muscular athlete.

Long, sustained aerobic exercise (longer than fifteen or twenty minutes) doesn't just burn off fat; it also makes your muscles smaller to increase efficiency. This decreases the lean body mass that actually uses energy, thereby lowering your overall metabolic rate. Even worse, sustained exercise of this nature causes your lung capacity and heart capacity to decrease, decreasing your overall health rather than improving it. I realize that this notion goes against our cultural dogma regarding exercise, but I urge anyone who is interested to read Dr. Al Sears' book on his *P.A.C.E.* program and the research on this topic.

Resistance forms of exercise are usually more effective for weight loss in general. These types of exercise include weightlifting, calisthenics (push-ups, sit-ups), plyometrics (jumping around) and even exercise like high-intensity yoga that fatigues the muscles. Athletes participating in sports like wrestling, gymnastics, football, sprinting, and others that focus on strength and power tend to develop impressive, lean, muscular physiques. While a wrestler or a football player does need considerable aerobic training, a wrestling match lasts only about six minutes, gymnastics routines usually last less than a couple of minutes, and a football play lasts a matter of seconds, so these aren't exactly endurance sports.

Mark Hyman's *Ultrametabolism*, as well as Al Sears' books on exercise physiology are useful references for this point of view. Dr. Hyman reviews the available research into exercise for weight loss and it shows that mild or moderate aerobic exercise is ineffective for most people because they burn some extra calories and then tend to eat more and rest more. Aerobic exercise, such as walking at a brisk pace on a treadmill for an hour, may burn a few hundred calories, but they are quickly replaced by the mocha or doughnut, soda, cookie—you fill in the blank with your own favorite reward—that you buy yourself as a treat for doing such hard work. You may feel tired from the expended effort and spend more time sitting the rest of the day because, after all, you already did your exercise.

If you start reading food and beverage labels, you will see how easily you can put three hundred empty calories back into your system. I want to stress this idea of "empty" calories in food again, because if you focus on eating nutrient-dense whole foods, you can usually eat your fill without becoming overweight or obese. Healthful food doesn't have all the empty calories that just tend to settle around your belly and butt.

Adapting to stress

So what types of exercise should you do to lose weight? You need to do something that forces your body to wake up and take notice that you are putting greater demands upon it and that shows you have high expectations about performance. You also need something that will increase your muscle mass. If you walk or jog, you will be making the movements as easy as possible for yourself and straining your muscles as little as possible in order to sustain the activity for longer. You can keep up this type of activity a long time, even if you're in poor shape, and it is not what you want.

As I mentioned before, try walking around your house a couple times while taking very long steps and doing a half lunge each time, rather than your usual little steps. If you can sustain that type of walking for half an hour I'll be very impressed. You can also try jogging while leaping as high and as far as you can with every stride, rather than pitter-pattering along as if you needed to keep it up for miles. You will get more effective changes in your body from five or ten minutes of the lunge-walking or leap-jogging than you will from a full hour of regular walking or jogging. Try it, and you'll feel the difference.

The point of effective exercise is to make things difficult for yourself, forcing your body to adapt and meet your new demands. Feeling the difference is the key here. Effective exercise burns. "Feel the burn," "no pain no gain," and other clichés are true to some extent. If you haven't broken a sweat, you aren't breathing hard, and you don't feel any degree of burning in your muscles from your exercise, then you probably aren't benefitting much from it.

I have seen many people in the gym (usually very out-of-shape people) strolling along on a treadmill, casually pedaling a bike while reading a magazine, or maybe lifting weights that are obviously too easy for them. You're wasting your time—and lack of time is one of the most common complaints I hear. If you're going to do it, do it for real, and stop fooling around! Get in, get sweaty, get out.

This is where a personal trainer or a good workout partner comes in. Many people need someone to kick them in the butt or push them in the spirit of competition to get them to do what's good for them. If there weren't drill sergeants in the military, the troops would be softer and weaker; it just isn't a natural instinct to make things difficult for ourselves, which is why our population has morphed toward obesity and sloth since our lifestyle has "improved." You have to find the will, whether it is within yourself or from someone else's pushing, to motivate you to make things hard on yourself a few times per week.

So what happens when you make things hard on yourself? When you push your cardiovascular system, your body adapts by increasing the capacity of blood vessels and blood flow to tissues, improving your heart's pumping efficiency and your cells' oxygen utilization efficiency. This kind of exercise puts less demand on the heart because the whole system becomes much more efficient. This is why athletes and people in good cardiovascular shape have lower resting heart rates; their body tissues have become much more efficient at using oxygen, so the whole system gets to relax when they aren't exercising. If your resting heart rate is in the eighties or nineties, you are either very out of shape or something else is causing it, like caffeine, illness, stress or anxiety.

When you strain your muscles, they respond to the increased demand by increasing the protein-derived muscle fibers and the number of energy-producing organelles (mitochondria), strengthening tendon attachments and getting stronger. Increasing your muscle quality in this way, as well as the eventual increase in muscle mass and size, will make the biggest favorable changes in your metabolism. Many women voice fears they will get big, ugly muscles if they lift weights, but you'd need steroids and ten hours per week in the gym to do that, unless you have a particularly muscle-building set of genes or unusual hormone levels.

Resistance training (weights, kettle bells, tension bands, push-ups, sit-ups, and so on) increases your lean body mass, which is the best way to increase your total energy expenditure. Your fat tissue, which does not burn any energy to speak of, works against you metabolically, while your muscle tissue does work and helps you burn off that stored energy.

I explain this to people as being similar to putting a bigger engine in your car. If you have a bigger engine, it consumes more gasoline with the same amount of driving, which means your car consumes more energy faster. This would not be desirable in your body if you still lived in the wild and food was hard to come by, which is why your body is so resistant to the idea and it takes so much work to get yourself "in shape."

People who are very muscular and who have very little body fat are not in a condition conducive to survival in the wild. They have a lot of tissue that requires energy to run and very little stored energy, which is like driving a huge pick-up truck with a three-gallon gas tank that gets only eight miles per gallon. Your body does not want to be like that because it is a bad idea under natural conditions, which is why elite athletes have to work so hard to maintain their performance. Your body breaks down that muscle tissue quickly when you decrease your exercise because we are geared toward energy efficiency.

Ideal exercise for physical fitness

The best type of exercise for weight loss and optimal fitness is probably an alternating combination of resistance training (anaerobic) and cardiopulmonary (aerobic) exercise. Both need to be performed at high intensity and for brief durations, alternating with short periods of rest, which is called interval training. This concept mixes things up for you and keeps your body guessing, stimulating the most rapid changes in your physiology.

If you prefer, you could achieve the same concept with a single form of exercise, such as walking alternated with short periods of running or sprinting. You could also use light to moderate weights with many repetitions in 30–60 second bursts of activity. If you have a treadmill, an exercise bike, or another piece of cardio equipment that has programs in it, there is likely to be an "interval training" selection you can try. If you don't have the program or you like to jog outdoors, go along at an easy or moderate pace for a minute or two and then kick it into high gear or sprint for thirty seconds to a minute; keep alternating between those two for a total of 12–15 minutes and you'll be finished!

The research presented by Dr. Hyman and Dr. Al Sears suggests that you need to do only about fifteen minutes of this type of exercise a few days per week to get better results than you would from doing five hours of mild to moderate aerobic activity per week. If you don't like to exercise or don't have much time to devote to it, then interval training is your answer. I tell my patients that this concept gives you the "biggest bang for your buck" in terms of time spent exercising. Some people love to run, bike or swim for long distances, and I find it pointless to try and convince them to reduce their exercise duration.

Of course, your results will depend on the effort you expend. You can't just stroll on a treadmill at the gym, eat a doughnut on the way home, and expect to lose weight or get in shape. What's more, it probably took a long time to get where you are, and it may take a long time to get healthy. A journey of a thousand miles may begin with a single step, but there are sure going to be a lot more steps before you finally get there! Be patient and persistent.

Psychological barriers to success

I have made some general observations about human behavior after working in health care for more than fifteen years. One thing I've noticed about many people who are trying to lose weight is they tend to put out some effort at first, but if they don't see rapid rewards, they quit. Some people are clearly more driven and will be much more successful, but they're in the minority as far as I can tell. Of course, the more driven and healthy people seldom need to come see me.

How many times have I seen someone start on some diet plan and get a gym membership, just to drop out in a month or less? How many of you have joined Weight Watchers off and on multiple times, done the Atkins or South Beach diets repeatedly, or bought a treadmill or other exercise machine you now use only as a coat rack?

You can't blame this problem on our "culture," as a culture is a collective of people who all have individual responsibility. I blame the individuals. Yes, I used the word "blame" even though our culture doesn't like to blame individuals or ask them to take responsibility for much; we are too worried about hurting someone's feelings. There is no emotion involved in my use of the word blame, just an indication of responsibility. Many of us would rather feel we are being oppressed by some outside force and that there are so many reasons outside of our control why we "can't."

However, if you don't assume responsibility for the problem, how can you believe you can be responsible for the solution? I think that is the main problem: belief. If we aren't immediately successful in our endeavors, we don't *believe* we can achieve our goals, and we stop. If you truly *believed* you could lose all the weight you wanted to lose if you kept up your program for a full year, you would probably stick with it. If you *believed* you had to put in ninety days of hard work before it paid off, but then it would make all the difference in the world for you, you would probably stick with it. That's often the reality in terms of adopting a new healthy lifestyle: you may not see real benefits for ninety days.

One problem is the persistent negative attitude many in our culture have. There is far too much "I can't" going on here. You may be surrounded by people who always say things can't be done or complain that things are going badly. These people seldom do what they could do to change things; they would rather sit around and complain. You may even be one of those people yourself; if so, you should get your hormones checked, clean up your diet, start exercising, and stop watching the news, reality television, or listening to talk radio.

Why is it that, when things don't improve with our first effort, we don't all want to try even harder? That kind of persistence and determination is a characteristic of successful people, as it turns out. I think a key part of persistence is *believing* you can get what you want if you just try harder. Start *believing* more in yourself and stop being a quitter! Don't listen to your father, boyfriend, mother, wife, brother, co-worker, or whoever it is poisoning your mind with negativity. Ignore them! The best revenge or counterargument to their oppressive attitude is achievement of your goals.

I've seen people do amazing things with themselves by way of their own efforts, although it does have to be your own effort; no one else can exercise or eat for you. I've seen many cases of success and believe every one of you can be successful as well. If you try hard for ninety days and still get nowhere, seek an appropriate medical practitioner to look for metabolic problems like hormonal imbalances, allergies, yeast overgrowth, and environmental toxicity problems.

Of course, you must be honest with yourself and your provider. Don't tell your doctor you have been eating healthfully when the fact is that you still grab fast food for lunch every day and eat cold cereal in the morning. Ordering a salad with your unhealthy dinner does not constitute a good diet. Don't say you're exercising when you're just strolling on a treadmill at the gym. Give the principles outlined in this book a real try before you go looking for help or some sort of artificial fix. You may be surprised.

Practical issues with exercise

In the first section of this book, I offered a list of common excuses people give for not following a healthy lifestyle, along with some brief rebuttals. Exercise is probably the subject of the greatest number of excuses I hear in my office. Here I would like to offer some helpful suggestions to increase your chances of success with exercise.

1. Find a type of exercise you enjoy, at least a little.

Not everyone likes to run or lift weights. If possible, find some sort of activity you can really get into so it doesn't feel like a chore. Just make sure you do it with enough intensity to get sweaty and out of breath, to feel some burning in your muscles. Get your whole body involved somehow. I realize many of you may hate any form of exercise, but you'll just have to suck it up. You may find that if you try something new, you'll learn to like it.

2. Don't get a gym membership if you aren't going to go or can't afford it.

I find it easier to exercise more often if I do it at home, so I dropped my gym membership many years ago. You don't need much in the way of equipment to get in shape, and if you exercise at home, it is much easier to find the time. I'm now finished with my workouts in less time than it used to take me just to drive to the gym and back. If you have lots of free time, you have no kids to care for, or you just like the gym atmosphere, then go ahead and hit the health club. If your life is busy, however, you may not have the extra twenty minutes or hour per day it takes you to prepare yourself for the public and drive to and from the gym. If you don't have the money for a gym membership, you can buy a good treadmill for less than a year's membership dues, and push-ups and jumping jacks cost nothing.

3. "Make" the time, don't try to "find" the time.

If you lie to yourself enough, you'll eventually start believing the lie. You have twenty-four hours in a day like everyone else, and I don't believe for a second that every minute of your day is accounted for and you can't find three minutes three times per week to do some push-ups and sit-ups, dumbbell curls, go for a half-mile walk or do a hundred jumping jacks. This is important enough for you to make time. Schedule yourself time during the week, at least in your mind, but preferably in your planner or calendar. Make it a priority.

4. Stop saying "I'll start exercising when"

So many patients come in after a year or more and tell me they kept moving their exercise start date back for some reason: "I was going to start after New Year's, but then I got busy." "I keep meaning to get my treadmill out, but I'm just too busy." Those excuses are nothing more than what they are: excuses. If you don't like to exercise, just admit it to yourself, make the choice to improve your health, and stop making excuses about it. We don't like to pay the bills, but we do it because there are consequences. We don't like to work, but we do it because we need the money. You have to figure out what it will take to motivate you to exercise. Start exercising right now, if you're ever going to! Put down the book and do some jumping jacks, push-ups, sit-ups, or knee bends. You will never do something if you're always going to start "tomorrow."

5.   Multitask.

I almost never do exercise by itself. I like to watch movies and television, but it's a sedentary activity, so I try to do some exercise while I watch. You can ride an exercise bike while you read (I did that for countless hours in medical school) and do sit-ups, squats or knee bends while you watch TV or listen to music or recorded books. The next time you find yourself just sitting as you watch television or listen to music, get up and do some kind of exercise. If you don't want to get up, grab some light weights and do arm exercises. Don't make excuses.

6.   Lie to yourself about something positive for a change.

Tell yourself you like exercise. Think about it in a positive light and convince yourself you are looking forward to exercising because you know how good you feel afterward and how much it will improve your health. There is a lot to be said for positive visualization and optimism. If you keep mentally framing exercise in a positive way, it may eventually become something you enjoy, look forward to, and refuse to go without. Sometimes you've got to "fake it 'til you make it," as my wife likes to say.

CHAPTER 17 – NOURISHING THE MIND AND SPIRIT

I discussed mental exercise briefly in the preceding chapter, mainly referring to the concrete cognitive functioning of the human brain. However, there is much more to our minds than just that aspect, and I don't think we currently come anywhere close to understanding the true potential of the human brain. This whole idea is very important to your complete health, as your mind can sometimes be a powerful force in healing what seem to be purely physical ailments.

Definitions

For my purposes here, let's say that "mind" refers to the part of you that thinks, feels emotion, senses, processes information, and makes decisions. This is the part of your "self" that talks inside your head, communicates verbally and non verbally, feels physical pain, dreams while you sleep, and so on. You have a great degree of control over this aspect of yourself, and it largely defines who you are in terms of philosophy and personal interactions.

"Spirit," on the other hand, is that less tangible aspect of who you are inside. It is defined on a more metaphysical level than the mind, so it is more difficult to comprehend in mental or cognitive terms; that's why there is so much debate as to its nature or even existence–arguments we will dispense with here. For now, we'll understand your spirit as a form of energy at its essence. It isn't electricity like the impulses from your heart or brain, which can be traced by EKG or EEG machines, but something on a more subtle level energetically.

Your energy field interfaces with the energy or life force of the organisms around you and the universe itself. You may view it as being based in physical energy as something placed inside you by your god or as something somewhere in-between—whatever fits into your personal spiritual faith, religion, or metaphysical framework. These distinctions and the arguments that inevitably ensue when people from different camps discuss them are not important to my discussion here (nor are they often very productive). The spirit aspect I'm referring to is difficult to characterize and describe. Your concrete physical senses and mind may not be able to observe the existence of your spirit because they are on a totally different plane of existence. For these purposes, I hope you'll just believe a spirit exists within you, whether you can "feel" it or not, as it is an important part of my discussion of health.

How your mind and spirit influence your health

Your mind and spirit are so important to your health that Harvard Medical School created a center for mind-body medicine. Numerous studies have researched positive visualization and how it can be used to overcome illness. You may have noted how your own attitude or mood can affect whether you fall ill or how you cope with an illness.

Some of this can be explained in terms of physiological processes. For the purpose of this discussion, let's make the distinction that all of the effects that can be explained physiologically are related to "mind" issues, while those that cannot yet be explained physiologically are attributed to "spirit" issues.

Stress and grief are two good examples of how your mental state can adversely affect your health. When I was in college, I tended to get a bad cold or bronchitis during or just after finals week every semester, and I later suffered terrible acid reflux when I was going through a divorce. Granted, some of the immune system suppression I experienced may have come from sleep-deprivation after late nights cramming for tests or writing last-minute papers, but some of it was related to the chemical effects of stress itself.

Scientists have described all sorts of changes in hormones like cortisol and neurotransmitters like serotonin during periods of psychological stress. The resulting chemical cascades can do a lot to weaken your immune system, interfere with sleep rhythms, alter appetite and gastrointestinal functions, and influence heart rate and other automatic functions of the body. You may feel there is nothing you can do about this, but there are ways to manage stress in order to avoid these consequences.

The effects of grief are similar to those of stress, but grief tends mainly to suppress normal systems rather than to include the initial up-regulation you may see with stress before the burn-out sets in. I have seen many examples of elderly men or women who die within six months or so following the death of a spouse. They may have been in good health prior to losing their partners but they soon get a cancer diagnosis, come down with pneumonia, have an unexpected heart attack, or experience some other kind of rapid decline after the loss of their spouse. One could make the argument that this example is largely rooted in the spiritual side of things.

I have also seen young adults with long-term health problems that begin after a period of intense grief, such after the loss of a child or other close relative. Adrenal or thyroid burnout, immune system dysfunction, or other physiological failures are often due to severe psychological or emotional stress. There is a spiritual wounding that I think most people can appreciate related to this type of loss and grief.

It is difficult to separate the effects of mind and spirit in terms of health problems because most of what we think we have explanations for starts with mind-related events. It is much harder to come up with examples that originate purely on the spiritual side because a spiritual source would mean that the problem had no observable characteristics in a practical or physical sense. These problems are often left unexplained or, in medical terms, "idiopathic."

Some of these issues may arise because of a lack of nurturing. Some children with emotional, psychological, or physical problems may have developed abnormally because they never received sufficient love and nurturing as infants. Early experiences and environmental factors have a major impact on the way we are wired neurologically and psychologically, and it is likely that those factors affect our spirit as well.

Studies, typically discussed in introductory psychology texts, done with monkeys have shown that if a baby had an artificial "mother" (a doll) that was padded and comfortable, the baby monkey would eat and grow pretty normally, while if it had a "mother" model made of hard material, it would eat much less and would usually do very poorly or even die in short order. This result may be explained by physiological mechanisms like pressure receptors in the skin sending different messages to the brain and causing changes in emotion and behavior, or perhaps the baby monkeys' spirits were broken by a lack of proper nurturing.

I have a personal example to share that may apply here. My fourth child, who was born a couple of weeks early, probably had too much Fentanyl (a narcotic my wife received for labor pains) in his system when he was born. When he finally came out after laboring for five to six hours, he didn't want to breathe and had to be resuscitated briefly. He was sent to the neonatal intensive care unit for short-term observation, and I went with him. He lay there looking pale and puny, breathing laboriously, and seeming generally out of sorts, but he was stable from a medical standpoint. I tried to put on a happy face for him, but I was a little worried.

He lay like that for five or ten minutes, but then his three older siblings came into the room and crowded around him in his little warmer. They stood shoulder-to-shoulder but made no physical contact with him at first. They just smiled down and cooed at him with genuine love and happiness, showing no shred of concern (because they hadn't been traumatized by medical training as I had). Right before my eyes, his breathing and muscle tone relaxed, he turned from pasty white to rosy pink, he started to look around, and his gaze softened. He no longer seemed distressed and sickly, though nobody had physically touched him. I was amazed.

It's experiences like that that make me wonder about the true nature of our spirit-energy and how we all interact with each other and the universe.

A few minutes later I told my wife's mother, whom had come in to check on things, that my wife could come see him if she was allowed to. I don't think it was a minute later that I heard a nurse say, "Crazy lady coming through!" and my wife rushed into the room, tears streaming down her face, moving like she was in a speed-walking race. A nurse pushed/carried her IV pole behind her, practically running to keep up. This time it was my wife's turn to be spiritually healed and balanced; she needed to see her baby.

I hope you have all felt something of this powerful spiritual nature yourselves. It's the way you feel around your children or the one you love when things are good. I know this can be described to some extent in terms of mental or cognitive reaction, neurotransmitters, and hormones, and other physiological processes, but there is something occurring on another level as well. Everything interacts and interrelates on multiple levels to some extent, which makes it difficult to understand what the spiritual side is.

The work of Edgar Cayce and others suggests that some of us can achieve the ability to sense and even influence what happens to other people a great distance away. I myself have training in Reiki, a form of energy healing, which allegedly enables skilled practitioners to send healing influence to others anywhere on the planet. Some studies have shown that intercessory prayer can help heal an individual some distance away, though a 2007 meta-analysis on the subject showed no consistent effect (Masters, 2007).

In a way, I think these ideas are the future of health and medicine, as well as the solution to many of our other problems as a global community. If you can heal a person's energetic essence, perhaps you can override most physical and psychological problems. I have met true energy healers and it is a powerful reality in my opinion. Every one of us may have the underlying ability to heal ourselves, and those around us. We may be able to transcend our current concepts of reality in terms of human health, existence, and potential.

For intriguing reading on this subject I suggest *The Celestine Prophecy* series by James Redfield, *The Life and Teaching of the Masters of the Far East* by Baird Spaulding (a six-book series), and *Mutant Message Down Under* by Marlo Morgan. There are also new writings and movies regarding quantum physics and how it relates to the energy within us all; some of these are *The Secret, What the Bleep Do We Know,* and *Down the Rabbit Hole.* If you have any interest in these ideas, I encourage you to pursue them because the more people who begin to put their positive intentions out there the sooner things will get better for us all.

Lessons from the water

In earlier sections of the book, I mentioned Dr. Masaru Emoto's *The Hidden Messages in Water* and his research. This simple research involved photographing water on a microscopic level while it froze into tiny crystals. What Dr. Emoto found was that the crystals formed different patterns depending on what sort of emotional environment the water was in or what feeling was expressed to it. I strongly urge you all to look this research up online or to buy the book; the power of seeing these images for yourself is much greater than any description I could offer.

What this research suggests to me is that there is a real, tangible interaction among living things, which are all comprised mostly of water, on an energetic level. The water molecules don't contain chemical hormones or neurotransmitters; they don't experience consciousness or emotion in the classic sense. There is something about our emotional expression that transcends the mere physical and has a powerful effect on the living and non-living systems around us. I think that may relate to the spirit.

You can take Dr. Emoto's research and extrapolate it to imagine how alterations in your emotional and spiritual state of health may translate to changes in your physical and mental health. Your body is roughly two-thirds water; if some negative external influence can affect your water molecules in a physical way, it may certainly affect your health negatively as well. Conversely, being loved and nurtured and having positive interpersonal experiences may greatly improve your health. Perhaps this is why happily married people tend to live longer.

I have tried to pay attention to this in my own life and have found that if I focus positive feelings toward my children and my wife, they are in better moods and return positive energy back to me. Your reaction is especially important when your significant other is being irritable and irrational. You may want to react defensively or negatively because you feel he or she is being unreasonable, but that approach never serves to improve the situation at my house. I've found that I can't always make things better, but I sure as heck can make them worse.

If I control my own reactions and stay calm and positive before I say anything, I find I can focus positive feelings and thoughts toward the other person and get a far better reaction. Smiling at people causes a different set of reactions than frowning at them does. Again, it is difficult to separate the metaphysical from the psychological or mental aspects of these human interactions, but part of it seems to occur on a spiritual level.

Researchers in energy medicine have found that energy healers can manipulate the activity of enzymes in solution to achieve significant improvements in what would be health-promoting chemical activity in the body. They can also influence the growth rate of plants by focusing energy and intention on the plant (Oschmann, 2000). Acupuncture theoretically works based on an energy network in the body; scientific studies of acupuncture have demonstrated effects that are not explainable by our current understanding of the nervous system and human physiology. I have witnessed acupuncture working by me own hand many times (though certainly not all the time).

The spiritual aspect of who you are is extremely important to your health, regardless of whether you understand it or believe in its existence. Methods of healing on an energetic level may not yet be understood by medical science, but that does not mean they are bogus or will not be understood eventually. Just because scientists and philosophers are not satisfied with any offered proof of God's existence does not prove there are no gods. The truth is the truth, whether people can measure it or not.

We just tend to make up our working definitions and explanations for everything as we go along.

Improving the health of your mind and improving your health with your mind

The confusing topic heading I offered here relates to the interconnectedness of the body, mind, spirit, and all aspects of who we are. If you improve the health of your mind, it will improve your physical health. If you improve your physical health, it will improve the health of your mind. Therefore, you have so much opportunity to improve your health! Techniques used to focus the mind's attention on physical problems can achieve improvement in physical health, and physical activity or healing can improve mental and psychological states.

We have plenty of data showing that physical exercise is a very effective overall treatment for depression and anxiety (Strohle, 2009). Exercise effectively lowers depression scores even at low to moderate volumes, around one to two hours per week (Annesi, 2011). There are certainly physiological reasons for this result that include measurable changes in serotonin levels with exercise, but there are also very likely to be energetic factors at play. It may be even more effective to get someone suffering from depression started on a fitness routine than to prescribe a drug; superiority of exercise over pharmaceuticals in depression and anxiety has been demonstrated repeatedly in clinical research (Carek, 2011). This is not disputed in psychiatry even though the drug companies have a death grip on that field of medicine these days. The problem is that most people in this country are much more willing to pop a pill every day than to devote time and effort to their health.

Mental exercises like crossword puzzles may improve cognitive function and delay or prevent dementia. Those mental exercises are ways to address the *physical* aspect of your brain, to keep the neurons firing and the neurotransmitters involved in learning and cognition in proper balance. However, there are other aspects to the "mind" that may not be adequately addressed by those methods. The psychological side of your mind is separate from the physiological side of the brain. Certainly, physiological factors, such as alcohol or drug use, nutritional deficiencies, hormone imbalances and allergies, can alter your psychology, but it is also possible to improve the physical and physiological part of your brain by focusing on the psychological. Let's look at some examples.

Psychological counseling methods, such as cognitive-behavioral therapy, have been shown to be consistently as effective or more effective than prescription drugs in the treatment of mood disorders like depression and anxiety (Hoifodt, 2011). This shows that you have the power within your mind to correct some of the problems going on with your brain and psyche. Again, the problem lies in the time and money people are willing to spend on their problems. Good therapy costs hundreds of dollars per week, while a drug costs only that much per month at the most, and some are available for just a few dollars per month now, even in the U.S. Insurance payers do not cover therapy as well as they do drugs, and they don't typically pay for a gym membership or personal trainer at all.

Meditation and other yogic practices appear to improve many chronic medical problems including both physical and psychological disorders. Proposed mediators of this effect include nervous system activity, cell trafficking, circulating signal molecules and bioelectromagnetism (Kuntsevich, 2010). Many patients recount examples of having recovered from an illness well because of how they framed it psychologically or what they did mentally (e.g., meditation, positive visualization, guided imagery).

So how do you use your mind to heal itself and the rest of you? You can meditate on an issue, focusing your attention on it calmly and peacefully, being mindful of all aspects of what is going on and how you are responding to it. Classic meditation involves emptying your mind, but that refers to meditation for spirit rather than mind. Mindfulness, becoming acutely aware and focusing your attention, is becoming an important field of study and is gaining attention for its application to health and healing.

Of course, mindfulness is nothing new, just somewhat new in the western world. In eastern philosophy and medicine, mindfulness has been in practice for millennia. A good modern source on mindfulness is Thich Nhat Hanh, a Vietnamese Buddhist monk who was nominated for a Nobel Peace Prize by Dr. Martin Luther King Jr. in the 1960s. Another is Jon Kabat-Zinn, Ph.D., the founding director of the Stress Reduction Clinic and the Center fo Mindfulness in Medicine, Health Care and Society at the University of Massachusetts Medical School. Numerous books, videos, and recordings by these men and others are available on the subject.

The practice is simple and takes almost no time; you can practice mindfulness all throughout the day. Just take ten seconds whenever you think of it to pay attention to something your senses are bringing you. Take a moment now to realize your breathing; pay attention to the feeling of the air moving in and out through your nose, throat and lungs. Feel—really feel—your chest expanding, your ribs swinging upward and outward, your belly passively distending forward and outward as you inhale. Become aware of how it takes no effort to exhale as the elasticity of your tissues pulls everything back to the beginning. You can repeat this for three breaths, ten breaths or a hundred breaths—whatever time you have.

You may notice you are not allowing your belly to relax outward with inhalation, as is very common in our society, where we expect bellies always to look flat. You may also note that there is excessive tension in your shoulders and neck muscles and possibly your upper back and chest. You have to breathe from somewhere; if you aren't using your belly as you're supposed to, you are probably anchoring your ribs abnormally from above and pulling them upward with too much force. You've been breathing all day and have likely never paid attention to it, even though it is so vital to your existence.

Spend at least a minute every day paying attention to how you breathe. Consciously relax your neck and shoulders. Feel the air move down into your chest and allow your belly to push outward, using your diaphragm muscle to breathe rather than pulling the ribs upward with your neck and shoulders. You will likely find that you feel more relaxed both physically and mentally, that the constant tension and pain you may experience in your neck and shoulders abates, that your mood is more even and your mental focus improves. Mindfulness is a very simple thing, but it is powerful. I try to do it at red lights while I'm driving, at various times through the day, and when I lie down to sleep at night.

One of the most powerful, not to mention quickest and easiest, things you can do for yourself is positive visualization, which takes no special training at all! Positive visualization, such as merely focusing on the concept of "appreciation" or some idea that makes you very happy and content, has been shown to be far superior even to trained meditation in generating healthy biorhythms and achieving a very high state of "coherence" (McCraty, 2010). Coherence occurs when multiple biorhythms such as breathing, blood pressure, heart rate variability and brain waves all resonate with each other. A highly coherent state is thought to be associated with improved health in a variety of ways; the entire July/August 2010 issue (vol. 16, no. 4) of *Alternative Therapies in Health and Medicine* was devoted to the concept of coherence.

When you have a moment when you don't need to focus your attention on what's in front of you, focus your mind on something positive. Think of something in your past that made you the happiest you ever felt or maybe something coming up in the future that brings you great happiness. When you focus your mind on something positive, you will notice widespread relaxation of your mind, muscles, breathing, and other functions. This result is measurable and powerful–and so simple!

If you want to become more advanced in your meditation skills, you certainly can. Some people spend hours each day in quiet meditation, but I simply don't have time for that at present—maybe when I retire. My point is that you can use simple, brief techniques like those I have described to keep yourself in mental, energetic, psychological, and physical balance all day and likely make every aspect of your life much easier and better.

Improving your spiritual health

Since the mind, spirit, and body are so closely connected, some of the practices I've discussed, such as physical exercise, mental exercise, and meditation, are good for spiritual wellness too. I firmly feel people benefit from doing things that are focused on the spiritual and energetic side of who they are. Most spiritual/energetic activities also involve both your body and your mind; in fact, I can't think of many examples that may use only your spirit—perhaps transcendental meditation and astral projection.

There are very diverse philosophies about the nature or existence of the spirit, soul, essence, energy, chakras, kundalini, or whatever you may choose to call it, and there are those who think the very idea is nonsense, and that is completely fine. In my mind, there is a vast difference between spirituality and religion, but for many people the two are intertwined, and that is okay too. No matter what sort of terminology or philosophy you choose, I hope there is some idea you can embrace because it is important to your health.

If there is some sort of spiritual practice you already perform, such as prayer, meditation, or journaling, keep it up. If you currently do nothing in this realm, the easiest way to get started is to practice simple mindfulness exercises and basic meditations similar to what I have described. They involve both the mind and the body in practice, but some positive effects also trickle through to the spiritual and energetic side.

You can learn a simple breathing exercise in just a few minutes, which is a quick sort of meditation. I call it "square breathing" because I tell people to visualize a square while they do it. Close your eyes and imagine a square of some color there in the darkness. As you breathe in, trace the square with your mind (perhaps the line can become brighter in your mind in the area you are tracing as you go around it) from the lower left corner up to the upper left corner. Then hold a full breath in your chest for three or four seconds while you trace across the top of the square to the upper right corner. Let the air out passively as you trace down the right side of the square to the lower right corner. Hold your lungs empty for three or four seconds as you trace across the bottom of the square. Then take in your next breath and go up the left side again.

You can use your heartbeat to count the time you spend on each side or just the top and bottom. Your square can become a rectangle if you find you take more time to inhale and exhale than you feel comfortable holding in or out. You can do whatever you want with it; it's *your* meditation. The point is to focus your intellectual mind on this simple, repetitive task so the other aspects of your mind and spirit can do other things. At first, all of your attention will be taken up by tracing the square in time with your breathing, but as you practice, that part of the exercise will become automatic and you can focus some attention on consciously relaxing the muscles all over your body.

Progressive muscle relaxation is another common simple technique of mindfulness meditation. Lie down or sit down, and starting at the top of your head or the tips of your toes, intentionally relax every muscle from there to the other end of your body. If it helps your focus, you can first tense the muscles as you go and then relax them; just move sequentially along your body from one end to the other and allow yourself to sink into the floor, chair, or bed.

The distractions and stresses of the physical world can fade away from your awareness as you practice these exercises. Notice how every part of your body feels; you may feel more than the usual physical stimuli. You will almost certainly find that simple exercises like these improve physical, mental, and psychological problems. Your day should become easier to navigate, and life should be easier and more enjoyable in general. It helps if you keep your thoughts in a positive optimistic light and think about positive goals if you don't have other goals for your meditation.

You may find at first that you can't shut off your mind, as stress and concerns come unbidden into your mind and awareness. You will probably feel stressed that you are thinking about these concerns while you are trying to meditate. This is totally normal and part of the process. While you do your simple meditation, allow whatever thoughts you have to come into and out of your awareness. Try to view these thoughts as if they were playing out on a TV screen and you are just observing them in order to be detached from the emotions these thoughts usually trigger for you, becoming objective in regarding them during this time. As you practice, you will find that your problems and concerns come into your awareness less often and more briefly and that they bother you less throughout the day. It will be easier to see solutions to your problems and to deal with adversity in your life.

One more topic to mention here is music. Most of us agree that music can invoke emotions and be very moving. In just a few moments, it can change our attitudes and moods. I believe that there is something about music that taps into the spiritual. Try listening to music when you are in need of an emotional or spiritual lift. Even better may be to learn an instrument or to sing. Try different kinds of music to see what works best for you. If no one else likes your music, it doesn't matter; it's yours.

Physical forms of energetic exercise

Meditation is not very physically active, and it does not appeal to everyone. Some systems of physical exercise from eastern cultures are designed to improve energetic and spiritual balance. These include yoga in its various forms, *tai chi*, and *qi gong* (usually pronounced "chee gung"). You can also get some energetic balancing and spiritual healing from repetitive, rhythmic exercises like walking, jogging, cycling, or rowing.

Tai chi and *qi gong* have been proven effective in treating chronic pain and fatigue issues such as fibromyalgia, more typical rheumatologic problems, such as inflammatory arthritis forms and skin disorders such as psoriasis (Wang, 2011). A 2011 study of *tai chi* demonstrated improvements in self-efficacy, mood and overall quality of life in patients with moderate congestive heart failure (Yeh, 2011). Another 2011 study, from Hong Kong, showed significant improvements in lung function and exercise tolerance for patients with chronic obstructive pulmonary disease (COPD) undertaking a *tai chi/qi gong* program as compared to patients in a standard exercise program (Chan, 2011).

These forms of exercise involve simple, flowing body movements performed in a standing position. Almost anyone can do them, as they require no great degree of strength or flexibility. You can find videos to follow along with or group classes in your area. You can easily incorporate some simple short routines into your morning or evening routine, and I can tell you from personal experience that regular practice does a lot for your overall mental and physical health.

Yoga is one of the forms of exercise I recommend most often to my patients. It is excellent for physical health in terms of increasing strength, flexibility, and resistance to injury. It is wonderful for nervous system function and balance. The breathing and meditative aspects of yoga practice are also good for the mind and spirit; they calm you, help you maintain psychological health, relieve stress, and improve your mental resilience.

Kundalini yoga is a form of yoga that specifically targets the energetic aspects of your body, the flow of energy and spirit within you, and your balance in the universe. It's not for everyone, because it seems strange to many westerners, but it can improve many health problems if you embrace it. Many people in our culture have negative feelings about these forms of exercise and their unusual types of movement, especially middle-aged men, because they see them as strange, against their religion for some reason, or just plain silly.

I frequently hear patients say, "I'm not flexible enough to do yoga," which is ironic because one of the purposes of doing yoga is to improve flexibility. Get past any irrational, negative feelings or misconceptions about these forms of exercise and try them; you won't be sorry.

My advice to patients about these types of exercise, particularly yoga, is that they first find videos to watch and follow along with at home, rather than going to a group class as their first experience with yoga. They won't know the terminology and may not be able to see the instructor clearly when they're in certain positions, and they're likely to get confused, frustrated, embarrassed, and discouraged. You can check out a video for free from your local library or buy some beginner-level programs to watch and practice at home. If you have the means, you can also ask for a couple of private beginner lessons from a yoga instructor.

From a video or private lessons, you can learn all the names of the poses and movements and gain some comfort with the exercises in privacy. After you have practiced for a while, you can attend a class where an instructor can give you advice about body position and movement. You can't see yourself well while you do yoga or tai chi, and a third party may be helpful in teaching you how the right position is supposed to feel so you can do it correctly on your own from then on. If you never go to a class, that's okay too; you will get a lot out of going through the motions with these exercises to whatever extent you are able or comfortable.

Attitude and mood

The last thing I want to discuss in this chapter is the effect of your attitude and mood on your health. I think this topic belongs here because, even though I can demonstrate many ways in which chemical neurotransmitters and hormones control your mood, attitude, and even personality, this is where the spirit manifests itself to you and those around you. Just think of phrases like "he's a spirited young man" or "she was such a happy soul." This spirit or energy within us is not visible or available to our physical senses, but we can appreciate it in the speech and behavior of another.

It is difficult to prove whether any one type of mood or attitude has better health value than another, but we have some cultural beliefs and some limited scientific evidence related to the effect of attitude and mood. Cultural sayings like "he was too mean to die" suggest that you may live longer just by being tough about it, but it is probably more likely that happiness and contentment will earn you a longer life. Some modern research has demonstrated that happier people—those who have a high level of enjoyment and life satisfaction—live longer and healthier lives.

We do know that happily married people and those who have more sex (which aren't always the same people) seem to have decreased risk of cardiovascular disease and live significantly longer lives than others do (Maggi, 2011), perhaps because they tend toward less risky behavior (the married folks), but I think it's because they are in a better place in terms of happiness and energetic balance. I've seen a number of cases myself in which an elderly person dies within six months of the death of their spouse, even though they seemed to be in good health up to that point. This is called the "widowhood effect", and has been shown to be more common for men than for women after losing their spouse (Maggi, 2011).

This doesn't mean I think the key to long life is to get married and stay married; I don't even believe humans are a biologically monogamous species. My point is that being happy and content does a lot for you in terms of your spiritual, mental, emotional, and physical health. If that means being in a loving, supportive relationship, which I think is important for many of us, then you should be ready to recognize it when it's offered. However, if being happy and content means being on your own or traveling the world without a permanent residence, then do it. Happiness and contentment does not come from the same source for everyone.

One thing you can do in your everyday life is just to stop periodically and recognize how you feel inside. Do you feel tense, upset, fearful, angry, or frustrated? If so, why? Is there anything you can do about it? If there is, then do it; if not, you may be in a place where acceptance is the best option for now. If you can't afford to take a vacation this year and that is upsetting to you, just accept it. If you lost your job, look at it as a new adventure or chance for a long-awaited career change. If you hate your marriage, perhaps you should get out of it; and if you hate your job, start looking for a different one or start training to do something new.

Acceptance can also work against you, so be rational about what you choose to accept. You don't have to accept the things that cause you suffering or turmoil. You don't have to accept being beaten or mentally abused. You don't have to accept being overweight and out of shape. You don't have to accept staying at a job you hate with a boss who treats you like an idiot. Success begins with the belief that you can make things better than they are right now.

Acceptance can also work for you in a very positive way, by not wasting angst and energy on something you can't change, by letting you move on or focus your energy in a new direction. If you love your spouse but you simply cannot get him or her to stop leaving dishes in the sink, accept it and find some way they can make up for it. If you love your job but don't like being required to work on Saturdays, accept it and restructure your weekend. I can tell you from personal experience it makes a huge difference. The number of little things I allow to bother me is much smaller than it used to be; as a result, I have much more space for happiness and contentment.

Positive visualization and positive expectations are growing ideas in our culture. Movies like *What the Bleep Do We Know* and *The Secret* have turned many people on to the idea that we may be able to influence or "create" our own reality and future to a certain extent. This is grounded in quantum physics theory, and if the premise presented in these movies is real, it is likely to have a strong metaphysical or spiritual basis as well. I prefer to believe in all the ideas presented, to maximize my chances of success. This kind of thinking is extremely powerful but difficult for many Americans because of our ingrained attitudes.

Our culture tends to be so negativistic that it's a wonder we can survive at all. We love to see people fail and to read the covers of the trash magazines at the checkout line at the grocery store. Our media focuses far more attention on people's failures than their successes. Our television shows have become more negative and even depraved, with idiotic "reality" shows about people overturning tables and throwing punches at each other popping up all over.

Depression has become something of a national pastime, with multiple antidepressant drugs ranking among the top ten medications sold in the U.S. There used to be a major stigma attached to depression, but it seems now we've come to think we're entitled to be happy all the time without any effort on our own parts. If we aren't spontaneously happy and content, maybe we need a drug to correct that? I think a bigger problem is that our lives have become too soft; we have so many conveniences and amenities we've lost sight of reality.

This attitude has become so ingrained that when some Americans go to poor countries where there is famine, disease or a recent natural disaster but people are smiling and singing and children are playing, our reaction is "What's wrong with you? Don't you know you're supposed to be depressed?" In reality, it is those people who understand what life is all about. If they have shelter, food for the day, and their health, then it's a good day.

After the devastating earthquake at the beginning of 2010, the children of Haiti were were depicted in our magazines and news broadcasts laughing and playing, having made simple toys out of garbage and rubble. Contrast this with American children over the age of four—until that age kids are just as likely to play with an empty box as the toy inside it—they act like they must have the latest electronics, video games, remote control cars or planes, television, and movies. Our commercialism has convinced them they can't be happy without all this, so they aren't. They complain if they don't have the latest fashion in clothing or the newest iPod. Our materialism has poisoned our minds; our kids, along with most adults, don't know how to occupy themselves without all sorts of external electronic stimuli, and we don't know how to be happy unless we have all kinds of "stuff."

It seems we've set our expectations at unrealistic levels in terms of material goods and what it takes to be happy. We no longer look to nature for fulfillment, and have forgotten how to be happy unless something external triggers it for us. When did we stop lying in the grass, smelling the flowers, listening to the birds sing, and watching the clouds roll by? Probably when we replaced the grass with concrete, traded the real thing for plastic or fabric flowers, and killed off the birds with pollution. In many ways "depression" is a luxury of affluent society; we mourn over a lack of things we don't even need.

I've gone way off track here, but to recap, I think part of why we no longer know how to be happy and content is that we have altered our material expectations as a culture. We need to get back to understanding what simple but true contentment and happiness is. We need to learn to see the positive aspects of our lives and to focus less on what we think is missing and more on seeing the opportunities in front of us.

Since I've adopted more positive attitudes and philosophies, most of what has happened to me has been positive–or maybe I'm just wearing my rose-colored glasses. But when you think about it, what's the difference? My view of positive visualization and thinking is that the greatest benefits derive from the simple act of deciding to think differently about your situation. It's not magic; you aren't "manifesting" things out of the ether. It's just that you are not as bothered by the little things that don't go your way as you once were, and you are more likely to recognize good things when they happen.

I have suggested that we can't appreciate the spiritual with our senses or minds very well, so this is the path—the path of mindfulness and positive visualization and expectation—that we have to walk to get there. If you pay attention, you will note how different you feel inside using a sense other than those you use to observe the physical world. Learn to improve your own spiritual health in whatever way works for you. Sometimes all it takes is an attitude adjustment.

CHAPTER 18 – AIR AND BREATHING

It may seem inappropriate to put air toward the end of this section when it is the one thing most vital to your existence. I put it here because we do pretty well breathing on our own without having to be told, while most of us need instruction in regard to our diets and exercise. The important issues to review here are air quality and *how* you breathe. This section focuses on the problems you may encounter with your air, rather than its nourishing properties.

Outdoor air quality

Everyone knows how it feels to be outside in the "fresh air," somewhere clean and clear, where there are no toxins in the air to poison your body or damage your lungs. Unfortunately, most places in the industrialized world now have somewhat compromised air quality. I encourage you to look online for current information regarding the air quality in your region at websites such as www.airnow.gov or www.weather.com/activities/health/airquality.

Sometimes there are natural causes for poor air quality, but the problem is usually man-made. Hawaii has problems with air quality that are due to toxic gas from some of their volcanoes. Ash mixes with mist to create "vog," or volcanic smog. We also have volcanoes in Alaska that erupt periodically, or forest fires that force those with respiratory problems to stay indoors or wear masks outdoors for up to months at a time. Dust, pollens, mold spores, and other natural airborne irritants also pose health problems for people all over the world.

In the Matanuska-Susitna valley where I live, the wind sometimes blows to hurricane strength from the direction of the glaciers at the east end. This wind carries a fine glacial dust all through the valley, giving some people runny noses, congestion, headaches, and wheezing. After Hurricane Katrina, the air around New Orleans became so full of mold spores that the EPA deemed much of the region uninhabitable. Forest fires create temporary problems with outdoor air quality as well, and liberate tons of mercury into the air and environment.

A great deal of outdoor air pollution is generated by humans, and it has become a global problem. Automobiles, trucks, trains, airplanes, lawnmowers, ATVs, other small vehicles, factories, houses, schools, and other buildings that use fossil fuels for power cause toxic air pollution. Power plants are a major source of air pollution, especially those that burn fossil fuels like coal. Coal burning has been called the major source of mercury in the environment worldwide. There is no such thing as "clean coal" because all of its toxins have to go somewhere; even if most of it is trapped in the scrubbers, it is still dumped into the environment later.

The outdoor air pollution problem is a global problem. Some sources, such as coal-fired electrical plants, spew so much toxicity into the air that some of it is carried all over the world. The mercury, PCBs, pesticides, and other toxins end up in our oceans and are carried by currents all over the world and into the food chain. America still produces some toxic chemicals, such as certain pesticides and industrial chemicals, which were banned for use here but not in many developing nations. We export them to other countries and get measurable amounts of them back into our own environment because of the global movement of air and water.

Storms in dry regions such as parts of Africa and Australia generate huge dust clouds that span the globe in the higher atmosphere, carrying toxins, chemicals and diseases to all parts of the world (Vidal, 2009). The air and ocean currents carry persistent organic pollutant chemicals (POPs) to every continent on the globe, with warm air and water moving from the hot equatorial and tropic zone toward the north and south, where toxins are deposited in the colder regions. While it seems as though the Arctic and Antarctic regions at the poles must be very clean and pure, they are not because of these global circulation patterns.

People are surprised to hear about the high levels of PCBs and other POPs found in our polar bears, walrus, seals, and fish here in Alaska because it's not on the news too often, but the data is there (Colborn, 1997). There are concerns about polar bear infertility's being caused by accumulation of these man-made chemicals, and these chemicals must have certainly contributed to the rising infertility in humans.

Indoor air quality

Indoor air quality is a surprisingly common and severe problem. Brand-new buildings have many toxins from paints, adhesives, sheetrock dust (which is usually the leftovers from burned coal, called gypsum), formaldehyde from new carpet, and other sources. It takes months for these chemicals to "out-gas" from your new home, and in that time you can easily develop neurological, respiratory, immune, skin, cardiac, or metabolic problems. If you burn natural gas, oil, wood, or other fossil fuels, you are exposed to toxins from your heat source and stove. Biological sources of indoor air pollution, such as dust mites and mold, pose a major threat as well.

Cigarette smoke is an important indoor pollutant because it is completely avoidable but is often inflicted on people against their will. Many smokers these days understand that their habit may cause harm to others and are considerate enough to smoke outside, but some smokers don't believe that second-hand smoke causes health problems in others and indignantly and insistently smoke around whomever they please, especially in their own home. If you are a nonsmoker, you can probably detect smokers from twenty feet away, though they may have no clue that you can. All you have to do is clean the walls or the windows inside a smoker's house to be convinced of the pollutant load there. Cigarette smoke contains toxic chemicals like formaldehyde and benzene and heavy metals like cadmium.

Humans put many other chemical toxins humans into their indoor air. Cleaning chemicals, hair spray and other cosmetics, perfumes, scented candles, and chemical air fresheners all pose potential health risks to those who are susceptible and add to the total toxic load we have to deal with in our environment.

You can smell some toxins, such as the new paint and adhesive in new construction and after renovations. Most people can detect excessive dust or mold in the air as well. Others you can't smell, such as carbon monoxide, which is produced from incomplete combustion of fossil fuels (natural gas, heating oil, engine exhaust) and causes deaths every year, often killing entire families while they sleep in their homes. Another odorless toxin is radon gas, which can leak from the ground into poorly ventilated basements and represents the second-leading cause of lung cancer. Low levels of chemicals and mold spores may not be detectable by most people, but they may be enough to cause illness. In that event, it often takes a long time to figure out the cause of the illness.

If you live in a cold climate like I do or in a very hot climate, you may spend most of your time indoors for half the year, where you are exposed to toxins from heated or air-conditioned air. I personally feel like I'm being physically attacked when I am near an air conditioner unit, even in my car. There must be some refrigerant chemical residue coming through in that air because that is how my body reacts to it.

Health consequences of air quality issues

Many people don't notice outdoor air pollutants unless they are stuck behind a big diesel truck in traffic or near a factory, forest fire, or erupting volcano. However, changes in air quality that our senses cannot detect have been found to cause significant problems for human health.

I mentioned above that carbon monoxide and radon gasses are silent killers inside homes, but there are some such silent killers outdoors as well. Some people are very sensitive to the toxins given off by aircraft, especially when there are visible jet trails in the sky. Those "contrails" as they are termed contain condensed water vapor with sulfur or nitrogen oxides, unburned jet fuel, metal particles and soot (Rossmann, 2011). Sensitive people may have headaches, respiratory problems, or other symptoms and have to retreat indoors. Multiple studies have shown that heart attack rates are significantly (by a small margin) higher when the outdoor air quality is worse in terms of pollutants and particulate matter (Nuvolone, 2011).

You can look up current the current air quality index at websites like www.airnow.gov or www.weather.com/activities/health/airquality unless you live in Alaska. These sites have maps of the continental U.S. and Hawaii, but not Alaska. Your own state may have more detailed air quality monitoring that you can find online. Alaska's state Department of Environmental Conservation (DEC) website posts air quality warnings only when they are of great significance, rather than current general information. This discrepancy seems ironic to me, since Alaska has more unpopulated "environment" to conserve than most of the continental U.S. collectively.

These studies and informational sources consider only particulate matter in the air, such as dust and smoke, which have been studied and shown to increase rates of asthma attacks and heart attacks (Nuvolone, 2011). These sources do not monitor heavy metals or chemical toxins in the air. Airborne chemicals tend to affect small local regions, such as those near factories or power plants, busy roadways, or other places where there are many running vehicles or machines.

If you have respiratory problems or are at increased risk for heart attack, you may want to look up your local air quality before venturing outdoors without a mask. People can have other adverse health effects from air pollution, especially indoor air, the symptoms of which may be very diverse and confusing to most, so I suggest you see a good holistic or integrative health practitioner with experience in environmental medicine if you suspect these issues.

Respiratory problems are probably the most obvious problem related to air pollutant problems. Chronic runny noses and congestion, coughing or wheezing, frequent respiratory infections, and asthma problems may be commonly linked to air quality issues. People can also experience headaches or other neurological symptoms, including those that may appear to be behavioral issues. Cardiovascular symptoms, skin problems, digestive issues, bed-wetting, and others may be less obvious problems linked to indoor pollutants.

The most important non-chemical sources to suspect if you have relevant chronic symptoms are mold, dust, pet dander, smoke, and other airborne irritants. You can usually find and abate these sources in your home without much difficulty. A notable exception is mold, which may be so infested in your walls that you must all but rebuild your house to eradicate it.

Combating indoor air quality problems

If you suspect you have indoor air pollution, you can get your house checked for some sources, get carbon monoxide detectors and radon detection kits cheaply at any hardware store to prevent lethal problems from these silent killers, get mold spore counts done by local agencies or get your own kits to calculate mold counts in your home, and have a friend with multiple allergies and chemical sensitivities go through your house like a drug-sniffing dog.

Even if you aren't aware of any chemicals present, they will accumulate in your body and may eventually cause problems. If you have radon in your basement, all you need is a simple ventilation pipe and fan set-up to take care of the problem. If you have elevated levels of carbon monoxide, you may need to have your furnace serviced or replaced. If there are new renovations or your house is new, you may be able increase the ventilation for a while to help the toxins dissipate faster.

If you have problems with pet dander you can get rid of your pets (though I understand why many people won't do this), replace your carpet with wood or tile flooring, bathe your pets more often, or have your allergies cleared by techniques I describe later. If you have mold, you may have a very big problem since mold is often deeply rooted within your walls and can't often be cleared up simply. However, it should not be ignored; indoor mold infestations can cause many adverse health problems (Seltzer, 2007). The quick and easy solution is of course to move, changing environments, although if you own your home, you will not be able to sell it with an existing mold problem. If your child is having problems with his or her room at school, you may be able to get your child into a new section of the school—maybe a room that was remodeled a year or two ago or a portable building outside the regular school—or even change schools. You may be able to move out of the "sick building" in which you currently live, or maybe not.

Sometimes changing your environment is not so easy. The school your child is in may be full of indoor pollution, but it's the only one he or she can attend. (Dr. Doris Rapp has a video called *Sick Schools* that I encourage you to watch if you have a chronically ill child). Your apartment may be old and full of mold, but any apartment you could afford in the same area and price range would likely be decrepit and toxic as well. The unfortunate fact is that you or your child may be stuck in an environment that directly causes sickness. In this case, there are ways to improve your body's resistance to these problems and to get rid of allergies (as I discuss later), and there are some measures you can take to reduce the indoor pollutant burden as well.

Removing things that hold pollution is a very important step. The most important step is to rip out old carpet and padding. If you have ever done this with carpet more than a few years old you were likely shocked and horrified by the amount of dirt and debris under it, and if you didn't wear a mask, you may have gotten sick afterward. If you can't afford to put new floor covering down, don't. Just paint the plywood underneath and use area rugs (which also trap some pollutants but are easier to keep clean) until you can afford a better floor covering, such as laminate, wood or tile. Vinyl is much cheaper, but has a lot of glue under it that is toxic.

Throwing out old pillows and replacing mattresses can also be very important. Those items can hold dust, dust mites, pet dander, and chemicals like formaldehyde and flame-retardants. New mattresses may have more chemicals, so consider putting a hypoallergenic bag around your old mattress instead of buying a new one. You may also want to choose a new mattress made from more health-friendly materials, such as soybean oil rather than petroleum. Controlling humidity in your house is very important for reducing mold levels; installing a good HVAC system or getting a dehumidifier can help a lot.

The way your house is constructed has a lot to do with indoor air quality and mold control as well. Using plywood instead of particle board or OSB reduces the chemical load, since particle board and OSB have huge amounts of glue that contains formaldehyde and other chemicals. These two types of boards also dramatically increase the chances of mold growing in the walls because they are made of ground up trees including the bark, where the mold spores reside; adding a little moisture grows mold right from these materials like a fertile field. Conversely, if plywood gets wet with moisture from the air, it doesn't grow much mold because the bark was peeled from the trees prior to making them.

It is important to have a proper vapor barrier (thick plastic sheets) in your walls to prevent moisture from getting to the wood. This can be done from inside the walls at the time of construction or after mold abatement. A good ventilation system is invaluable as well; just make sure it gets air out of the house effectively, rather than just re-circulating it. If you are chemically sensitive, it is important to use chemical-free materials as much as possible, such as tile or wood floors, granite or other hard solid countertops, and low-chemical paints (or wooden walls with no paint at all).

A natural way to improve indoor air quality is to use house plants. Plants recycle the carbon dioxide exhaled by animals and generate clean, pure oxygen. In addition, some varieties such as the spider plant, bamboo palm and others have been shown to be excellent natural filters for some common airborne chemical pollutants. NASA studies in the 1980's conducted by research scientist Bill Wolverton showed a number of plants to be excellent chemical detoxifiers and air purifiers; the top three were palm plants (areca, lady palm and bamboo), followed by the rubber plant, *dracaena* varieties, English ivy, the dwarf date palm, *ficus alii,* Boston fern and peace lily (Kuznik, 1999). Plants can also produce excessive moisture in the air, so try to find a balance.

Air filters and purifier systems can also help to clean up your indoor air problems. They are less effective than some other measures I've discussed, but they can be helpful in reducing the pollutant burden. If you get an air filter system, make sure it has a HEPA filter and a fan that circulates the air actively through the system. Change your air filters in these devices and your installed HVAC system regularly.

Some people believe that ionic air purifiers are effective. I don't like how they smell because they give off some ozone, which is an effective tool for cleaning your indoor air environment, but is also a toxin itself. Ozone causes chemical and organic pollutants to be disrupted to some extent and to settle on surfaces in your house, where you can clean them off.

You can purchase ozone generators at hardware stores or through specialty companies. Use them on some regular basis, depending on your air situation, make sure you are not in the house while they are running or for an appropriate period afterward (based on the time it was running, size of the area, and ventilation), and carefully clean up surface debris afterward. You need to do this only weekly, monthly or even less often depending upon your circumstances, so consider sharing the cost of an ozone generator with multiple families and taking turns.

Of course, the ideal approach is to plan your own home construction, but this is not often possible. Second best is to remodel your indoor environment as much as possible. Third is to do your best to ventilate and clean up the indoor environment you're stuck with.

Combating outdoor air quality problems

You have much less control over the outdoor air quality as an individual than you do over the indoor air problem. The solutions here lie mainly with relocation or public action. If you have asthma or other respiratory sensitivity problems, you probably should not live in a big city where there is a high level of vehicle and building exhaust. If you are allergic to hay, you may not want to live in farm country. If you're allergic to juniper, you will have problems in the southwest United States, and if you're allergic to birch trees, you do not want to visit south-central Alaska in May or June.

About 80 percent of us live in large cities, where the vast majority of man-made air pollution is found. Since our culture has become dependent on mass-produced foods, goods and services, people crowd together in large metropolitan areas where they work to earn money to buy the things required for survival. We spend inordinate amounts of time driving, producing even more pollution from our vehicles, to perform the duties modern society dictates are important. We have developed a global economy that demands bananas and tomatoes in the winter, spices from the other side of the world, and electronics made in China. This global trade system consumes fossil fuels, creates pollution, and wastes resources, time and money.

Our modern industrialized society may be unsustainable unless we change our energy sources to those that do not create toxic pollution. An even better solution would be to return to regionalized production, where most everything you need is produced within a small radius of a couple hundred miles. There is so much unused land in the United States that if everyone could spread out a bit, it would improve the air quality overall tremendously. While we can't control the wind or the volcanoes, we can control is our consumer habits and our voting for public officials and policy. We can do what we can on an individual level to control pollution through our own behaviors (e.g., stop smoking, ride a bike or mass transit, recycle, use green power in our homes) and clean up our air little by little.

I mentioned houseplants in the discussion of indoor air quality control; the same concept applies to outdoor air. You can plant trees, but you may make an even bigger difference through your behavior as a consumer. Buy recycled paper products as much as possible, revitalize old furniture or housing rather than buying new, and purchase products that help sustain the rain forest rather than promote its destruction (certain brands of chocolate, yerba mate, other goods and produce from Central and South America). Repair, reuse, repurpose, recycle.

If *you* don't start to make a difference, why should anyone else? John Mayer sings that he's "waiting for the world to change", which I find annoying and unhelpful. We *are* the world, so we're the ones who can change it! Everyone needs to embrace their own roles in this mess and do what they can to fix it if we are to have a world worth passing on to future generations. As Ghandi said, "*Be* the change you wish to see in the world."

Proper breathing

We can't finish talking about air without talking about breathing. Having clean air is pointless unless you use it to your advantage. I mentioned how most people in our culture breathe sub-optimally, so let's review proper breathing technique. I know breathing is an involuntary behavior, but we still develop habitually poor patterns or practices in breathing that can be turned to good behaviors with practice, awareness, and mindfulness.

Every cell in our bodies needs oxygen to generate energy efficiently, to kill bacteria and other invaders, and to detoxify chemicals and other substances. Our lungs and respiratory system have to extract oxygen from the air (which is only 20–21% oxygen) so our cardiovascular system can deliver it to our cells. Your circulatory system is vital to this process; you can breathe all day, but if your heart and blood vessels don't get the oxygenated blood around the body, the whole breathing process is pointless. Fortunately, these two processes are intertwined.

Most Americans want their belly to look small and trim, so they suck it in and try to hold it there. Most men want their chest and shoulders to look big—at least bigger than their bellies—so they hold their chest out and shoulders up. This is terrible breathing mechanics; it leads to substandard ventilation of the lungs and chronic muscle tension in the shoulders and neck.

Your chest is surrounded by ribs that operate like bucket handles; they swing up and out a little when you inhale, expanding the volume of your chest, because they are being pulled upward by a series of muscles that connect the ribs together and are anchored at the top by muscles attached to the collarbones. Your collarbones are suspended from muscles that originate in the neck, the muscles you shrug with. You can pull your whole chest up using your shoulder muscles, and many of us do this unconsciously. You can breathe this way, but it's very inefficient.

Our culture has engendered this bad breathing behavior for many generations. Your mother or other older relative may have barked at you to sit up straight, put your shoulders back, and "don't slouch!" Why do they say that? Is there any evidence that people who slouch have back problems? No. This is just Western culture. Your spine is very flexible, and the best way to keep it healthy is to move it through its full range of motion, rather than holding it rigid and straight. Relax, slouch if you want to when you sit, stretch, and move your body around.

Only about 40 percent of your inhaling action is supposed to be accomplished through those shoulder/neck/rib muscle actions pulling your ribs up and out. The majority (about 60%) of your inhalation is supposed to be accomplished by your diaphragm, that big, dome-shaped sheet of muscle that attaches inside your lower ribs and separates the chest from the abdomen. The diaphragm is supposed to contract and push downward, pushing your guts down and out to create space for the lungs to expand downward from the chest cavity. You breathe in by pulling your chest cavity open in these various directions, creating negative pressure in the chest, which sucks air in through your upper airways.

Most people breathe with a dysfunction about as bad as that of the 2009 U.S. senate under President Obama's first year in office. The diaphragm has a sixty-vote majority but is too passive to accomplish its duty. The forty-vote minority steers the ship by being rigid, and the insecure diaphragm just lets it happen. This causes all sorts of problems, as we've seen. What we need is good bipartisan coordination here; the diaphragm should pull down and out smoothly, while the chest and shoulder muscles hold just firmly enough from the top to keep things grounded, pulling gently in the opposite direction.

When you breathe, your belly should be relaxed and should move out considerably when you inhale. You don't have to sit up straight and rigid; just maintain a comfortable position, with your spine relatively straight horizontally. (It's hard to breathe when you are bent to one side, but leaning forward a bit is fine.) Don't force things; just push your belly outward until you have achieved a comfortable breath, and then let everything relax back inward on its own.

There are several reasons why it is important to breathe through your nose, rather than your mouth. One is that your nose has a filter system in it to prevent germs and debris from getting down into your lungs, where they may cause illness or irritation. Another is that your nose has irregular passages that cause moisture to condense on the way in and out, conserving water; you can demonstrate this when it is cold enough to see your breath outside. Note that if you breathe out through your nose, you don't see the mist because your nose retrieved most of the water from your breath.

I think another reason that it is important to breathe through the nose, although this view hasn't yet been supported by research to my knowledge, is that it stimulates your central nervous system. Air passing through your nose gets very close to the brain, and we know the sense of smell is transmitted from nerves in the nose directly to the brain. (There's another reason to breathe through your nose: your sense of smell is important in guiding your actions, and you can't smell through your mouth.) I suspect your brain and the autonomic nervous system functions better when you are passing air back and forth through your nose. This may be part of why hyperventilating through the mouth causes psychological distress to escalate. You may have noticed that people can't or don't breathe through their nose just look wrong on some level. (We use the term "mouth-breather" colloquially to indicate low intelligence.) Mouth-breathing dries you out and lets bad things into your lungs, so save it for when you are exercising and out of breath.

Why should you care about how you breathe? Isn't it obviously working out fine if you are still alive? Proper breathing can alleviate chronic complaints, including some medical conditions. If you improve your breathing and take a few deep, relaxing breaths, you may feel your neck and shoulder muscles loosen. You can reduce chronic severe headaches and other forms of chronic pain with proper breathing, both through proper muscle mechanics and through improved oxygen delivery to struggling tissues.

Proper breathing and breath exercises, such as periodic deep diaphragmatic breathing (take in as much air as you can slowly, letting your belly way out, then passively exhale for ten beats), have been shown to reduce problems like anxiety, asthma, high blood pressure, pain problems, and stress-related symptoms. There is even an FDA-approved device for lowering blood pressure called "Resperate" that guides your breathing with a tone heard through headphones and a simple strap around your belly; this device has been shown to work as well as a prescription drug to lower blood pressure.

You may be able to reduce your risk of heart attack significantly through breath training as well. Heart rate variability is the best measurable predictor of heart attack risk, and you can watch yourself improve it with simple computer programs like "Heart Math" or "Freeze-Framer." The simple breathing exercises I've discussed will visibly improve your heart rate variability and overall biorhythm coherence when you use these biofeedback programs.

Your cultural biases may mean that the idea of mental and spiritual balancing seems weird. You can try these exercises out in private, or you can do whatever works for you; it doesn't have to be any of the things I've described here. If you attend to your mental and spiritual health, you will reap benefits in terms of your physical health and longevity as well as overall life satisfaction.

Hyperbaric Oxygen and Ozone Therapy

The therapeutic use of oxygen is an amazing tool, given the importance of oxygen to our cellular and physiologic function. You may be familiar with the use of supplemental oxygen delivered by mask or a tube under the nose to those with some medical emergencies or chronic lung disease. Much more powerful ways to introduce oxygen include hyperbaric oxygen therapy and ozone therapy.

Hyperbaric oxygen therapy (HBOT) entails placing the patient in a pressure chamber and compressing the air with or without supplemental oxygen added. You can deliver tens of times more oxygen to the tissues in this way using room air than you could by putting a tube into your lungs with pure oxygen at normal pressure. The difference is the amount of oxygen that is dissolved in the liquid portion of your blood, rather than being bound to hemoglobin; oxygen bound to hemoglobin becomes saturated easily and cannot be increased. The amount of oxygen dissolved passively into the water portion of your blood however, can be increased dramatically relative to the pressure applied to the system.

HBOT has been shown to improve many medical conditions. The FDA-approved uses, which are limited, include only such conditions as diabetic foot ulcers and other wounds, carbon monoxide poisoning, diving injury ("the bends"), and a few others. Those types of treatments require a "hard" hyperbaric chamber that can reach high pressures, to above three atmospheres. These can usually be found only at hospitals or outpatient hyperbaric centers, and not typically in private doctors' offices.

Integrative practitioners have found low-pressure HBOT to be useful for many other conditions. Low-pressure treatments can be performed with soft portable chambers that reach only 1.3 atmospheres of pressure. These types of chambers may be used more commonly in private clinics, rented out for home use, or purchased directly by the consumer. The scientific evidence for what these chambers can do is quite limited, but the companies that sell them make lots of impressive claims. Be sure to do your homework and ask lots of questions before using one of these for a medical problem; they are not adequate for the serious medical problems mentioned in the preceding paragraph.

Conditions that are often treated with soft low-pressure chambers include acute respiratory problems, cardiovascular disease (atherosclerosis), inflammation of various types, chronic fatigue, chronic pain, and all sorts of chronic neurological problems. The potential neurological and brain effects are some of the most exciting; benefits may be seen in autism, stroke, Parkinson's disease, multiple sclerosis, dementia, traumatic brain injury, recovery from concussion, and possibly others. These are conditions for which there is often nothing else that is helpful. For more information on HBOT, a good resource is *The Oxygen Revolution* by Paul Harch, MD.

Ozone therapy can be performed in a variety of ways. You cannot safely breathe ozone, but it can be bubbled into your GI tract rectally to decrease colon inflammation or total body inflammation since some will absorb into the bloodstream this way. Wearing a suit with ozone pumped into it that keeps your head excluded can help most with skin conditions.

Ozone may also be bubbled into a drawn sample of your own blood and then injected back into your body, a process that has been used with success for many types of chronic infections, inflammatory disorders, chronic fatigue syndromes, and even emergency conditions. Ozone may also be bubbled into liquid solutions and injected directly into inflamed joints for various arthritis conditions. The two latter-mentioned uses of ozone must be performed only by trained medical practitioners, while the rectal and skin approaches are done by people at home with their own ozone machines.

If you want to try one of these oxygen therapies, you can look for a practice that includes hyperbaric oxygen or ozone therapy, purchase or rent your own portable HBOT chamber for home use, or find your own ozone machine and a source of oxygen. If you want injected ozone, your best bet may be to look for a naturopathic office since many medical doctors stay away from treatments so far off the mainstream because of concerns about actions by state medical boards. Naturopaths can perform these procedures more freely because the conventional medical boards don't rule them.

CHAPTER 19 – SLEEP

Sleep is extremely important to your health—even to life itself. If you tried to go without sleep, you would begin to show signs of psychosis or hallucinate after a few days (Gove, 1970). I use sleep quality as one of four overall markers of general health for my patients to rate on a scale from one to ten when they come in. Sleep is a vital process that should occur naturally to provide rest and revitalization. Sleep is an extremely important and too often overlooked aspect of overall health.

Why we need sleep

Sometimes it upsets me that I need to sleep at all. I don't know about you, but I always still have plenty to do when it comes time to go to bed, and I could use an extra six hours or so of productivity per day. However, I also know that if I don't get five or six hours of sleep, I can't think as clearly as I could otherwise, which is probably why in 2003 the government restricted the amount of hours a medical resident can work. Unfortunately, despite the fact that numerous laboratory studies have confirmed that sleep deprivation definitely reduces cognitive performance and increases mental errors, that regulation hasn't been shown to reduce medical trainee mistakes at all (Kramer, 2010). This lack of demonstrated benefit is probably because doctors are humans who err like they are supposed to, trainees don't know what they're doing yet, it decreases how seriously the trainee takes their role in patient care and residency faculty don't provide proper oversight–but I digress.

We need to sleep so we can recharge or reset our brain and central nervous systems, although the system doesn't exactly "rest" while we sleep. Functional studies of brain waves and brain activity show that our brains are metabolically very active during sleep; for some of us, they are even more active than when we are awake. Our eyes move side to side rapidly during part of it, although no one knows why; we dream, sometimes crazy vivid dreams; and there is activity in brain regions we don't otherwise use.

Hormonal processes also rely on proper sleep rhythm and amount in order to promote optimal health. Growth hormone is largely secreted during sleep, as is testosterone. Cortisol levels normally drop low while we sleep, allowing our system to relax and recharge from an adrenal standpoint. Melatonin levels are typically high at night, which is part of how we go to sleep, but those high levels of melatonin are also needed to help prevent and fight cancer. The balance of sex steroids (progesterone, estrogen, and testosterone) also has a major impact on sleep.

Our immune system and general repair processes must require sleep as well. Studies have shown significantly increased blood levels of inflammatory markers like C-reactive protein, interleukin 6 and tumor necrosis factor alpha in humans with even just the mild intermittent sleep deprivation associated with rotating night shift work (Khosro, 2011). Animal models of induced shift-work sleep dysregulation, without loss of overall sleep time (just circadian rhythm disturbance without actual sleep deprivation) have been shown to interfere with normal innate immune system functioning and lead to a more than four-fold increase in the death rate following experimentally-induced shock using a bacterial cell wall particle (Castanon-Cervantes, 2010).

It does appear that we can adapt to chronic sleep deprivation to some extent, and that our brains may in fact become more resilient to certain types of chemical stress. One animal study allowing test subjects to sleep only four hours per day for thirty days showed their brain neurons became resistant to injection of an endogenously produced (normally made within the brain) excitotoxic neurotransmitter. The test animals actually experienced *less* brain cell damage than the control animals that had not been partially sleep deprived (Novati, 2011). This probably represents an adaptive response to being awake more of the time, and not a truly "beneficial" effect of sleep deprivation.

Sleep is still a bit of a black box in the medical world; we don't understand as much about how it works and why we need it so badly as we want to. What we do know is that we need to sleep and that many things can go wrong with it, resulting in adverse health effects. Poor sleep can lead to fatigue, accidents, poor mental function, depression, anxiety, pain problems, weight gain and all its attendant consequences, high blood pressure, and cardiovascular complications.

How much sleep do we need?

Most studies say adults need an average of six to eight hours of sleep per night. Babies can sleep most of the day, but our teenagers often want to sleep all day too. Children and teenagers require more sleep than adults because they are growing and developing, but an adult's need for sleep depends at last in part on his or her level of mental and physical activity. I find I need a little more sleep when I exercise more vigorously am under more mental or psychological stress than usual, but I also find that I feel foggy and dysfunctional if I sleep more than eight hours.

As people age, they often seem to need less sleep and may have more trouble sleeping. Perhaps they are less active and need less restoration, or perhaps it is a sign of gradual system dysfunction like the decreased thirst and hunger responses I discussed. An individual's need for sleep is variable for many reasons, but if you don't feel rested with eight hours of sleep per night, something may be wrong.

I have had repeated arguments about the required amount of sleep, and whether you are likely to live longer with *more* sleep or *less* sleep. My stance has always been that you live longer if you sleep *less*, plus you get to experience your life more because you're awake more, and I have encountered a few studies confirming that. The most recent study I found evaluated elderly Brazilian people in the Bambui Health and Ageing Study. This study reviewed the sleep habits of 1512 elderly individuals and found a linear relationship between sleep time and mortality rate; those who slept nine hours per night had a 53% increase in death rate, over the nine year duration of the study, compared to those who slept seven hours per night (Castro-Costa, 2011).

Numerous other studies have been done looking at sleep duration as it relates to mortality over the years, and it is clear that short duration of sleep (less than six hours) is related to increased death risk as well. One large meta-analysis found short sleepers to have a ten percent increased mortality risk over those sleeping six to eight hours per night, but a twenty-three percent increased risk of death for those sleeping greater than eight hours as related to the "medium" sleepers (Gallicchio, 2009). Therefore, excessive sleeping still appears to be the bigger risk. In that same meta-analysis, this difference was even more pronounced for cardiovascular and cancer-related deaths in particular; cardiovascular disease deaths were increased thirty-eight percent for long sleepers and only six percent for short sleepers, while cancer deaths were increased twenty-one percent in long sleepers and actually were *decreased* one percent in short sleepers (Gallicchio, 2009).

These epidemiologic studies, as discussed previously, do not indicate causation. That means we still don't know whether sleeping longer than eight hours per night is in some way harmful to a person. It is just as likely, or perhaps more likely, that people who are sleeping more than eight hours per night have some sort of metabolic problem, toxicity or deficiency that is making them sleep excessively, and *that* problem is the root cause of their earlier demise. It is easier to believe that sleep deprivation is an actual cause of death, because it may lead to increased accidents (and, since it was shown not to really increase cardiovascular or cancer deaths, accidental death becomes one of the most likely forms). Another serious limitation of all the epidemiologic studies on sleep is that the amount of time people slept was simply estimated by the people themselves, and we are in general somewhat poor at estimating how much we sleep.

The best recommendation from all this is probably to try and get at least six hours of sleep per night as often as possible, and to avoid night shift work if at all possible. If you are sleeping less than six hours per night you may be over-worked, overly stressed, or have detrimental habits interfering with your sleep. If you find you need more than eight hours of sleep per night consistently you may have something metabolically wrong with you, and may want to consider a thorough evaluation from a naturopath or integrative practitioner.

Sleep hygiene problems

The term "sleep hygiene" refers to general lifestyle habits and nighttime rituals or practices that interfere with sleep for psychological or physiological reasons. Many people with sleep problems can fix them by improving their sleep hygiene.

Caffeine intake is a big one. As I mentioned before, caffeine stays in your system more than twenty-four hours, and many people have trouble sleeping even though they have just one cup of coffee in the morning. One of the first things I tell people who are having trouble sleeping is that they should avoid coffee, tea, energy drinks, and sodas with caffeine. Most resist this suggestion because they have become somewhat psychologically and physically dependent on the caffeine and don't think they can function without it. Most people sleep far better without the caffeine.

Alcohol is another big problem. It may well help you relax and fall asleep (or "pass out", which is not the same thing) more readily, but alcohol causes abnormal brain wave patterns, and most people who drink alcohol before sleep have physiologically poor sleep rather than restful, restorative sleep. Many people also experience early morning waking, depriving them of some needed sleep.

Inactivity is a problem for some. People who are sedentary all day may not tire themselves out enough to fall asleep easily. If you have a sedentary job and lifestyle, do some sort of vigorous exercise in the evening, but not late evening, to promote tiredness and get you to sleep more easily.

Stimulation late at night is a common problem. If you want to go to sleep, turn off the lights, turn off the TV, stop playing video games or surfing the internet, turn off the music or make it something relaxing like classical or easy listening, put down the book unless it is something restful rather than stimulating, get comfortable, and go to sleep. Don't go to the doctor for a prescription sleeping pill when the real problem is your own behavior. If you stay up late playing video or computer games, watching movies, working or playing on the computer, reading exciting books or doing something else stimulating and you can't go to sleep, you don't have a medical problem; you just have bad habits.

My two-year-old daughter stayed up one night until midnight playing games on my wife's iPhone. She was so tired that she was crying, but the game was so stimulating that it kept her from going to sleep. If you have the TV on in your room, it may seem to help you fall asleep, but most people are kept up later as a result.

Some people say they need the distraction of a television because their mind will race otherwise, but relaxation techniques, meditation, or natural sleep remedies are usually better than having the TV on. "White noise" in the form of fans, classical music, or devices made to generate bland, repetitive sounds can help you sleep. They drown out random noises, or reduce the perceived sudden difference of noise events that can disturb your sleep by arousing your central nervous system (Stanchina, 2005). Even with white noise, various noises may cause your brain to wake you because of survival or child-rearing instincts. Women with young children are particularly sensitive to sounds, and they wake up even when their baby's breathing pattern changes or they make the slightest whimper. (Men can usually sleep through the baby's crying.)

If you avoid caffeine or other stimulants (cocaine, meth amphetamine, Ritalin™, and others should be obvious) and avoid stimulating your mind with electronic or printed entertainment at bedtime, and you start winding down your day hours before you plan to go to bed, you should have less trouble sleeping. Another important suggestion is that you turn the lights off or way down when you are trying to wind down for bed. Our sleep cycle is very much influenced by light, so you should turn the bright lights on in the morning to help you get up and turn them down to dim at night to help you get sleepy.

Some people will shuffle around in the morning, keeping the lights dim and feeling tired so they can "wake up slowly." These are not "morning people"; they are the people who can't do anything more than grunt until they get their first cup of coffee. Instead, they should really turn the lights on as bright as possible and use that stimulus to help them wake up. If you wake up more vigorously in the morning, you may have an easier time with your sleep rhythm at the other end of the day.

Another important bit of advice is to get up out of bed if you can't sleep. If you have lain there, wide awake, for more than fifteen minutes, get out of bed and sit somewhere else; read a book in low light, rock in a chair in the dark, or listen to relaxing music until you feel ready to fall asleep. Go back to bed and try again when you feel ready. People can develop a psychological anxiety about their bed as a place where they fail to fall asleep, so it is important to be successful when you try to go to sleep.

Anxiety and worry

One of the most common complaints I hear from people regarding insomnia is they just can't seem to shut off their mind and relax. All sorts of things tumble around in their heads: issues related to work, finances, politics, family, or their personal lives. Sometimes these issues are minor and don't keep you awake for long, but other times the issues are severe or traumatic and they keep you up most of the night.

Acute stress reactions with resulting insomnia problems are one of the reasons I will prescribe sleep medications. Losing sleep for days at a time just worsens the stress and psychological problems those people are having, and sometimes it takes a drug to break the cycle and get them to sleep. However, I usually suggest people try natural, drug-free ways to improve sleep first.

Medical conditions that affect sleep

Sleep apnea is a growing problem in our culture, mostly because of obesity, but it sometimes occurs in thin people as well. If you sleep alone, you may notice that you wake up frequently in the night or that you feel exhausted all day even though you thought you slept all night. At first, you may wake up in the night feeling as though you are starving for air, but over time your body and brain get used to not having enough air and stop trying to alert you. Some people have apnea because of drugs that suppress their central nervous system (e.g., sleeping pills, pain medications, alcohol), and some may have apnea because of nervous system problems involving a lack of normal stimulation; it is not always related to obesity.

If you sleep with someone else, he or she is likely to tell you that you seem to stop breathing in your sleep, and it probably freaks them out. You need to take this kind of report seriously because sleep apnea can lead to high blood pressure, mental fatigue, cognition problems, heart dysfunction, and eventually heart failure or sudden death. A sleep study, while expensive, is often required before you can get a C-PAP machine, which forces air into your lungs and keep you breathing during sleep. These machines are life changing and life saving for those with sleep apnea.

If you think you will never wear one of those sleep masks, think again. I have seen so many obese, middle-aged men swear they will never be able to tolerate these masks, but when we finally convince them to have a sleep study and try it, they feel so much better they declare they will never sleep without their machine again.

Hormonal problems are common medical causes of poor sleep. Thyroid or adrenal deficiency can cause you to be tired all day but still have trouble falling asleep at night. Progesterone deficiency, which is practically universal after menopause, frequently causes insomnia. Poor melatonin production from the pineal gland definitely causes insomnia; pineal gland damage can be caused by fluoride accumulation (Connett, 2010).

Iron deficiency may cause insomnia, anxiety, restlessness, and restless legs syndrome. Iron deficiency is most common in women with heavy menses, people who have had gastric bypass or stomach removal surgeries, people who donate blood frequently, and those who use chronic-acid-suppressing medications. Magnesium deficiency, which is very common, can cause similar issues with sleep. Magnesium is a frequent ingredient in natural sleep aid combination products.

Depression often affects sleep; I find it is best to first look for organic causes of depression rather than simply medicating it, but treating the depression problem often resolves the sleep issues. Any source of pain is another very common medical reason for poor sleep, so treating pain is often important in improving sleep. Some people self-medicate with alcohol for depression, pain, anxiety or sleep problems, which is a terrible idea.

Medications for sleep

Dozens of drugs are marketed to help you sleep, and there are some instances when they may be the best solution for short-term sleep problems, such as acute stress or trauma, acute pain, jet lag, or travel. In my opinion, they are not a good idea for chronic sleep problems. Medications you use induce sleep artificially probably do not replicate the brain rhythms that promote normal restful sleep. In addition, most people rapidly become dependent on them because of their addictive properties, and many get rebound insomnia when they discontinue use. Frequent use also creates a psychological dependency when you begin to think you can't sleep without them; I see this in my own practice frequently.

Some sleep aids have dangerous side effects as well. Older sleep aids can disturb the heart rhythm, and some of the newer ones cause memory loss and may lead to cooking or driving while asleep. Many can cause a hangover effect the next day or give you subtle problems with thinking and memory. My general philosophy is that sleep is a vital natural phenomenon so you should be able to sleep without a drug. If you can't, something is wrong that must be sorted out.

You should not simply cover up a potentially serious problem with a drug that knocks you out, especially if you have sleep apnea, since taking a sedating drug may increase and lengthen the episodes during which you stop breathing. This is often a difficult decision to make in clinical practice. We know people need to sleep, but we also know there are risks associated with prescription sleep medications. It is somewhat similar to the treatment of pain in that respect.

Natural remedies for sleep

When people see me for sleep issues, my primary goal is to figure out why they can't sleep. If they are going through a divorce or grieving a death, I do often prescribe a drug to help them sleep because natural remedies are typically not sufficient in those situations. If they have pain, I address the pain. If they have poor sleep hygiene because they drink too much caffeine or alcohol, I try to help them to resolve those problems. Sometimes I identify hormonal problems, toxicity issues, allergies, or other underlying causes of insomnia and work on those.

Hormonal support is often important. Many of my patients sleep better with adequate vitamin D supplementation, progesterone replacement (for postmenopausal women), thyroid replacement, cortisol/adrenal balancing, testosterone, DHEA support if needed, or possibly pregnenolone (available over the counter). Testing for heavy metals and undergoing detoxification therapy (e.g. chelation) may also be important. Food allergies or indoor allergies can be found and dealt with.

While we are working on these underlying causes—or if we can't find a cause—I suggest some natural remedies. A great many products in combinations or individual forms are marketed for sleep, some of which I list here, but feel free to try something else if you are having trouble.

Taking vitamin D, iodine, B complex vitamins, magnesium and omega-3 fatty acids (fish oil, flax, hemp or krill oils) every day helps quite a bit to keep your sleep normal. Eating a proper diet and getting adequate, vigorous, regular physical activity are also important in promoting normal sleep. I believe that a healthy dose of physical romance at bedtime is the best natural sleep aid, but if that doesn't work or you're sleeping alone, try some sort of exercise in the evenings, but not too late in the evening. This is also a good time to practice your deep breathing and progressive relaxation techniques.

Melatonin is usually my first choice among the sleep-promoting natural agents because, in balance with cortisol from your adrenals, it is the normal means by which your body regulates the sleep-wake rhythm. Melatonin should be taken every night around the same time, about an hour before bedtime, to establish a pattern. Many patients have told me they have tried melatonin for a few nights and that it didn't work, so they gave up on it, but these patients did not give it an adequate trial.

Find melatonin in a capsule or sublingual (under-the-tongue) product that is high quality, not some cheap hard tablet. Begin with 1mg melatonin nightly and increase gradually as high as 20mg, though most people don't need to exceed 5mg. Melatonin overdose can cause you to wake in the middle of the night feeling anxious or having heart palpitations, so watch for those symptoms and reduce your dose if they occur. Some people may have a mild hangover effect from melatonin, but that usually improves with continued use.

You can also try magnesium 500–600mg nightly at first. Magnesium should always be taken with vitamin B-6 because they usually work together metabolically; get at least 100mg B-6 per day, up to 200mg. It is fine to get your B-6 in the morning, with your B complex vitamin; you don't have to take it at the same time as the magnesium, it just has to be in your system.

5-HTP is a form of the amino acid tryptophan and the precursor to making serotonin and melatonin in the body. It is very useful for sleep, especially in people with anxiety or depression and pregnant or nursing women because they are donating tryptophan to the baby. I often suggest taurine, another amino acid, for sleep, as it calms agitated neurological activity, such as anxiety or worry, and helps you fall asleep; you can take 1,000mg to start and go as high as 5,000mg nightly.

Phosphatidylserine is a lipid extract from soy that helps settle cell membrane activity in the brain and often works well for insomnia, especially for those with high cortisol levels at night because of stress or other reasons. Doses are usually in the 200–500mg range. Pregnenolone can help improve sleep via adrenal balance in doses ranging from 50–100mg. Phosphatidylserine and pregnenolone also are thought to help with memory and general mental function.

GABA, a modified amino acid that is the major inhibitory neurotransmitter in the brain, can be found over the counter as a supplement for sleep and anxiety and can be taken in doses from 250mg to more than 1000mg nightly. Glycine is another simple amino acid, also the main inhibitory neurotransmitter for the spinal cord. I prescribe it for sleep and for muscle spasms, including the severe spasms of cerebral palsy. Dosing can range from 1,000 to 5,000mg nightly for sleep, or a few times daily for muscle spasms.

Valerian and Kava are common relaxing herbs found in many herbal sleep remedies. Chamomile tea works well for some, and 200 mg of theanine, an amino acid found in tea (green or black), has been used with some success for relaxation and sleep. One other herbal remedy for sleep that bears mentioning is marijuana. Many people use marijuana for sleep, anxiety and pain problems with great success and far less risk than manufactured prescription drugs. Marijuana is legalized for medical use in some states now, including Alaska and the other three West coast states.

Various homeopathic preparations made for sleep may work for some, and you can try some of the electronic devices, wristbands, special pillows, and other items made for sleep as well. Many products are marketed for sleep, and many of them may work, but the ones I've mentioned here are those with which I have some personal experience in clinical practice.

CHAPTER 20 – SUMMARY OF SECTION III

I covered a lot of information during this section, and here and there, and I probably tended to run on and give more information than needed to make a point. Therefore, I think it would be useful to offer a recap of the chapter to review the key points. You can tag this chapter in your book as sort of a "quick reference guide" to what is most important to manage your health. This time I'll go in order of importance; we'll start with air as the most critical factor, and then move to water, food, and mind/body nourishing.

Air

You need to find clean air.

If you live in a place with terrible indoor air quality because of dust, mold, old carpet, past occupation by pets or smokers, or some other problem, you should move.

If you have lung problems or other respiratory problems, you should not live in a big city or near a source of significant pollution.

If you can't move, clean up your indoor air environment by removing old carpet, abating mold, and using ozone or air filtration.

Work toward influencing the global air pollution problem through your consumer behavior. Buy local produce and products as much as possible, use mass transit whenever you can, conserve energy in your home, and recycle.

Vote for effective and sensible clean energy legislation and remember that there is no such thing as "clean coal."

Plant some trees outside. Get some plants inside.

Breathing

Breathe with your belly instead of your neck and shoulders. Breathe "down-loose" rather than "up-tight."

Pay attention to your breathing for at least a minute every day and do some focused breathing exercises or try a breath-training device.

Practice "mindful" breathing. Pay attention to how your body responds to breathing.

Water

Find clean water sources.

The best water is from a natural spring or well, but make sure it has been tested for heavy metals like arsenic and for harmful bacteria.

The second choice is filtered water. Filter it yourself or purchase it, but buy water in glass bottles rather than plastic since it is likely *all* plastic contains toxic chemicals.

The third choice is distilled water, which you can generate yourself if there is no safe water around.

Drink about one eight-ounce glass of water for every fifteen to twenty pounds of body weight daily.

Anything with caffeine or alcohol in it works against you, so replace the volume of coffee, tea, colas, energy drinks, and alcoholic beverages you drink with an extra amount of water greater than the volume of those drinks.

If you're elderly, find a way to remind yourself to drink because you lose the sense of thirst. If there's an elderly person in your life, help that person remember to drink water.

Ionized alkaline water may be beneficial for you. Consider trying some if you have chronic health problems, and pay close attention to how your body responds. The long-term effects are not known and there is not adequate research showing ionized water is clearly beneficial or safe for use long term for healthy individuals.

Salt

Don't be categorically afraid of salt. We need it for survival and many body processes.

Make sure your salt is real, unrefined *sea salt*, a granular product with lots of colors in it, not a white or clear product.

Avoid manufactured, processed food products that contain large amounts of added sodium, which throws your electrolytes way out of balance. Read labels.

If you have issues with fatigue, dizziness, dry skin, excessive thirst, frequent urination, high blood pressure, or dry mouth, eyes and nose, take about half a teaspoon of sea salt daily in a quart of water and see if the condition improves. Be cautious if you have high blood pressure, and monitor it closely for the first week or two.

The blood pressure of a small percentage of hypertensive people who are salt sensitive will rise with even moderate intakes of real sea salt, and those individuals may do best with a diuretic for their hypertension.

Food types

Try to eat only organic or wild whole foods.

Avoid manufactured or processed food items with long lists of ingredients on the label. Avoid foods with labels altogether if you can.

Avoid grain-based foods (wheat, corn, barley, and others).

If you eat dairy products, make sure they are organic and grass-fed products only. Look for local producers of raw, organic dairy.

Try to eat strictly organic produce, and focus on local produce as much as possible.

This kind of food can be expensive and hard to find, but so is medical insurance and the care you will need when you develop diabetes, cancer, or heart disease from eating poor-quality food. If we all buy primarily organic, whole foods, they will become cheaper and more plentiful.

The battle for your health is often won or lost at the grocery store or restaurant; make good choices.

If you live where no healthful food is available, you should move.

Super foods and things you should eat

Try to eat several items on the super-food list every day.

Eat wild animals whenever available.

Avoid poultry unless you know who raised it and that the bird was raised outdoors with wild natural food sources. If you do buy some at the store, at least make sure it's organic.

Eat dark fruits and berries liberally; blueberries and prunes are good examples.

Eat apples and have some apple cider vinegar every day.

Eat organic vegetables liberally, but don't overcook them. Seek out crucifers, kelp and kale specifically.

Broccoli sprouts are one of the most "super" of the vegetables.

Corn is *NOT* a vegetable; it is just excess sugar.

Raw organic nuts and seeds are excellent snacks.

Get healthful sources of fat in your diet, including wild or naturally produced animal products (e.g., grass-fed bison or beef; truly free-range organic eggs; raw, pasture-fed dairy, such as butter and cheese; wild fish and seafoods, and fish oil).

Seek out other healthful fat sources like olive oil (extra-virgin), coconut oil, pasture butter or ghee, flax oil, chia seeds, and avocados.

Use herbs like turmeric, cilantro, oregano, basil, and cinnamon liberally because many have medicinal properties, and they make your food taste better. Turmeric in particular appears to have profound health-promoting properties; consider taking it as a supplement as well.

Chocolate is a wonderful thing, but should contain at least 80% percent cocoa.

Green tea is a very good drink, but don't overdo it and don't over-brew it.

Red wine is on some lists of healthy foods, but keep it to one glass per day.

Healthy bacteria are extremely important in your diet, whether obtained through fermented foods (yogurt, kefir, kimchi, sauerkraut, kambucha and others) or supplements.

Nutritional supplements

Make sure your supplements are high quality, in dissolvable or digestible forms, and screened for toxins and impurities.

The supplements I urge most people to take are vitamin D, iodine, magnesium, and fish oil. Vitamin D is likely the most important of them all.

Vitamin D dosing is based on size and latitude (where you live on the planet). Infants should get 1,000–2,000iu per day, no matter where they live; school-aged children can usually take 5,000iu daily; older kids and adults can usually take 10,000iu per day without risk of toxicity, but they should have their blood levels checked after a few months on that dosing. Shoot for a blood level (25-OH vitamin D) of 90–140ng/mL, which is likely to be different from the reference range on the lab report.

More than 90 percent of us likely have some degree of relative iodine deficiency, meaning we would probably benefit from supplementing. Take several kelp capsules daily or iodine supplements equivalent to at least 1,000mcg iodine daily for school aged children and adults, at least 500mcg for infants and smaller children.

Magnesium is safe taken orally, and most of us are deficient to some degree. Take 500–1000mg daily for most adults, but watch for diarrhea.

Fish oil supplements should be molecularly distilled to remove toxins.

Dose them based on EPA content and try to get 800–1000mg daily. If you eat salmon or other cold-water fish twice in a day, you may skip your supplement.

Take a good multi-mineral supplement with amino acid-chelated forms of zinc, selenium, and other minerals because our food supply is largely depleted of minerals.

Probiotics (healthy bacteria) are important supplements for many. Make sure the product is a refrigerated capsule with mixed strains of bacteria totaling 25 billion or more organisms per day.

Most of us need extra vitamin C to help detoxify and to support our adrenals and other functions. Try to get at least 1,000mg daily.

I also suggest that most people take 500-600 mg of N-Acetyl Cysteine daily because it is the key to making glutathione, your body's most powerful antioxidant.

General dietary habits

Eat a mixture of animal and plant foods, but keep everything in moderation. You don't need meat every day but you must incorporate clean, healthy animal foods into your diet on a regular basis.

I suggest you don't go totally vegan. If you have cancer or some other serious disease condition, make sure your animal products are strictly wild varieties.

Eat raw and unprocessed foods as much as possible.

Eat whenever you are hungry and stop when you begin to feel satisfied. Eating just what you need rather than eating to excess promotes longer life. Eat breakfast, preferably with fat and protein, but no cereal, pancakes, waffles, doughnuts, pop-tarts, or other processed carbohydrates.

Try not to eat within three hours of bedtime.

Remember, if we all buy only organic and properly produced foods, the dangerous stuff may go away and the good food will get cheaper.

Produce your own food whenever possible, and support local food producers.

Physical exercise

Do it. Find a type of exercise you will do, and do it.

Don't try to "find time"; make time.

Schedule at least a couple of hours per week total to exercise.

Real exercise makes you sweat, breathe hard, and feel a burning in your muscles.

Ease into it and don't hurt yourself. Be sure to stretch and warm up.

Do a variety of exercise: some repetitive, low-impact exercise like walking, swimming, or cycling, and some more strenuous exercise like lifting weights or doing plyometrics.

Interval training is the best in terms of both results and efficiency.

Multitask. Exercise while you watch TV or read. Put the treadmill in front of the TV.

Exercise with a partner or friends to help with motivation.

Tell yourself you like to exercise and look forward to it. Fake it until you make it.

Mental exercise

Use it or lose it. Do activities that make you think and stimulate your brain.

Consider continuing to work in some capacity rather than retiring; or stay active with hobbies, music, volunteering, learning new languages, and traveling.

Teach others your trade or do some mentoring.

Do crossword puzzles or other puzzles, read books, or play strategic games.

Spiritual balance

This is a very commonly overlooked but vital part of your health.

Find your own path to enlightenment and inner enrichment.

Pray, practice your religion, meditate, or go out and become one with nature.

Take up energetic forms of exercise like yoga, *tai chi*, or *qi gong*.

Get some videos or attend a class to help you learn how to do the exercises.

Practice mindfulness and breathing exercises.

Try to get in touch with who or what you are inside; escape inward from all the chaos around you in the physical world.

Happiness

Be happy whenever possible.

Your attitude and state of mind are usually a personal choice for the most part.

Be happy and focus on positive thoughts, especially when things are toughest.

In most situations, choose to contemplate rather than to react—although this advice doesn't apply when you're driving!

No one else can make you feel bad about yourself; only you can do that.

If you find it difficult to achieve happiness or to find any pleasure in life, see an integrative or alternative health practitioner to be evaluated.

Sleep

You will go crazy and increase your risk of death without adequate sleep; it's important.

Practice good sleep hygiene. Don't watch TV in bed, and don't just lie there if you're not truly ready to fall asleep.

Exercise in the evening to wear yourself out.

Practice your breathing or meditation when you go to bed to help settle your mind. Practice progressive relaxation to prepare for sleep.

Try to get at least six hours of sleep per night, but probably not more than eight hours on a regular basis.

Try melatonin, 5-HTP, taurine, magnesium, phosphatidyl serine, valerian, kava or other natural remedies before trying a chemical agent for sleep.

If you are not adequately rested with eight or nine hours of sleep, something is probably wrong and it's time to be evaluated.

Consider a sleep study if you suspect sleep apnea, restless legs, or some other medical problem. Try the C-PAP; you will love it if you need it.

Words of encouragement

Don't let yourself feel hopeless or resign yourself to failure or to remaining in your current condition.

Don't let anyone else tell you what you can and can't do.

You have to believe you can achieve before you are likely to be successful.

You are usually the biggest obstacle to achieving your goals; you may have to discard some of your prior beliefs in order to move forward for your own health.

See yourself succeeding in improving your health; then make it happen.

Manifest your own reality every day, and make the future you want come to you.

Start today, not tomorrow or the next day; tomorrow is always a day away. Tomorrow therefore never arrives.

Next...

This wraps up my suggestions concerning how to achieve ideal health through your own actions. The following section addresses some of the most common underlying causes of chronic complaints and disease, some of which may require the assistance of a skilled medical provider. I hope you find much there that is relevant and useful to your own health or the health of your loved ones.

SECTION IV

ADDRESSING THE UNDERLYING CAUSES OF ILLNESS

Now it is time to address some factors important to individual health that go beyond lifestyle issues. What follows is a discussion of what I consider to be many upstream causes behind the great majority of chronic diseases people face today in the industrialized world and beyond. This list is by no means exhaustive, nor is this discussion all-inclusive, because I cannot pretend to have all the answers and because each category could itself comprise an entire text if there were a complete discussion of the topic. What I have tried to cover are the most common underlying issues I find in my own practice, which I suspect addresses more than 90 percent of the chronic disease problems faced by primary care doctors in the United States and other industrialized nations.

My goal with this section is to help shift your way of thinking about illness and disease and to provide a new framework to aid understanding of medical problems so you can work toward solutions. After all, if you don't know what you're treating, you are not likely to succeed. As I often tell my children, "If you don't ask the right questions, you probably won't get the right answers."

It is also important to understand that a given chronic illness usually has multiple causes, such as nutrient deficiency, hormonal imbalance, allergy, and infection together. Just as one problem can cause many different diverse symptoms, one symptom or disease condition can have multiple causes. To complicate things further, these "causes" can influence each other as well, making it difficult to decide where to start or how best to intervene.

The practice of medicine is extremely complicated, and this book is not likely going to equip you with the clinical skills to figure everything out for yourself. My hope is that the book will greatly improve your understanding of illness so you can dramatically improve your own health and the health of others by gaining and sharing knowledge.

CHAPTER 1 – GENETICS AND EPIGENETICS, CONGENITAL PROBLEMS

You can't change your genetics, but if you can understand the specific genetic or epigenetic factors involved an individual's problems, you may be able to influence the condition in some positive way.

Origins of genetic and epigenetic problems and possible solutions
Let's talk about the causes of the causes. We think of genetic problems as purely spontaneous occurrences brought about by chance, but they frequently are not. Genetic mutation or epigenetic shift is dramatically influenced by environmental toxins, nutrient deficiency or sufficiency, and environmental stress.

Once a human being has been conceived, he or she can't change his or her underlying genetic code, but the epigenetic factors can still be influenced, and one may overcome many genetic mutations through nutrition. The toxins and nutrient balance a to which a fetus is exposed in utero dramatically affect its future health in many ways, including its expression of genetic traits. Detoxification of reproductive-aged women, prior to conception, may therefore improve genetic expression.

If the conditions while a fetus is developing are poor, there can be disastrous results in how the fetus is formed or even in whether it survives. Some of these factors are nutritional, some toxin-related, and some the result of hormonal influences. Enough environmental influence over time will even change genetics or at least genetic expression. One frightening modern example is in autistic children; more than a dozen gene mutations have been identified that influence this condition; many autistics persons

435

have some of these mutations in common, even when they have no close familial relationships.

It is likely that these mutations were caused or influenced by the pressures of environmental toxins and nutrient deficiencies, so it is conceivable that detoxification and nutrient supplementation could improve the condition. This improvement is much more likely to be observed in future generations, if our young people start making appropriate changes prior to having children of their own, than in individuals who are already afflicted with autistic spectrum disorders.

Recessive gene mutations that cause illness

Most of us can think of a number of purely genetic examples of chronic disease conditions, such as sickle-cell anemia in African populations and cystic fibrosis in Caucasian populations. These two are examples of recessive genetic diseases, which means the individual received a defective gene from each of his or her parents. How common the condition is depends upon how frequently the particular gene mutation occurs in the population. In the majority of cases, the parents themselves are unaffected by the disease and have no idea they carry the trait.

Since environmental pressures tend to drive mutation in our genetic code, it follows that there is a reason for these common genetic mutations' persisting or increasing in the population. It so happens in the two genetic disorders mentioned above that having just one copy of the disease mutation does provide an environmental advantage without disease or illness. Having a mutation in both genes is devastating but having one copy of the mutation was, at some point in time, a major bonus under the circumstances.

Sickle cell anemia is a horrifying condition, and its victims rarely live to adulthood. The disease involves a single base-pair mutation (out of thousands) in the gene for one of the proteins within the hemoglobin in your red blood cells. This means that just one amino acid is different out of a long string of amino acids comprising that protein. The problem is that, when your hemoglobin is changed in this way, the blood cells change from a bouncy doughnut shape to a flattened crescent shape (like a sickle) when they're depleted of oxygen after passing through tissue.

As a result of this change in shape, they stack up on each other and plug the small blood vessels. This causes tissue in that location (e.g. the spleen, lungs, or limb muscles) to suffer infarction, where the cells are no longer getting blood flow. Therefore, that tissue is deprived of oxygen, and the toxins produced by metabolism are not carried away. The tissue in question begins to die, causing intense pain, organ dysfunction, and a place for infection to set in. Even with modern medical care it is uncommon for individuals with sickle cell anemia to survive very far into adulthood. So how did this horrible genetic condition become so prevalent in certain populations?

The sickle cell mutation in *just one* of the two genes for the hemoglobin subunit confers resistance to malaria without causing the sickle cell illness itself. Since malaria has long been perhaps the greatest killer in parts of Africa and surrounding areas, this mutation became very common in those populations because individuals with the trait had a far greater chance of surviving to reproduce. Statistically, sickle cell disease will be present in one out of every four children born to parents who both have the trait. In the high-malaria environment of Africa, that was an acceptable risk as these children would be resistant to malaria and have the trait to pass on but no disease; one out of four would have no trait at all but be susceptible to malaria and one in four would have sickle cell disease. Half of their children would have a better chance at survival.

Cystic fibrosis involves a defective chloride channel in all cell membranes, again caused by a single point mutation in a particular gene. The problem is that chloride passage through cells influences water excretion from various tissues. If the chloride can't move, neither can the water, which negatively affects the bowels, pancreas, lungs, and other organs. If there is no water excreted into the lungs, the normal secretions will be too thick for the child to cough out, setting up conditions that promote recurring respiratory infections and worsening lung damage over time. These recurrent severe lung infections are generally what ultimately lead to premature death in these individuals.

The bowels may be very sluggish because of decreased water in the stool; many affected kids are diagnosed in infancy because of bowel obstruction at birth or shortly thereafter. The pancreas is progressively destroyed because there is not sufficient fluid excreted to carry the digestive enzymes it produces out into the intestine. Those enzymes therefore just passively "digest" the pancreas itself. (This is where the condition gets its name since biopsies of the pancreas show numerous cysts and fibrous scarring.) Destruction of the pancreas leaves the child unable to digest food or absorb nutrients properly.

Like kids with sickle cell anemia, most kids with cystic fibrosis do not live past the age of twenty. Why does this disease exist at such high frequency in the white population (1 in 25 people of European descent)? Just as sickle cell confers an advantage against malaria, having just one cystic fibrosis trait tends to confer resistance to cholera, an intestinal infection that quickly dehydrates the victim and frequently leads to death. There have been worldwide outbreaks of cholera in modern history that may have led to dramatic increases in the prevalence of the CF trait in afflicted populations. Individuals "lucky" enough to have mutated *just one* of their chloride channel gene copies in this way could resist cholera better than those who did not have the mutation; and they would not have the cystic fibrosis disease condition with just one copy.

What is the point of my discussing these two genetic conditions? What can we do about them, and why pick these two when there are so many others to choose from? I chose them because they are common, they are devastating, they can be screened for, and they show how understanding the genetics of a problem can help you treat it.

It is now possible to have genetic testing for these diseases before you have children. If you happen to carry one of these genes and you plan to have children, you can try to make sure your prospective mate does not have the gene, or you can do in vitro fertilization to ensure you implant only those embryos without the genetic disease. While this process prevents the disease's occurrence, it doesn't help those already born with the condition.

From a medical provider's perspective, understanding the biochemical aspects of a genetic disease greatly improves our ability to treat it. Doctors know to give kids with sickle cell supplemental oxygen when they are sick and to give kids with cystic fibrosis pancreatic enzyme replacement. They should also support salt intake for kids with CF because they lose it through their skin at a high rate and provide N-acetyl cysteine to help thin secretions and improve infection clearance; unfortunately though, neither of these treatments are typically considered by conventional doctors. Stem cell transplants may have a chance at curing sickle cell, and there are new cures in the works for kids with CF that reintroduce normal chloride channels to their cells through genetic therapies.

Certain other recessive genetic conditions are largely or completely correctable with nutritional intervention; examples include phenylketonuria (PKU) and methylene tetrahydrofolate reductase (MTHFR) mutations. Many others have been identified genetically that have a wide range of clinical manifestation and severity. Treatment is possible if the underlying biochemical causes are understood. There are likely to be thousands more out there we know nothing about and certainly many mutations that confer some type of advantage, since mutation isn't all bad. After all, we're all mutants to some extent; it's what makes each of us unique.

Dominantly inherited genetic diseases

Dominantly inherited genetic diseases are genetic problems that occur even if only one of your two gene copies has been altered, so every individual with the mutation is affected in some way, with some degree of diversity likely based on nutrition and other environmental factors. Statistically, each child of an affected individual has a 50/50 chance of getting it. That makes one much more likely to inherit a dominant genetic disease than a recessive one, even if only one parent carries the mutation. The upside is that if you don't manifest the disease you usually don't have to worry about passing it on to your kids.

If, however, the disease in question does not show itself early in life, before reproduction, those affected may pass it unknowingly to the next generation. Some common dominant genetic diseases that don't manifest as disease problems until adulthood are Huntington's chorea, adult polycystic kidney disease, Marfan's syndrome, colon polyposis (which predispose the carrier to colon cancer), and BRCA1/BRCA2 mutations (which predispose the carrier to breast and ovarian cancer). There are many of these diseases, and some of them can be tested for genetically.

My own family (maternal side) has a dominant genetic disease that is not well known but statistically affects as many as one in ten thousand, which is relatively common as such things go. It's most commonly called *Stickler's Syndrome* (because it was described by a doctor named Stickler), but its technical name is hereditary arthroophthalmodystrophy. Involving a defect in type 2 collagen formation, the disease most commonly causes severe near-sightedness, retinal detachments, and early-onset severe arthritis in almost all joints.

My mother, her father and brother, and other affected family members all required numerous joint replacements beginning in their forties or so. My older sister has had both hips replaced at around age thirty. I won the coin toss (remember, it's a 50/50 shot at having a dominant disease), and was deemed unaffected after being poked and prodded at the Mayo Clinic when I was ten. (I'll never forget the horror of having an attractive young female doctor examine my genitals - when I thought they were supposed to be concerned with my joints. They certainly are thorough at Mayo.)

At one point, we also thought our family had Huntington's disease because my father's mother developed a tremor and signs of dementia in her late sixties, and all four of her siblings had died of Huntington's. The odds of all five kids in a family being affected are one in thirty-two, so not very likely, but we were freaked out for a while, and she was tested three times. Huntington's is one of the worst of these types of diseases to have: the nervous system slowly shuts down, but your brain usually remains fully functional, so it's like being trapped inside your body as it slowly stops functioning. Many family members of Huntington's patients don't even want to be tested, because they don't want to live their lives knowing what is going to happen to them later.

Most of these genetic disease conditions are pretty much unavoidable if inherited, due to their nature of being dominant genetic traits. Only one of the two gene copies need be altered for a person to suffer the consequences. In some diseases certain treatments may alter the course of the condition, but it is important to know the underlying biochemistry of the condition in order to devise a treatment that will favorably influence the condition.

You may have caught the fact that my sister needed joint replacements more than a decade earlier than our mother and other family members needed their joints replaced. This early joint replacement was probably incurred because she was the only one who smoked cigarettes and because she exercised fanatically through her teenage years and into her twenties, both of which may have accelerated her joint destruction. That the disease can be made worse by lifestyle choices implies that it may also be improved or ameliorated through lifestyle choices. This observation leads to the most important discussion of this chapter: how we can influence our *health*, within our genetic framework, through our *behaviors*.

Knowing the specifics of a genetic condition may help to delay or prevent the disease's negative manifestations. In some cases, early surgical intervention, such as removing the colons of patients with the familial colon polyp and cancer conditions or doing preventive early mastectomies in women who test positive for the BRCA1 or 2 genes, may be appropriate. Such interventions would be a great use of the human genome project data.

I have found nutritional support and reduction of other inflammatory influences to be very helpful in treating my family's arthritis condition. The supplement MSM has made huge improvements in joint pain and has even visibly shrunk damaged joints in some family members. Identifying food allergens (which I address in detail later) and eliminating inflammatory foods has also made a major difference. The point is that, even though your genetics may be working against you, there may be much you can do to improve your health outcome if you understand what is going on biochemically.

Epigenetic problems

Epigenetic problems, it seems to me, are likely to be much more common than purely genetic problems. Think of it as reading a book: It is less likely that the book has typographical errors (genetic mutations) than that people will make mistakes when reading it (epigenetic changes). Reading errors caused by formatting problems, such as the margin's being chopped off or a missing page (structural problems), food or ink stains on a page (environmental toxicity), ink faded in places (aging through hormonal decline or nutrient deficiency), or the stress level of the reader (psychological or mind/body problems) are far more common than typographical errors.

Many factors have to go just right for this metaphorical book to be read exactly as intended, and it's the same with our genetic code: the "words" may all be there like they are supposed to be, but a great number of factors between the genes and their manifestations, including nutritional status, hormonal balance, and environmental toxicity, can alter those manifestations.

How many people today are the first in their families to have some kind of disease or problem? How many have physical features very different from those of their parents and other family members? How many of our new "mutations" are not true mutations at all but variability in gene expression? These mutations are arguably a much more common driving force behind human change than is specific gene mutation, and they can certainly occur more quickly. The good news is that these changes are also reversible over generational time.

Dr. Pottenger showed that cats became more physically diverse and developed more illness problems when they were born several generations into eating cooked food (instead of *raw* meat and milk). He then showed that a "normal" cat could be recreated by feeding several generations perfectly once again. The changes they exhibited could easily have been seen as genetic alterations, but they weren't; instead, they were alterations in the way the genetic code was being read or interpreted. Very few of the changes Pottenger observed could be seen as *positive* adaptations, as most involved some sort of deficiency or illness.

Dr. Roger Williams found many dramatic examples in which

individual animals with the same genetics (twins, triplets, quadruplets) expressed markedly different physiological capacities and functions. It is not clear to what degree these differences were explained by altered gene expression from nutritional or other intrauterine inequalities vs. other epigenetic factors, but they certainly weren't explained in genetic terms. They had to be epigenetic differences.

How many of our common problems today may have arisen under the pressures and processes of epigenetics? Dr. Pottenger described how problems like allergies, asthma, and arthritis arise alarmingly in animals, along with other alterations, afflictions, and ailments. The cause of these problems was insufficient nutrition alone—not even contending with the environmental toxicity issues that we humans face every day.

Do you know anyone with any of those problems mentioned above? Allergies are only the most common reason for visits to primary care doctors in the United States for some time now, and people seem to think of arthritis as a normal consequence of aging after age fifty or so. These problems were not seen in the isolated populations studied by Dr. Weston Price prior to their adoption of food processing and deviation from a purely natural diet.

The concepts of epigenetics, coupled with the work of Price and Pottenger, suggest to me that many of our common disease problems today are our own fault and that they could be eradicated from our future generations. While this is an amazing concept, and sounds very encouraging, it will take a great deal of work and some committed and widespread participation to make happen!

We will have to work "backward" as we go forward in time, moving the health of our future descendants toward that of our ancestors. As people who are alive today, we can alter our own personal fates only a little compared to the impact our behavior may have on our children and future generations. We can't make ourselves perfect specimens (all that plastic surgery aside) in this lifetime. What we can do is to change our habits and our world to help each future generation get progressively closer to the ideal. Our own good behavior, until we reproduce anyway, is a necessary investment in the future.

Cheating your genetics or epigenetics and overcoming the challenges

This section involves something of a "nature vs. nurture"—or perhaps more appropriately "nature vs. torture"—discussion. Many of our health problems are related in some way to our parents' and other past generations' behavior as the result of environmental changes and pressures, which may have altered our genes or gene expression to predispose us to certain health problems.

A predisposition to a health problem does not mean that the problem is a certainty. Common examples of diseases to which we may be genetically predisposed include some of our major health problems in industrialized society, such as heart disease, cancer, high blood pressure or type 2 diabetes.

Some of these problems have become increasingly common in our society, and many people are at risk regardless of whether the condition runs in their families or not. Many of us have become genetically or epigenetically predisposed anew in our own generation, most likely because of nutritional and environmental factors prior to our birth. Heart disease is our number one killer, and it doesn't matter if neither of your parents ever had a heart attack. Breast cancer risk based on family history used to seem important, but now reportedly over 70 percent of women with new breast cancers have no family history of breast cancer or other notable risk factors. The American Cancer Society states that now only 5-10% of breast cancers are thought to be hereditary.

The genetic factors behind breast cancer seem to be having greater expression over time, probably because of our diet and lifestyle's creating an epigenetic shift. Dr. Mary Claire King, the woman who discovered the BRCA1 and BRCA2 genes underpinning breast cancer rates in some families, found that "the lifetime risk of breast cancer among female carriers (of the BRCA mutations) is 82 percent. Risks appear to be increasing with time because before 1940 similar risk is extrapolated to have been only 24 percent. Lack of physical exercise and obesity in adolescence may be important modulating factors for risk carriers" (King, 2010)

Identical twins provide a good way to understand epigenetics. Identical twins may have subtle differences in appearance, major differences in personality, and different susceptibility to diseases. Some of these issues, such as the fact that twins have different fingerprints, are not genetically related at all; the "friction ridges" on our fingertips form randomly and aren't genetic traits. Other, actual physiological differences are probably better examples.

The difference in hereditary patterns for the two types of diabetes mellitus is a good example. It has been observed that if one identical twin develops type 1 diabetes (the kind where the immune system attacks the pancreas, and insulin production is destroyed), the second twin will also develop it about 35 percent of the time; but the second twin is likely to develop *type 2* diabetes (the kind related to obesity) more than 90 percent of the time when it is present in one twin.

Both of these occurrence or concordance rates are much higher than the rate of these diseases in the general population, which suggests that some degree of genetic predisposition is involved. What is surprising is that the obesity-related, later-onset type 2 diabetes is clearly more strongly genetically related than is the childhood-onset, more intuitively genetic-seeming type 1 diabetes. Does this mean that if your twin develops type 2 diabetes, you may as well accept that as your own fate? No! This just reflects an inherent (i.e., genetic) tendency or predisposition to the condition, not a certainty, because type 2 diabetes is still essentially a lifestyle and environmental disease.

The Pima Indians of the Southwest have proven the lifestyle association of type2 diabetes. The Pima who live in Mexico live very hard-working and underfed lives, are typically thin, and have maybe a 5 percent or lower rate of type 2 diabetes. Meanwhile the Pima who live on reservations in the United States eat our horrible processed food and lead very sedentary lifestyles. Pima Indians living in the U.S. are often very obese; and they exhibit the highest rate of type 2 diabetes seen in any population. Roughly half of them have diabetes as adults, according to the CDC.

Researchers are studying the Pima for genetic links to type 2 diabetes, but this effort seems misguided to me. I believe they want to develop new drugs to combat type 2 diabetes by understanding the predisposing physiologic and genetic factors, but why don't we just learn how to eat and live differently instead? Diet and exercise clearly makes the difference between developing the disease or not in this population. That would be far simpler and certainly healthier; it would also cost exceedingly little (possibly nothing). Of course, the pharmaceutical companies couldn't make a profit.

This is a perfect example of how you can overcome genetic predisposition with lifestyle, but research is not looking at it in that way. Why don't we look at what is in the food the Pima in the United States are eating that may be poisoning them in some way, or the effects of exercise on diabetes risk in this population? It's because the drug companies want to make another billion dollars by developing a drug they can market with the false promise that those with type 2 diabetes can continue to be sedentary and eat trash rather than eating a healthy, whole-food diet and getting some exercise.

There is no quick-fix solution to the enormous lifestyle problems of obesity, type 2 diabetes, cancer, heart disease, and these diseases' risk factors. No drug company is going to produce a magic pill that allows you to misuse your body and flout your genetics or epigenetics. We must live cleaner and better in order to live healthier longer; I'm sorry, but there's no shortcut. The real benefit of understanding your genetics is discovering how you, as an individual, have to live in terms of diet, activity, and environmental exposures; knowing your genetics is not a ticket to individualized drug therapy as Big Pharma had hoped. I believe this is why we don't hear much about the results of the much-anticipated *human genome project*.

Type 2 diabetes is an excellent example of genetic predisposition that is modifiable with good behavior, and so are heart disease, cancers of many types, obesity, emphysema, and many other common chronic problems. I have found that many people justify their conditions by telling me that it runs in the family, so the problem was unavoidable, but that is simply not the case for most diseases. That excuse is a total cop-out that most doctors also buy into because it's the easy way out for them too.

One of the most important points of this book is that your health is largely in your own hands and that your behavior (as well as our behavior as a national and global society) can modify your health for better or worse. Just because your parents both had heart attacks in their forties doesn't mean you have to. Just because everyone in your family is obese and has type 2 diabetes doesn't mean you are destined to be that way too. If you teach your kids to live healthy lives, each successive generation in your bloodline can be better off than the last.

I know someone, for example, who believes that since his mother had a heart attack at an early age his own cardiac disease (he underwent a 7-vessel bypass in his mid-fifties) was genetic and *unavoidable* as a result. He continues to smoke and drink excessively, believing that these lifestyle choices don't really influence his condition. It would be great if we could smoke and drink all we wanted without any repercussions, but we can't. This man's genetics may have made it most likely for him to die of heart disease, as opposed to something else (we all die at some point after all); but his smoking and other lifestyle issues may have caused his disease to manifest in his fifties instead of his seventies.

What those familial trends do mean is that, if you want to avoid their fate, you have to behave better than they did. It means you may have to eat better, exercise more, laugh and love more, detoxify yourself, and take certain nutritional supplements. It is part of the "life isn't fair" principle, which also applies when some people seem to be able to eat anything they want without gaining an ounce.

Faced with this kind of "unfair" issue, you have two options or maybe more: you can do whatever you want in the short term—eat bad food, live a sedentary lifestyle, and accept your fate—or you can put down the doughnuts, get off the couch, live your life in a healthy and fulfilling way, and beat the odds. Fight your genetics! Reject those DNA messages telling you "you can't," scrape up some hope and some audacity, and say, "Yes, I can!" (Okay, so I stole a catch phrase from President Obama.)

Some people say you shouldn't blame yourself if you're overweight and develop diabetes or some other lifestyle-related disease. That's a nice nod to your self-esteem, but it's not helpful; in fact, it's often the opposite of helpful.

I don't think absolving people of their personal role and responsibility in their problems is a good idea. If your weight problem could be resolved through your own good behavior, I'm certainly going to point that out and encourage you to fix it, rather than coddling you in order to protect your self-esteem. The best thing for your self-esteem is to stop wallowing in self-pity, get up, and lose that extra fifty pounds! Of course, I offer some understanding and tools to help people overcome those genetic hurdles and improve their own health, despite what happened to their parents or their DNA. You can't change your DNA, but you can certainly affect the expression of your genes.

Summary of issues related to genetics

Your genes likely play a role in the development of any chronic disease.

Some of these conditions are unavoidable because of the nature of this genetics, but in most cases, your future may be modified by your behavior.

It is important to learn as much as you can about the nature of any genetic disease or disease predisposition you may have, in order to live the longest and best possible life.

A dismal family history can be the impetus to live better and cleaner than those around you, rather than resigning yourself to the same fate.

Take charge of your environment, diet, and lifestyle to make the most of the DNA you were dealt.

CHAPTER 2 – NUTRITIONAL CAUSES OF ILLNESS

There is not space enough here to give a comprehensive review of all nutrients and the various conditions they may improve, as that would fill several volumes. My goal in this chapter is to reinforce the idea that, while poor food and deficiency of nutrients are common causes of chronic disease issues, good food and proper nutrients have great potential to overcome illness.

Overeating

A famous rat study published in *Nature* more than seven decades ago showed that restricting calorie intake to only what was needed would extend an animal's life span significantly. This intervention was the only one ever shown to extend life until recent studies showed some similar effects from mega-dosing animals with resveratrol. A more recent study demonstrated this effect in a primate species as well, showing that calorie restriction in rhesus monkeys significantly extended life spans and reduced the incidence of age-related disease issues like cancer, cardiovascular disease, diabetes, and brain problems (Kemnitz, 2011)

A more appropriate way to say this is that over-consumption of calories shortens your life expectancy. This suggests that eating more than you need may stress the body in some way such that your cells will not function as well or for as long as they should. We know from biochemical studies that caloric intake influences the expression of genes called sirtuins, which regulate the function and life span of individual cells in various ways. Eating too much doesn't necessarily cause a toxic accumulation or place excessive metabolic stress on your cells; after all, this effect is shown with the consumption of typical healthful food by test animals.

The sirtuin genes seem to represent a system in place in our cells to regulate population control. If there is abundant food, individuals will eat their fill, reproduce effectively, and be robust; however, they will live shorter lives in order to prevent or reduce overpopulation. If food is in short supply, individuals will tend to be leaner and less robust, possibly have decreased fertility—we see this clearly in the female athlete who loses her menses when her body fat drops too low—but live significantly longer. Thus, the individuals surviving a relative famine can perhaps raise more offspring by surviving longer.

We certainly have abundant food available in our modern society—in fact, we have more than ever before. People are bigger than ever, fertility is decreasing in both sexes, chronic disease and age-related dysfunction are increasing and occurring at younger and younger ages, and people born today here in the U.S. are now expected to live a shorter life span than their parents do; though this decline in life expectancy is not being observed in Europe, where they spend far less on health care (Brown, 2011). What if all you had to do to prevent that was to stop eating when you first feel satisfied, or even just before? Combine that with a purely natural diet, and you may well live past a hundred years.

This kind of dietary restriction is hard for most people to do because we have innate mechanisms in place telling us to eat, and keep eating, when food is readily available. Our evolution/adaptation early on was not in a setting of abundance, but one involving a struggle to find food. Those instincts to find food that developed through hardship still persist in most of us it seems, so a person must be highly disciplined to stop eating at the first sign of satiety. Exercising enough to stay at an acceptable weight despite overeating is not the same thing as restricting food because exercise creates free radicals and cellular damage. This means that eating more, but exercising enough to maintain the same healthy weight, cannot be expected to result in prolonged life span similarly to caloric restriction.

The priceless work of Price and Pottenger

There have been many pioneers in the area of nutritional medicine, but I encourage everyone to read two seminal works on the subject by Dr. Weston Price (*Nutrition and Physical Degeneration*) and Dr. Francis Pottenger (*Pottenger's Cats*). Dr. Price, a dentist who traveled all over the world in the early 1900s studying recently discovered populations that had only experienced the introduction of modern processed foods within the last generation or so, published a book with hundreds of pictures illustrating malformations of the face, jaw, and dental arrangement that were clearly related to this dietary change. He also documented many other health problems that showed up in the populations only after they adopted modern processed foods in their diets. These "malformations" Dr. Price observed have become the norm for industrialized nations now for generations; and nobody seems to find it unusual if a child has cavities or needs braces.

Dr. Pottenger's book documents his elegant but simple experiments on cats. He showed that by eating cooked food cats incurred myriad developmental anomalies and chronic health problems—many of the same health issues now common in industrialized human populations. He also described vast differences in the health and ability between children raised on farms eating almost exclusively healthy, whole foods and children raised in metropolitan areas eating mainly processed foods. These two books and their authors are powerful in content and obvious truth, rare in today's world.

Few people can read these two books and still deny the power of proper food and nutrition in your health. You can get copies of these books and many others on the subjects of nutrition in health, detoxification, disease prevention, and treatment through natural means and other similar topics from an educational organization for the general public called the *Price-Pottenger Nutrition Foundation*. The foundation also publishes an excellent newsletter for which you can sign up. It is one of the better sources of current nutrition information available.

These publications all show how eating a proper diet obtained in a natural state promotes optimal health and how failing to eat this optimal diet promotes the development of all manner of physical and mental health problems. The distinction must be made here between severe individual nutrient deficiency conditions described in the classical conventional medical literature and more subtle chronic health issues that are survivable but that cause moderate ongoing problems or dysfunction. For example, severe vitamin C deficiency causes scurvy, but long-term moderate deficiency leads to easy bruising, poor resistance to infection, impaired detoxification, and increased risk of heart attack. If you look only for the signs of scurvy, you will miss the importance of vitamin C in terms of *optimal* health.

Specific examples of nutrient deficiency

Severe single-nutrient deficiency diseases have been described for most of the known vitamins and minerals. These conditions have often been taught to modern conventional physicians as the only relevant issues related to nutrients. The more subtle chronic effects of relative nutrient deficiency are not taught but are treated symptomatically with drugs instead. This is a significant oversight in modern medical training and a big part of the reason health is so poor in industrialized nations. It is a deadly mixture of ignorance and arrogance in medicine that leads doctors to cover the symptoms of nutrient deficiency with chemical medications as dictated by the *standard of care.*

I offer a series of common examples here, but the topic is too large to cover completely. I urge you to continue your own research using some of the books and publications I have mentioned, as well as any other sources you may find.

Most B vitamins have their own well-described severe deficiency diseases. Thiamin (B-1) deficiency causes beriberi or Wernicke's encephalopathy; niacin (B-3) deficiency causes pellagra; cobalamin (B-12) deficiency causes Korsakoff's psychosis, macrocytic anemia and peripheral neuropathy; and so on. These severe deficiency conditions are rare in modern civilization, and most doctors never see them. The problem is there is a great deal of milder dysfunction with moderate deficiencies of these vitamins that also goes unnoticed. Many Americans are walking around with mild *functional* deficiencies of vitamins B-6, B-2, B-3, B-5, B-12, and others.

Most of the B vitamins are involved in energy production to some extent, and many people have discovered on their own that taking a B complex vitamin every day does a lot for their energy and mental alertness. Riboflavin has been shown to be very helpful in preventing migraines (Schiapparelli, 2010), niacin has been shown to help reduce cholesterol and cardiovascular disease events (Duggal, 2010), and B-12 shots are a common treatment for fatigue even in the absence of documented major deficiency. These are examples of orthomolecular medicine, but they also probably represent some chronic problems associated with moderate deficiency of these specific nutrients.

The realization that lower intakes of folic acid during pregnancy leads to a risk for neural tube defects (i.e., spina bifida) sparked the fortification of all bread and grain products in the United States with folic acid and recommendations for increased folate during pregnancy in prenatal vitamins (which, unfortunately, nauseate most pregnant women). Now we also know that folic acid supplementation helps to lower blood homocysteine levels, a molecule that is important in the development of cardiovascular disease. Unfortunately, there are meaningful genetic differences in the way humans metabolize and utilize folic acid; this causes some to benefit by seeing prevention of cardiovascular problems with folic acid supplementation, but others to actually see *worsening* of their atherosclerosis with that same therapy (Mazur, 2012).

Modern biomedical research has now shown us that it is not homocysteine itself, but the proper metabolites of folic acid, that determines cardiovascular disease risk. Homocysteine is seemingly just an indirect indicator, or surrogate marker, for the level of active folic acid metabolites such as 5-methyltetrahydrofolate (5-MTHF) (Antoniades, 2009). This all leads me to believe that folic acid supplementation should all be in the form of 5-MTHF rather than folic acid or folinic acid, which are the common forms found in supplements. Two of genetic mutations involved in this issue with folic acid metabolism can be tested for through major labs now (MTHFR mutations), and that is a worthwhile thing to do for anyone with early cardiovascular disease in the family.

An association has also been found between folic acid levels and depression. The biochemistry involved is that folate is involved in the production of serotonin and other neurotransmitters. Folic acid supplementation as adjunctive therapy has been shown to make large improvements in the success rate of treating depressed patients with antidepressant medications. Unlike cardiovascular disease, the effect on depression does not appear to involve the MTHFR mutations; therefore, it does not seem necessary to use 5-MTHF in place of plain folic acid for the treatment of depressed patients in general (Lizer, 2011). Lastly, folate also improves genetic expression and detoxification via the methylation cycle and many other biochemical processes involved in common chronic disease problems.

Vitamin B-6 is involved with arguably more biochemical processes in the body than any other single nutrient, so it's logical that it might be useful in treating chronic disease complaints. But do you think doctors receive any training in identifying patients who may benefit from added vitamin B-6? Are we taught in medical school that we should supplement with B-6 those patients with anxiety, seizures, insomnia, muscle spasms, depression, autism, neurological problems of most varieties, various metabolic disorders and other conditions? No, but we are certainly taught that you can get nerve damage from too much B-6.

Vitamin C has many benefits and is inexpensive, but doctors usually scoff at supplementing with it, perhaps other than to reduce cold symptoms. Medical professionals are taught that vitamin D deficiency causes rickets, but are usually not taught about the myriad other conditions with which vitamin D has been proven to be involved. Doctors are told vitamin D can be toxic with supplementation, so they prescribe pitifully low doses even though vitamin D deficiency is one of the most common and important deficiency problems we have today. Many people are also deficient in zinc, which is important in resistance to infection and in skin and tissue integrity, wound healing, hormone regulation, brain function, and many other aspects of health, but few doctors suggest supplementing with zinc either.

Iodine insufficiency is probably one of the most common nutrient deficiency problems worldwide, including in the United States. Iodine deficiency leads to lower IQ scores, thyroid deficiency problems (with or without the huge goiters common in photos from indigenous cultures where severe iodine deficiency is endemic) with all the attendant clinical problems, increased rates of heart attacks and breast cancer, and other problems (Brownstein, 2004 and Derry, 2001). The public, including doctors, typically believe they get plenty of iodine from our standard American diet, but that is far from the truth.

The World Health Organization recommends iodine supplementation prior to and during early pregnancy for women, and also supplementation for infants, living in areas where less than ninety percent of households use iodized salt, and school age children have low-range levels of <100mcg/L urinary iodine concentration (Zimmerman, 2009). Subtle, functional iodine deficiency is present in up to 90–95 percent of our population based on urinary challenge testing (Brownstein, 2004), but that form of testing is not the mainstream standard, and those notions are very controversial at this point. The problem of iodine deficiency is so easy and inexpensive to correct that it is inexcusable, in my view, if we fail to do so.

Magnesium deficiency is also extremely common, and contributes a wide array of disease or illness conditions. Magnesium is involved in more than three hundred different biochemical reactions in the body, so there are many symptoms and chronic complaints associated with magnesium deficiency. Our food supply is deficient in magnesium because of depleted soils, and common issues like the use of caffeine, alcohol, and diuretic drugs and emotional stress accelerate urinary loss of magnesium.

I see chronic problems, such as high blood pressure, anxiety, muscle spasms or tension, headaches including migraine, insomnia, rapid heart arrhythmias, asthma, and chronic constipation improved significantly or totally eliminated through magnesium supplementation. Magnesium is inexpensive and widely available, and moderate diarrhea is its only significant toxicity. It seems a serious shortcoming to me that few doctors prescribe magnesium for these complaints.

The brainwashing against nutritional medicine in conventional medicine is pervasive. I once went back to my residency program to give a lecture on integrative medicine, where I discussed all the benefits of magnesium. I asserted that we should be suggesting supplemental magnesium to most of our patients—in high doses for those with deficiency symptoms (which is most people). Many of the residents suggested, some with obvious hostility, that was bad medicine because I hadn't proven that the patient needed magnesium, and any perceived benefit of magnesium on my part might just be a placebo effect.

I was so disgusted I haven't been back since. I explained I know they all *need* magnesium because you'll die without it–it's not like a drug, it is an essential nutrient. The benefits of magnesium in various ailments have been shown in numerous scientific studies, but residents typically don't read anything without a drug ad on every other page; and conventional journals don't tend to publish positive studies on nutritional interventions. I also informed them that they also never know if a prescription drug's perceived benefit is from the placebo effect or the drug itself, since the placebo effect often improves up to 30% of people. If a blood pressure drug improves BP in 60% of people in one group and the placebo to which it is compared improves BP in 30% of that group – that suggests that 30% of the people in the "real drug" group were likely improved just due to the placebo effect, and only 30% were actually improved by the drug. You don't know whether any given individual benefitted from the drug or the placebo effect; and they are somehow okay with *that*, but not if that is related to magnesium or some other nutrient – it's total hypocrisy. At least magnesium doesn't kill people and it's inexpensive! It's amazing to me that the attitude of even our young conventional doctors is so galvanized against using safe, natural, and potentially effective therapies first; they want to jump straight to drugs because that's "real" medicine.

The nutrient deficiency problem doesn't stop at vitamins and minerals. It also includes essential amino acids from proteins and healthy fats, as well as other macronutrients.

The amino acid tryptophan is the precursor for serotonin and melatonin. Deficiency of these neurochemicals leads to common problems like depression, anxiety, insomnia, constipation, and irritable bowel syndrome. Supplementing with 5-HTP is inexpensive and can frequently resolve these problems by addressing the actual cause, but our doctors don't do that, preferring instead to prescribe antidepressant drugs, anti-anxiety drugs, sedatives, sleeping pills, and counseling, but no amount of talk-therapy is going to overcome the fact that you need more tryptophan! I have seen many of my patients derive a great deal of benefit from taking 5-HTP for depression, anxiety, insomnia, panic attacks, appetitie control and sugar cravings.

Essential fatty acid imbalance is another common and pervasive nutritional problem in our culture, but our health care providers are not educated about it. If we could get the omega-6 to omega-3 ratio back down from 20:1 to 3:1, we would likely see tremendous drops in cardiovascular, inflammatory, degenerative, and neurological problems, but that would mean changing our diets. Fish oil supplements have been proven to help treat cardiovascular problems like high cholesterol, hypertension, and cardiac arrhythmia and to decrease stroke and heart attack risk, improve arthritis pain, decrease inflammatory bowel disease symptoms, and treat depression, anxiety, and ADD. The list goes on. A drug company has put out a prescription fish oil capsule, so why aren't more doctors suggesting people take fish oil supplements or change their diets to get the fatty acid ratio back in line?

Biochemical Individuality

The concept of biochemical individuality bears mention here. Roger Williams, Bruce Ames, and others helped pioneer the understanding of this concept but it is not taught to modern doctors with proper emphasis. We all say things like "everyone is unique" and "treatments affect everyone a little differently," but the concept is not put into practice as a clinical tool often enough.

There are more than thirty thousand suspected single-nucleotide polymorphisms (point mutations) in genes that can alter an individual's requirements for any given nutrient. A woman may need ten times the amount of folic acid during pregnancy that her mother needed in order to prevent spina bifida in her children. Another individual may need fifty times as much vitamin B-6 than the average person in order to prevent epilepsy. Yet another person may have a poor ability to make serotonin and require a much higher intake of tryptophan than usual in order to prevent chronic depression or anxiety.

These differences are the *rule* rather than the exception. Most of them will not reach clinical significance or cause discernable disease as long as those individuals eat a balanced, healthful diet that is high in all essential nutrients. It's when you eat a nutrient-poor diet (i.e., the typical American "die"-et) that these problems begin to show up in most people. Unfortunately, conventional doctors are not likely to see these complaints as being related to nutrient deficiency, so they bring on the drugs.

Adept medical application of this knowledge includes the ability to test individuals for specific nutrient insufficiency based on their own unique biochemistry. Some of this uniqueness is genetic or epigenetic, while some of it is circumstantially related to the patient's environmental stresses, toxic or infectious burden, nutritional status, and other issues. In any case, there are ways to assess the metabolic needs of the given individual.

I usually decide what to supplement patients with based on their spectrum of complaints and symptoms and possibly some physical signs. If they want a more scientific approach or if the initial guess doesn't seem to work, there are various testing options to help get things right. You can test directly for specific nutrient levels in a variety of ways, and there are effective urine test panels called *urine organic acids tests* that can often point the way.

You can measure vitamin levels in the blood and sometimes in the urine. These tests can indicate dietary intake and absorption capacity, but they don't always tell you whether the individual has enough vitamins for their unique biochemistry. You can measure mineral levels in the blood (but they should be RBC levels rather than dissolved serum levels), the urine, or even the hair, but these tests don't tell you whether the individual has enough of those minerals for them specifically. Hair analysis can be particularly skewed by genetic factors and other variables, so I never suggest that test.

Measuring a direct nutrient level is not always going to give you the right answer. Finding a blood level of vitamin B-12 in the middle of the reference range doesn't tell you whether the individual has enough B-12 to meet their unique genetic or other circumstances. The urine organic acid panels measure a wide array of metabolic byproducts and compounds that may indicate a pattern of relative biochemical insufficiency of many nutrients.

If you are relatively deficient in vitamin B-12, you will have elevated levels of MMA (methylmalonic acid) in the blood and urine, even when your blood level of B-12 is high-normal, suggesting that you have a genetic or circumstantial need for more. If you need more magnesium to meet your specific situation, there will be elevated levels of various organic acid compounds in your urine. A lack of adequate vitamin B6 will cause elevations in other compounds. Functional deficiency of many vitamins, minerals, and amino acids can be determined in this way.

The standard conventional labs run a very limited organic acids panel that is geared toward identifying a couple dozen rare genetic diseases in newborn infants or young children. There are not as many or diverse analytes tested in these standard conventional panels, the reference ranges do not have the specificity to pick up subtle problems, and you do not get a very useful interpretation in your lab report. There are several independent labs used primarily by integrative or alternative medical providers that run much more comprehensive and useful panels with excellent interpretations and informational support. You can ask your provider to order test kits from *Great Plains, Metametrix, Genova*, and other such companies at no cost to themselves; you take the kit home, collect the sample, and send it off yourself. The provider doesn't even have to know anything about the biochemistry because the lab provides an excellent interpretation. The kits are free to your provider (so they have no excuse), and your doctor just has to send them a copy of his or her medical license to order tests. Of course, you are best served by a practitioner who is familiar with these tests and how to help interpret them in the context of your clinical picture.

One down side is that you usually have to pay for these tests up front directly to the company. Sometimes they will bill insurance for you, but they usually do so at a notably increased cost. Many insurance plans don't pay for them anyway, so we always suggest that patients pay the lower direct price and then submit the receipts to their insurance companies. The typical price range for these is $200–$300, which may be cost-prohibitive for some. I most commonly order these tests for generalized fatigue, psychological disturbance, seizures, and other neurological problems, but they are also a great tool for many other conditions and for those who want to optimize their diets and nutrition for wellness and prevention purposes.

Other areas where individual biochemical differences apply include immune system function and susceptibility to toxicity. Some people have much stronger or weaker immune systems than others, or they are not very good at handling specific infectious viruses or organisms. (Have you ever noticed that just one or two people in the house get cold sores or warts when you know everyone in the family must be harboring the virus also?) Some people are the proverbial canaries in the mineshaft in terms of common environmental toxins like heavy metals and various chemicals.

My final thoughts on this subject are that you should not assume that what is good or adequate for those around you is also enough for you; you should not assume everyone in the house can do well on the same diet; you should not assume something safe for most will not be toxic to you or your child. Remember that everyone is different, which explains why only one person in a group will get sick when all have the same environment and diet. These issues can be very challenging to figure out, but you can be persistent with your own provider and move forward to optimize your own or a loved one's health.

Congenital malformations and conditions

Many people think birth defects like cleft lip, clubbed foot, and heart defects are genetic issues. The reality is that, in most cases, these problems are not genetic at all. Just because something is present at birth does not make it genetic; the word "congenital" refers to conditions present at birth, but not necessarily genetic conditions. Remember that your baby was made from *food*, just as you are; the diet and environment of a pregnant woman influences the health and status of the baby. Embryology and fetal development are complex processes, and a great many things have to go just right in order to make a fully functional human.

We have only described a few specific examples of nutrients that are related to birth defects, but there have to be thousands not yet worked out. We know that spina bifida and other neural tube defects like anencephaly, where a baby is born without a brain, are related in many cases to deficient folic acid. We know that cleft lip and palate are sometimes due to biotin deficiency. (Recall that biotin is largely made for you by your intestinal bacteria; so taking antibiotics may deplete pregnant women of biotin.) We know that iodine deficiency causes small heads and low IQ or even profound mental retardation.

We know about a handful of other conditions related to nutrient deficiency, but still the only standard recommendation for pregnant women is to take a low-potency, sure-to-make-you-nauseous prenatal vitamin! There is no thorough discussion of diet, nutritional supplementation, environmental toxin avoidance, detoxification, or other vital issues before or during pregnancy other than to tell the women that they need to eat more than usual and that they should take a prenatal vitamin. If they are obese, they may be put on calorie restriction, which doesn't usually lead to better food choices than what made them fat in the first place and which has the potential to deplete them of nutrients even more. When women develop gestational diabetes, at least they are told to avoid sugar, which should have been a standard suggestion from day one!

Weston Price described how most indigenous cultures had special diets for women who were pregnant, breast-feeding, or trying to conceive. They either knew instinctively or through generations of observation that increased intake of specific foods were needed to nourish a child through their early development and to replenish a woman after pregnancy, that early development starts even before the sperm fertilizes the egg, that the womb needs to be a clean and happy place biochemically, that the sperm needs to be swimming straight and to have intact DNA, and that the egg needs to be uncontaminated and to have good DNA.

The infertility and miscarriage rates we see today are staggering when you think how important reproduction is to any species. The whole point of being alive from a purely biological perspective is for an organism to make more of its kind. If ten to fifteen percent of couples can't conceive, there is something drastically wrong with the population, and this problem is just going to get worse the way we are headed. In my opinion, the problem is a combination of bad nutrition and environmental toxicity. Francis Pottenger showed that cats' fertility came to be greatly impaired just from eating cooked food, suggesting a general connection between nutrient depletion and infertility.

Prenatal and preconception nutrition and other issues that affect a child's overall health are some of the most important concepts to our survival as a species, but they are largely ignored by our conventional obstetricians, perinatologists, neonatologists, and pediatricians. Our culture's idea of improving prenatal care is to increase the number of visits to an obstetrician during pregnancy. Of course, if your provider doesn't know how to improve your health and the health of your fetus, visiting him or her more often doesn't help a bit! All that most doctors do at those frequent visits is screen for impending problems like gestational diabetes and preeclampsia, with little or no attempt to *prevent* these or other complications. You can prevent those problems with nutritional interventions, but that isn't what's done. Most other industrialized nations post beter pregnancy outcomes with few prenatal visits than here in the

U.S. For more on this topic I suggest reading the book *Expecting Trouble* by Thomas Strong, MD.

Our rates of pregnancy and birth complications would likely be dramatically decreased if we improved the quality of our food supply, counseled young people and pregnant women about proper diet and nutrition, cleaned up our environment, and worked on detoxifying women prior to conception. Unfortunately, those concepts are not part of our cultural view in the general population or the conventional medical community at large. Instead of taking simple steps to prevent problems, we watch for them to occur and then take drastic steps to save the mother and child when catastrophe strikes. And now autism is reported to affect one in eighty-eight children overall in this country, with one in fifty-four boys affected. The road to autism begins before conception, involving the nutrient and toxin status of our women.

If you are pregnant or thinking of becoming pregnant (or if you are of child-bearing age), I suggest you follow all the nutrition and environmental suggestions in this book and take supplements, including at least vitamin D, iodine, magnesium, and fish oil. I also suggest we all raise our children with sound ideas about health so each generation can be healthier than the last. It's up to our current younger generations to start moving our species back toward optimal epigenetic health, but this is going to take a hundred years or so. As it is now, we have been *de*-volving as a species for several generations.

Overcoming genetics with nutrition

Understanding the biochemistry of a genetic problem can help you prevent its manifestation. We screen for *phenylketonuria*, at birth because modifying the baby's diet can prevent the retardation and neurological damage would occur on a typical diet in babies with this genetic condition. There are many other examples of preventing the appearance of rare genetic diseases in children, but it is much more difficult to modify clinical problems in adults since our brains and tissues were fully formed a long time ago, and some tissues do not turn over much once we're adults.

One example of a specific dominant genetic disease is my family's genetic arthritis condition. My mother has improved dramatically by taking MSM, a simple nutrient component of joint cartilage. Some of her formerly enlarged and dysfunctional finger and hand joints have shrunk to normal size and returned to their normal range of motion, which I would not previously have thought possible. Her ankles are no longer swollen or painful, although she had previously considered having them replaced because they hurt so badly. She was on glucosamine and chondroitin for decades before we started the MSM, and those supplements never made this kind of difference.

Hereditary hemochromatosis, the most common genetic disease in Caucasians, is simply an iron-management problem that leads to iron accumulation in the tissues. If this condition is identified, all the person need do is go donate blood on a regular basis. One can also avoid iron-rich foods and limit foods with vitamin C when eating foods with iron, possibly eliminating the need for frequent blood draws. Other common genetic diseases, such as cystic fibrosis, can improve markedly with nutritional changes, such as avoiding dairy, increasing high-antioxidant fruits and vegetables, taking optimal doses of vitamin D and other supplements, and taking N-Acetyl Cysteine. There are also special diets for those with Down syndrome that have been shown to improve cognitive function dramatically.

The effects of hereditary hyperhomocysteinemia, which often leads to increased rates of cardiovascular disease and depression, may be modified by taking high doses of folic acid (*methylated* folate in particular). Celiac disease, which has a strong genetic component, can be completely prevented if the person avoids eating gluten. A genetic predisposition toward developing type 2 diabetes can be mitigated almost completely through diet.

Many of our chronic diseases have genetic components that are usually multifactorial rather than single-gene in origin. Nutrition can modify almost all of them to some extent. If your family has a predisposition to heart disease, check your homocysteine, take extra folate (at least 1mg of 5-MTHF), eat an organic diet with no processed sugar or grains, and strict avoidance of nonorganic grain-fed animal products; and also take vitamin D, iodine, magnesium, fish oil, turmeric, N-acetyl cysteine, and perhaps other supplements. If your family is prone to cancer, try to live as chemical-free as possible, eat a pure diet full of plant foods with anti-cancer compounds (e.g., green tea, cruciferous vegetables, dark fruits), and use some general detoxification methods regularly. Also be sure to take vitamin D in therapeutic amount, to improve immune function against cancer.

Autism is a rapidly rising problem with some degree of multi-gene genetic predisposition. It appears to be related to altered genetics in the areas of detoxification and immune system function; these children are generally at great risk from before birth because of all the chemical exposures in the womb and the nutrient-poor diet most pregnant women have. Gluten sensitivity is also very common in these kids (and the entire human population). The genetic markers associated with celiac disease itself may be tested through some mainstream labs (HLA-DQ8 and DQ2), but *anyone* can develop serious problems with other forms of gluten-sensitivity, regardless of their genetics.

There is usually a final trigger for these kids, such as an infection, adverse vaccine reaction, or other environmental exposure that sets their immune system afire and starts the process of chronic systemic and brain inflammation. But these kids were generally very much at risk before that event, so it is not possible to prove that these events actually "caused" the condition; there are too many underlying variables. Autism should be largely preventable with the nutritional and detoxification measures discussed in this book, although these measures won't help the purely genetic causes that afflict about one in two thousand children. In any case, women may need to start "preparing" a year before conception in order to make a meaningful difference.

Many people seem to be the proverbial canaries in our environmental mine shaft; they are made ill by minor environmental exposures that do not bother most of us. These people often have genetic mutations that make it difficult for their livers and other organs to clear environmental chemicals. There are many nutrients with which they can load their bodies to help aid internal detoxification. Of course, dietary habits, such as eating nutrient-rich foods and avoiding toxin-laden foods, are very important in preventing illness as well. Genetic tests for mutations in genes like glutathione methyl transferase and others, by certain specialty labs are now commercially available; these tests can help individuals determine what supplements they need and what chemical substances they should avoid.

Fundamentally, we are all supposed to be made out of food, although many of us today are composed of large amounts of petroleum derivatives and other chemicals as well. Our genes just tell all those food particles where to go and what to do. Even our DNA is made of food. If you can understand which genetic signals have changed and in what way, you can often alter the nutrient environment to create more positive clinical outcomes. It just requires that you or a good health practitioner understand the genetics and biochemistry, have a good working knowledge of nutrition and physiology, are disciplined with the program, and structure your life a bit differently.

Curing "medical" problems with nutrients: Orthomolecular medicine

Orthomolecular medicine uses high doses of specific nutrients to alter your physiology favorably and correct disease processes. It is similar to pharmaceutical treatment in that you are using a single agent in a powerful way to force a change in the body. However, it is different from pharmaceutical treatment in that the treatment used is a natural substance that *belongs* in the body anyway and has a more predictable and consistent effect. Generally, the risk of adverse side effects is far lower with nutrient therapy than with drugs.

Magnesium is one of the best and broadest examples of orthomolecular nutrient therapy. Magnesium relaxes smooth muscle, the type of muscle that contracts blood vessels and airways and moves your intestines. Magnesium helps to normalize heart rate and rhythm because it is important electrically in the body. It also relaxes all your skeletal muscle, the big, bulky muscle tissue that moves your limbs and that you control voluntarily. Magnesium often helps because we are replacing a significant deficiency, but other times we use the properties of magnesium to encourage a physiologic change and treat symptoms.

We give some patients who come to our office with migraine headaches 2,000-3,000mg intravenous magnesium pushed in fairly quickly. (If you go too fast, you can drop a person's blood pressure precipitously and make him or her pass out, so don't try this at home unless you know what you're doing.) This usually breaks a migraine or tension headache and leaves people feeling refreshed and alert, in contrast to the groggy stupor with which they generally leave the ER after they give you narcotics and anti-nausea drugs for the same thing. We do a similar injection to break severe muscle spasms in the neck, shoulders, back or other areas. This therapy works well with very little risk.

Clinical medical research shows that intravenous magnesium can improve asthma or COPD exacerbations, improve the outcome of an acute stroke, and break some cardiac arrhythmias (it is a necessary intervention in the critical heart rhythm disturbance called *torsades de pointes*, as we are all taught in critical care). Intravenous magnesium is still the only proven effective treatment for severe preeclampsia during pregnancy, and in my opinion, it is the best and safest treatment for preterm labor as well.

I use Vitamin C in our office intravenously in an orthomolecular fashion as well. We give high doses (50,000 to 100,000mg) of vitamin C intravenously to patients with cancer because it has been shown to help the body kill abnormal cancer cells in a natural way, without doing damage to normal tissue. Recent published research is finally establishing intravenous vitamin C in the conventional literature as a viable anticancer therapy, through the creation of hydrogen peroxide and direct selective killing of cancer cells (Chen, 2012). Vitamin C often works synergistically with chemotherapy and radiation to kill cancer while at the same time protecting your healthy tissues from the adverse effects of the conventional therapies. Unfortunately, most oncologists don't know about this; even worse, they believe the vitamin C will negate the effects of their chemotherapy drugs, even though there is scientific and clinical research to the contrary. Conventional doctors still tend to caution patients not to try such a "foolish" treatment as vitamin C, which has no demonstrated toxicity (Monti, 2012) and has mounting evidence in its favor.

If you wish to try vitamin C therapy in this fashion, make sure you see someone who has had training in this area of integrative medicine. It should not be given at the same time as many types of chemotherapy, while that drug is at therapeutic levels in the body. It can be given up to a few hours prior or a day after chemo in most cases. The NIH is actively studying the effects of vitamin C in cancer treatment with the help of integrative practitioners, so more information should be forthcoming.

Other common uses for high-dose IV vitamin C are in acute viral illnesses and other infections and with toxic exposure problems. We have helped many of our patients recover quickly from influenza, bronchitis, mononucleosis, and even viral meningitis with one or two infusions of 25-50,000mg vitamin C with some other additives (glutathione, B vitamins, and magnesium, among others). Recent research has shown improvements in pain, fatigue and skin rash in patients with shingles, even using fairly small doses of IV vitamin C (Schencking, 2012). We have also treated a number of patients with acute exposure to toxic chemicals, such as solvents and machine engine exhaust, using vitamin C, glutathione, B vitamins and other nutrients with significant observed recovery.

Many other examples are common practice for integrative physicians. High doses of vitamin A can help clear stubborn acne, zinc can help clear infections and speed wound healing, and high doses of fish oil (or other sources of EPA) can improve inflammatory symptoms in diseases like arthritis and inflammatory bowel disease, as well as psychiatric problems like depression and anxiety. Fish oil has also been shown to drive down high cholesterol and to improve various cardiac arrhythmias dramatically.

Many of the B vitamins have been used in an orthomolecular fashion as well. Niacin has been used to lower cholesterol; and the work of Dr. Abram

Hoffer showed that it can be used to treat schizophrenia. Recent study has further elucidated that patients with more severe cases of schizophrenia have physiologically decreased response and sensitivity to niacin, suggesting a greater biochemical need for the vitamin in those individuals (Messamore, 2012). B-12 shots have long been used successfully for generalized fatigue. High doses of B-12 often improve language in autistic children; and some children with autism have been shown to have improvement in behavioral and other symptoms, as well as reduced oxidative stress, through the use of injected methyl B12 (Bertoglio, 2010). Riboflavin can help reduce migraine frequency, folic acid has been shown to improve depression, and there are many other examples.

Most of this information has been known to integrative and alternative (i.e., naturopaths) practitioners for decades. I read about using magnesium for asthma and acute hypertension in my grandmother's nursing physiology textbook from the 1940s. When I used intravenous magnesium successfully for an ICU patient with acute airway constriction and blood pressure elevation symptoms during my first night on call as an intern, my attending, a doctor who had been practicing for thirty years, told me the next day that he had never heard of using magnesium in this way. What's more, when he looked it up, it was listed as "new and innovative." He was intrigued, because it had worked.

I have seen many patients' high blood pressure controlled with magnesium, vitamin D, and fish oil (along with diet, exercise, and relaxation techniques) rather than multiple prescription drugs. Sometimes this treatment simply replaces a deficiency, but there is an orthomolecular effect as well. In my opinion, it is always better to use biologically normal substances before trying drugs; doing so eliminates a great deal of toxicity risk and prevents dependence and withdrawal problems. Our doctors too often prescribe toxic drugs for problems that could likely be fixed far more cheaply and safely using simple nutrients available at the grocery store.

Let's not forget about the importance of salt and water. For all my talk of food and its macronutrients and micronutrients, your body mass is composed mainly of water, and you need proper salt and electrolytes to keep the water where it belongs. Fish can't swim anywhere without enough water to move through, and your body's necessary chemical and physiological processes can't operate normally without enough hydration in your cells and tissues. A great many health complaints could be improved by increased intake of clean water and possibly some raw sea salt.

Summary

This section addresses the *causes* of illness, so let me make the point one last time regarding food and diet: Nutrition, primarily in terms of *nutrient deficiency*, plays a role in almost every form of illness. Resolving any type of disease process involves the action or reaction of your own tissues, which all ultimately involves having adequate amounts of the proper molecules on hand. All of the molecules that make up your body tissues, hormones, and other chemicals have to come from food and water.

Many disease and illness conditions are a direct result of nutrient deficiency, and a great many more can be treated by supplementing with certain foods, macronutrients, or micronutrients, even if deficiency was not present as a contributing factor (orthomolecular medicine). Some may suggest that improvement through nutrient supplementation indicates there was a "relative" deficiency; this may certainly be the case for individuals with genetics that result in a greater need for a given nutrient compared to the general population. In many cases, drugs can be replaced by nutritional interventions, to achieve or resume normal physiology.

Now that you know you can treat various ills with some foods and that you have potent cancer prevention on the shelves of every grocery store, have an apple or two every day, eat some cruciferous vegetables and curry, chase it all down with a cup of green tea, and you should be in better shape. You can try buying a bunch of expensive supplements instead, but they won't work as well if you are still eating a poor diet; it's like buying flowers to cover up the smell of your garbage and poorly kept house.

Additional nutritional supplements may help when you are dealing with specific nutrient insufficiencies that are causing chronic problems and when you are trying to treat certain symptoms or conditions. Just make sure you know what you're taking and use quality products. Educate yourself as best you can from a variety of sources, and don't hesitate to seek the help of a good health care provider if you aren't sure about what you should do.

CHAPTER 3 – HORMONAL DEFICIENCY AND IMBALANCE

Introduction-

This chapter poses a particular challenge for me because I would prefer to write an entire book about the subject; in fact, others have written entire books about just one hormone, such as thyroid or testosterone (two of my favorites). There are numerous hormones to discuss, each with its own potentially interminable discourse about the intricacies of clinical symptoms, diagnosis, testing, and correction of problems, not to mention the complex interaction of many different hormones with one another.

If you have strong academic interest in the subject or you are a health care provider looking for information about hormonal therapies, I encourage you to find old endocrinology textbooks that are biochemistry-based (not drug-company-propaganda-based) or perhaps the *Hormone Handbook* by Thierry Hertoghe, MD, which is an excellent resource for both busy clinicians and interested lay people.

My goal in this chapter is to cover the most prominent hormones I deal with in clinical practice in order to provide a useful overview of the symptoms, testing, and treatment relevant to problems associated with each hormone. I also comment on the most common hormone interactions relevant to each hormone. This chapter is not a comprehensive treatise on each hormone, but it should give you most of what you need in order to recognize a possible problem in yourself so you can get it checked out. After reading the chapter, you will likely have a better understanding of these hormones than most doctors have, and you can use that knowledge to help direct your treatment even if your provider offers different advice and opinions.

Hormone replacement or therapeutic intervention is one of the most common tools I use in clinical practice because hormones are powerful molecules that *belong* in the human body and that therefore have fairly predictable biological behavior, side effects, and toxicity in most individuals. Hormones are the little project forepersons that tell your cells what to do and determine how resources are used and directed in the body. Without the adequate amounts and balance of hormones, things don't "go"—or at least they don't go right.

Vitamin D

Identity

I am always excited to talk about vitamin D, but since I realize I have already given much of the story away earlier in this book, I will try to be brief. Because I live in Alaska, vitamin D is easily my favorite thing to prescribe and to talk about. I have given countless mini-lectures on vitamin D to patients, medical colleagues, strangers at the park, helpless passengers in neighboring airplane seats, and many others.

Recall that "vitamin" D is not a vitamin at all but a hormone. I make this statement based on its chemical action and the fact that it is produced and processed in the body in typical hormonal fashion. The proper bio-identical form of vitamin D is *cholecalciferol*, so remember that when you are looking at bottles on the shelf of a store or online purchasing supplements. The alternative choice, which should really not be a choice at all, is *ergocalciferol*, which is a synthetic version made by exposing a fungus to radiation and artificially forming a molecule from sterols in the organism's cell wall into something that behaves much like—but not exactly like—cholecalciferol.

Ergocalciferol is referred to as vitamin D-"2", while the bio-identical cholecalciferol product is termed vitamin D-"3". To confuse everyone further, there is no D-"1" version. D-2/ergocalciferol is far more expensive than D-3; it is available by prescription in a 50,000iu dose that is sixteen times more expensive than the same dose of cholecalciferol capsules I carry in my office. D-2 has only about a third the biological potency, in terms of absorption and maintenance of blood levels, of D-3 (Laura, 2004). D-2 also has less than one fifth the physiological activation potential of D-3 (Holmberg, 1986)), making D-3 therefore at least fifteen times more effective at similar dosages compared to D-2 at similar dosage. D-2 may cause allergic reactions in those sensitive to molds and fungi, and it is suspected of having mild liver toxicity in some individuals (several European and Russian articles in PubMed allude to this in the title, but they are old studies and none of them have abstracts available). Therefore, ergocalciferol is inferior to cholecalciferol in every possible way. There is no reason for it to exist, other than pharmaceutical company profits.

I can't think of a single reason why anyone would want to use D-2 over D-3 but it is the form most doctors give you because it is available by prescription in a 50,000iu strength. However, you can get D-3 in the same strength at much lower cost on the internet, at a health food store, or possibly at your provider's office if you ask them to carry it. Some people want to use the prescription form because their insurance covers it, but at $4 per pill versus 25 cents per pill for a better form of D-3, that is extremely poor value for the health care system. Most commercial D-3 these days is derived from sheep's wool and is not synthetic in any way; but be vigilant for any adverse reaction if you are highly allergic to wool or sheep.

Biochemically, vitamin D (which hereafter refers to the *D-3/cholecalciferol* form) is a version of a steroid hormone. "Steroid" means it is derived from cholesterol. In a natural setting, we produce a pre-hormone molecule in our skin that is converted to the partially active form of vitamin D, called 25-OH vitamin D, upon exposure to proper sunlight or UVB rays. If you live in the tropics, you can activate vitamin D in your skin with sun exposure all year; the farther you are from the tropics, whether north or south, the harder it is to activate vitamin D in your skin in this manner. As you approach the Arctic or Antarctic circles, you have no chance of making any vitamin D, at any time of the year.

Based on years of testing patients and some self-experimentation, I am convinced we make no significant vitamin D in south central Alaska at any time of year, and it can only get worse going further north (well, it can't really get worse than zero). I have seen no seasonal variation in my patients' vitamin D levels in blood; and my being sure to get lots of direct sun exposure through the month of June yielded no increase in my own blood level. This point is important because the general public and many physicians believe that you can make plenty of vitamin D by getting just fifteen minutes of sun on your hands and face every day, no matter where you are.

Researchers have now determined, for example, that you cannot make vitamin D with sun exposure even in Atlanta, GA, from November through February, which is a third of the year. Researchers in France have noted significant increases in cancers and other vitamin D-related causes of death at higher latitudes, and suggested that vitamin D supplementation should significantly decrease this burden of disease (Grant, 2010). This problem is due to the increasingly tangential angle of the sun's rays striking the Earth at higher latitudes, passing through a thicker slice of the ozone layer, which tends to absorb the UVB rays peferentially. No UVB rays mean no vitamin D. Of course you can still get burned by the UVA rays, which do get through. I suggest that if you want to make vitamin D using a tanning bed, you must use a bed with full-spectrum UVA/UVB bulbs.

25-OH (hydroxy) vitamin D is the main circulating form and reservoir for vitamin D activity in the body, the form that should be measured in blood to determine adequacy. This molecule is converted to 1,25-OH vitamin D in the kidneys for circulation of this, most highly active form, in the body. Some of its systemic effects, such as calcium absorption from the intestine, are dependent upon the 1,25-OH form. Measuring the 1,25-OH form is reasonable only if you're trying to assess kidney function in terms of vitamin D conversion, or investigating abnormal calcium levels.

Do not let your medical provider base your vitamin D status on a 1,25-OH level; make sure it is the 25-OH level. The 1,25-OH level is very inconsistent in the blood, changing significantly from hour to hour; that is why it is a poor means of monitoring overall status. The 25-OH level is far more constant and has a much longer half-life in the blood, making it far more useful for assessing nutrient status of vitamin D. Also, it is very important to note that the 1,25 form is available as a prescription drug, called *calcitriol* (generic) or Rocaltrol™ in the brand name. Make sure this is NOT the form your provider prescribes for you, unless you have chronic kidney disease and cannot make that biochemical conversion yourself from cholecalciferol. I have seen this happen, and giving people high doses of calcitriol can cause hypercalcemia and kidney damage, or even death eventually.

Because it's fairly new information, most practitioners don't realize that your other tissue cells also convert vitamin D to its most active form for use inside that particular cell or tissue, based on its particular needs. We now know that this conversion influences every tissue in the body directly and that it has far-reaching effects. This is why there is no need to supplement with the active form in the absence of kidney disease. Vitamin D has been shown to influence the expression of roughly two thousand genes, which is about half of all your genetic code! I think that proves that sunlight is a vital need for our species and that vitamin D is important.

Actions of vitamin D

On a molecular biochemical level (for those nerds like me out there who like to know that sort of thing), the function of vitamin D is often to modulate gene activity and expression. This means it provides a signal to the cell to turn certain genes on or off, resulting in more or less of a particular protein or enzyme and altered biochemical activity. Some of these important such gene products for which vitamin D increases production are called *cathelicidins*. These proteins function in such a way as to increase dramatically cellular defense against bacteria and other infectious agents. They directly kill germs like an antibiotic. If you have adequate vitamin D you will even produce large amounts of cathelicidins onto the palms of your hands. Because of cathelicidins and numerous other immune system effects, vitamin D supplementation has been shown to decrease the rate of colds, flu, and other common infections, and also to help your body contain chronic infections such as tuberculosis and HIV (Khoo, 2012).

Many of the actions of vitamin D influence the movement and actions of calcium in your cells and tissues, including the absorption of calcium from food and deposition of calcium into the bones; the use of vitamin D for patients with or at risk for osteoporosis is well known. Calcium is also a common messenger molecule in every cell; it affects many different cellular processes. Vitamin D exerts various control mechanisms over the actions of calcium as a signaling molecule within cells; it tells calcium where to go and what to do. This magnifies the physiological role of vitamin D in the body.

Vitamin D can also act as something of a neurotransmitter and a cellular messaging molecule. It directly stimulates certain serotonin receptors in the brain, which improves mood, energy, and mental acuity. It also affects multiple other neurotransmitters in terms of regulating production and secretion (Stumpf, 2012). Vitamin D promotes energy use, growth, and the normal development of tissues like nerves and muscles, as well as bones. It appears to have some degree of activity and importance in virtually every tissue in the body. Many more mechanisms of vitamin D activity are probably still unknown and this is an area of ongoing research, so stay tuned.

Symptoms of deficiency

The first symptoms of vitamin D deficiency people tend to notice are depressed mood and decreased energy, mental alertness, and physical strength to varying degrees. Patients may present with complaints of fatigue, excessive sleepiness, depression, irritability, weakness, and chronic muscle or back pain. One study in Minnesota showed that more than 93 percent of patients with low back pain had severe vitamin D deficiency. These are just the early observable symptoms for most people; the long-term consequences are legion. One fundamental problem in clinical medicine is that people don't ever really know how they are *supposed to* feel; this means they often don't realize they have a problem with vitamin D deficiency; instead they think it is just "normal" for them. Once we supplement them, then they can tell the difference.

The concept of biochemical individuality is important as it regards vitamin D. You live at the same latitude as everyone else in your area, but we all may have different places of origin, ethnicities, skin color, and biological thresholds for vitamin D deficiency. I lived in the cold, dark North for more than thirty years before I ever started taking vitamin D supplements, and I never felt I experienced fatigue or any other relevant symptoms. If I had been raised in Honolulu or Miami and later moved to Alaska, it may have been a very different story. I have seen this scenario in many of my patients who moved to Alaska from more southern latitude, and they can tell the difference in how they feel after making this tremendous "latitude adjustment."

Dr Jonathan Wright likes to ask, "Does a fish know it's wet?" We don't know what "normal" feels like if we've always known the same "abnormal" state, and we don't know how a given variable affects us unless we change it. I'm sure a fish that has been caught, held thrashing in the air for a minute, and then returned to the water, gains a greater appreciation for being wet. Similarly, I am sitting in an airplane seat in coach, on a six-hour flight, working on this book en route to a conference. Since I have had an opportunity to sit in first class a couple of times in the past, I now have new appreciation (or discontentment) for how cramped I am here in coach, typing with my shoulders hunched and elbows tucked tightly to my sides.

It is common for one individual in a family to be far more affected by deficiency than are others in the household, perhaps because that person's system developed in a setting of greater vitamin D adequacy, because they have toxins that break down vitamin D, allergies, or infections that consume it rapidly, or because of genetic reasons. In any case, vitamin D deficiency contributes to many fatigue, depression, chronic pain, allergic, infectious, autoimmune or tissue degeneration conditions.

Therapeutic and preventive uses

The symptoms I have mentioned as the most common usually quickly improve with vitamin D replacement. There are many other more chronic degenerative or pathological conditions for which I routinely prescribe high doses of vitamin D and many common causes of death or chronic disease that early implementation of vitamin D therapy may help to prevent or mitigate.

Osteoporosis and osteopenia are the chronic conditions for which most conventional providers prescribe vitamin D because the association of vitamin D with bone formation has long been accepted. Other degenerative conditions in the body—muscular decline associated with aging, neurological degeneration like peripheral neuropathy or dementia syndromes (i.e., Alzheimer's), growth and developmental abnormalities in children, and even other hormonal deficiency problems—should also be supplemented with vitamin D because of its regenerative effects on every tissue.

Immune system problems should also be treated with vitamin D therapy. Vitamin D has a highly positive influence over the immune system in every direction. It increases immune function in terms of fighting infection of all types and modulates immune function so as to decrease systemic inflammation and also the effects of allergic or autoimmune conditions (Youssef, 2011).

Vitamin D has been shown to lower blood pressure and cholesterol and to reduce the risk of cardiovascular disease including death. Vitamin D is far better at decreasing heart-related death than any drug therapy in my opinion. Repeated studies have shown dose-dependent decreases in sudden death, heart failure and all-cause mortality that are greater and greater at higher levels of vitamin D in the blood (with no plateau, because they don't supplement high enough). One recent study, the Ludwigshafen Risk and Cardiovascular Health (LURIC) study, followed more than 1,800 patients with metabolic syndrome (a pre-diabetic condition that predisposes to higher rates of cardiovascular disease) for an average of 7.7 years. 92% of the patients studied had suboptimal (<30ng/mL) levels of vitamin D. Those with "optimal" levels (still far, far below the levels to where I supplement my patients) had a 75% relative decrease in all-cause death and a 67% relative decrease in cardiovascular death compared to those with severe deficiency (<10ng/mL). There was an 85% reduction in sudden death and 76% reduction in congestive heart failure. These results were all dose-dependent, suggesting that further benefits would be expected with even higher vitamin D levels (Thomas, 2012).

Vitamin D has been shown to decrease significantly the risk of developing many types of cancer, including prostate (Gilbert, 2012), pancreatic (Baggerly, 2012) and colon (Pereira, 2012) cancers. Deficiency has also been linked to the risk of developing autoimmune diseases such as type 1 diabetes, multiple sclerosis, and schizophrenia as well as allergies and other immune-related conditions (Radlovic, 2012).

In short, we have conclusive evidence that vitamin D can help prevent or even treat the most common causes of death and disability in our society. The top three categories of disease are cardiovascular, cancer, and autoimmune conditions, and vitamin D supplementation should be a part of treating them all. Neurodegenerative problems, allergies, infectious issues, and other disease categories that are influenced by vitamin D add to the seriousness of the widespread vitamin D deficiency problem as an important public health issue.

In short, the answer to the question concerning for whom we should consider vitamin D testing and supplementation is "everyone", unless they have a contraindication.

Dosing and toxicity

Vitamin D is one of my favorite examples of the vitamin toxicity paranoia because I encounter resistance to my recommended dosing so often, especially from other physicians and conventional health providers (who usually have no training in nutrition). It has been widely taught that vitamin D is dangerous in large doses and that it can cause hypercalcemia (too much calcium in the blood), potentially leading to heart rhythm disturbances, muscle pain, kidney failure and even death. That is true, but extremely rare, and vitamin D toxicity of any degree is very difficult to induce in the typical person.

The RDA for vitamin D was set a few decades ago at only 400iu per day (10 micrograms or 0.01mg in terms of weight) for both newborn babies and adults of all sizes. It should be intuitively obvious that if you weigh 150 pounds, you might need more of something than if you weigh only 10 pounds. Do you know where the magical 400iu number came from? It was found that children who had a teaspoon of cod liver oil forced upon them every day by caring mothers or grandmothers did not develop rickets. Analysis of typical cod liver oil samples yielded about 400iu (10mcg) of cholecalciferol, so that's where the level was set. Since rickets doesn't develop later in life, it was not thought important to increase the dose for adults, but we now know that many chronic diseases can be ameliorated to some extent through vitamin D supplementation and that the doses required for adults are much greater than 400iu per day, especially if you live some distance from the equator. People must keep thinking and learning instead of clinging to old guidelines and dogma!

The U.S. Institute of Medicine (IOM) published an extensive report on vitamin D in 2010. Their report downplayed the importance of vitamin D in health and disease, suggested that deficiency is not as common as recent research has implied, and that we (those who are excited about vitamin D supplementation) were making a big deal about nothing. At the end of this predominantly negative report, they paradoxically suggested *increasing* the RDA by 50%. There have been many critical reviews written about this report since its release, including an excellent analysis by the Alliance for Natural Health. Criticisms have included statements that the "study" was funded about 80% by pharmaceutical companies, there were more than a dozen vitamin D researchers interviewed for the IOM report whose statements were conspicuously absent from the final report (and all of these researchers reportedly had much more *positive* things to say in support of vitamin D supplementation at higher doses), and that the IOM report clearly focused on the limited available negative vitamin D research rather than the far greater amount of positive research. In my opinion, this report should be ignored in its entirety as biased and irrelevant.

Multiple studies have now demonstrated that adults can take 10,000iu per day safely, regardless of where they live, for several months or longer. This amount of vitamin D is produced within about thirty minutes of full-body sun exposure near the equator for a light-skinned individual. To my knowledge, that much vitamin D from the sun never hurt anyone.

Vitamin D is a fat-soluble molecule that can, with sustained use at high doses, accumulate to high levels in the body; this is a greater concern than toxicity from a single high dose. The case reports of vitamin D toxicity I have found in the literature, which are quite rare, typically involve use of supplement products that contain more than 500,000iu vitamin D, often manufactured in error and labeled as having only 1,000-5,000iu. This extreme level of over-dosing can certainly cause toxicity within a few months or less; this is why I suggest people have their vitamin D level checked within a few months into a supplement regimen. Some cases involved persons who were taking significant supplemental doses over a long period while also avidly sunbathing.

The Merck Manual, one widely accepted repository of conventional medical knowledge, states that a typical adult would need doses of 100,000iu or greater daily for several months to risk significant toxicity. Of course, there is variability in that amount, and this considered only severe toxicity. Vitamin D toxicity is usually assumed to be related strictly to excessive calcium absorption and to the effects of the resulting hypercalcemia rather than to the high vitamin D level itself. To date, there has not been described direct toxicity of vitamin D itself.

From extensive personal experience with vitamin D, I believe that the first symptom of overdose is insomnia, but I have not seen this reported in the literature. I once took 50,000iu every day for seven months just to see if I would suffer toxicity, and the only problem I developed was trouble sleeping. It was a highly functional insomnia because I felt energetic and very good in general, but I stopped taking the high dose because I was starting to get dark bags under my eyes, and I could get along on four or five hours of sleep per night for only so long. The insomnia must have been a direct effect of vitamin D rather than a calcium effect because I had normal calcium levels (even with a 25-OH level near 474ng/mL, more than three times the established safety limit). I have also seen others develop insomnia within a week or two at high doses, long before any significant calcium elevation would occur.

To test your vitamin D level, have the 25-OH level test done, *not* the 1,25-OH level test. Remember that the reference range on most lab reports is going to be *wrong*; this is one time when you may need to be better informed than your doctor is, because most doctors don't know that the range is wrong, and the correct range is very important.

The No Observed Adverse Effect Level (NOAEL) for 25 OH vitamin D is 150ng/mL, which means that a "normal" person should not incur any toxicity risk at that level or lower, so 150 is the *proper* upper limit of the reference range on a lab report. However, most laboratories have set their upper ranges at 100ng/mL; this is likely to build in an extra margin of safety, but it could be at the expense of potential health benefits for some. Having a level above 150 ng/mL does not mean you will have toxicity—far from it, in my opinion; it means only that no science has suggested toxicity risk up to that level. NOAELs are usually fairly conservative designations in medicine.

Since doctors don't generally know the NOAEL for 25-OH vitamin D, they don't know any better than what the lab report says. If you are taking 10,000iu per day (or 50,000iu twice per week, my preferred regimen for adults because of the much lower cost and better chance of compliance), you may achieve a level of 120–140ng/mL, which is the therapeutic range I aim for in the average person. A blood level that high will scare most medical providers, and they will tell you that you are "toxic." I have held my own level up around 200ng/mL for years now without consequence, just to prove a point, though I cannot recommend that to others. We don't as yet know the consequences of maintaining very high levels of vitamin D, if there are any.

There is a wide variation in how well oral vitamin D is absorbed and assimilated, especially if you've had a gastric bypass (which I strongly feel is a horrible idea), so if you don't get your vitamin D level to your goal, you should simply increase your dose until you do. However, see the section below on special circumstances for added safety.

If your level exceeds 100 and your provider isn't educated about vitamin D, he or she is likely to call in a panic and tell you to stop or reduce your vitamin D supplement because you have vitamin D toxicity. Of course, this not true if you are still in the accepted safe range below 150 and your calcium level is not elevated. I held my own 25-OH level far above the safe range with my 50,000/day experiment and held it there for several months without my calcium level's ever going above the normal range. I didn't develop kidney stones or bone spurs, and I didn't have a heart attack.

I have seen patients with levels above 600ng/mL with no calcium elevation or notable symptoms. They kept taking 50,000iu per day for over a year and felt good on it, despite my instructions to reduce their dose. I have seen others with mild widespread muscle pain at levels in the 300s; this was also without calcium elevation in the blood, but was likely a symptom of true toxicity. People can have a wide range of responses to almost everything, so be careful and don't go above 120-140ng/mL, unless guided by an experienced health provider. This is an area where you can help educate many of our more open-minded conventional practitioners.

Special considerations for vitamin D toxicity risk

There are at least four circumstances when hypercalcemia may be a consequence related in some fashion to vitamin D supplementation, indicating the need to avoid vitamin D or lower the dose. The first is therapeutic use of excessive vitamin D, resulting in a true overdose. This can occur by accident because of improper manufacturing, because of individual variations in absorption, or because of cavalier supplementation practices. Vitamin D is a hormone replacement therapy, so it is not like vitamin C or other true vitamins in terms of safety. If you are using it at high doses, you should have a 25-OH level and a calcium level checked in your blood *after two to three months of consistent supplementation* because your level will not plateau until then.

As I mentioned previously, there is a prescription form of 1,25-OH vitamin D, the "activated" form, which is normally systemically produced by your kidneys. It was created for patients with kidney failure, who cannot make enough circulating 1,25-OH from other tissues. It is a necessary prescription for almost everyone on renal dialysis and many others with advanced kidney disease; without it, their calcium levels drop very low and they suffer from muscle cramps as well as possibly fatal cardiac arrhythmias. However, this prescription form is highly potent. You need less than one microgram per day to achieve normal calcium absorption; more than that can cause chronic calcium overload and destroy what is left of the kidneys, among other kinds of damage.

This detrimental effect occurs because the therapeutic range for the *activated form* of vitamin D is so tight; a little bit works well, but just a little bit more may do damage. It is far safer to dose large amounts of D-3 (cholecalciferol) and let the body convert it to calcitriol as needed. Doctors often don't understand this difference between D-3 and calcitriol. An endocrinologist, a "hormone specialist," recently told one of our pregnant patients that she should stop taking D-3 and take Rocaltrol™ instead; this was because the endocrinologist thought the D-3 was a pregnancy category C drug (that is, of questionable safety for pregnant patients). That was incorrect, of course, because we make D-3 in our own bodies. The well-meaning physician had gotten their information backward; D-3 is a category A (believed to be safe) drug, and Rocaltrol™ is the category C drug! Make sure your provider does not prescribe you the 1,25-OH form of vitamin D by mistake!

The other three special circumstances, to which I alluded at the beginning of this passage, when hypercalcemia may be a consequence of vitamin D supplementation, are medical conditions that can cause hypercalcemia on their own and where the use of typically-safe doses of vitamin D may trigger unacceptably high levels of calcium even with normal-range levels of 25-OH vitamin D:

One category of these conditions is certain types of cancer. The most common types of cancer to cause hypercalcemia include lymphomas, or squamous cell forms of cancer found in the lung, skin, esophagus, and some other organs. Sometimes, patients manifest hypercalcemic problems as the first symptoms of their cancer.

Another medical condition that may cause hypercalcemia is hyperparathyroidism. The parathyroid glands, which are embedded in the back of the thyroid gland at the base of the neck, produce parathyroid hormone (PTH). PTH causes calcium to be released from the bones, where it is stored, for use in metabolism around the body. Patients who have a tumor in one of these glands or whose glands are overactive liberate excessive amounts of calcium from their bones, leading to accelerated bone loss, osteoporosis, fractures, and the attendant symptoms of hypercalcemia if the calcium level itself rises as a result.

Many of these patients have no idea they have the problem, and their blood calcium level may be normal or only barely above normal for years, rather than rising to an abnormal value that would attract attention. They may have vague bone aches, fatigue, odd feelings of disequilibrium, or vague generalized mental suppression. Most people have subtle symptoms for years before ever being diagnosed; they finally realize that all their little complaints were due to the parathyroid problem after they've had surgery, when they feel so much better.

When someone with occult hyperparathyroidism is put on a decent dosage of vitamin D, his or her blood calcium will generally jump up above the normal range. The upper limit is around 10.5 by most labs, and you should definitely suspect it at levels above 11.0. If this increase in calcium occurs after initiating vitamin D therapy, levels of PTH and both 25-OH and 1,25-OH vitamin D should be checked. If those are all normal, the PTH-related peptide (PTH-rp), an indicator of cancer, should also be checked.

I have diagnosed in this manner a number of patients with primary hyperparathyroidism, who had likely suffered mildly with the problem for years. You could call it a "vitamin D challenge test" for the condition. This possibility is why it is important to have your calcium level tested within a few months of starting vitamin D at a significant dosage. However, if you're just taking a multivitamin with under 1,000iu, there is no need for a test; that dosage is too low to be significant in my opinion.

Infections with a category of bacteria called *mycobacteria* have been shown to trigger hypercalcemia in some cases. Well-known diseases such as tuberculosis and leprosy are caused by bacteria in this genus; and those with impaired immunity or lung function can develop chronic lung or other infections with common forms of these organisms that are everywhere in the environment (you likely inhale some every time you take a shower, because they tend to colonize shower heads). Chronic infection with these organisms causes a peculiar reaction in some individuals, whereby some of their white blood cells begin actively converting cholecalciferol to calcitriol on a systemic basis. This leads to a dramatic increase in the blood 1,25-OH level, resulting in elevated blood calcium as well. These infections are difficult to test for; they should be considered if the other tests are normal.

The last medical condition I will discuss here that may cause hypercalcemia is a complicated one that is disturbingly common where I live, as it's increasingly common the farther you get away from the equator. *Sarcoidosis* is a condition in which affected individuals develop unusual granulomas (nodules comprised of inflammatory tissue and immune system cells) in various tissues; in fact, it can involve literally every tissue in the body and lead to disease in any organ. It usually starts in the lungs and may be picked up on a routine chest X-ray. It looks a lot like tuberculosis or a fungal infection of the lungs; and it is my belief that it is caused initially by an infection of one of those types, with a deranged and disorganized immune response following. It took centuries to figure out that tuberculosis was caused by an unusual type of bacterial infection; it is caused by a pathogen in the category of mycobacterium (a name that denotes similarities to fungi), and close cousins are the organisms that cause leprosy and the one suspected of causing many cases of Crohn's disease and ulcerative colitis. I suspect someone will eventually prove sarcoidosis is similarly caused by a mycobacterium.

This condition is rare in the tropics, but it becomes increasingly common as you move north and south from the tropics, and it is most common in dark-skinned people living at higher latitudes (displaced tropical individuals). These two factors—prevalence in regions with less sunlight and prevalence among dark-skinned people native to tropical areas—point to vitamin D deficiency as a likely contributing factor; but the problem in sarcoidosis is that these patients may spontaneously develop dangerously high calcium levels. It seems that the immune system cells within the granulomas noted in this condition mutate in some way to convert vitamin D to its active form in the manner normally only performed by the kidneys. This dramatically increases the circulating 1,25-OH form of Vitamin D and can cause life-threatening hypercalcemia, even in individuals who are not supplementing with any vitamin D.

Does this mean you cannot under any circumstances take vitamin D if you have sarcoidosis? In my opinion you can still take vitamin D, but must be extremely cautious and have labs checked repeatedly. Doctors successfully treated tuberculosis with sunshine and/or vitamin D therapy before we had antibiotics for it, and I try to do the same thing with sarcoidosis patients because I believe it has a similar microbial cause. My suspicion is that high doses of vitamin D may actually help your body kill and potentially eradicate the infectious organism that I believe is causing the condition we call sarcoidosis. None of this is proven however.

In spite of my cautions about treating sarcoidosis patients with vitamin D, the doses I use are as high as those for cancer or MS. I cannot suggest that anyone out there try high doses of vitamin D for sarcoidosis without being closely followed by a medical provider who can order labs and interpret them for you. The problem is that some patients with sarcoidosis develop hypercalcemia even without vitamin D supplementation, and adding more vitamin D to the equation can become extremely dangerous in a hurry.

Calcitonin

Identity and action

Calcitonin is a comparatively obscure hormone that most of you are unlikely to have heard of. I am discussing it here because it is involved in calcium metabolism in some ways that are similar to vitamin D, and I may as well put it here while calcium management is fresh in your mind. Calcitonin is a simple peptide hormone produced by the medullary cells within the thyroid gland (but don't confuse it with thyroid hormone). The medullary cells are in the structural matrix tissue of the thyroid gland, rather than in the follicles that make thyroid hormone. You may recall that the parathyroid glands are embedded in the thyroid gland and are also involved in calcium metabolism; the body may have some reason for keeping these antagonizing cells in close proximity. I say "antagonizing" because calcitonin does the opposite of what parathyroid hormone (PTH) does: While PTH leaches calcium out of bone, calcitonin puts it back in. While PTH can raise your blood calcium level, calcitonin can lower it. While PTH can cause bone loss and osteoporosis, calcitonin can strengthen bone and help heal fractures.

Therapeutic indications and usage

There aren't too many reasons for using calcitonin. The most common reason—perhaps the only reason—for deficiency is surgical removal of the entire thyroid gland. I have a few dozen such patients in my practice but have needed to put only a couple of them on calcitonin for chronic hypocalcemia, so it still isn't common to need calcitonin even in this population. That's good, because the stuff is very expensive.

The reasons to consider using calcitonin therapeutically are osteoporosis, other evidence of accelerated bone loss, bone fractures such as vertebral compression fractures, and calcitonin deficiency with related symptoms, such as fatigue and bone aches. Calcitonin, which is available only by prescription, comes in either nasal spray or injected forms, and you usually cannot use it if you're allergic to salmon.

Thyroid

A great many books have been written on thyroid problems and thyroid deficiency, and I have hundreds of patients on thyroid replacement. I will try to cover what I think are the most important aspects of thyroid disease or deficiency—at least enough for you to identify whether you or your loved ones have reason to get a thyroid evaluation or to manage it in a different way. If you want to know more about this topic, head to the bookstore or find a good integrative provider.

Thyroid hormones and their actions

"Thyroid hormone" is really a small group of small peptide (meaning that they are made from a short string of amino acids) hormones with the same amino acid structure and varying numbers and positions of iodine atoms attached. (Iodine is necessary for the production of thyroid hormone if you recall from earlier.) These hormones are all produced by the thyroid gland, which is situated low in the front of the neck, just above the collarbones, and is wrapped around the windpipe below the Adam's apple. You should not be able to feel a normal-sized thyroid gland if you probe with your fingers in that region, so don't worry if you can't find it.

The most abundant form of circulating thyroid hormone is T4, or *levothyroxine*; in humans, T4 comprises about 90 percent of the circulating thyroid hormone. T3, or *triiodothyronine*, the second most abundant, comprises about 9 percent of the circulating pool, but it is several times more potent in biological action than T4 is, so it is more important in terms of clinical effect (i.e., how you feel). T3 is derived primarily from T4 via the enzymatic removal of one iodine atom in the proper location.

There is also a T2 hormone, which has only two iodine atoms. T2's biological activity is poorly understood, so it is presumed to have none of significance. There must be a T1, but no one discusses it. I have seen

481

mention of aT7 as a possible lab value, which doesn't make sense to me unless it is comprised of a T4 and a T3 stuck together. Let's forget I even mentioned T7 for now. (Just watch: T7 will be all the rage next season.)

Besides T4 and T3, the other type of thyroid hormone I'm interested in is called *reverse* T3. It is here, among other places, that conventional medicine and I dramatically part ways on matters related to the thyroid. Most conventional doctors have never heard of reverse T3, and they wouldn't know what to do with the results if they ordered the test. There's a good chance that knowing about reverse T3 is important to you or someone you know.

Reverse T3 is created from T4 by removing a different iodine atom than that removed to create "normal" T3. It was thought that reverse T3 was some sort of anomaly or that it had no biological purpose because the hormone seems to cause no cellular effect when it binds to the thyroid hormone receptor. However, that's precisely the problem: it binds to the receptor and then does nothing but act as a thyroid blocker, preventing the normal thyroid hormones from binding to the receptor and getting things done. It's a thyroid obstructionist.

So why do we have it? There's usually a purpose for the molecules your body produces. It is my view that reverse T3 is supposed to prevent you from starving to death by lowering your metabolic rate in times of famine so you don't burn your fuel too fast. Normal thyroid hormone activity turns on energy production and cellular activity in all of your cells, causing all sorts of things to happen and generating heat as a byproduct. Reverse T3 blocks that process, thereby slowing down your fuel consumption and preserving energy when needed. Studies have shown significant increases in reverse T3 fraction over time as an animal is deprived of food (Abdel-Fattah, 1991).

Individuals with elevated reverse T3 production are functionally hypothyroid and can suffer all the same symptoms and metabolic dysfunctions as a more "classically" hypothyroid person, even when their commonly tested thyroid labs appear to be normal. Elevated levels of reverse T3, as evidenced by a lowered T3/reverse T3 ratio, are associated with poorer surgical outcomes and decreased survival in critical care situations. This has been known since at least the mid-1980's (Calvey, 1986; Peeters, 2005), but most practitioners today are still not aware of reverse T3 and do not appreciate its clinical usefulness.

When there is little food around and your mineral levels, particularly zinc and selenium it seems, decrease, the enzyme activity that affects thyroid conversion switches to decrease your normal T3 production and increase the reverse T3 so your metabolism slows down. The presence of this little bit of biochemistry has likely saved many lives throughout history. In our culture the vast majority of us aren't starving. If you're not starving, why should this information matter? I'll answer that below.

Signs and Symptoms of thyroid deficiency

Hypothyroid symptoms can occur directly from the absence of enough thyroid hormone, but other symptoms can occur when other hormone systems try to overcompensate and in various organ systems because of long-term tissue dysfunction or changes related to prolonged deficiency. This can make the clinical symptoms of thyroid deficiency very diverse, and confusing to many.

The most common symptoms involve the immediate lack of cellular energy production: generalized fatigue and sluggishness, muscle weakness or a feeling of heaviness, and mental suppression manifesting as poor attention, memory impairment, poor cognitive function, depression and low mood, and eventually coma may result in extreme cases. The lack of energy in the heart can cause a low pulse rate, but other stimuli can bring the heart rate up above normal in spite of hypothyroidism. Low energy in nerve tissues can lead to symptoms of numbness, tingling, electrical shocks, or twitches in your limbs. Low energy in the muscles and other peripheral tissues can lead to painful muscle cramps and widespread pain felt in the muscles, joints, or skin. Patients with these symptoms are frequently diagnosed with "fibromyalgia"; this diagnosis enables their doctors to forever ignore their complaints or just tell them they are depressed, which is neither helpful nor correct.

The three most common overall complaints are fatigue, mental suppression, and pain without apparent cause, but you don't have to have any of those symptoms to have hypothyroidism. Some people with very low thyroid levels have no major complaints at all, which likely has to do with the level of sensitivity to thyroid hormone and many other factors. After all, we are very complicated organisms.

Some other common primary complaints of those with thyroid deficiency are intolerance to cold, hair loss (from the head, diffusely); constipation; dry skin, particularly thick, dry, cracking skin at the heels; insomnia, despite being very tired; heart palpitations, usually when lying down at night; ADD symptoms; hyperactivity in kids; recurring infections like bronchitis, sinusitis, sore throats, and pneumonia; allergies of any kind;

acid reflux and heartburn; plantar fasciitis (chronic heel and foot pain); carpal tunnel syndrome; and many others. At one point in my practice, I put almost everyone on a little thyroid replacement just to see which symptoms would improve. I took some myself and gave some to each of my three oldest children, as an experiment, around that time as well.

Common clinical "signs," meaning they are objectively visible or perceivable, as opposed to "symptoms," which are purely subjective statements from the patient, of hypothyroidism are dry hair and skin; a thickened tongue, perhaps with scalloped sides; a slow Achilles tendon reflex; a generally heavy and sluggish look all around; and changes in the skin and subcutaneous tissues called myxedema. Myxedema occurs in hypothyroidism because the cells don't have the energy to dispose of their cellular waste properly. It's like your house filling up with trash because you don't have the energy to walk it out to the curb; over time, you add more rooms to the house in order to store the mounting garbage. How this usually displays in humans is what looks like fat but is really thickened skin. It usually begins at the upper arms and shoulder areas, later spreading to the ankles, face and neck and eventually everywhere.

You can identify myxedema by trying to pinch and lift the skin away from your lower shoulder/upper arm area. If you get a fold of skin that is only about ½ inch thick, you're likely normal or haven't manifested this sign (because everyone develops their own constellation of symptoms). If you can't even pinch and lift anything you very likely have had impaired thyroid function for some time. Then, of course, there's every possibility in between. If you don't have this particular symptom, it doesn't mean your thyroid function is normal, just as the absence of a goiter is not indicative of normal thyroid function.

A goiter is an enlarged thyroid gland; in some cases, there is visible swelling in the lower front area of the neck. You may have seen pictures of people with enormously swollen goiters that are due to total iodine deficiency in their region. In the United States, we get just enough trace iodine in our diets to prevent that extreme symptom. What most practitioners don't remember or weren't properly taught is that any thyroid gland you can even feel *at all* with your fingertips is too large and is technically a goiter. You may try to feel this on yourself, but it is difficult to feel your own thyroid because the angle of your fingers will be all wrong.

It's better to have someone stand behind you and place his or her fingertips on the sides of your trachea, down between the Adam's apple and collarbones. If the person presses in gently and can feel all the cartilage rings on both sides within that stretch of windpipe, your thyroid is likely of normal size. If instead the person feels smooth tissue adherent to the trachea (it might be soft and mushy, firm and smooth, hard or lumpy), there is likely abnormal enlargement of the thyroid or the nodules within it. If you swallow while the person's fingers are in place, he or she may feel your thyroid move up and down, confirming its identity, as it moves with the trachea.

If your thyroid is big and lumpy or too small to feel, it may still be working adequately or not working at all. It's size and texture have absolutely nothing to do with how it is functioning at the moment. A goiter is its own separate issue to some extent, as it generally indicates either significant iodine deficiency or an autoimmune process. Unfortunately, taking iodine may not shrink it to normal, and adding thyroid hormone may not either. It is important to have someone feel your thyroid to look for thyroid cancer, one of our most rapidly increasing cancers in recent decades. If a distinct lump is found on one side, you should have an ultrasound and then a needle biopsy if the nodule looks suspicious. A nodule larger than one centimeter in size with internal blood flow should be biopsied, unless perhaps there are a whole bunch of them.

Diagnosing hypothyroidism

As with every other aspect of medicine, the most important part of diagnosis is what the patient tells you, the patient's "history." Our "history," of course, includes the present, and I can often identify hypothyroid patients by how hard they try to convince me that their present condition is poor. Hypothyroidism is one area in modern medicine where laboratory testing has been adopted as a standard over patient history, physical findings, and overall clinical evaluation, which I believe is to the detriment of most patients.

I don't know how many times I've had patients tell me that they looked up the symptoms of hypothyroidism online, found they had nearly all of them, presented them to their prior doctors (who agreed that they appeared to have classic hypothyroidism), then had a blood test that revealed that their thyroid hormone was within the reference range and were then told that they did not have hypothyroidism after all. Why aren't doctors taught how poorly those blood tests correlate with the original means of diagnosis and the patients' response to treatment? Until the 1960s, hypothyroidism was identified by clinical history and physical examination, usually followed by either temperature testing or basic metabolic rate testing (BMR). BMR was used first, but it was difficult to do because the patient has to lie very still for a long time while they measure how much how much carbon dioxide comes out in the breath. It was later found that basal body temperature (BBT) was just as good as an indicator and far simpler (Barnes, 1976).

You can test yourselves for hypothyroidism to some degree at home with a simple thermometer (preferably a glass thermometer). Place it next to your bed and set your alarm for ten minutes earlier than usual. When you wake up, put the thermometer deep in your armpit and just lie still for ten minutes before reading it. (If you have a digital thermometer, put it under your arm for a minute before you turn it on so it can equilibrate with your body better.) Any temperature lower than 97.5° is potentially abnormal, and lower than 97.0° is definitely suggestive of thyroid impairment, in my opinion. Older cutoffs were 97.8° or so (Barnes, 1976), but I think that some modern factors, such as environmental toxins that impair metabolism and other hormonal deficiencies or imbalances, often lower our temperatures as well.

I still sometimes have patients check their BBTs, especially if they don't have insurance or money to cover $200-300 in blood tests. Labs are useful to help guide treatment, and their most important use, I believe, is to look for overdose in those taking thyroid hormone. The initial labs I always get are the TSH (which, in my opinion, should be below 1.0), free T3 (ideally between 350 and 440, or 3.5-4.4 depending on your lab; this one changes some with age, as teens and growing children need free T3 up to 600, or 6.0), and free T4 (ideally 1.2-1.8, for anyone).

If a patient has very typical symptoms, I may give him or her a trial of thyroid hormone replacement without doing any initial thyroid tests. Laboratory tests have not been proven to correlate with clinical diagnosis well, so I still consider clinical suspicion to be more important, as I was taught. If the patient responds well, this may confirm the diagnosis, but his or her *not* responding does not rule out the diagnosis. If a patient has relevant symptoms and their initial thyroid levels (T4 and T3) are in the lower half of the reference range (regardless of their TSH level), I often treat that person with thyroid hormone replacement and see how they respond.

Response to treatment is the best "test", in my opinion. If you give enough thyroid to someone who has low thyroid hormone, he or she will feel significant improvements, and someone who doesn't need it will usually feel symptoms of overdose. Unfortunately, there are factors that prevent effective response to thyroid replacement even in those who really need it, some will not feel symptoms of overdose, and some will feel overdosed even when they are still deficient. The factors that cause these problems include adrenal imbalance, nutritional deficiencies (iodine, selenium, zinc, vitamin D and vitamin C) allergies (gluten in particular), heavy metals and other toxins; and yeast overgrowth or sensitivity.

If a patient doesn't respond favorably to treatment, or if he or she seems to have toxicity issues and multiple kinds of dysfunction at baseline, I check a *total* T3, which includes the "free" T3 plus that which is bound to protein in the blood, and *reverse* T3, which comes only in a "total" form, driving the need to measure total T3 for comparison. I then calculate a ratio of normal T3 to reverse T3, making sure to convert the units to the same kind. If the ratio is less than 10, nutrient deficiency or toxicity may be barriers to success. It is important to note here that anyone taking synthetic T4 products, such as levothyroxine, will likely have elevated reverse T3 and a low ratio; this may also be seen to some extent in patients who are fasting and haven't eaten in ten hours or more.

Monitoring patients on therapy should involve periodic blood testing to rule out overdose, for which the blood tests are the most useful. Overdose of thyroid may be evidenced by elevated free T4 or free T3 levels. A low thyroid stimulating hormone (TSH) does not by itself indicate overdose; many of my patients have been seen by other providers or in the ER where they had a TSH that was very low. They were told they were toxic on their thyroid replacement and should cut their dose way down or even stop it. These patients have seldom had T4 and T3 levels checked at the same time, but even if they were checked and were normal, the doctor often told them they are "overdosed" simply because of the suppressed TSH. This is a major flaw in our standard conventional training regarding thyroid supplementation and management, in my opinion.

A low TSH by itself does *not* satisfy the definition of hyperthyroidism. The problem is that the TSH is what we are all taught to use in assessment of thyroid status, but it is not produced by the thyroid gland and is not a direct indicator of thyroid function. It is an indirect indicator of thyroid function, but has a number of variables that may make it unreliable in terms of understanding the overall thyroid metabolism of a given individual. If a patient gets more thyroid hormone than his or her pituitary gland "thinks" he or she needs, the TSH will go down below our usual parameters. But, if this person's brain had things figured out correctly in the first place, perhaps the person wouldn't be in their current state of functional thyroid deficiency. You have to give many people more thyroid hormone than their pituitary glands think they need in order to correct their thyroid deficiency symptoms. As long as their actual thyroid hormone levels (T3 and T4) are not high, they are *not overdosed*! Several of my patients have had below-range thyroid hormone levels *and* a low TSH; by conventional standards of just checking the TSH, they were *hyper*thyroid when, in fact, they were actually *hypo*thyroid.

Another common test, which I never use myself, is an iodine uptake scan. Which is done by giving the patient a small amount of radioactive iodine and then scanning the thyroid gland to see how much radioactivity it is giving off. In my opinion, this test is usually interpreted backward: if the reading is high, the report will state that the patient has high thyroid output, when the test is really measuring "uptake," which is a completely separate idea. A high uptake is diagnosed as hyperthyroidism, but what it really indicates most of the time is iodine deficiency. If the thyroid gland is starved for iodine, it will soak up a much greater amount of the dose taken. This result does not necessarily mean the gland is putting out excessive amounts of thyroid hormone; that is assessed easily and more accurately with simple blood or urine tests for T4 and T3.

In addition, I just don't like the idea of putting radioactive iodine into the body since doing so could, at least theoretically, increase the risk of thyroid, breast, and other cancers. No study of which I am aware has shown such a connection, but there are long-standing recommendations to give everyone near a nuclear accident or blast a load of iodine (the non-radioactive variety) in order to saturate their thyroid gland and decrease the chances of the gland's absorbing radioactivity. This is to prevent them developing thyroid cancer in the future. Why should we intentionally inject people with radioactive iodine if there are other options?

Causes of hypothyroidism

There are some common, long-standing causes or contributors, as well as some more modern ones, to the high numbers of hypothyroid people in our culture. A major and still under-appreciated factor is iodine deficiency. Common contributors to the iodine problem are the environmental toxins that displace iodine from the body, such as bromine (from breads and other flour products, hot tubs, medications) and fluoride (medications, water, processed beverages). Those toxic halides are smaller than iodine atoms, and therefore displace iodine from its usual binding sites. Iodine deficiency results in the inability to produce adequate thyroid hormone.

Autoimmune attack on the thyroid gland is considered the most common cause of hypothyroidism in the United States, but iodine deficiency may be a bigger factor. Autoimmune thyroiditis (inflammation and resulting destruction of the gland) can be in the common form called Hashimoto's thyroiditis (diagnosed by biopsy or elevated anti-TPO antibodies in blood), Grave's disease (which causes hyperactive thyroid first and is usually treated with thyroid gland destruction), or less common forms of thyroiditis.

Gluten (a protein from wheat, barley, rye, malt, and other grains) is thought by many to be the primary trigger for autoimmune attack on the thyroid gland. I recommend that everyone with diagnosed (or suspected) immune reaction to thyroid stop eating any foods that contain gluten. Doing so may enable some people to recover thyroid function and get off their thyroid replacement if the gland hasn't been totally ruined.

When the thyroid hormone is somehow blocked from binding to its cellular receptor, or the thyroid receptors themselves are not functioning properly, clinical hypothyroidism will result, but blood tests will be normal. Dr. Mark Starr refers to this condition as "Type 2 Hypothyroidism" (Starr, 2005), similarly to how we describe insulin-resistant physiology as "Type 2 Diabetes". In addition to reverse T3, what typically interfere with thyroid receptor functions are environmental toxins like heavy metals, pesticides, plasticizers and flame retardant chemicals. We virtually *all* have at least trace amounts of these toxins in us today.

Adrenal gland deficiency causes symptoms of hypothyroidism without the person's being hypothyroid at all. We need adequate circulating cortisol, the main adrenal hormone of concern here, in order for our cells to express the thyroid hormone receptor. If we have adrenal deficiency, our normal levels of thyroid hormone are not "sensed" by the cells, and we will have all the relevant symptoms. The treatment here lies in identifying the adrenals as the real cause, and addressing that deficiency. I get a clue that this problem is present if I have to give a patient an excessive amount of thyroid hormone before they can feel any change at all, or if they have a high T3 level but relatively low T4 level.

The factors that seem to increase reverse T3 production include heavy metals like lead and mercury and probably other toxins as well. Deficiency of zinc, selenium, and possibly other trace may be a factor as well, but this is easier to correct than the presence of heavy metals.

Of course, many of my patients are hypothyroid because of well-meaning doctors who either surgically removed the gland due to goiter or suspected cancer or destroyed it with radioactive iodine because of Grave's disease or other thyrotoxic states. In my opinion, many of these extreme treatments were not necessary and may have been avoided with proper nutrient replacement, detoxification, and thyroid replacement therapy. Of course, some of the cases were too advanced to correct in that manner, but by the time I get them, it no longer matters.

Some patients have had the thyroid gland removed because of cancer, which is well justified of course. If it's possible to remove just half the gland, it will be easier to get the patient back in proper balance than if they have no thyroid hormone production of their own at all. The patient is also less likely to have to contend with calcium-management issues related to calcitonin and/or parathyroid hormone deficiencies. We try to get our local surgeons to just remove the half with the cancer, rather than the entire thyroid gland, as often as possible.

Treating hypothyroidism without thyroid hormone replacement

Even though I have hundreds of patients on thyroid hormone replacement, I will certainly tell you that it is probably better to try to correct hypothyroidism by other means. Of course, other means are not options if you don't have a thyroid gland, and many cases of hypothyroidism may not be correctible without thyroid replacement even if the gland is intact. Still, it's worth a shot to try to correct thyroid production through iodine replacement, detoxification, energy medicine, and diet, including adequate protein intake and relevant vitamin and mineral replacement.

A typical adult nutrient regimen is iodine (as a mixed iodine/potassium iodide formulation, not just potassium iodide alone) 25-50mg per day, vitamin C 2,000-3,000mg (many can't absorb and assimilate the iodine without it), vitamin D 10,000iu per day typically, zinc 25-50mg per day, selenium 200-400mcg per day, and possibly some magnesium and fish oil thrown in for good measure. Protein intake is important because the core molecule in thyroid hormone is the amino acid tyrosine. About ten percent of patients may recover their own thyroid function on this sort of regimen within about a year, in my experience.

Glandular extracts or homeopathic agents can sometimes help patients who still have a partially functioning thyroid gland. These extracts are likely acting as a form of energy medicine taken orally that guides the body to respond more appropriately to the thyroid hormone that is present. Acupuncture, craniosacral therapy, Reiki, healing touch, bioenergetic devices, kundalini yoga and other energy therapies may also work well.

Dietary modification is often critical to success. In most cases, gluten elimination must be total for real success to occur because even a little bit here and there (like half a cracker once a month) may trigger the immune response, inflaming the thyroid. This issue is especially important for those with Hashimoto's or any form of thyroiditis. Other foods that have been shown to impair thyroid function include soy and broccoli. I don't think many people eat enough broccoli or any of the other foods on the list to cause them trouble. Some people may consume enough soy to block thyroid function, especially since it is in so many prepared foods these days, and some vegetarians depend heavily on soy foods as a source of protein. Of course, the amount that could cause problems is different for everyone.

Detoxification, a major topic, is discussed in the next chapter. Heavy metals and various chemical compounds are of concern to the thyroid and many other areas of your physiology and may be cleared by methods described later. Bromine and fluoride are problems somewhat more specific to the thyroid because they cause thyroid problems by displacing iodine. They are also likely to be a problem for estrogen-sensitive conditions, including breast cancer, because iodine aids estrogen conversion and metabolism.

Iodine replacement is the main way of ameliorating and eliminating the toxic halide problem. Elimination of toxic halide takes time because the toxic halides are smaller than iodine and bind better to the receptors than iodine does. Clearing these elements may be a long, slow process, and the patient may have to take large amounts of iodine for years to do it. Iodine replacement has been shown to eliminate fibrocystic breast disease (especially with the complete nutrient regimen listed above) and has also been associated with a very significant decrease in breast cancer rates among hypothyroid women (Derry, 2001).

Thyroid hormone replacement
If these measures don't work, you don't have the patience, or you want to feel better while you are detoxifying and working on your diet, you may want to use thyroid hormone replacement. Thyroid hormone preparations have been among the top selling prescription substances for more than a hundred years now. There is a long track record of use, experience and safety with these substances. For over 120 years we have used biological thyroid replacement products derived from mammalian thyroid glands. The commercial preparations are strictly pig-derived in the modern era, but cows and sheep were once used as sources as well. These sources may

have been discovered by accident when people who ate thyroid tissue from livestock or game experienced symptoms of thyroid overdose. A condition listed in old medical diagnosis coding books, called "hamburger thyrotoxicosis", was caused by eating ground beef that included high amounts of thyroid tissue.

Porcine (pig-derived) thyroid products on the market today include Armour Thyroid™, Westhroid™, and Nature-Throid™, as well as generic Thyroid-USP. These desiccated (dried) thyroid (DTH), products are all considered equivalent to one another by pharmacists, but about a third of our patients seem to prefer one brand over the others. If you use these products, consider trying them all to see which one you like best, since you never really know how you're "supposed" to feel. I usually start people at one-half or one grain (roughly 30-60mg) each morning and gradually increase their dose by 30mg per day every couple of weeks up to around 120 mg (two grains) or until they feel a definite response. At that point I usually check the basic labs (TSH, free T4, free T3) to see if they need a dose adjustment. Some may go a little higher if they made it to 120mg without noting improvement in their symptoms. There is a lot of trouble-shooting to be done with thyroid replacement, so it may not be this simple. As usual, find an experienced provider to help manage your care, and ask questions about how they plan to evaluate you. If it's just by checking a TSH level, find someone else.

Most conventional physicians and practitioners will put you on synthetic thyroid hormones rather than the biological ones. These were made first in the 1960s, many decades after biological thyroid products were implemented. Synthroid™, the brand name of the primary synthetic hormone used, is a synthetic T4 product. Cytomel™, a synthetic T3 product, is not used by many conventional providers. Generic T4 is called *levothyroxine*, and generic T3 is called *liothyronine*. It is possible to have a compounding pharmacy put them together for you into one pill if you like, and I have a small number of patients who feel best on this type of product.

The standard of care in conventional medical training is to use levothyroxine alone, starting at small doses and increasing perhaps monthly based on repeated blood tests more than patient response. If I do have to put someone on the synthetic hormone for some reason—pork allergy, religious exemption against pork, unavailability, or because the synthetics work better for them—I typically add some T3 to the T4 therapy in order to achieve proper balance. In some cases, all a person needs is a little supplemental T3 because he or she isn't converting his or her own T4 correctly; this may qualify as "Wilson's Thyroid Syndrome", if any are familiar with that term.

Most of the new patients I see who have been diagnosed as hypothyroid are on Synthroid™ or generic equivalents from previous providers. The synthetics were heavily marketed to physicians as "the latest and greatest" when they came out, and the practice has stuck. Most providers must not have read the available data on these products; if they had, they would know that the synthetics have poor results in terms of symptom relief compared with the DTH products. (See the research reviewed in Mark Starr, MD's *Hypothyroidism Type 2*.) Part of the problem is the egos of most humans; you often just have to suggest that "all the really smart doctors are using our product now" to get a prescriber on board.

Another part of the problem is that, by this time, physicians were using the TSH test to determine the effect of thyroid therapy, rather than patient symptoms. The synthetics may not correct symptoms very well, but they do bring the TSH down to normal. What you get as a result of most modern thyroid treatment now is cold, fat, tired, mentally foggy, achy people on an ineffective dose of synthetic T4, but with normal TSH levels to show for it. In all fairness, though, 20–25 percent of people will feel just fine on the synthetics; they are valuable tools, and a percentage of my patients prefer to use them instead of the DTH products.

The big problem with the synthetic products is that they don't fit well into our biological enzymes and hormone receptors. The synthetic *levo*-thyroxine is much more likely to be converted inappropriately to reverse T3 than the biologically identical thyroxine (biological T4) in DTH products. When I get a new patient on high doses of Synthroid™ or its equivalent who still has significant hypothyroid symptoms, I usually switch him or her laterally to a roughly equivalent dose of a DTH product instead. We then make adjustments as necessary, based on clinical response and follow-up lab testing.

Your ideal thyroid dose will change based on stress, activity, ambient temperature (i.e., the season), food intake, your state of nutrient replacement or detoxification, changes in body weight, pregnancy, menopause, other hormone replacement, and various other factors. It is important to pay attention to how you feel and to make small adjustments (within 30mg of DTH, 25mcg T4, or 5mcg T3 per day) up or down if you feel you need to do so based on symptoms and circumstances. For example, a significant proportion of my hypothyroid patients need 15-30mg more DTH daily from October through March or so in Alaska, presumably because they need to generate more body heat in the cold temperatures.

Symptoms of thyroid excess

Patients with Grave's disease, acute thyroiditis after an infection or during pregnancy, toxic goiter, or those who take too much prescribed thyroid hormone may experience symptoms similar to those of caffeine overdose, with which many Americans are familiar. These symptoms result primarily from excessive energy production or excitation of cells in the heart and nervous system.

Patients with thyroid excess may have rapid heart rate or palpitations (especially with exercise or even minor physical exertion), a fine trembling of the hands (holding the arms out straight and laying a piece of paper on top of the outstretched fingers is the most sensitive way to see it) or more intense tremors, agitated feelings or mood, anxiety, insomnia, and/ or diarrhea. I generally suggest to thyroid patients that they not drink much caffeine in order to avoid greater risk of these side effects. People with hyperthyroidism or thyroid overdose will often become very fatigued as well, similar to if they had low thyroid. Patients with Grave's disease may notice a distinctive gradual protrusion of their eyeballs from the sockets (exophthalmos), which unfortunately does not resolve after medical treatment such as radioactive iodine ablation, and requires surgery to correct.

Sometimes I suggest that patients slowly increase their thyroid dose until they start to feel some of these overdose symptoms, and then cut their dose back down to the previous slightly lower dose. I then check their labs to make sure they aren't still "subclinically" overdosed. It's one way to find what is probably the optimal dose for each person, and it teaches him or her what sort of symptoms to watch for in the future as he or she detoxifies and improves his or her nutritional status. Some patients will just feel tired and foggy again, without the other more typical signs of overdose. This is why it's important to stop at some reasonable level and check labs.

Diagnosing and treating hyperthyroidism

Diagnosing hyperthyroidism is much easier than diagnosing hypothyroidism, but treating it is often trickier unless it is caused by thyroid hormone overdose. Hyperthyroidism generally presents with at least some of the typical symptoms, a low TSH and elevated T4 and/ or T3 levels on blood tests. This is clear and straightforward for people who are not on any thyroid treatment, and are checking baseline labs for diagnosis.

For those who are on thyroid replacement, the timing of their test relative to taking their dose is critical. It is important to mention that if one is taking thyroid replacement and having blood levels tested, they should be sure *not* to take the thyroid product within six hours or so of testing, as the T4 and/or T3 levels from the blood test may be notably higher and erroneously suggest overdose. I advise having labs drawn in the late afternoon, after taking the thyroid replacement at least six hours prior. Alternatively, someone may do their labs first thing in the morning, about twenty-four hours after their prior dose, but those levels are not as meaningful in my opinion.

If I see someone with mildly elevated T3 or T4 who says he or she feels good on the current dose and doesn't want to cut it down, they do not have an elevated heart rate and exhibit no tremor, I run tests to look for evidence of excessive bone breakdown. I check their *deoxypyrodinoline* (Dpd) level in the first morning urine to look for excessive bone collagen turnover, which could lead to osteoporosis with prolonged thyroid overdose. Some labs do not run Dpd levels, so either *N-telopeptide* (NTx) or *C-telopeptide* (CTx) may be used instead. If these tests are not elevated, the patient may have high peripheral thyroid resistance and need to stay on the high-range dose, at least initially, in order to have appropriate clinical response. This will change over time in most cases, so there should be continued monitoring.

The situation is more difficult if someone has full-blown Grave's disease or another internal cause of hyperthyroidism. Most of these patients may be corrected over time with measures like the nutrient replacement for hypothyroidism; in this case, however, it is important to hold off on the iodine at first, load with the higher dose of selenium (400mcg per day), zinc (50mg per day), vitamin C (3-4 grams per day) for a while, and also take lots of magnesium with the regimen. I suggest phasing in the iodine perhaps in a couple months, starting at around 6mg per day, and working slowly up to 50mg daily at the most. Even though Grave's disease presents with thyroid excess, the condition may actually be related to iodine deficiency. (See Dr. David Brownstein's books on iodine and thyroid disorders.)

The problem can be imminently dangerous in some with hyperthyroidism, making this a much more difficult problem than thyroid deficiency. These patients may lose a lot of weight, stress their heart to the point of heart attack, developing arrhythmias or heart failure, suffer the eyeball protrusion problem, and have other serious issues. It may take months to correct the condition using nutrition or it may not work at all, and taking that kind of time to treat the condition may be unwise for some. Some patients should use medications that block or blunt the abnormal thyroid activity to get by safely while they correct underlying problems or pending more definitive therapy. These drugs include *methimazole* and *propylthiouracil* (PTU), which should be managed by an experienced practitioner.

The definitive conventional treatments for serious hyperthyroidism are surgery to remove the gland or destruction of the gland using radioactive iodine. I've already told you how I feel about using radioactive iodine, and this is a much bigger dose than what is used in testing thyroid uptake. I have also mentioned that it is often more difficult to treat those without a thyroid gland. Unfortunately, hyperthyroidism can be imminently dangerous and *should* be treated this drastically in some cases. This condition is worthy of a visit to the emergency room and an endocrinologist.

Final thoughts/summary on thyroid disorders

Thyroid problems, especially hypothyroid conditions, are very common and are often not properly diagnosed or treated. They occur many times more often in women than in men, probably because of the increased need for iodine in women as well as increased susceptibility to autoimmune disease. Therefore, I treat women who come in with mild relevant symptoms at a lower threshold than men with similar symptoms. Correcting thyroid problems is not a simple matter in many cases.

You may be able to improve your thyroid function with diet, nutrition, herbs, glandulars, homeopathics, detox, and other methods, or you may not. You can have labs checked on your own at local outpatient labs in many places, without a doctor's order. If your symptoms or blood tests aren't improving, seek out a good provider. If you have hyperthyroid symptoms, seek conventional medical help first to avoid disaster. Thyroid management is one area in which integrative doctors run into lot of trouble with their peers and state medical boards; in my opinion, it is worth the fight to provide what I see as the best care, but you may not find a provider in your area willing to see things your way on this one.

Cortisol

Adrenal deficiency is very common in our culture. The adrenal gland generates dozens of hormone metabolites, and we don't even know the function of many of them yet. The one to which we pay the most attention is cortisol, for which we can prescribe specific replacement with good results in most cases. Lifestyle, nutritional, energetic, and herbal interventions probably improve all those other adrenal hormones, so they comprise the mainstay of therapy, rather than just replacing cortisol.

Causes of adrenal dysfunction

The functions of the adrenal hormones include retaining salt and water in the body, producing energy on a cellular level, releasing sugar from the liver for use as energy, maintaining blood pressure, and stimulating the immune system. Hormones like cortisol and adrenaline (epinephrine) are key chemical intermediaries of the "fight or flight" response.

The most common cause of adrenal problems is related to the discrepancy between what our adrenals are designed for and what we do to them or how we use them in modern society. Our adrenals were designed for a life of sitting around quietly most of the day and performing mild, sustained exertion here and there or occasionally an intense burst of energy to settle a dispute, compete for a mate, run after dinner, or run away from a predator. Our lives are supposed to be 90 percent "down" time and 10 percent "go" time. However, today's American lifestyle does not fit that model.

We are seemingly designed to go to bed around 9:00 or 10:00 p.m. and get at least six hours of uninterrupted sleep. We are supposed to eat a nutrient-rich diet that provides all the myriad vitamins, minerals, and healthy fats we need to make hormones like cortisol and DHEA. We are also supposed to be happy and content with life the majority of the time, which keeps our adrenals set to "low" and doesn't put added demand on them from emotional and psychological stress.

However, the typical American lifestyle now involves a great deal of physiological and psychological stress. Just the commute to work is enough to meet the stress quota for the day in terms of adrenal output for some people. Throw in a boss you don't get along with, a job you don't like, an unhappy marriage, stress over what your kids are or aren't doing, the activities you must run your kids to after your work day, financial problems, and despair over your possible future, and your adrenals are in trouble just from psychological stress.

The standard American diet does not help since it is deficient in many of the essential nutrients used in making the adrenal hormones, and many of the nutrients that are ingested are diverted to other strained body processes like detoxification, neurotransmitter production, calming inflammation, and other issues common to our toxic existence. Eating sugar and highly processed foods increases the inflammatory response, putting more demands on our adrenals because cortisol is a vital anti-inflammatory. Sugar is also a strain on the adrenals because cortisol has to save us from the hypoglycemic crash we get after eating excessive amounts of sugar.

Caffeine and alcohol seem to be directly toxic to the adrenal glands. They not only deplete essential nutrients, they also interfere with normal adrenal function and create a special sort of dysfunction. Caffeine drives the adrenals artificially and then leaves them exhausted when the effect wears off; this is part of the development of caffeine dependence or addiction. Alcohol depresses adrenal function; it may calm you down and help you fall asleep initially, but then you are likely to wake up early in the morning or the middle of the night because of the resulting adrenal swings. Some people even break out in a sweat in the middle of the night because of this effect.

As if that weren't enough, any type of illness or disease tends to strain the adrenals and deplete reserves as well. Any inflammatory condition, such as allergy, asthma, arthritis, and chronic infection, speeds the decline in adrenal function and then worsens the inflammatory symptoms. Many environmental toxins, such as heavy metals and chemicals, are damaging to the adrenals as well.

Let's not forget doctors. We doctors have caused the dysfunction of many a person's adrenal system by prescribing high anti-inflammatory doses of prescription corticosteroids (a term that describes these drugs' similarity to the hormones derived from the adrenal cortex, such as cortisol, and separates them from sex steroids like estrogen and anabolic steroids like DHEA and testosterone). When prednisone and other synthetic corticosteroids were developed decades ago, they were thought to be the miracle cure for conditions like rheumatoid arthritis and other unrelenting inflammatory diseases, but the unacceptable side effects found later led to these drugs being used with much greater caution or not at all.

Your pituitary gland gets lazy when you take exogenous (from outside the body, like a pill or injection) steroids, and the signal (adrenocorticotropic hormone, or ACTH) the gland normally sends to your adrenals, triggering the release of cortisol and other hormones, is shut off via negative feedback regulation. When you stop the artificial steroids and your adrenals aren't getting the message to put out product like they should, you can have quite a crash. This is a very important phenomenon, and one fairly unique to adrenal steroid therapy. You don't see this type of dependence develop with supplementation of other hormones such as thyroid or the sex steroids.

Patients on corticosteroid therapy for more than a week or two may need to taper off slowly. Those on therapy for years or even months may never successfully get off steroid therapy. This is yet another example of why it is important to find the real cause of the illness and correct it, rather than covering up symptoms with potentially dangerous drug therapy.

Adrenal testing

A patient's adrenal steroid levels and ACTH level should be tested in most cases before deciding how they should be treated. The problem is that a patient with adrenal excess can look just like a person with adrenal deficiency and vice versa, partly because adrenal hormones interact in so many ways with so many other hormones and partly because of a U-shaped response curve with cortisol, called hormesis, wherein many of the same metabolic problems occur at both very low and very high ranges of adrenal output.

I usually do not try to just guess what someone's adrenals are doing from history and physical exam. I may offer a trial of therapy in some patients when I really think they are on the deficient side, giving them 5-10mg of oral hydrocortisone (prescription form of bio-identical cortisol) first thing in the morning so they can see if their symptoms improve (or perhaps worsen). This test works pretty well because the effects are usually seen within a few hours and are usually obvious. Adrenal problems can have almost all the same symptoms as thyroid problems, so I usually end up testing both.

There are various ways to test adrenal function because cortisol and other adrenal steroids can be measured in blood, saliva, and urine. The best overall assessment of daily production is a twenty-four-hour urine collection because you get a whole day's output, and cortisol levels cycle dramatically throughout each twenty-four-hour cycle. We have expected reference ranges for blood levels at various times of day, but our modern cycles are far too often royally screwed up, and a single blood sampling is just a snapshot in time with potentially misleading results. To make matters worse for the blood draw idea, cortisol, which is part of the immediate stress response, often rises to a "normal" level in a mildly deficient individual when he or she is approached with a needle.

My preferred test is a salivary panel with four collection times spaced throughout the day. This test not only shows production throughout the day, but it also provides a look at the cortisol "rhythm," which is just as important as production clinically. The four-part salivary cortisol is the only way to assess this pattern, unless one submits to multiple blood draws throughout the day, and sometimes the rhythm disturbance is the only problem.

Cortisol levels are supposed to be high in the morning, then taper off throughout the day, and then low at night. Many people I see with adrenal "dysregulation" problems will have low levels in the morning, with a flat line across the day; this makes that same absolute level "normal" in the afternoon and too high for nighttime normals. These patients will feel exhausted in the morning, may have adequate or low energy in the middle of the day, and then not be able to go to sleep at night. These people will have normal twenty-four hour urine cortisol totals. Several labs in the country offer this test, which is collected at home. Your practitioner may provide you with a test kit, or sometimes you can find one at a compounding pharmacy without a doctor's order.

Blood testing is useful to rule out extremes of deficiency or excess. One useful method for determining critical or severe adrenal deficiency is the ACTH stimulation test. In this test, the patient is injected with a sample of the hormone signal from the pituitary (usually a synthetic analog, called Cortrosyn™), which tells the adrenals to crank out more cortisol. Blood cortisol levels are drawn before and after the injection to determine whether the level rises by a sufficient proportion (it is expected to rise by 50-100% by about an hour after the injection); if it does not, the patient's adrenal glands are not working properly. This test has to be performed in a doctor's office or hospital, and it isn't done very often.

Symptoms of adrenal deficiency

The most common symptom of adrenal deficiency is fatigue. While fatigue is a common symptom of many conditions, the pattern and quality of fatigue can be different in different conditions. Most with hypothyroidism have fatigue starting as soon as they get up, but may get a bit better through the day, and they may feel a bit invigorated if they do some kind of physical activity. Those with adrenal deficiency, on the other hand, usually feel better when they first get up and then become exhausted when they try to do anything active because they don't have the cortisol reserves to support physical activity.

Of course, there is a great deal of overlap here, and I do not try to diagnose people just by their pattern of fatigue. Thyroid hormone and cortisol depend upon one other to work in the body, so a deficiency of one may look much like a deficiency of the other. I frequently test both hormone systems in patients with fatigue complaints because they are frequently both deficient in our culture.

People with significant adrenal deficiency also complain of mental suppression and trouble concentrating, finding words, and remembering things. They often feel anxious or depressed and can't go to sleep at night even though they were exhausted all day. These individuals' four-part cortisol levels often show low-range levels all day and then above-range at bedtime because the normal range falls very low at bedtime, and it's the only time their production is able to exceed expectations.

Since cortisol is responsible for keeping salt and water in the body, those with low cortisol may complain of thirst, salt cravings, frequent urination, and water passing right through them when they drink it; they may suspect diabetes because of this. They may also crave sugar because cortisol normally provides sugar release from liver between meals. They are prone to hypoglycemia because of this, which causes shaking, sweating, heart palpitations, hunger, and anxiety when they go too long between meals, or perhaps occurring an hour or so after eating excess sugar.

The immune system is often weak in those with adrenal deficiency, and they may have frequent illnesses, such as sore throats and bronchitis, or they may never seem to get sick at all. The latter instance occurs because we need a functioning immune system to mount the typical symptoms of the common cold or flu; symptoms such as fever, runny nose, sore throat, and cough, are caused by our immune systems rather than the viruses themselves. These people often get "their first cold in years" after we put them on adrenal support or replacement; if I haven't counseled them that this is a good sign, they may feel I have made them sicker rather than better!

Any sort of inflammatory problem may be worse in those with adrenal deficiency because it is the body's most important natural anti-inflammatory force. Arthritis pain will be worse, allergies will be more noticeable and numerous, rashes will flare more, and pain may seem out of proportion to injury. Just think of all the medical conditions we treat with "steroids" (which usually refers to corticosteroids, rather than anabolic steroids like testosterone); those conditions may all be worse in the face of internal cortisol deficiency.

Some with low adrenal production have chronically low-range blood pressure, below 100/60 or so. If that is present in someone who is not an athlete or on medications that lower blood pressure, I may suspect adrenal deficiency Blood pressure is not a reliable marker overall because some people with chronically low cortisol have excessive adrenaline production in an attempt to compensate. These individuals may have normal or even high blood pressure in spite of their low cortisol, and they may have constant anxiety rather than depression, frequent heart palpitations, and trouble sleeping. Those without the reflexive adrenaline production are more apt to feel depressed and tired and may sleep excessively. There are many other factors that affect blood pressure as well, so a normal or high blood pressure certainly does not rule-out relative adrenal deficiency.

Some patients with low cortisol lose weight and muscle mass, while others will gain weight and put on extra belly fat. We are more used to those with high cortisol putting on belly fat, which I discuss below, so it makes it difficult to determine who is high and who is low in cortisol production based on this factor as well. Again, it is very difficult to determine adrenal status based on the clinical picture alone; I often resort to testing.

A number of books address adrenal deficiency or thyroid and adrenal problems. You may still not get it right, no matter how educated the guess, and you may just need a simple saliva or urine test to have your answer. If you suspect you have adrenal deficiency, have it checked in some manner.

Treatment of adrenal deficiency

The ideal treatment is to get the adrenal glands functioning better on their own if that's at all possible. This may not be possible because of autoimmune destruction (Addison's disease) or some other drastic condition, in which case we have to use hormone replacement with prescription corticosteroids. In most cases, however, the most important long-term solutions lie in lifestyle changes and nutritional and herbal supplements to support normal healthy adrenal function.

Excessive stress is bad for our adrenals, so reducing stress is particularly important. This may mean changing jobs in order to work less, drive a shorter distance, have a safer work environment, enjoy work more, or have better job satisfaction. It may mean finding a new partner, going to marriage counseling, or even getting a divorce (especially for those who are being mentally or physically abused). It can be very helpful for some to do mind/body/spirit exercises like yoga, qi gong, tai chi, meditation, or prayer.

Getting adequate sleep is very important, which leads into the importance of eliminating caffeine and alcohol, substances that put tremendous strain on your adrenals. You owe it to yourself to try eliminating caffeine and alcohol if you want to be healthier. You may feel that you "need" the caffeine to get moving or keep moving, but that is false energy that wrecks your adrenals. You may believe your coffee, tea or soda is keeping you going, but it's probably oppressing you to some extent. I have the hardest time getting people off coffee because they just won't believe it is a problem for them, until perhaps they get a headache when they try to stop it (a clue that they have a chemical addiction). Those dark circles under your eyes may vanish after a couple weeks off caffeine, saving you money on under-eye makeup (which my wife calls "fake awake").

Be sure to also watch out for caffeine in pills, beverages and other over-the-counter products that claim to give you energy. The caffeine or other stimulants (e.g., ephedra, ma huang, guarana, orange peel extract) in some of these products can affect your adrenals negatively. Short-term use of caffeine on an intermittent basis may work out just fine, and maintain its effectiveness without becoming an addiction or dependence. Many caffeine users drink some every day however, and become heavily dependent upon it for even normal daily function.

Alcohol, as mentioned earlier in the book, interferes with your sleep pattern and adrenal function. You may feel you can't fall asleep without a drink, but alcohol causes abnormal sleep rhythms in the brain with midnight and early-morning arousal, and deranges your adrenal function far worse than if you had just taken longer to fall asleep. Alcohol used for sleep can become a vicious, self-perpetuating cycle just like caffeine use to get up and going. Within a couple weeks, you will feel better off alcohol, and after you're healthy, you can probably go back to having a social drink now and then.

Sugar, another adverse part of the diet, has to go if you want your adrenals to work for you again. Eating sugar or processed carbohydrates (e.g., bread, pasta, crackers, baked goods made from white flour) spikes your blood sugar and then your insulin and then crashes your blood sugar. When your blood sugar crashes, your adrenals have to churn out cortisol in order to release more glucose from the liver to bring your blood sugar back up and prevent seizure or death. If your cortisol production is weak, your adrenals substitute epinephrine (adrenaline), which makes your heart pound and causes you to shake and sweat. Most people have felt this, either

503

due to eating sugar and crashing later or going too long without eating. It doesn't feel good, does it?

Eating only complex carbohydrates (nuts, beans, vegetables, starchy fruits, and limited whole grains) and ensuring you have some protein with every meal or snack balances your blood sugar and keeps the stress off your adrenals. Eating healthful, whole foods rather than processed foods is also more likely to provide the nutrients you need to support proper adrenal function. Be sure to limit liquid sources of sugar, such as juices, milk or milk substitutes, sodas, energy drinks, and sports drinks. Liquids with sugar absorb even faster and crash your blood sugar even harder than eating foods with high sugar.

This brings me to artificial sweeteners. You may think that switching to "diet" forms of sodas, soft drinks, juice, and energy drinks is a good choice, but it is not helpful at all. Products with artificial sweeteners like aspartame, acesulfame potassium, sucralose, and saccharin or even natural sweeteners like xylitol and sorbitol spike your blood insulin levels and cause a crash of your blood sugar also, because just having the sweet taste in your mouth causes insulin release from the pancreas and a resulting drop in blood sugar. This crash may be even worse because there isn't any real sugar in what you consumed, and intense hunger may then ensue along with a craving for carbohydrates.

Artificial sweeteners become neurotoxic chemicals after digestion, and some people can develop physiological addictions to them (Patel, 2008). It is a good idea to stop consuming them completely. For heavy consumers, doing so may be just as difficult for many people as getting off caffeine, alcohol, or real sugar because of how these substances affect brain. I've seen people go through nasty withdrawals from their artificial sweetener habits, so be strong!

Nutritional support is important in the function of your adrenals. Cortisol itself is made from cholesterol, so getting healthy fats in your diet is important. Sources may include naturally produced eggs, butter, cheese, wild meats and fish. Grass-fed beef or bison are acceptable alternatives to wild game. B vitamins are needed to improve the function of the enzymes that manufacture the hormones, as is vitamin A. You can get B vitamins from brewer's yeast or in a B complex vitamin (B-50 or B-100 strength) and vitamin A from pasture-fed butter, cod liver oil, or a supplement (5,000iu to 10,000iu daily).

B-12, which is particularly important, requires eating meat sources and using a good sublingual supplement or possibly a course of B-12 shots to start. Vitamin B-5 (pantothenic acid) is also very important for adrenal function, and it improves many fatigue syndromes. The best "food" source of B-5 is royal jelly, which may be obtained from health food stores. You should get at least 1,000mcg B-12 and 500mg B-5 daily.

Vitamin C, which is present at very high concentrations in the adrenals, plays an important role in adrenal function. Make sure you get at least 2,000mg daily when you're trying to revive your adrenal glands. The mineral chromium is also found largely in the adrenal glands and is very important for regulating blood sugar levels (as a key part of "glucose tolerance factor"); you can get it by itself or in a multi-mineral product with other important nutrients (zinc, copper, magnesium, manganese, selenium). Be sure to get at least 200mcg chromium daily, and it may be better to go up to 2,000mcg at first.

Several herbs show promise in improving adrenal problems. Licorice is one specific to *low* cortisol conditions (and is not to be used in those with possible adrenal excess) because it blocks the degradation of cortisol, thereby maintaining higher levels. Other herbs act more directly on the adrenal glands themselves to optimize adrenal output and regulate function. We term some of these "adaptogenic" herbs because they seem to lift your adrenal function up if you need more or hold it down a bit if you're producing excess cortisol. In short, they help you adapt to adrenal stress and help correct dysfunction. Adaptogenic herbs include *rhodiola*, *ginseng* (American, Korean, or Chinese), *eleutherococcus* (Siberian ginseng), *cordyceps* (mushrooms), *schisandra* and *ashwaganda*.

One particular product from Europe, which contains a mixture of rhodiola, eleutherococcus and schisandra, has been demonstrated to significantly improve attention, speed and accuracy during stressful cognitive tasks in human volunteers as compared to placebo (Aslanyan, 2010). You can find various other herbal combination products that include these herbs, but avoid any with licorice unless you have been tested to verify your cortisol is low rather than high. Bee pollen and royal jelly are helpful as well. I find all these supplements particularly useful for people who work night shifts or who have other causes of chronic sleep deprivation (e.g., infants at home, medical residency).

If the lifestyle changes, nutritional support and herbal supplements are not sufficient to improving symptoms, I move to pharmacologic replacement or support for patients with proven low cortisol. Of course, I implement this treatment early on in those with severe symptoms of deficiency so they feel and function better while working on their lifestyles and diets.

It is very important to pay attention to lifestyle and diet for long-term health, rather than relying on supplemental cortisol. Elimination of any food allergens from the diet, particularly gluten, is extremely important for many as well.

Cortisol itself can be made into pills at a compounding pharmacy, and some people prefer a long-acting or sustained-release form produced in this manner. Prescription hydrocortisone pills may be obtained from any standard pharmacy. Hydrocortisone, which is generally cheaper and more likely to be covered by insurance, is bio-identical cortisol and no different from compounded cortisol except that it does not come in a sustained-release form. Dr. William Jeffries' comprehensive text, *Safe Uses of Cortisol*, demonstrated that the vast majority of people can use up to 20mg cortisol or hydrocortisone daily without shutting off their own adrenal function, so one should try to stay within that range (Jeffries, 1996).

You want to front-load cortisol replacement first thing in the morning, when your body would naturally be at its highest levels. Keep it by the bed and take it before you get up if you wish; this may help you get out of bed if that is a struggle. You may try a single dose of sustained-release cortisol first thing in the morning or take hydrocortisone 5-10mg first thing upon waking and a second, equal or smaller dose around noon. There are also synthetic corticosteroids, such as prednisone and Medrol™ (methylprednisolone), that are dosed once per day and that may work better for some individuals. You shouldn't exceed 4mg of Medrol™ or 2-3mg Prednisone in this setting of mild adrenal insufficiency; greater doses may suppress one's own adrenal function.

Some people use topical cortisol preparations, which must be obtained through a compounding pharmacy, which may work because the hormone is lipid-soluble so it will absorb through the skin. It may be difficult to find the proper dose because of the variability in skin absorption between individuals, and the topical version is likely to cost more than oral forms. I'm not sure why anyone would prefer this route unless they just hate taking pills or can't swallow. Follow the directions on the label to stay within the safe maximum dose for topical cortisol.

Those with severe adrenal failure who fail the ACTH stimulation test, such as in Addison's disease, should work with an endocrinologist or other experienced physician to determine an optimal corticosteroid replacement regimen. They will need to use steroid replacement for cortisol and possibly something to replace other hormones more associated with retaining salt and water (i.e., Florinef™). Patients with this severe degree of adrenal deficiency should wear a medical identification bracelet and understand how to dose higher levels of steroid when they are ill or under excessive stress.

Symptoms of adrenal excess

You may see symptoms of adrenal excess if you are taking a product with licorice or adrenal steroids you don't need, if you have a tumor in your pituitary gland or adrenals that is producing excessive corticosteroids (i.e., Cushing's syndrome, which is not very common), or if you have excessive ongoing stressors in your life and you still have enough reserve adrenal function to run high corticosteroid levels. This can be seen in those who haven't decompensated into adrenal burnout yet (which is the most common scenario eventually).

The symptoms of adrenal excess may be very similar to those of adrenal deficiency, especially in milder cases. People may gain weight around the belly, as they may also do in adrenal deficiency. Those with Cushing's classically get very large bellies with red-violet stretch marks on them, accumulate fat around the back of their necks and above the collar bones, and lose muscle mass in their buttocks and elsewhere. Those with adrenal excess may also lose weight at first because of psychological stress, and many will run high blood sugar levels, especially if they have diabetes.

Most people with high cortisol levels have elevated blood pressure above their usual, but it may not be clinically high. Some may feel anxious, while others may feel depressed or irritable, but there is often some sort of emotional disturbance and sense of unease. Sleep is often decreased, with trouble falling asleep or staying asleep or both. These people will be unhappy the majority of the time.

Some of the pertinent symptoms that may help differentiate those with low cortisol from those with high cortisol are the urinary and hypoglycemic symptoms. Those with high cortisol usually do not have frequent urination or the typical hypoglycemic symptoms because they tend to retain salt and water and run higher blood sugars. Those with adrenal excess also tend to have normal to high blood pressure, and almost never have low-range blood pressure.

Causes and treatment of adrenal excess

If you have severe symptoms suggestive of Cushing's syndrome, such as very high blood pressure, weight gain, acne, stretch marks and headaches you should be evaluated by a physician. Those with pituitary or adrenal tumors generally require surgery to remove the tumors. Many with these symptoms may have just been overdosed with prescription steroids for some inflammatory condition, such as rheumatoid arthritis, and the cure lies in stopping the steroids; although doing so may not be entirely possible in these situations.

The vast majority of people with elevated cortisol do not have severe problems, and their cortisol levels can be corrected with lifestyle and dietary changes. Just as with cortisol deficiency, the most important efforts are those that reduce stress, eliminate caffeine, sugar and alcohol, and ensure adequate sleep and a healthful diet. There is a continuum of adrenal function as it relates to stress and adverse influences: first the cortisol levels (and DHEA levels, which we will discuss shortly) go up, because the adrenals have plenty of reserves with which to respond; the body adapts to these changes just fine for a while; over time, the person will start to run out of nutrients and adrenal reserves, with the eventual depletion of cortisol and other adrenal products. The nutrients described for support of adrenal function help to prevent or delay the eventual burnout of one's adrenals; the adaptogenic herbs are helpful as well.

Some less common activities that may be helpful in reducing cortisol levels for some, especially those with high levels at night that prevent sleep, include drinking chamomile tea, which can reduce cortisol levels slightly and which may improve relaxation and sleep. Phosphatidyl serine is a lipid from soy that can help directly lower cortisol levels in some people; get it from a health food or supplement store and take 200-500mg nightly. There are many "cortisol-controlling" combination products on the market, but many of these have licorice or other components that may actually raise adrenal production, so be careful.

Summary of adrenal problems

I spent a lot of time on the topic of adrenal problems because they are so common in our society and because the proper diagnosis can be difficult to make. The most important factor by far in treatment is lifestyle-related in the vast majority of cases. That means you can't expect your doctor or alternative practitioner to "fix" this for you, unless you have a tumor or complete adrenal failure. You generally have to fix it yourself.

It is much easier to prevent these adrenal imbalance problems through pursuit of a healthful lifestyle, diet, and regular moderate exercise. Once your adrenals are out of whack, it may take you more than a year to get them working right. If you have mild symptoms suggestive of adrenal imbalance, start addressing your diet and behavior right away.

However, if your symptoms are severe, see a conventional medical doctor, such as an endocrinologist, internal medicine physician, or family practitioner immediately to rule out life-threatening adrenal dysfunction. If you don't have an extreme case, most conventional providers have nothing to offer, so you may then need to work with a competent integrative practitioner (naturopaths are particularly good with adrenal problems) to get you back on track.

DHEA

DHEA stands for "dehydroepiandrosterone" (which is why people usually just say "DHEA"). DHEA is a steroid hormone that is produced by the adrenal gland but is not considered a corticosteroid because it is produced by cells deeper inside the adrenal gland (not in the outer "cortex") than those producing cortisol. It has primarily "androgenic" properties, which means it tends to promote typically masculine processes and features like muscle mass and strength, body hair growth, increased energy and sex drive.

Both men and women need DHEA, and it plays a key role in physical development in children, especially early in puberty. It is responsible for the development of pubic and armpit hair, body odor, and vertical growth (height) to some extent. It helps deepen the voice, strengthen the muscles and the resolve, increase the sex drive and mental alertness, and improve mood. People who are deficient in DHEA notice a decrease or loss of all of these factors, and those with excess DHEA, such as those with an adrenal tumor that produces DHEA, may notice increases in all these factors.

DHEA is often prescribed for depression, fatigue, low sexual function, weakness, or loss of muscle mass. DHEA is highly regarded as a useful tool in anti-aging; it is available over the counter because it is assumed to be generally safe, and many natural or alternative practitioners recommended it in comparatively large amounts for both men and women. Studies have shown that oral DHEA can prevent various types of cancer in test animals (Schwartz, 1986), but this effect has not been studied in humans to my knowledge (no articles to that effect in PubMed).

However, in my opinion, DHEA should not be available over the counter, and it should not be given to anyone unless they have been tested and shown to be truly deficient. DHEA is a precursor hormone for both testosterone and estrogen. If a woman takes DHEA, it may significantly increase her testosterone, and if a man takes DHEA, it may significantly increase his estrogen levels. Neither of those is a good scenario. DHEA is also converted to at least a dozen other metabolites, the function for some of which we don't even understand. Some of these downstream hormone metabolites appear to do wonderful things for the immune system, while others may cause more adverse effects; we just don't know yet.

DHEA might convert to the hormones you really want, but it is just as likely to convert to hormones you don't want. A woman may grow a beard or a man may see his breasts enlarge if they take too much DHEA. Excessive estrogen is a problem for both men and women, as I discuss later.

That said, I do recommend DHEA to people with symptoms of deficiency. I test them first to verify whether the deficiency is DHEA alone, testosterone is deficient, or both. DHEA levels can be tested with saliva, blood (which should test the "DHEA-sulfate" level, not plain DHEA), or a twenty-four-hour urine hormone profile. This last is perhaps the best because it shows a daily total and several of the metabolites. Saliva is the cheapest, but the results can be very inconsistent in my experience. Blood levels (of DHEA-sulfate) are consistent and the only test likely to be covered by insurance.

If a patient does have low DHEA, it is important to replace it because it performs some vital functions. You can use oral forms available over the counter, starting at 5-10mg daily for women and 15-25mg daily for men. Morning dosing is recommended. The most a woman should take is 25mg daily, and the most a man should take is 50mg, unless they are still relatively deficient upon repeat testing. Topical DHEA cream can be made through compounding pharmacies by prescription; some prefer this option, as topical forms bypass the liver and may avoid the conversion of DHEA to some of the other hormones. However, this may not be desirable after all because some of the metabolites appear to be beneficial. The topical form is also significantly more expensive than the oral form, making it a less attractive option.

Sometimes I use DHEA without testing when the patient has general adrenal deficiency and is on cortisol replacement. The adrenals make DHEA along with cortisol, so DHEA is often low after periods of intense stress (which is very common in those with PTSD) or other adrenal burnout conditions. I sometimes give patients a little DHEA without testing when I suspect adrenal deficiency. If you are taking cortisol replacement, you should probably also take some amount of DHEA because the signal from your pituitary (ACTH) may be depressed by the cortisol and result in lowered DHEA production via negative feedback loops. I still prefer to test people in this instance, but you can expect those on significant amounts of cortisol or synthetic corticosteroids to be deficient in DHEA.

My final words on DHEA are to be careful with it. Don't go out and buy some just because you read about it in an anti-aging or natural health publication. It is a tricky hormone to use and it's use should be monitored clinically by a trained provider.

Testosterone

Testosterone is probably my second-favorite hormone to prescribe and discuss—vitamin D, of course, being number one. Testosterone promotes healing, strength, energy, mental alertness, memory and focus, physical stamina, sex drive, increased sexual performance, improved mood and pleasure overall. It reduces the effects of aging on almost all tissues, and it promotes tissue maintenance and health of muscles, ligaments, tendons, and bones. Testosterone deficiency has become extremely common in American men; one recent review found that thirty percent of men aged forty to sixty-nine had significant testosterone deficiency (Traish, 2011).

Without adequate testosterone, men and women experience similar deficiency symptoms. In addition to the complaints noted above, they may develop medical problems like osteoporosis, anemia, poor wound healing or recovery from injury, more frequent illness and orthopedic problems like muscle or tendon tears, chronic low back pain, and generalized muscle weakness. Men with low testosterone have been shown to be much more prone to obesity, type 2 diabetes, cardiovascular disease, and have a higher risk of death in general (Cattabiani, 2012). Hypogonad men also appear to have a higher risk of prostate cancer in general, and greater risk for more aggressive prostate cancers (Raynaud, 2006).

Causes of testosterone deficiency

Testosterone deficiency has increased drastically in our society over the past several decades. Some estimates suggest average testosterone levels and sperm counts in thirty-to-forty-year-old men are only half what they used to be fifty years ago or so. My own experience supports this contention; even I had to start using testosterone replacement at age thirty-five after finding my own level to be low.

A study recently reviewed more than two thousand men over the age of forty-five found more than 38 percent had hypogonadism, which is the name for significantly low testosterone (Mulligan, 2006). Estimates reported in places such as *healthcommunities.com,* a physician-developed and monitored database, suggest there are roughly thirteen million men in the United States with hypogonadism and that less than ten percent have been diagnosed and are receiving treatment. These estimates are probably too low because I regularly find hypogonad males in their twenties and have even been diagnosing a growing number of later teenage males with symptomatically deficient testosterone. The problem is clearly getting worse for each generation; it may have an epigenetic component as well as an environmental toxicity influence.

Women don't seem to have problems with testosterone deficiency as often as men do, probably because their testosterone is made by converting DHEA from their adrenal glands, and perhaps that system is not as fragile as the testicular production in males. (This is just my theory.) That said; I certainly do find significant testosterone deficiency in women now and then.

More than 300 men in my practice—as of early 2012—are on testosterone replacement. Between myself and my physician's assistant, we start on average probably three new men on testosterone every week. Clearly, testosterone deficiency is a common problem, but conventional medical training does not teach doctors to manage it properly. In fact, my conventional medical training in optimal hormone replacement therapy was easily as lacking as the training in nutrition.

Men may have testosterone deficiency for reasons related to testicular damage or removal for cancer, trauma leading to removal, or torsion. Others were born with undescended testicles inside their abdomens; if they don't travel normally out into the scrotum, they often don't work right. Injury to the blood supply for the testicle during surgery, such as vasectomy or hernia repair, can also be a factor.

I personally think the most obvious and most prevalent cause of the apparent epidemic of hormone deficiency in men is environmental pollution. Men born after the 1940s have experienced an increasingly complex and toxic soup of chemicals. We are exposed to more than eighty thousand manmade chemicals in our environment, and a growing number of these chemicals have been found to disrupt hormone systems. Most of the men I've seen with hormone deficiency have no history of the more obvious causes such as testicular injury, this means their deficiencies are caused by some more obscure forces.

Narcotic pain medications deserve special mention here as a cause. The opiate (e.g., morphine, oxycodone, hydrocodone, codeine) painkillers appear to shut off the pituitary signals (LH, FSH) that normally stimulate testosterone production from the testicle. This effect may last long after the pain meds have been stopped, and could be permanent for some. Many men continue taking the medications, partly because their resulting testosterone deficiency worsens their pain. I have seen a number of women on chronic pain medications with low DHEA and testosterone as well, but I don't know if they have the same causal relationship because their testosterone is made from adrenal steroids, rather than testicles. I feel that all men who have been on narcotic pain relievers for more than a few months should be screened for low testosterone, even if their period of use was years prior since the body does not always rebound on its own.

Testosterone for men: Diagnosis

Symptoms of testosterone deficiency in men begin with the psychological manifestations. They often first start to lose interest in doing the "manly" activities they used to enjoy and look forward to, such as fishing, hunting, working on their cars, and riding dirt bikes, motorcycles, and snowmobiles. These activities begin to feel like too much effort because these men get tired more easily than they once did. They have a general feeling of unrest and discontent, which they may describe as depression or disinterest. They typically become irritable and angry more often, or they may become relatively passive and submissive.

Hypogonad men may feel like crying at times for no reason, but they will usually never tell anyone that (because they are men, and our culture frowns on that sort of thing). Men with low testosterone can slowly become pathetic shells of their former selves in terms of the psyche and personality. They may lose interest in sex and have erectile dysfunction at some point—every man who asks for Viagra™, Levitra™, or Cialis™ should have his testosterone checked—but that is often the last thing to go. Doctors who believe that a man with normal sexual function couldn't be hypogonad are sorely mistaken.

Physical decline manifests gradually, and most will just blame how they feel on "getting older". Men note that they aren't as strong as they once were, and they don't seem to be able to get much stronger even if they work out. They don't have the physical stamina they used to have, and they seem to get injuries, aches, and pains with what seems like minimal strain. They may develop spontaneous low back pain and other muscle or joint aches in the shoulders or other places that never seems to heal. They may lose some body hair, starting at the lateral lower leg. The ones who have been hypogonad for many years often have no hair on their legs at all and may exhibit small varicose veins or mild ankle swelling; these are signs of excessive estrogen influence relative to their testosterone. It's all about the balance.

Eventually, men with severe testosterone deficiency may develop anemia, osteoporosis, and easy fractures. There is growing evidence that hypogonad men are at greater risk for cardiovascular disease, obesity, neurological degeneration and dementia, certain types of cancer, and other age-related diseases than other men are. What we do not know yet is whether giving these men their testosterone back will decrease the occurrence of those medical problems and chronic disease issues.

Men often do not go to the doctor because they blame themselves for feeling tired and think they are being weak if they complain about it. We feel that we just need to work harder and put more effort into it, but we'll start next week or maybe after a nap. About 80 percent of the hypogonad men I see were either sent or physically dragged in by their spouses or girlfriends (which may suggest why married men seem to live longer). I identify others at routine physicals because I screen most men over age thirty for testosterone deficiency these days.

Testing is simple and very straightforward. A blood level of total testosterone below 300ng/dL, which is way too low, may be correlated with increased death rates at earlier ages from a variety of causes (Cattabiani, 2012). The optimal range is from 700-1000ng/dL, in my opinion, and I seldom find a man in that range (though I don't test the big, healthy, muscular ones too often). I encourage treatment for any man who tests below 300 and often treat men with levels from 300-500 if they have relevant symptoms or physical signs of hypogonadism. Everyone is different; one man may function normally at a level of 301, while another needs a level of 500 to achieve the same degree of benefit.

Saliva testing is another option, but its results are not as reliable, in my opinion, because saliva does not measure the total level of testosterone, more than 95 percent of which is bound to circulating proteins (sex hormone binding globulin, or SHBG) and does not get into the saliva. Therefore, only the "free" portion of the hormone is assessed by saliva testing, which reflects less than 5 percent of the total pool. Some people feel that the free portion of the hormone is the important part to measure, but I disagree because it is like looking in the man's wallet to determine his total net worth, just like checking a serum magnesium rather than an RBC magnesium.

There are instances when checking both the total and free testosterone levels is of great value. A small percentage of men will have decent total testosterone, but a relatively low free testosterone. This generates a low percentage of free testosterone, and can cause symptoms in men who seem to have adequate levels if you just check the total hormone level.

The only reason I do saliva hormone testing is for cost reasons, but that is my bias. Saliva testing generally costs only about a quarter of what blood testing costs for the same tests; the saliva test panels also provide estrogen levels, dihydrotestosterone, and other hormones in the same panel, which saves even more money if you want those levels tested. Insurance never pays for saliva testing however, so those with good insurance coverage will actually pay less out of pocket for blood tests than for saliva.

The third testing option is a twenty-four-hour urine hormone profile. The urine panels are quite a bit more expensive than saliva, and are also not typically covered by insurance. These test panels can assess a far greater number of hormone metabolites than measured in blood or saliva, but many of those levels have little or no known clinical usefulness. Urine panels are much more useful in women, who have many more hormones of interest represented on the panels; frankly, I have never run one of these test panels on a man.

I also check DHEA levels in men with hypogonad symptoms because low DHEA can cause all the same symptoms as low testosterone. The DHEA test can be a separate blood test at the same lab draw, or it can be included on the saliva panel or in a twenty-four-hour urine test. Remember that a blood test should be for the DHEA-sulfate metabolite. The desire to know the DHEA level can steer your testing decisions toward the saliva test because of costs considerations, but I find the saliva test's DHEA levels to be somewhat inconsistent and less reliable.

Testosterone deficiency in men: Treatment

Treatment is simple and straightforward; you need testosterone. The synthetic oral form isn't safe, it is known to cause liver toxicity, plus it is incredibly expensive. I suggest using a topical form, an injected product, or possibly implanted hormone pellets. Topical therapy is well accepted by men who don't like the idea of injections, which is the only reason to use it because it is clearly second best. The down side to topical therapy is that it has to be used every day, even twice per day for some men. (It lasts only twenty hours or so in the blood after application.) It is a little messy, and you must be careful not to rub any onto your wife, as a little testosterone can go way too far in a woman, or children.

The best way to get topical testosterone is in a cream made by a compounding pharmacy; I prescribe a twenty percent cream (200mg per mL) to be used at 1mL (200mg) daily, rubbed onto the sides of the torso or some other relatively hairless area. It absorbs the best when applied to the scrotum, but that is not necessary, and it can create more problems with conversion to other hormones if applied there. Also, there may be greater exposure to testosterone in the prostate gland if you apply to the scrotum, another reason not to put it there.

I suggest that men use their dose at night if possible so they don't wake up with a hot flash as it wears off, and so their levels will peak in the late morning, which seems ideal physiologically. Some men need 100mg or less per day, some need 300mg per day, and others need somewhere between these two levels. I find that 200mg per day works well for the great majority of men, so I start there and adjust the dose if needed.

Manufactured topical testosterone products made by pharmaceutical companies are available at every pharmacy. I never use them unless the patient insists on trying them first because they don't usually work, and they are much more expensive (like most products made by pharmaceutical companies). The goals of therapy are symptom relief and to get the peak testosterone level up around 1000 (800-1200). The testosterone level rises and falls dramatically in the blood every twenty-four hours with topical therapy, and it takes a significant dose to get it to 1000 at peak and keep the levels in an acceptable range up to the next dosing.

Androgel™ is a prescription topical gel made in only very low concentrations. It is made in 1% and now 1.62% strengths. The product comes in a 5mL packet, yielding only 50mg or 81mg testosterone per packet. This means you have to apply five times as much gel to get only a quarter to two fifths the amount of testosterone compared to the 200mg I usually prescribe. Testim™ is another 1% gel, packaged in 5mL tubes. Axiron™ and Fortesta™ are newer manufactured testosterone gels, made in 2% strength and sold in a pump.

The gel preparations do seem to absorb better than the compounded creams, but I still find that most men must double the standard dose—10mL of gel at least—to see clinical response; this usually means rubbing it all over the torso and limbs, a real mess. Few men stay on these gel forms, both because of the mess and because it costs around $700 per month to use them at an effective dose versus $25-30 per month for the compounded cream.

Androderm™ is a testosterone patch also made by a drug company and available with insurance from any pharmacy. The problems with it are similar to those with the manufactured gels—it doesn't work well at all and it is very expensive—without the messy application issue but with the added problem of a potential rash from the adhesive. The glue on these patches causes an itchy, red rash in the large majority (I'd say around 80%) of the men for whom I have ever ordered them. Alternatively, the patches may not stick well to some men at all. The patches come in only 2.5mg and 5mg doses and must be changed every day. When you consider that you may need at least 100mg daily, that's a lot of patches and a lot of itchy red circles.

Injections are superior to all of the topical forms in terms of effectiveness, and equal to the low cost of compounded creams. There is variability in how men absorb topical products through their skin, but much less variability in dosing by injection. Getting the testosterone through injection, right into your tissues eliminates some variables and offers a more rapid and predictable response to therapy. The shots usually have to be given only once per week, but some men metabolize testosterone more quickly and need to do injections every five days perhaps.

If a man opts for injections I prescribe either testosterone "enanthate" or "cypionate"; these are the two forms currently available. It doesn't seem to matter what form you use, no matter what you may read on the internet. The second chemical word there (enanthate or cypionate) is just an organic molecule attached to the testosterone to make it soluble in the injection solution; it has no relevant effect itself. I suggest using an intramuscular injection (into the thigh or buttocks) of 100mg per week to start with, which is the most common dosing, regardless of body weight. I always prescribe the more concentrated 200mg/mL preparation so you can inject less volume. (Don't let your doctor give you 100mg/mL if you can help it, because you have to inject a full mL instead of just 1/2mL.)

Using shots, most men will feel the effects within the first week or two, while it might take a full month for topical therapy to have a similarly noticeable physical effect. It is not uncommon for men to start feeling *psychologically* better within the first week, regardless of which form they use; it gets right to the brain and starts improving attitude and motivation right away for many of us. The increased muscular strength and stamina should be more evident after a month or two. In my opinion, it is critical that men start exercising as well, so their testosterone gets used by the body properly. Increased sex drive may be noted in the first week or two, but erectile function may not improve for months if it has been gone for a long time; sometimes it doesn't improve at all with just testosterone replacement because there are other causes.

Another method of testosterone replacement one could consider is implanted pellets. A small incision is made in the skin, some number of little white testosterone pellets is stuffed inside and then the wound is sutured shut. The benefit is that you don't have to receive your "dose" very often, and don't have to do anything on your own at home. This approach is catching on here and there around the country, but I have not used them myself.

You can't adjust the dose quickly if needed, and it requires an invasive procedure every few months to use it, or to get it out if you need to (e.g., for a rising PSA level). The manufacturers claim the pellets can be placed just every four months, but patient forums I read online suggested that the benefits seem to wear off by just two or three months for many men. Even if your doctor puts more pellets in the dose wont last longer, it will just peak higher and then crash harder, because the pellets all dissolve at the same time and rate. Many people apparently do well with the pellets, so don't let my personal trepidation keep you from trying it out.

I mentioned that some men will have normal total testosterone but low free testosterone, and may have hypogonad symptoms. These men may benefit from testosterone replacement itself, bringing up both the free and total testosterone levels, but their insurance may not pay for therapy because they do not meet the criterion of having low total testosterone. Passionflower extract, probably via the active chemical *chrysin*, is a potential treatment for these individuals. Chrysin causes increased dissociation of testosterone molecules from SHBG, thereby increasing the bioavailable (free) testosterone level without impacting the total. Animal studies with passionflower extracts have shown significant increases in libido, sexual performance and sperm counts (Dhawan, 2002).

Many combination herbal products online claim to boost testosterone naturally, and some hormonal precursors are suggested as well. Some of the herbs worth trying include *Tribulus terrestris* and ginseng (the Korean, Chinese, or American forms), which may increase production a bit in some. You may hear about a number of other herbs as well, and some of them may work. If the problem is the inability to produce testosterone because of testicular damage or toxicity, then this approach will not work at all of course. My experience with this approach is that it works only to a small extent, and in only a small percentage of men.

Some men also try hormonal precursors, such as DHEA or pregnenolone, which have the potential to become testosterone downstream. They may increase testosterone levels only a little because a man may need much more testosterone than he needs of either of these precursors, and there is no guarantee the supplements will actually become testosterone. DHEA is just as likely to become estrogen or one of another of fifteen or so metabolites as it is to become testosterone, and this can cause more harm than good. Pregnenolone is arguably more likely to become an adrenal steroid like cortisol, and it can help those with adrenal deficiency but generally not one with testosterone deficiency.

Testosterone replacement in men who need it is usually *life changing.* Give men testosterone replacement is one of the best parts of my job. So many happy men and their wives return feeling like they have their lives back; it's very gratifying. If you think you or a man in your life may have low testosterone, get it checked out and treated early. Don't wait until life has obviously deteriorated in quality and things are falling apart physically. There are a few complications and caveats to watch out for, however, so keep reading.

Testosterone in men: Monitoring and maintenance

Once you're on hormone replacement, you must make sure nothing ill comes of it. The most common side effects noted in men are acne, oily skin, new body hair growth, loss of head hair with receding hairline, testicular shrinkage, and an increase in assertiveness. (I say "assertiveness," rather than "aggression," because at the physiologic doses we use for replacement you don't see the "roid rage" phenomenon you hear about in bodybuilders and other athletes that use testosterone because those individuals are often using ten times the dose we use for hormone replacement.) You are unlikely to get big muscles either unless you intentionally work out very hard.

Infertility may be an issue for some men who still want to have children, but it may be a blessing for those who don't want more children and were thinking about having a vasectomy. Testosterone injections have been shown to be 98 percent or more effective at shutting off sperm production because of feedback to the pituitary gland and resulting shut-off of the signal hormones (LH and FSH) that promote sperm production. This is also why the testicles often shrink with testosterone replacement.

Testosterone replacement does not make you sterile permanently because, when you stop using testosterone, your pituitary will turn back on and signal your testicles to make sperm again. A Chinese study published in 2009 showed that a monthly injection of 500mg was highly effective in shutting off sperm production and preventing pregnancy, and that infertility was virtually 100 percent reversible when the men stopped therapy. I suggest weekly 100mg injections or 200mg injected every two weeks, rather than the 500mg monthly approach, in order to avoid the roller coaster effect.

Topical HRT (hormone replacement therapy) probably works as well for birth control as injections, but we aren't sure about the dose yet. It is important to note that a man will still be fertile for about three months after starting the testosterone; and one should consider laboratory confirmation of sterility before stopping other forms of birth control. If you do want to have children, consider trying to conceive before starting HRT. You may also try using HCG therapy (discussed below) to achieve fertility while remaining on testosterone.

The most important monitoring issues for men on testosterone are to watch out for estrogen-conversion problems, excessive blood cell production (the opposite of anemia, called "polycythemia"), and prostate issues including cancer. After a few months of HRT, I check a blood count, PSA (prostate cancer screening blood test), cholesterol, liver enzymes, and estrogen in one way or another. I often also check a dihydrotestosterone (DHT) level; DHT is a metabolite of testosterone that can cause male pattern baldness and enlargement of the prostate.

I check testosterone levels at this first reevaluation and periodically until I feel the individual's dose is correct. I check the blood count and PSA on an ongoing basis, usually once per year. I don't keep checking estrogen or DHT levels into the future unless there was a high level the first time or relevant symptoms develop later on. DHEA should be tested initially, and also checked at the first follow-up to make sure dosing is adequate, similar to checking testosterone levels.

The over-conversion of testosterone to estrogen (which can also occur with DHEA) is called aromatization. It can cause weight gain, water retention and ankle swelling, emotional swings, prostate gland enlargement and possibly prostate cancer (this is not yet proven), breast tissue development, and nipple soreness. Some of these breast tissue changes are permanent so I screen every man for estrogen elevation two to three months into therapy by checking total estrogens in a blood or a saliva panel that includes estrogen.

I believe that producing too much estrogen because of HRT puts men at increased risk for prostate enlargement and/or cancer—this connection is being studied right now—and of course negates many of the expected benefits of HRT. I find that this occurs in 20–25 percent of men on testosterone or DHEA replacement. The symptoms may not be seen for a long time, so I screen everyone for it at follow-up testing.

It is generally easy fix rising estrogen levels, but it usually requires a drug. The prescription drugs Arimidex™ (anastrozole) and Femara™(letrozole) are expensive, but they work by far the best in blocking the estrogen conversion problem. I only have experience with anastrozole, because it has gone generic and is far less expensive now. Most men can take anastrozole at 1mg just a couple of days per week to keep their estrogen under control. These drugs can have some dangerous side effects, primarily chest pain and cardiovascular events, but those are very uncommon and most likely to occur only in those at high risk for cardiovascular problems to begin with.

Various herbal products are on the market claiming to reduce estrogen for men on testosterone. Some may work to a small degree for some men, but I have been extremely unimpressed by the results I have personally seen from the most highly regarded of these products. Herbal products are not cheap either; it is cheaper to take generic anastrozole twice per week than to take one of these herbal products at the suggested dosage. The herbal product with the best success (still a minimal effect in my experience) costs forty dollars every three weeks and requires taking nine capsules per day; while taking two tiny white tablets of anastrozole per week only costs about twenty dollars per month.

The prostate cancer issue is an important one. Testosterone itself does not appear to cause prostate cancer, but it may theoretically "feed" certain types of prostate cancer if it does develop. This has been called into question by recent study however. A small series, of just thirteen men, showed that giving testostcroue to hypogonad men with untreated prostate cancer resulted in no progression of their cancer (Morgentaler, 2011). Prostate cancer is known to be very diverse in its physiologic behaviors and responsiveness to various hormones, and this was a very small study, so the standard caution would still be to avoid testosterone in men with prostate cancer until we know more.

The point is that men on testosterone or DHEA hormone replacement therapy (HRT) should be vigilant about screening for prostate cancer with PSA testing within six months after starting HRT and then annually. If the PSA goes up to worrisome levels, the HRT should probably be stopped right away and further testing initiated.

Aside from looking for potential complications, men should be evaluated for appropriate clinical response and testosterone levels at two to three months into therapy. They should be feeling happier, stronger, more energetic and more "manly" by this time. If a man is not seeing these benefits he may need a dose increase or perhaps switch to injections if he is not responding to topical therapy. A man on injections may improve effectiveness either by increasing the dose of each weekly injection, or by increasing the frequency of their injections to every five or six days perhaps. Repeat testing can help determine what is going on.

It is important to do repeat testing with the proper timing relative to dosing of their type of HRT or you will just be confused. The timing of testosterone measurement is one area of HRT management in men I have often seen done wrong; frankly, my own bio-identical hormone training did not address it either and I had to figure it out on my own. Luckily, I guess, I ended up on testosterone myself and could readily experiment on a willing participant.

Most doctors prescribing testosterone in my opinion make the mistakes of using too low a topical dose, too infrequent an injected dose (often every two to four weeks rather than weekly, making men come to their office for shots rather than teaching them to do it themselves), and their doing repeat testing at the *wrong time relative to testosterone dosing*. Most doctors don't know to check estrogen levels either, another major failing.

I have found that testosterone levels fluctuate dramatically every twenty-four hours when men are on topical therapy. (My blood level was 1100 at six hours and only a little above 100 at twenty-four hours after a single 200mg dose application.) Therefore, I prefer to test men twelve to eighteen hours after their last application, and I want their total testosterone to remain at 600-1000 range during this time. Men who use injections do not have the same dramatic daily fluctuation in blood levels; their levels peak around day two to three after their shots and are not usually gone until day seven or eight usually.

I prefer to test men who are using injections on day five or six following an dose, and I want to see their total testosterone still at 700-800 on day five or 500-700 on day six. If their dose is wearing off too soon, they may need to shift to a five or six day shot cycle. If their levels don't rise enough in the first place (below desired range at their mid-week peak, and inadequate clinical response) they should increase their weekly dose amount.

"How long do I have to do this?" It's a common question from men who are undertaking HRT. The correct answer is, "I don't know; maybe forever." I used to say: "Use it until you want to feel like crap again" because I didn't think men could resume their own testicular function and endogenous production of testosterone. I have since learned that some men can in fact resume adequate production of testosterone on their own.

If a man's testicles have been removed or damaged, he will certainly need HRT for his lifetime. But if a man has just become fat and sedentary with resulting decline in testosterone, or his testicular function was suppressed by narcotics usage, his testicles may resume production after using HCG or a temporary period of testosterone replacement with significant lifestyle changes. If the man ate a poor diet or was obese, his testicles may resume more normal production on their own with weight loss and vigorous exercise. If environmental toxins are the biggest factor, a man may be able to detoxify and see some resumption of testosterone production.

I find that most men feel much better and more motivated to eat better and start exercising if I put them on HRT first to perk them up and increase their energy. We may be able to stop the HRT after six to twelve months, and they may carry on just fine afterward if they have started eating healthfully and exercising, and if they have lost some fat and done some effective detoxification. Using the testosterone for any length of time does not "commit" one to having to use it forever. I frequently use up to several months of supplemental testosterone for people trying to heal an injury or recover form surgery as well (both men and women); you do not see dependency develop.

I now believe that a significant percentage of men may get off their testosterone at some point, but they are still a minority of the group overall. This has not been the case for me; whenever I stop my injections my levels drop very low again and I feel terrible by day nine (the levels stayed low even when I've tried to stick it out for several months). Most men like their HRT so much that they won't bother trying to quit.

Testosterone replacement to optimal levels has some potential major health and anti-aging benefits and contributes to overall quality of life, but because of its risks, the decision to use HRT should be made with careful consideration and should be monitored by a suitably trained and experienced physician or prescribing naturopath. Testosterone is a controlled substance, and a provider can't prescribe it without a DEA license.

The bottom line is that testosterone deficiency is a common and underappreciated problem, and testosterone replacement therapy is highly rewarding the vast majority of the time. As always, find the right prescriber. Don't stick with someone who just wants you to come to the office for shots every two to four weeks, because that schedule really doesn't work. Make sure the right monitoring is done (testosterone, total estrogens, CBC, PSA, lipids), and you may have to demand that your estrogen level is checked, since there is likely to be some resistance to that one from many practitioners (they wont understand why a man should have their estrogen checked).

Testosterone for women

Women may present with the same complaints as men when they have significant testosterone deficiency. They may experience fatigue, weakness, depression, loss of sex drive or enjoyment, vaginal dryness, and musculoskeletal pain, particularly if they have chronic pain treated with opiates. Sometimes I empirically treat (without testing) women with vaginal testosterone purely to improve sexual function, such as in those with vaginal dryness or inability to reach orgasm, but it also helps many women with stress urinary incontinence (e.g., when they pee a little every time they cough or sneeze).

If women have many of the symptoms I test them, via blood, saliva or urine panel, just as I would a man. Of course, women have much lower testosterone levels than men do; for example, a blood level below 25ng/dL is a good threshold for considering treatment in women (compared to 400 or so in men). Women also need a much smaller dose of testosterone for replacement than men do. Most of a woman's testosterone is produced by conversion of DHEA from their adrenals because they don't have testicles. The ovaries normally produce only a very small amount of testosterone and are not a significant source; therefore a woman's testosterone level is not expected to drop off significantly due to menopause or surgical removal of the ovaries.

Using DHEA for women with testosterone deficiency (and low DHEA as well) is the best first-line treatment, rather than putting them on testosterone itself. DHEA replacement covers both bases in one stroke and often works well because low DHEA and low testosterone look much the same in women. If a woman happens to have normal DHEA but low testosterone in isolation, or if she has sexual or urinary issues, testosterone replacement itself may be better. The doses are much lower than for men, of course, and the topical form is the only realistic option, in my opinion.

Oral testosterone forms are out, for the same reasons mentioned with men. Shots are unnecessary for women because the doses are so low and because the shots, typically given only once every month or so by most prescribers, may cause large swings in testosterone. Topical therapy works well and it is inexpensive and well received by most women. Vaginal placement of a compounded or manufactured cream product absorbs well for treating sexual or urinary problems (applied directly to the clitoris for improving orgasm) but, in general, testosterone deficiency may be treated by rubbing the HRT cream into the skin anywhere, just as with men.

I usually start women on doses of just 1-2mg daily (far less than the 200mg most men require) and go from there, based on response. Some women may need up to 5mg daily—10mg daily in rare instances—but most don't need more than 2mg per day. Some may find they need it only a few days per week to control their symptoms once they note a positive response.

As for the downsides, women may convert the testosterone to estrogen with relevant side effects such as mood changes, headaches, weight gain, breast soreness or water retention. They may also of course have direct overdose effects of testosterone itself. The masculinizing or "virilizing" effects of testosterone (or DHEA) in women may include growth of facial or body hair, acne, oily skin, deepening voice, male-pattern baldness, and an enlarged clitoris. They may also experience increased anger or aggression (much more often than men do on their typical doses in my experience). In fact, with enough testosterone, you can turn a woman into a very convincing "man," so testosterone replacement is a key part of transgender medicine for women who are undergoing gender reassignment.

These overdose symptoms shouldn't scare you off; they are easy to spot when they start, and you can just stop or reduce therapy long before they become permanent problems. Testosterone replacement in women can be a very rewarding and life-improving treatment, and it is my opinion that a trial of therapy should be considered for every woman with relevant symptoms. Again, just find someone with experience in this area and a good compounding pharmacy to make your product. If you don't have a local compounding pharmacy, there are many of them in the country that will send your product directly to you with a faxed prescription from a licensed provider (who has a DEA number).

Women may experience signs of testosterone excess even if they are not using any DHEA or testosterone replacement, and this indicates some sort of hormonal or metabolic problem in most cases. If a woman is experiencing acne, weight gain, growth of facial hair, and other typical symptoms of androgen excess, she should be tested for elevated internally produced androgens (male-predominant hormones) including testosterone and DHEA. These sorts of symptoms are normal, to some mild extent, in women from certain parts of the world. If her testosterone level is very high, it may be coming from an ovarian tumor, and she should have an ultrasound.

If the DHEA level is high, with or without elevated testosterone as well, the androgen excess may be related to an adrenal tumor. If the testosterone is only mildly or modestly elevated and the ultrasound shows the possibility of cysts on the ovary, then polycystic ovary syndrome (PCOS) is likely. This syndrome is often associated with metabolic syndrome (pre-diabetes, obesity, abnormal cholesterol) and infertility problems. The cysts on the ovaries are just a symptom, not the cause. Various metabolic processes are disturbed here, and the condition is usually relieved by dietary changes, thyroid correction/replacement, weight loss, clearance of yeast, therapeutic vitamin D dosing, inositol supplementation (4000mg daily), and possibly progesterone.

Estrogen

Women have suffered for centuries at the ignorant hands of a male-dominated medical profession. Any complaint from a menopausal woman was summarily treated with estrogen without doing any testing to verify that she needed it. To make matters worse, the "estrogen" of choice since the 1940s has been Premarin™, which is derived from horse pee (the brand name is derived from the source: "pregnant mare urine") and which contains at least a couple of forms of horse-derived estrogen that don't exist in humans and that appear to have unpredictable negative effects. When women still complained after being put on estrogen they usually received Valium™ or another sedative, a hysterectomy (to get their "hysteria" out), or even a lobotomy. Granted, these practices are no longer standard of care, but it really wasn't all that long ago if you think about it.

The most common practice among gynecologists and conventional primary care physicians is still to put women directly on estrogen of some sort, although now it is more often estradiol, a real human estrogen, rather than Premarin™, immediately after a hysterectomy (if the ovaries were removed too) or with the onset of typical menopause symptoms like hot flashes and night sweats. This kind of treatment is unnecessary the majority of the time, as becomes apparent if women are tested first.

Testing considerations

The reason that it is so important to test women before putting them on estrogen is that estrogen has far more bad effects than good. Estrogen promotes cancer in the breast and uterus and increases the risk of blood clots. Synthetic and equine estrogens appear to also increase cardiovascular events like heart attack and stroke; this became common knowledge following the publication of results from the *Women's Health Initiative (WHI)*. This NIH study was started in 1991 and then stopped prematurely in 2002 because it became evident that the subjects receiving Prem-Pro™, a combination of the horse-pee estrogens and a synthetic progesterone analog called Provera™ (medroxyprogesterone), had a greater incidence of coronary heart disease, breast cancer, stroke, and pulmonary embolism, than subjects receiving placebo (Writing Group for the Women's Health Initiative Investigators, 2002).

Aside from the above life threatening complications, estrogen also causes weight gain, water retention, psychological disturbance, and migraines or a serious headache condition called *pseudotumor cerebri* in some. Even natural or bio-identical estrogens have these effects. There is generally a very low concentration of estrogen in the body even in women, and the liver has very active mechanisms for "detoxifying" estrogen because it is such a potent influence.

A little bit of estrogen goes a long way, and my view is that it should not be given to a woman unless she is tested and proven to be deficient. Progesterone deficiency can cause many of the classic symptoms of menopause, so it should be used first, before estrogen replacement is considered. There are three different forms of estrogen in humans that we know of, and two are used commonly for replacement.

Women produce estrogen from the ovaries to some extent, so after the ovaries fail and menopause begins, some women do become clinically estrogen deficient. However, women also make estrogen via conversion from the DHEA produced by the adrenals, which occurs mainly in the body's fat cells. This secondary production source for estrogen maintains adequate levels for most women. Many women with true estrogen deficiency will be thin, lacking the body fat to produce adequate estrogen. Most women in the United States are not thin, and they may produce plenty of estrogen even after menopause. This does not mean overweight or obese women are immune from estrogen deficiency by any means; I have seen plenty of women with symptomatic estrogen deficiency regardless of their body fat content.

Testing should be done if a woman has relevant symptoms of estrogen deficiency, including vaginal dryness, often accompanied by dry mouth or eyes; fatigue and poor stamina; low libido; loss of breast tissue or muscle mass; and various emotional complaints. Hot flashes and night sweats are common, but they are also often related to lifestyle, progesterone, or adrenal issues, which should be treated first before estrogen is considered. Intake of caffeine, alcohol, and sugar in excessive amounts (which sometimes means any intake at all) can trigger hot flashes and sweats in many women. If a woman has some of these complaints and has not responded to dietary changes or progesterone replacement, she should be tested for estrogen deficiency or possibly treated with a conservative trial of estrogen replacement.

Testing can be done via blood, saliva, or urine just as with men. I preferred blood testing by far in men but use a lot more saliva or urine testing in women. Estrogens are not as highly bound to proteins in the blood, so the "free" portions are higher and are more accurate in the saliva than are testosterone or DHEA. Saliva and urine test panels include all three forms of estrogen: estrone, estradiol and estriol. Blood tests do not accurately assess estriol levels via the blood in nonpregnant women. Salivary panels also generally include progesterone, testosterone, and DHEA, along with the three forms of estrogen, all for one low price, which can save more than a thousand dollars on testing.

A twenty-four-hour urine profile is the test of choice for women in some cases because the test measures all of the above-mentioned hormones plus many more hormone metabolites, and women's bodies are much more complicated than men's. In addition, women's risk of breast or uterine cancers is influenced to some extent by the way they metabolize their estrogen. The relevant estrogen metabolites are currently only available through urine tests.

The three types of estrogen, once again, are estrone (E1), estradiol (E2), and estriol (E3). Estradiol is the most cancer promoting form and estriol the least. Estriol does not appear to increase breast or uterine cancer at all in fact, and recent research has even suggested that vaginal estriol supplementation is likely to be safe in women who have had breast cancer and are on estrogen-depleting drugs such as anastrozole (Pfeiler, 2011). We can calculate from saliva or urine an "estrogen quotient" by dividing the estriol level by the sum of the E1 and E2 levels. It is commonly suggested that this quotient should be one or higher for lower cancer risk, meaning at least as much estriol as there is estradiol and estrone combined.

There is really not convincing data on this in my opinion, with most of the studies I reviewed exhibiting various confounding issues and showing weak "associations", which of course do not prove cause and effect. A recent study of *pre*-menopausal women, evaluating urinary estrogen levels and metabolites from more than 18,500 women enrolled in the Nurses' Health Study, showed the exact opposite of what is commonly believed in bio-identical hormone therapy (BHRT) circles: they showed that *high* urinary levels of estradiol and estrone were associated with *lower* risk of breast cancer. These were not small differences either; those with the highest quartile of excretion showed nearly fifty percent reductions in relative risk of breast cancer for both estradiol and estrone compared to those in the lowest quartile of excretion (Eliassen, 2012).

What the above study calls into question is what exactly you can deduce from urinary estrogen (or anything else for that matter) levels. When something is elevated in the urine it could indicate that there is too much of that substance in the body, or that the body is "dumping" that substance at a high rate. The latter instance could lead to low or normal levels being left in the body. In the case of urinary estrogen levels this means you don't know whether a woman with high urine levels has high estrogen in the body, which puts her at increased cancer risk; or just excretes her estrogen at a high rate and leaves lower levels in the body, which would effectively decrease her risk for breast cancer. As I've said repeatedly: knowledge in medical science is constantly growing and evolving. I try not to get too bonded to what we currently "think" we know. Checking both urinary and blood levels together should help discern what is really going on for a given individual; but this makes one question whether the urinary levels are even necessary, or useful at all.

How the estrogens are being metabolized as they are broken down is also thought to be important. As estradiol is degraded in the liver, it is "hydroxylated" (a hydroxyl, or –OH, group is added to the molecule) at one position or another. The 2-OH estrone metabolite is believed to be protective against cancer, or at least may have the lowest potential to cause it, while the 16-OH and 4-OH levels may be increasingly cancer promoting. Research has suggested that the 2-OH/16-OH ratio should be higher than 2:1 and the 2-OH/4-OH ratio should be higher than 3:1 for the lowest theoretical breast cancer risk. The human research suggesting this relationship is very limited, it is observational and not treatment based, it shows only fairly weak associations and tends to have numerous confounding issues in my opinion.

I've looked into this question extensively, because I would dearly love to believe we have a tool for accurately predicting breast cancer risk and possibly even intervening on some of these causative hormonal metabolites.

My research has thus far, unfortunately, led me to feel that these tests are of little value. One study of premenopausal women in the Nurses' Health Study showed no predictive value of urinary 2- or 4- hydroxylated metabolites in terms of breast cancer risk. It did suggest increased breast cancer risk with higher urinary excretion of the 16-OH metabolites however (Eliassen, 2012). Additionally, I found a rodent study where they implanted female animals with pellets containing various forms and amounts of estrogens and estrogen metabolites. Females implanted with high doses of estradiol all (one hundred percent) developed breast tumors, while those implanted with 4-OH estrone (which is allegedly very cancer-promoting according to the current BHRT thinking) did not yield any breast tumors at all. Those implanted with the 2-OH, 4-OH, or 16-OH metabolites of estradiol also yielded no tumors (Turan, 2004). This proves that those metabolites of estrogen do not directly "cause" breast cancer formation, at least in rats.

If one is interested, the best way to measure these 2-OH, 16-OH and 4-OH estrone levels is with twenty-four-hour urine collection tests, which are performed by only a few laboratory companies in the country. The three major forms of estrogen involved in the estrogen quotient mentioned above may also be measured in saliva but not in blood. It is important to understand the limitations of each type of testing: Blood levels show "total" amounts of hormones; estriol the various –OH metabolites are not available. Salivary levels show only the "free" portion of hormones, which is a very small percentage of the total; they are also very affected by dry mouth, topical hormone use, and they just aren't very precise. Urine levels can give you a completely wrong idea about what is going on, because you don't know whether the urine level reflects what is left in the body or not. Any testing method performed needs to be evaluated in the context of the individual's symptoms and specific situation.

Treatment considerations

Since estrogen has many potential ill effects (blood clots, migraines, breast and uterine cancer to name a few) it is important to me that it only be given to those who really seem to need it and the likely benefits should outweigh the potential risks. When we replace estrogens at my office, for women with relevant symptoms and low levels upon testing, we often start with estriol by itself—usually as a vaginal preparation because it works great for vaginal dryness—or in combination with estradiol at from a 2:1 to a 4:1 ratio (more estriol than estradiol). Practitioners may prescribe a compounded (made special by the pharmacist, not at a pharmaceutical factory) combination estrogen called "BiEst," made as a cream with an 80:20 mixture of estriol and estradiol, respectively. I usually start women at 0.5mg or so daily of either form and work up (or down) from there based on response. You can also determine changes with repeat testing, but the clinical response is the most important thing in hormonal therapy. BiEst and other hormonal replacement products may be made into oral capsules, vaginal suppositories, sublingual solutions or other various forms as well.

We often prefer to use topical hormones rather than oral forms with the sex steroids because when you swallow something it is absorbed from the stomach and intestines, therefore going to the liver first for processing before being distributed around the body. The liver modifies or destroys 85–90 percent of most hormones on their way through, requiring larger doses to be given, which exposes the liver to large amounts of a potentially harmful substance in order to get the right amount into circulation. Oral testosterone has been associated with harm to the liver as a result, and taking oral synthetic estrogens can create benign tumors and blood vessel anomalies in the liver called hemangiomas.

Oral forms of progesterone, DHEA, and cortisol don't seem to have any direct liver toxicity, and it is actually preferable to use oral DHEA and cortisol over topical forms in my opinion. Each hormone is really a different situation. Bio-identical hormone therapy (BHRT) practitioners each have their own preferences in terms of how they use these tools. Cost can of course be of some consideration. Manufactured oral and topical forms of estradiol are readily covered by insurance, but if you want estriol or estrone included, the product has to be made by a compounding pharmacy. That is easily done, but it is frequently not covered by insurance. Compounded products are typically much cheaper than the manufactured forms however, so those without medical insurance are generally better off with compounded prescriptions in terms of cost.

The manufactured forms of bio-identical estrogen are all estradiol-only products. I prefer to use a compounded product that contains estriol for safety, but most of the world just uses estradiol, and the potential increased risks may not be great; we don't know for sure. I strongly suggest you do not use Premarin™ or any synthetic estrogen product because the behavior in the human body is unpredictable, the levels are not measurable for monitoring purposes, and significant adverse effects have been reported, often caused by the abnormal metabolites these products create once they're inside your body. There is no reason to use an artificial or animal estrogen product when biologically identical hormones are readily available; I don't even understand why the FDA leaves these things on the market (well, I do understand – but it's reprehensible in my opinion).

Estrogen should be handled with care because of the potential for overdose and serious long-term consequences. If estrogen is used at all, the lowest amount of the safest form should be used. Estrogen should never be given without also prescribing some form of progesterone, which tends to counteract many of the negative effects of estrogen. Progesterone should always be tried first for hot flashes and some other typical menopause symptoms in my opinion. Then, if necessary, estrogen may be added.

In my opinion, estrogen should be started at a low dose and gradually adjusted upward. My bias is toward using the lowest effective dose of pretty much any hormone, but this is most important with estrogen because of the potential risks. I usually start topical doses in the 0.5 to 1mg range, oral doses and vaginal doses about the same. Each does should be given at least a week or two before going up to higher levels. I suggest going up by 0.25 to 0.5mg per day in dose with each incremental increase. Once symptoms have been controlled for a few months, it is often possible to drop the dose a bit once again, which I encourage everyone to try in the case of estrogen.

Estrogen comes in an injected form as well, but this is rarely ever necessary. If there is no response to the other routes of estrogen replacement it may be prudent to try injections. Injections should be done weekly, just like testosterone for men; don't let your gynecologist give you just monthly shots, because they don't really last more than a week. Injection doses are completely different, and must be managed with an experienced provider.

Estriol should be the only estrogen used at first, unless estradiol levels are very low upon testing, in which case I would use BiEst. I would like to mention that some women will need to have just estrogen used alone for a couple weeks to get their hot flashes under control, then have progesterone added. If these women use progesterone first and their hot flashes don't improve, simply adding in estrogen will not fix their symptoms for some reason. The progesterone has to be stopped, and estrogen used alone for a week or two, then the progesterone may be resumed.

Despite all my concerns about estrogen, when a woman truly needs estrogen it can be a wonderful thing. The quality-of-life problems incurred in estrogen deficiency can be miserable on many levels. The only reason to deprive women of estrogen when they have deficiency problems is if they have had breast or uterine cancer or are at very high risk for them, as it may not be worth the risk to use estrogen if you have a personal or family history of these cancers. Natural, bio-identical progesterone itself does not appear to increase breast cancer risk, though the synthetic "progestins" used in manufactured birth control pills and hormone replacement products (e.g. the Provera™ used in Prem-Pro™) clearly *do* increase cancer risk (Seeger, 2008). Therefore natural progesterone may probably be used safely even in the presence of breast cancer.

If there is concern about the balance of estrogen metabolites I discussed above, these parameters can be manipulated with nutritional supplements. You can improve the estrogen quotient (bring up the estriol level) by taking iodine, one of my favorites, or of course by using estriol replacement. We often give iodine at 37.5 to 50mg per day for a few months and then recheck the estrogen levels. You can improve your 2/16 and 2/4 ratios by eating more crucifers (broccoli, cauliflower, cabbage, Brussels sprouts) or taking supplements derived from these vegetables. Supplements include products made directly from the vegetables, from broccoli seed extracts (probably the best options available currently), or as extracted single molecules such as *indole-3-carbinol* (I3C) or *diindolyl methane* (DIM).

For as much as I called into question the utility of testing the estrogen metabolites in terms of assessing cancer risk, the treatments (iodine, crucifer derivatives) are safe and likely to be effective. Therefore, I don't really care if the tests are correct; the suggestions that follow are virtually harmless and are likely good for everyone. Iodine has evidence for reducing breast cancer risk and as a breast cancer treatment itself (Singh, 2011). Sulforaphanes have been shown to inhibit breast cancer growth through various cellular mechanisms and inhibit breast cancer stem cells in a preventive fashion (Li, 2010). DIM and I3C have been shown to directly inhibit breast cancer cell growth through various mechanisms as well (Jin, 2011 and Marconett, 2011). This means to me that every woman should be eating crucifers and supplementing with these sorts of things, especially if she has family history or other increased risk for breast cancers. If a test helps to convince a woman to take these things, that is probably good; even if that test is truly irrelevant.

Estrogen for men
There is never a reason to give estrogen to a man. Never.

Progesterone

After all the cautions about estrogen, it is refreshing to talk about progesterone. I love prescribing or recommending progesterone, as I have seen it eliminate suffering in women of all ages, and it has saved many marriages and relationships in my practice. Progesterone creams are available over the counter almost anywhere, and women are often shocked, and disgusted at the same time, that the cure for their misery was right there on the shelf all along.

Sometimes the problem is low progesterone, and sometimes it is a relatively high estrogen level compared to their progesterone, a condition called "estrogen dominance." The term was coined by Dr. John Lee, who wrote a number of books about menopause, progesterone, and hormone balance in women that are very good references. There is a distinct lack of research or "evidence" regarding this use of progesterone in the conventional literature (the stuff is cheap and available OTC, so nobody pays for research like this). Correspondingly, there is a lack of understanding and belief in its value on the part of conventional gynecologists and primary care practitioners.

Myriad common conditions in women can be ameliorated or eliminated with progesterone therapy. The common symptoms of PMS, including irritability, emotional swings or rage, menstrual cramps, breast tenderness, water retention, bloating, migraines, and anxiety, are usually related to relative progesterone insufficiency. Asthma and allergies to foods or inhalants may be worsened by progesterone deficiency; these immune problems, as well as various autoimmune conditions, often develop or flare up after a pregnancy or menopause, when progesterone levels suffer a major sharp decline.

Application of topical progesterone to areas on women's faces where whiskers or hair is growing may decrease such growth because progesterone counters the adverse effects of testosterone or DHEA in women. We can often improve anxiety and insomnia with progesterone, especially in post-menopausal women. Migraines that cycle with the menses are almost always improved with progesterone. Endometriosis often improves with progesterone replacement, but may also flare up, so be careful in this situation. Fibroid tumors in the uterus have a more predictable beneficial response, and may shrink dramatically with the use of progesterone. Again, none of these benefits may be seen similarly with the synthetic *progestins*, because they are not at all the same thing.

Progesterone may correct most of the typical menopause complaints that have been thought to be due to estrogen deficiency. Hot flashes, night sweats, insomnia, mood changes, and weight gain associated with the onset of menopause are often relieved by progesterone therapy and generally don't require estrogen replacement in most women because progesterone decline is what defines menopause. Most of a woman's progesterone comes from the ovaries, and when they "burn out" at menopause, progesterone generation decreases. Women may continue to produce plenty of estrogen after menopause via conversion from DHEA in their fat tissue, which is particularly common in the United States where most of us have excess fat.

Progesterone has been shown to stimulate bone production and can decrease complications and risk of osteoporosis synergistically with estrogen (Seifert-Kaluss, 2010) even increasing bone density in some studies. (Lee, 2004). Again it is important to point out the difference between natural progesterone and synthetic progestins; depot medroxyprogesterone acetate (Depo-Provera™) use as a birth control measure has been shown to decrease bone mineralization and increase the risk of fractures later in life (Meier, 2010). Progesterone appears to have no effect on blood clotting or cardiovascular disease, whereas oral estrogen has been implicated in problems with both. It is important to note that transdermal estradiol has been shown to not affect blood clotting in the same manner, and has been shown to decrease heart attack risk (Mueck, 2012). This is another reason to preferentially use *topical* estrogen over oral forms.

Data from the Women's Health Initiative alerted the world to the fact that synthetic progestins may increase breast cancer formation (at least when taken orally). Natural progesterone has not been shown to similarly increase breast cancer risk, and there is no reason to suspect that it does, but this question has not been studied directly. This issue is very controversial still and most conventional practitioners are going to tell you with certainty that "progesterone" causes cancer, though they do not understand the distinction between bio-identical and synthetic forms. The studies showing cancer increase are invariably done using a synthetic progestin rather than real progesterone. I encourage you to do your own research into this issue and draw your own conclusions.

Further digression on synthetic hormones

These studies' use of a synthetic "progestins" rather than real bio-identical "progesterone" warrants some further discussion here. Progesterone is a naturally occurring hormone in the human body that has a specific chemical structure. Since it is naturally occurring, it cannot be patented, so it can't be sold for much money. Therefore, the drug companies have made half a dozen or more synthetic progesterone-mimics called progestins that have slight chemical alterations and may be patented because they are not natural compounds. I have mentioned this phenomenon and behavior of pharmaceutical companies repeatedly as it relates to vitamins, herbal compounds and hormones.

These progestins are what you get in birth control pills or injections (Depo-Provera™), implanted birth control devices (Norplant™, Implanon™), and the Mirena™ IUD (intrauterine device). These are what are in Provera™ (often used to stop excessive menstrual bleeding) and Megace™ (a synthetic progestin that dramatically stimulates appetite and promotes weight gain). The differences between progestins and natural progesterone are significant, so it is imperative that everyone understands the difference.

One of the best examples of this difference can be viewed in terms of fertility and pregnancy care. Just a tiny dose of a synthetic progestin absorbed from a birth control pill or patch or exuded from an IUD or contraceptive implant shuts off the pituitary signal for ovulation and creates a temporary infertile state. Conversely, giving women natural progesterone for the two weeks or more leading up to their menses (the *luteal* phase) significantly *increases* their fertility and their chances of having a successful pregnancy (Bjueresten, 2010).

Progesterone is often given in large doses to women with recurrent miscarriage in the first trimester or beyond because they have a poor internal progesterone response, which leads to miscarriages. The word "progesterone" can be translated to mean "for gestation" or "for pregnancy." Conversely, drugs like Provera™ are contraindicated in pregnancy because they cause potentially devastating effects including serious fetal abnormalities. Provera™ is pregnancy category "X", which means it should never be used in pregnancy; while natural progesterone is category "A" or "B", meaning it is believed to be safe – and it is often intentionally used during pregnancy. They are not the same at all!

The synthetic estrogens in birth control pills can cause known, although unusual, problems like benign liver tumors, blood vessel clusters, severe migraines (or *pseudotumor cerebri*), increased blood clots, and other issues. A synthetic estrogen made for pregnant women more than fifty years ago, called DES or "diethylstilbestrol," was advertised as improving pregnancy symptoms and ensuring a healthy pregnancy and delivery, even though there was no evidence that these claims were true. More than a decade after its inception, the product was found to cause infertility, rare cancers (clear cell vaginal cancer), and hormonal abnormalities in offspring.

The story of DES is important not just because it is a poignant example of terrible outcomes from synthetic hormones and subterfuge by pharmaceutical companies but also because of *how* it caused problems. It did not cause any notable problems for the women who took the pills, and it caused no discernible problems in the offspring at the time of birth, other than an increase in undescended testicles or penile abnormalities in boys. The devastating effects of DES were realized in an increase in what was previously a very rare type of cancer in young women, clear cell vaginal cancer.

The other problems increased by DES were fairly common occurrences on their own and were not noticed enough to spark investigation. It was only after years of retrospective review that all the other myriad problems caused by DES were realized (e.g., infertility and testicular failure and cancer in male offspring). Does this scare you? It should. Do we know what sort of effects all the other synthetic hormones in our pharmacies may be causing down the road? No. Is anyone going to look into it? Probably not.

Does anyone still take DES? No, but it took years to get it off the market even after some of these effects were known. We no longer give any synthetic hormones to pregnant mothers, and we are much more careful with every type of pharmaceutical during pregnancy, in no small part because of the experiences with DES and thalidomide, the best-known deformity-causing drug given to pregnant women. The cause of that tragedy was figured out quickly because its effects couldn't be ignored. (Children born missing one or both arms are pretty obvious.)

Did you know that the plasticizing chemical Bisphenol-A (BPA) looks much like DES in terms of chemical structure? BPA was initially created to be marketed and used as an oral estrogenic drug for pregnant women, similarly to DES (Janssen, 2010), and now we know about BPA and its ill effects on people and fetal development. Do you think any of those bad effects came as a surprise to the companies that produced BPA?

I'll get more into this in the chapter on environmental toxins, but for now keep in mind that there are myriad synthetic chemical toxins and some very dangerous ones that have been made to put directly in your mouth are covered by your health insurance plan.

That digression aside, natural progesterone is much safer than estrogen or synthetic hormones. I use it liberally for a wide array of female hormonal issues. I also suggest it as preventive medicine for postmenopausal women in general because of its potential to decrease the risks of osteoporosis and cancers of the uterus or breast.

Testing progesterone

Testing for progesterone deficiency is similar to testing for the other sex steroids in that you can do saliva, blood, or urine assessment. The twenty-four hour urine collection is probably the best overall, but it actually assesses a metabolite of progesterone rather than progesterone itself. I often do saliva testing because it's relatively reliable and far cheaper. Blood testing for progesterone measures only a total amount, including the free fraction and protein-bound fraction, without listing them separately. The free portion may be what we care most about with progesterone, as with estrogen, so many BHRT practitioners tend to favor saliva levels. That said, I do a lot of blood testing for progesterone because it's covered by insurance; and the results are useful the vast majority of the time.

One big problem with salivary hormone testing is that the levels go way up when one is using topical hormone creams for HRT. If a patient is on bio-identical hormone therapy (BHRT) with topical hormones, I think saliva testing should probably be done no less than sixteen hours after the last application, and I like to wait twenty-four hours in many cases. Blood levels will not be so affected by topical BHRT, and neither will the urine tests.

Another oddity of salivary hormone testing related to progesterone involves the testing of salivary *cortisol* levels. Bio-identical progesterone shows up as cortisol on modern saliva tests, causing the cortisol level to appear extremely high. Any woman on progesterone therapy wishing to test their cortisol by saliva panel needs to stop their progesterone for at least a few days before testing. Blood and urine tests for cortisol are not confounded by progesterone in this manner. This is yet another reason why I am generally a little skeptical about salivary hormone assessment.

Since progesterone has so little risk and offers so much potential benefit, I like to see levels at the high end or even above the reference range on lab reports. If a woman has symptoms typical of progesterone deficiency, whether she is at baseline or already on BHRT, and her level isn't at the high end of normal, I'll give her more. This is not true of estrogens, other than perhaps estriol. Once I have a woman on progesterone, I usually don't bother retesting for that hormone since it is easy to tell if she has enough or too much in most cases based on clinical response (i.e., her symptoms).

Repeat testing of a patient on BHRT can often just confuse the practitioner if he or she doesn't understand the inconsistencies of test results.

Forms of progesterone

You can get real, bio-identical progesterone creams right off the shelf at most grocery stores in the "natural food" or "health food" sections. Don't ask the pharmacist because he or she is likely to tell you it requires a prescription. Try to find an over-the-counter cream that is progesterone by itself, not mixed with a bunch of herbs or other ingredients. You should also make sure there is at least 200mg of progesterone per ounce in the cream and that the recommended dose (usually one eighth to one quarter teaspoon) provides 10-20mg of actual progesterone.

It costs a bit more to prescribe progesterone creams at a compounding pharmacy if you have one near you, but this offers a couple of advantages. One is that your insurance may cover it, and the other is the smaller amount of cream you have to apply to get your dose since the prescription can be made ten times more concentrated than the over-the-counter form.

Progesterone can be used orally as well, and sometimes the oral form works better. This is particularly true when it comes to helping with sleep, presumably because of the way oral progesterone is metabolized in the liver. One oral form of progesterone manufactured by a pharmaceutical company is called Prometrium™. It works well for many women but only comes in 100 and 200mg strengths, and many women don't need that much. It is marketed for short-term use to regulate an abnormal menstrual cycle or for use during pregnancy when progesterone dosages should be higher than at other times. A potential problem with this product is the potential for allergy in those allergic to peanuts, since it contains peanut oil. If a lower dose is needed, compounding pharmacies can make oral progesterone into capsules of any strength desired.

Progesterone (and other steroid hormones) can also be made into an oil form, for topical use if you don't like creams; troches that dissolve in your mouth; sublingual drops; vaginal suppositories; or even implanted pellets (which I discourage). We can be very creative in BHRT with a cooperative compounding pharmacist around. Just explain what you want to your provider.

Dosing for progesterone

In most cases, I start with 10 or 20mg of topical progesterone daily if I'm treating a younger woman who is still having menstrual cycles. It's usually 10mg if they have just very mild symptoms, probably 20mg or higher if they want to boost fertility. 20mg is the most common dose I use in my practice, but up to 80mg may be required by some women. For post-menopausal women I generally start at 20mg and may have to go up from there. If it is a woman with very mild symptoms or I'm just using it for preventive health reasons, I may give only 10mg per day.

Most do fine taking it all once daily, but some feel better if they split their dosing to twice per day. Some BHRT educators believe you should rotate the application sites of topical hormones and should take a day off every week or a three-day period off every month to give the body a "break" from the hormones now and then; I have not seen any relevance in these practices myself and am not aware of any scientific research on these issues. Most people forget to take their vitamins or medications or use their hormones now and then anyway, so I don't advise them to skip days intentionally.

My bias is that the lowest effective dose is what should be used. Some other practitioners (and some who are not practitioners but who have formed strong and otherwise educated opinions about BHRT and have achieved national notoriety) push doses of progesterone and other hormones way up because they believe we should be shooting for the levels of hormones seen in very young, healthy women. The rationale for this approach is the desire to try to create a hormonal state like that you had when you were "healthiest". The philosophical problem I have with this idea is that there are a great many physiologic changes that occur with aging, and it may not be desirable to have the hormones of a twenty-something in the body of a sixty-something woman. Another problem is that post-menopausal women usually don't want to start having periods again. Provided they still have a uterus, that's exactly what will happen on these high-dose protocols. In the first year I was doing BHRT, I had plenty of women on high amounts of multiple hormones because I was excited about all the possibilities, and some very unhappy women in their sixties were buying maxi-pads again. I learned my lesson.

Women in Japan and other countries have lived very healthy lives past the age of one hundred without having any menses for their last fifty years or more of life. They don't appear to suffer with symptoms of menopause, presumably because they don't drink so much caffeine, eat so much sugar, carry as much extra fat, or live such stressful lives as we do in our culture. Some studies have shown that these healthy one hundred-year-old Japanese women have significantly higher levels of DHEA, testosterone and other beneficial hormones compared to American women of similar age. Their healthier lifestyle may keep their levels of longevity-promoting hormones higher for much longer (Suzuki, 2001).

Side effects and trouble-shooting

Progesterone has few side effects at the doses I use. If a woman is particularly sensitive or pushes the dose up, she may experience nausea and fatigue in the short term and water retention and weight gain, along with some other more estrogen-like symptoms, in the long term. My wife scooped out way too much progesterone cream a few times and had to lie down for a nap an hour later because of the sedation. You can have your prescription put into a syringe for precise dosing, if using a compounded product. We frequently take advantage of the relaxing and sedating properties of progesterone and use it at bedtime to improve sleep. The oral form tends to cause more sleepiness than topical preparations do.

The nausea side effect bears more discussion because I think there is confusion about morning sickness during pregnancy being related to rising progesterone levels. When a woman becomes pregnant, her levels of estrogen and progesterone are both supposed to rise dramatically, but all the negative symptoms of pregnancy—nausea, weight gain, spider veins and varicose veins, irritability, food cravings, and so on—have been incorrectly blamed on progesterone rather than estrogen. We know that estrogen causes weight gain, blood vessel dilation, headaches, and water retention, and we know that progesterone can cause nausea in non-pregnant women, but many other hormones produced during pregnancy may be causing nausea.

Morning sickness and even the severe repeated vomiting some women experience during pregnancy (*hyperemesis gravidarum*) are more often associated with low levels of progesterone. These symptoms can often be reduced or eliminated with supplemental progesterone in my experience. I usually have women start with 40mg topically or 100mg vaginally or orally and go up from there until their nausea stops. It is completely fine to try this as an experiment since natural progesterone use is safe during pregnancy.

Many women today seem to have recurrent miscarriages because of poor progesterone production after conception, so it is common to prescribe progesterone for maintenance of pregnancy. Morning sickness was once thought to be a sign of a healthy pregnancy, which doesn't make a bit of sense to me because there's no reason that nature would want a healthy woman to be vomiting every day when she needs to be eating more food to nourish a fetus.

Weight gain, water retention, and estrogenic effects are quirks of progesterone that complicate its use over the long term for some women. Progesterone at lower doses seems to counteract the effects of estrogen, but when taken in higher amounts or over long periods at lower doses, it can begin to promote more estrogen-like effects. Some women notice that it accentuates their estrogen even early on and at lower doses; sometimes this is a desired effect, and it may partly explain why progesterone tends to clear hot flashes well for most post-menopausal women.

However, sometimes when we give menopausal women progesterone, their hot flashes get worse, which may mean that they need some estrogen itself or that the progesterone is antagonizing the estrogen they have. In such cases, we often stop the progesterone and use a low dose of estrogen replacement, phasing the progesterone back in a week or so later. This approach usually works well, and you can often wean off the estrogen later. Remember my advice never to use estrogen alone without progesterone to balance out the negative effects, even if it seems like estrogen was what you needed to relieve your symptoms. This is just suggesting a short term of use of estrogen alone; then adding back in some progesterone.

Some women react badly to progesterone even if their levels are low and all their symptoms indicate progesterone deficiency. This problem can be related to a sort of "allergy" or sensitivity to one's own hormones. One can become immunologically or energetically intolerant to one's own hormones, which is most common with estrogen and progesterone. This reaction may have something to do with all the chemicals that mimic those hormones, or perhaps with the sterols in yeast cell walls that look a lot like those hormones.

Because of those last two possibilities, one can often fix this problem through chemical detoxification of the body or eradication of yeast. Endometriosis, a particularly bad problem for an increasing proportion of women in our society, appears to be related to one or both of these issues. Many cases will clear up with yeast eradication and detox, but some won't. It may be possible to desensitize those women with paradoxically bad responses to what should be appropriate progesterone or estrogen replacement to those hormones and correct their symptoms through NAET, sublingual neutralization, bioenergetic devices or other allergy-elimination techniques.

Some of these confusing details about possible responses to progesterone exemplify just how complicated hormone replacement therapy can be. I will be the first to admit that there is no way for me to predict how a given individual is going to respond when I give them any particular hormone, no matter what sort of testing and evaluation I have done. The fact is that biochemical individuality, environmental toxicity, complex interactions between hormones, immunologic reactions to hormones and other factors create so much chaos with our physiology that it is a total crapshoot every time I give someone a hormone. This uncertainty is disturbing to many, but must be embraced philosophically if one is to do a good job with BHRT management. We as practitioners must always keep our eyes and minds open to what is *actually happening* during treatment, rather than "expecting" things too seriously.

Progesterone for men

Unlike estrogen, there are some possible occasions to use progesterone in men. Men with enlarged prostates are the most likely group to benefit from some progesterone because it may help counter the negative effects of estrogen and testosterone metabolites on the prostate tissue. Many integrative and BHRT practitioners use progesterone in this manner, but I was unable to find scientific data on the subject; it is therefore anecdotal and theoretical at this point. Some men get estrogen-dominance symptoms, including varicose veins, leg swelling, and breast enlargement, even though their estrogen and testosterone levels appear normal. These men may benefit from some progesterone as well. Again, there is likely not adequate scientific data on this practice either.

We men all have some progesterone to begin with, so nobody should feel too weird about this. You aren't likely to lose any "manliness" by using some progesterone. Typical dosing is only 2.5 to 5mg topical progesterone daily—maybe as much as 10mg—but you have to go by symptoms and effect because everyone is different.

Pregnenolone

Pregnenolone is a precursor hormone from which all of our other steroid hormones are made. If you look up the biochemistry of steroid hormone synthesis, you will see that they are all initially derived from cholesterol; cholesterol is then converted to pregnenolone, then progesterone or maybe 17-OH progesterone, and then it goes in various directions from there, depending on which gland is making hormones and for what purpose. A large number of our liver enzymes are devoted to making the various steroid hormones.

Supplementing pregnenolone can help significantly improve sleep, memory, and cognitive problems, as demonstrated in some studies. These properties have also been noted for DHEA and allopregnanolone; the trio is referred to collectively as "neurosteroids". It is unclear how these effects occur physiologically, and there is still much to learn about these effects (George, 2006). Problems with sleep, memory and intellectual function are the most common reasons I have used pregnenolone in practice; unfortunately I have never seen any dramatic clinical response myself.

Some integrative and alternative practitioners—primarily those who can't prescribe the hormones they want to use, such as testosterone and cortisol—use pregnenolone in the hope that it will be converted downstream to the hormone the patient really needs. That's a bit like spraying water up in the air and hoping most of it lands in your cup. Pregnenolone taken as a supplement usually becomes adrenal steroids like cortisol and its relatives, but there is really no predicting what it is going to do. I don't use it for this purpose because results are mixed and because I can just directly prescribe the hormone I really want, but sometimes pregnenolone is just the right thing.

I use pregnenolone in an oral form since it is readily available in that form OTC. I'm not sure whether it works well topically because, in this case, you're counting on the liver to turn it into other hormones. I generally start people on 25mg nightly and often go up to 50mg, or as high as 100mg. The benefits may not be seen for a few months, so you have to stick with it if you're going to give pregnenolone a fair shake.

You can test pregnenolone indirectly in saliva, by measuring 17-OH progesterone, which is just "downstream" in the steroid metabolism pathway, or a comprehensive twenty-four-hour urine hormone profile (using pregnanetriol or pregnanediol levels), but I haven't seen a direct test of pregnenolone itself. Therefore, pregnenolone assessment is something of a guess. Pregnenolone is available over the counter (OTC) at health and nutrition stores, and it can be obtained by prescription through a compounding pharmacy. There is no manufactured pharmaceutical form, and if you ask your conventional doctor about it, he or she will most likely not know what you're talking about.

Melatonin

Melatonin is a useful hormone for those with insomnia and those with cancer. It is a simple peptide hormone produced by the pineal gland that helps regulate your sleep cycle and antagonizes cortisol. It normally goes way up at night when you are going to sleep, dropping off by morning when your cortisol starts to surge in preparation for waking up. There is supposed to be a constant dance between cortisol and melatonin, both going up and down every twenty-four hours in opposition to one another to regulate normal sleep.

Some people may have a relative melatonin deficiency, which can be tested with a first-morning urine sample sent to certain specialty labs. The test measures a metabolite of melatonin since we can't measure melatonin directly yet. Some people implicate fluoride in melatonin deficiency since fluoride preferentially accumulates in the pineal gland (Luke, 2001) and may theoretically cause it to harden and stop working to some degree over time. Dr. David Kennedy, DDS has a fascinating audio CD about fluoride that mentions this concern and many others regarding fluoride, available through the Price-Pottenger Nutrition Foundation. Since fluoride has no proven beneficial role in your tissues, I suggest you avoid it.

Unfortunately, many features of modern society can interfere with the normal dance of melatonin and cortisol. Those who work the night shift, soldiers, doctors, fishermen, fire fighters, and others who are expected to stay awake and work more than twenty-four hours straight on a recurring basis have difficulty keeping their melatonin and cortisol straight. Staying awake in this way interferes with the normal circadian rhythm and disturbs normal melatonin and cortisol cycling. Traveling across multiple time zones will do this too, leading to the "jet lag" phenomenon.

Many people in our society have problems falling asleep for reasons other than their jobs, and these people often seek over-the-counter medications, natural remedies, alcohol, or prescription drugs to deal with it. Of course, one should first try the basic sleep hygiene practices, reduce stress, and eliminate caffeine and alcohol. If that doesn't work, I usually have patients try melatonin first.

There are many ineffective, poor-quality melatonin products on the market and no real regulation of it because it's considered a supplement, not a drug. If you buy the cheapest, hard-tablet melatonin preparation you can find, it probably won't work. Instead, try a relatively expensive capsule or sublingual form from a specialty health food or vitamin store. Some think the sublingual forms are the way to go, but I don't think it makes much difference. If the high-quality product works, then you'll know what to expect and can go to a cheaper brand.

Melatonin is not a sedative. It won't make you pass out like you might with alcohol or a prescription drug. Some people do feel quickly sedated from melatonin and even get a hangover effect the next morning, but those responses are in the minority. You should take it an hour or so before you want to go to sleep and be consistent about the time you take it. It may not work immediately. Melatonin is not a sedative but a way to regulate an internal system, so you need to imitate your normal melatonin cycle and use it consistently for a while to see the full benefits.

Take it nightly at the same time every night for at least a couple weeks before you give up on it. If you wait an hour or two and then take another sleep aide to get to sleep, that's fine, but don't give up on the melatonin too quickly. It helps you promote a natural sleep rhythm in most cases, so it is in my opinion superior to artificial drugs and even herbal sleep remedies. Patients often tell me they've tried melatonin and it didn't work; then I find that they don't know how much they took or what type of product it was, other than that it was inexpensive, and they took it for only a couple of nights.

Of course, dosage matters. I generally suggest adults start with 1-3mg orally per night and go up from there, as high as 20mg. Small children should use a liquid preparation and start with .25mg, probably not exceeding 5mg per night. Overdose often leads to mid-night waking and trouble getting back to sleep. Some who overdose have anxiety and panic attacks, heart palpitations, and general distress when they wake up, so watch out for those symptoms. In a child, it may cause them to cry inconsolably in the middle of the night for no apparent reason.

Melatonin doesn't work for everyone, and not everyone can tolerate it. It does not overcome major stress, anxiety, PTSD, heavy metals toxicity, chronic caffeine overuse, or other common problems that lead to sleep disorders. Some people who take it have disturbing dreams or nightmares, wake up with a feeling of panic, or feel hung-over the next morning. Overall, it works reasonably well for most people, and it is relatively harmless. It is particularly beneficial for autistic children; around 75 percent of more than 27,000 parents responding in an Autism Research Institute survey reported good efficacy (unpublished data), making it the product most often reported as helpful in that population.

Multiple clinical and scientific studies suggest melatonin appears to help with various cancers. Good sleep is critical for your immune system, nervous system, and other systems, but melatonin also appears to have direct anticancer properties. Melatonin has been shown to have some therapeutic effect against breast, liver, prostate and various other cancers. Its anticancer effect involves immunomodulating, antioxidative and hematopoiesis (blood cell stimulating) effects among others (Srinivasan, 2008). A recent biochemical study involving breast cancer cells showed melatonin inhibited Notch-1 and epidermal growth factor (EGF)-mediated signaling and decreased mitochondrial membrane potential and cellular energy production within cancer cells, altogether leading to cancer cell death (Margheri, 2012). Melatonin has not been shown to cause harm other than the side effects mentioned above, so the chance that it may improve cancer survival is extremely encouraging and should be common practice among oncologists (but unfortunately it is not yet).

Insulin

It may seem odd to put insulin here with a discussion of hormones, but insulin is a hormone and insulin deficiency—type 1 diabetes at the extreme—is becoming increasingly common. It was very rare in our society a hundred years ago and even when I was in elementary school in the 1970s and 1980s. Now there are diabetic children in just about every classroom, at least in the northern states like Alaska, because type 1 diabetes is generally caused by an autoimmune disease. Autoimmune conditions are much more common in the face of vitamin D deficiency. Type 1 diabetes is increasingly common the farther you are from the tropic zones, and there is a significant amount of epidemiological data suggesting a relationship between vitamin D deficiency in infancy and early childhood and the risk of developing type 1 diabetes.

Many children who develop type 1 diabetes also have gluten sensitivity, autoimmune hypothyroidism (also associated with gluten sensitivity), and high rates of celiac disease. In my opinion, the gluten reaction is likely to be a co-trigger for developing type 1 diabetes. The general theory is that a viral infection triggers the disease, though we aren't sure which viruses or other organisms are involved. (Doctors like to blame many conditions on viruses when we don't know their causes.) It is likely this disease occurs in a child with particular genetics, significant vitamin D deficiency and gluten sensitivity, probably genetically-driven, who then gets a certain viral infection and the whole process is set off to destroy their pancreatic islet cells. The only two factors in this equation that one may control are the vitamin D intake and gluten intake.

If you or your child has type 1 diabetes, it may be worth doing the genetic tests for gluten-sensitivity risk (HLA DQ-2 and DQ-8). The vast majority of those with type 1 diabetes have these same genetic markers, which is probably why the conditions are often seen together. I automatically tell all type 1 diabetics to eliminate gluten. I'm sure we don't know all the causes of type 1 diabetes yet, and people can debate them *ad infinitum*, but I believe that if we keep gluten away from our kids, feed them healthful diets, avoid chemicals, and give them vitamin D from birth we may make type 1 diabetes in pediatrics far less common.

So is insulin an important hormone? Absolutely! Prior to 1922, before insulin was made available as a treatment, the development of type 1 diabetes meant a quick and gruesome certain death. You cannot live long without insulin. That said, while type 1 diabetics must have exogenous insulin, I strongly recommend that they use the *least* amount of insulin required to maintain good blood sugar levels. Insulin is necessary for life but is also very dangerous in both the long and short term.

The job of insulin is to "control" your blood sugar by bringing the glucose level *down* in your blood. Insulin accomplishes this task by causing the glucose in your blood to turn into glycogen within your muscles and liver or fat to be stored in areas all around your body. If someone injects far too large a dose of insulin it will drive the blood glucose level down so low they may have a seizure and then die. The stuff is extremely dangerous.

Dieticians, diabetic educators, and conventional medical practitioners frequently tell diabetics that they can eat whatever they want and then just dose their insulin higher to keep their sugar levels down. ("Go ahead and have some cookies, just use more insulin.") That is terrible advice! Insulin lowers your blood sugar by moving it into cells and out of the bloodstream, but the sugar doesn't just magically "go away". If you eat more sugar than you need, and you have enough insulin on board, that extra energy is stored in your tissues in the form of fat. Insulin takes care of that extra cookie you ate by planting it squarely on your butt or somewhere else.

Is it good for a diabetic to get fat? No! It's even worse for a diabetic than for a non-diabetic person. Telling diabetics to eat what they want and just use more insulin to control it is expediting their death from cardiovascular disease, which is the number-one killer in the United States and far more common in diabetics than in the rest of the population.

You need insulin to live, but the best amount of insulin is the minimum you need to keep your blood sugar levels normal, whether you have a working pancreas or not. Non-diabetics' insulin production and levels go up if they eat sugar or excessive carbs, which results in obesity and increased cardiovascular disease risk in them as well. First control your diet and exercise more, and then you may be able to use the insulin more sparingly. A type 1 diabetic usually notices that when they exercise a lot in a day their blood sugar drops and they need much less insulin, so they can use their insulin requirement as a measure of how good their lifestyle (diet and exercise) is. The average adolescent or adult should need less than 40-50 units of insulin total per day; if he or she needs more than this to maintain normal blood sugar, he or she should reduce carbohydrate intake and increase the activity level.

All that said, if a diabetic does not control his or her blood sugar, blindness, kidney failure, nerve damage, and foot or leg amputations may result. A large meta-analysis including fourteen studies and more than 28,600 patients with type 2 diabetes (which presumes they still produce insulin but have significant insulin resistance, requiring larger amounts of insulin for effect) found that "intensive control" of blood sugar, utilizing more frequent testing of blood sugar and administration of insulin throughout the day, resulted in a small decrease of only borderline statistical significance in these "microvascular" complications (Hemmingsen, 2011). The idea of controlling the blood sugar tightly, with more insulin usage has been the dogma for some time, and is why there is so much emphasis placed on controlling the blood sugar level itself as much as possible, even though that is somewhat short sighted.

I say that idea is short sighted, and possibly misguided, because there is also evidence that attempted to achieve such "tight control" causes more harm than good. That same large meta-analysis found no difference in mortality rate with intensive control, a small but non-significant *increase* in cardiovascular mortality (some theorize that higher insulin levels may accelerate atherosclerosis), and a large (thirty percent) increase in severe hypoglycemia events (Hemmingsen, 2011). These results demonstrate the difficulty of using insulin safely while trying to achieve optimal blood sugar control. This hormone is certainly a double-edged sword and must be used with great care. Type 1 diabetes is a very difficult disease to manage precisely, because the pancreas normally makes moment-to-moment adjustments in insulin secretion, and you cannot replicate that with an insulin pump or injections no matter how many times per day you try to test your blood sugar.

Type 2 diabetics have insulin resistance, and most of these folks make a considerable amount of insulin on their own already, usually far more than a non-diabetic person of equal size and weight. A subset of type 2 diabetics will in fact have impaired insulin production, even "burning out" their pancreas completely over time in some cases. A certain group may also develop the autoimmune antibodies that eventually destroy the pancreatic islet cells and cause a total loss of insulin production. That is the same thing that causes type 1 diabetes, but when it occurs later in life in a person with type 2 diabetes initially, it is termed "latent autoimmune diabetes of adulthood" (LADA). It is possible for a person to have both insulin resistance and insulin deficiency; some authorities call this mixed situation "type 1 1/2 " diabetes. (I think it should be called "type 3" because one plus two is three.)

In terms of treating diseases based on their causes (the title of this section) it is very important to know exactly what is going on with the physiology of a person with diabetes, in terms of insulin production and the status of insulin receptivity. This is easy to determine if you check a fasting insulin level and blood glucose at the same time and then repeat those levels two hours after ingesting a large dose of sugar (the standard is a 75g dose of glucose). In this manner you can see what the person's insulin production and responsiveness looks like; then medical treatment can be prescribed more appropriately. Most type 2 diabetics are obese already, and adding insulin to their therapy usually leads to further weight gain. This is a huge failure if they are actually producing excess insulin already; it's the opposite of good medicine.

The real keys to treating and even curing pure type 2 diabetes are lifestyle control with diet and exercise, weight loss, detoxification of environmental chemicals and heavy metals, and eliminating chronic infections (especially yeast problems and gum disease). Following this type of comprehensive approach, I have seen many of my diabetic patients (type 2) rid themselves of this condition.

Occasionally, elderly or even younger persons have mild insulin deficiency, but not high blood sugar, therefore they do not have type 1 diabetes. Older individuals with this condition may be weak, tired, and thin with very low muscle mass. These symptoms are probably due to a corresponding drop in appetite and food intake, but without adequate insulin one cannot build healthy lean body mass. Small amounts of insulin supplementation may improve health in those individuals, but this scenario is not common, and most with these symptoms may more likely need thyroid, testosterone, DHEA, or growth hormone rather than insulin.

Some integrative physicians use insulin in cancer therapy. They perform what is called "insulin-potentiated chemotherapy", or IPT. This practice involves carefully administering insulin to drop the patient's blood sugar very low followed by small doses of chemotherapy and some glucose. The theory is that, since cancer cells take up glucose much more avidly than normal cells do, you can get the cancer cells to open up their glucose channels dramatically by lowering the blood sugar level. The cancer cells should then suck up the injected glucose at a tremendous rate and also preferentially take up the chemotherapy agents because of the resulting sudden increase in metabolic activity specifically in the cancer cells.

One last note regarding insulin is that it may be important to use products that are biologically identical to human insulin. There are some modified forms of insulin on the market that have become very popular because they have nearly a twenty-four hour duration of action and can therefore be used once per day as a form of general blood sugar control; those with poor or absent insulin production of their own must then also use fast-acting insulin doses with their meals. One popular type of long-acting insulin, insulin glargine, has been the subject of some concern. Some studies have suggested there is increased risk for certain types of cancers in those using insulin glargine. Other research has shown not such effect. Still other studies have shown increases in certain types of cancer, but decreases in other types (all statistically significant findings) with the use of this type of insulin (Ruiter, 2012 and Chang, 2011).

Growth Hormone

I hear a lot about growth hormone these days. It was discussed extensively at my own BHRT training in 2007, portrayed as something of a miraculous anti-aging treatment and cure-all. Growth hormone (GH) plays a large role in metabolism, maintenance and healing of muscle and bone, and promoting improved energy and psychological wellbeing. Those with true growth hormone deficiency in adulthood frequently suffer from intense depression, fatigue, muscle wasting, and prominent abdominal obesity. Their skin wrinkles and sags, arthritis may set in much earlier than usual, and other degenerative conditions may occur.

If you have this constellation of symptoms, it may be reasonable check the status of your growth hormone production. One caveat here is that you can't measure growth hormone (GH) directly because the levels are very unreliable, as GH doesn't last long in serum and it fluctuates throughout the day. GH levels are generally highest at night, which is when children usually experience their "growing pains." Instead of measuring GH directly, we measure insulin-like growth factor type 1 (IGF-1), which is the major downstream hormone/metabolite stimulated by GH. IGF-1 levels are much more constant in the blood and they provide a better overall assessment of GH status.

If your IGF-1 is low, your insurance may still not agree to pay for GH replacement therapy. Insurance companies usually demand to see a level that is actually lower than that associated with symptom onset, and they typically demand that you fail a stimulation test of some sort, such as the *insulin tolerance test*. In my opinion, this requirement is just a hurdle the insurance companies put in your way to ensure you don't get coverage for the treatment. Even if you reach an adequate GH level during the stimulation test, that doesn't help you produce more GH on your own. That would just suggest that the real problem was a poor signal from your hypothalamus, rather than pituitary failure. You still need GH replacement to ultimately improve your condition. These practices are consistent with the U.S. Endocrine Society's current practice guideline (as of 2012) regarding growth hormone replacement in adults. I've read their guidelines, and this requirement still makes no sense to me.

I have had two patients with low GH levels, and both of their insurance companies refused to pay for growth hormone. Why do they make it so difficult to get GH? Insurance companies don't want to pay for growth hormone because it is so expensive, costing more than $500 per month— and closer to $1000 if you need a larger dose. Wealthy people who want to combat the effects of aging at any cost can use some GH even if they don't need it, because they can afford it, while those of lesser means who may need it just to achieve normal health can't get it. I can't say that's wrong, just a bummer for those who really need it and can't meet the proper criteria.

There is not much risk associated with physiologic dosing of growth hormone, but it can certainly cause some side effects. Most adverse effects are the result of salt and water retention caused by GH; symptoms include joint swelling and pain, leg swelling, headaches and elevated blood pressure. GH administration can also cause dangerous intracranial hypertension, and leads to type 2 diabetes in some because it causes impaired glucose tolerance. There has been some worry about cancer incidence increasing, but that fear has not been substantiated by the literature. The U.S. Endocrine Society suggests avoiding the use of GH in those with active cancers just as a precaution, though they admit the available research shows no increased risk of new cancer occurrence.

I personally don't think GH therapy is all it's cracked up to be by its proprietors. Most people are not going to see much benefit from its use, unless they do have severe deficiency. Testosterone has almost all the same effects in the body as GH in terms of promoting optimal wellness and anti-aging, without the relatively high risk of side effects seen with GH; it also tends to promote better GH production. Therefore, I have very rarely ever needed to give anyone growth hormone; I just prescribe testosterone first. If a patient still had symptoms of decline or depression after trying testosterone, I would consider whether GH replacement were warranted. After all, if a person has a true GH deficiency, then replacement with GH is the only treatment that will address their symptoms.

If you do need it or if you are wealthy enough to afford GH treatment as a preventive, anti-aging therapy, you should find someone trained in bio-identical hormone therapy, anti-aging medicine, or functional endocrinology. Most conventional endocrinologists will berate you or look at you like you're crazy for asking—unless, of course, you are in bad shape with a severe deficiency.

You also should know that using real growth hormone entails giving yourself intramuscular injections at home every night at first and then several nights per week. It is not for those with a fear of needles! You may not notice an improvement for a while, so you have to be willing to keep up with the injections despite the apparent lack of immediate results. It's not for everyone.

The numerous prescription forms of "human growth hormone", or HGH, on the market are all biologically engineered from recombinant DNA technologies in bacterial cultures; there are no human-derived GH products since cadaveric pituitary gland extracts were banned around 1985. These expensive prescription products are the only things that work. There are many nutritional supplement products out there today claiming to be "growth hormone" or "HGH", coming in pill or cream form. These are not real growth hormone, or anywhere near it; they are at best what we term "secretagogues" for GH.

Secretagogues are substances that promote increased internal secretion of growth hormone from your own pituitary. These products typically include a compilation of vitamins, minerals, amino acids, herbs, bovine colostrum, or other ingredients. They may improve symptoms through their nutritional benefits and perhaps physiologic stimulation of internal hormone systems on some level. However, if you have true GH deficiency, these products are extremely unlikely to work for you. If you have used one of these products and felt some sort of positive results I suggest you look at the label and find a cheaper product or combination of products with the same ingredients that isn't marketed as "HGH" or HGH-promoting. If you find one that truly *raises your IGF-1 level*, please let me know.

HCG

You may have heard of using "HCG", which stands for *human chorionic gonadotropin*, for weight loss. Alternatively, that acronym may sound familiar because it is the hormone we measure in the urine or blood when identifying pregnancy. This is because HCG is a hormone that is typically only made by the placenta.

HCG appears to have many different effects on metabolism that are helpful in losing body fat. It seems to help effectively burn off the fat from all that storage tissue parked on your belly, thighs, and butt. The mechanisms of this have not been clearly worked out, but it is perhaps because of some direct effects on the fat cells as well as the HCG's increasing your tissues' sensitivity to or production of other hormones such as thyroid, cortisol, DHEA, estrogen and testosterone. The overall effect is that your body finally starts using that fat it worked so hard to store and never seems to want to tap into.

The protocol for losing weight with HCG involves administering the hormone every day via a daily injection, a twice-daily sublingual solution or pellets, topical creams, or possibly other forms. The other part of the weight loss protocol is to restrict your diet so your body is forced to use your stored fat for its energy. You are not allowed any sugar or starches to speak of, and most need to reduce their daily calories to just 500 or so total per day. That is very restrictive, of course, and critics say that you lose weight because you're starving yourself. If you've ever tried to starve yourself like this, you know that you lose muscle tissue just as quickly or quicker than you lose fat when you cut your calorie intake down, and that's not the goal.

The theory is that if you drastically cut your calorie intake in this manner while using HCG, you don't lose the muscle tissue because the body is preferentially utilizing stored fat for energy and is actively promoting the maintenance of your lean body mass. When it works properly, people feel very good and energetic and experience little hunger, unless they try to exercise.

There are not many scientific studies on using HCG in this manner, with a restrictive diet of such magnitude, and the ones that have been published are primarily negative or equivocal. One such study looked at twenty women receiving HCG and twenty getting placebo, with all following a low calorie diet. The authors reported finding no difference in total weight loss, psychological profile, body circumference or hunger level between the two groups. They concluded there was no rationale for the use of HCG injections in the treatment of obesity (Bosch, 1990). That study was out of South Africa, it is not clear whether they evaluated differences in body composition (i.e. whether participants lost fat or muscle) throughout the study, nor is it clear what the sources of funding were for the study. I also don't know what dose or product they were using, because only the abstract is available on PubMed.

Earlier studies also showed "no benefit" versus placebo when using HCG for weight loss by the protocol popularized by Dr. Simeons, which is the same protocol commonly used today. A study from the 1970's published identical weight loss and no significant difference in mood, hunger or body measurements in those using HCG compared to those getting placebo on the same diet (Greenway, 1977). These studies are surprising to me, and I'm glad I heard of them *after* I started using the HCG diet regimen with patients myself, so I didn't have a jaded negative opinion of the protocol. I have seen extremely good success overall using this regimen with over three hundred patients now. My experience causes me to doubt the credibility of those published "negative" studies.

I could find only one recent study in PubMed, that being the only one listed published since the 1990 study, regarding the HCG diet program. This study tracked only nine patients and did not compare HCG to placebo; it is therefore scientifically "lame". The participants did see drastic improvements in their cholesterol profiles, total body weight, body fat, basal metabolic rate (odd for people on a low calorie diet), and the number of stem cells in circulation. Most participants lost between ten and twenty *percent* (not pounds) of their total body weight by eighty days (Mikirova, 2011). The results of this study are extremely impressive and imply there is some meaningful physiological effect here, even if there was no placebo group. Hopefully larger and better studies will be forthcoming.

There was a study done with middle-aged men with relative testosterone deficiency, using HCG injections without a restrictive diet, that demonstrated a loss of 1kg body fat and gain of 2kg lean body mass over a three-month period. There was no caloric restriction or special diet. The participants in this study (forty total) were injecting either 5000iu of HCG (which is a lot more than we use with the modern weight loss regimen) or placebo twice per week. Participants receiving HCG experienced significant increases in testosterone and estradiol levels (Liu, 2002). This is a positive change though not nearly as dramatic as the loss of fat we see when the HCG is combined with a low-calorie, no-sugar diet.

It is well known that HCG increases testicular or ovarian function and hormone production, which likely explains some of the above findings. Men using testosterone have taken advantage of this fact for many years, using HCG as an adjunctive treatment in their HRT regimen to retain testicular size and function as well as fertility while on testosterone replacement. Typical dosing regimens include 500-600iu injected subcutaneously every two to three days. I have done this myself three separate times and seen it work first hand. HCG is clearly a powerful tool.

HCG for weight loss has become a popular therapy across the country, and there is a good deal of "information" about it online. However, there is a lot of "old" information about HCG out there, and people using it have learned a lot more about HCG in clinical practice these last few years. There are many weight loss clinics or places calling themselves "HCG" clinics because of the current interest. This tends to feed into the typical quick-fix mentality of our population too much in my opinion. HCG-based protocols for rapid weight loss are indeed effective, but if you don't address the underlying metabolic problem people have and they go back to eating badly after their forty days of HCG are past they are just going to regain all of their weight. This tool is best used as just a part of a comprehensive medical approach to correcting obesity and in conjunction with permanent changes in diet and lifestyle.

HCG is available online from many different sources, but some of those are bogus, so you have to be careful. There have also been places selling "homeopathic HCG" on the internet and from private shops or supplement stores all over the place. This is not real HCG, which may only be obtained with a prescription. The FDA has been shutting down the OTC sale of this so-called homeopathic HCG in recent years, so that may no longer be available. If you want to be safe, find a practitioner with experience in HCG and ask him or her to prescribe or provide pharmaceutical grade HCG for you.

I advise that people have their thyroids thoroughly evaluated before starting and take antifungals to eliminate any excessive yeast issues at the beginning of the program, as those two concerns are the most frequent barriers to success with HCG that I have encountered. Since HCG is available from pharmacies, there is FDA-approved indication for it. The brands Pregnyl™, Novarel™, and Ovidrel™ are available at the pharmacy— all are injected forms—the FDA indication for which is stimulation of fertility in women who are trying to conceive. It is the same HCG substance we use for weight loss, but the entire 10,000 units is given in a single dose for fertility, whereas we stretch the 10,000 units out over the course of forty days for weight loss. Sublingual solutions are available through compounding pharmacies around the country.

HCG is also used by men on testosterone replacement to resume fertility or restore testicular size and function. HCG imitates the pituitary gland signals that trigger testosterone and sperm production from the testicle (those same pituitary hormones stimulate ovulation in women). This promotes internal testosterone production and sperm generation in men on HRT. Many men also report that adding HCG to their testosterone regimen makes them feel better and more stable emotionally. Injection of 500-600 units every two to three days should have the desired effect.

CHAPTER 4 – ENVIRONMENTAL TOXICITY

Introduction

Environmental toxicity is such a large topic that I cannot possibly cover in one chapter all the different types of environmental chemicals and toxins you may encounter. I do not have the space here to review the physiological effects of individual toxins or even begin to list the more than eighty thousand artificial chemicals we have to worry about in industrialized America. I can't describe the thousands of ways you may come into contact with chemicals and toxins in your environment from day to day.

What I do try to do is to give you a sense of the overall problem, scare you, give you some specific areas of concern regarding categories of toxins and where they are most encountered, review some of the common physiological effects and symptoms of chemical toxicity to watch for, and most important, offer some advice about how to detoxify yourself and treat chemical illness or other biological toxicity.

If you want more information on this topic, there are a great many books written on the subject; you can also check out the EPA website if you want the watered-down, corporate-influenced version.

At least the problem is not going totally unnoticed by the current administration. President Obama's Cancer Panel issued a press statement in spring 2010 stating that the scope of environmentally induced cancer is grossly underestimated in our country and that exposure to carcinogenic chemicals is widespread. The report included the need to move toward removal of toxic substances from our everyday environments, but we'll have to wait and see if any action comes of this.

Categories of environmental toxins

We often think of chemicals and artificial substances as the only major toxins of concern in human health, but there are many naturally occurring toxins as well, and some of them are bigger problems than the man-made chemicals. Toxic elements like heavy metals and toxic halides, biological substances like mold and bacterial toxins, ozone, and forms of toxic energy all bear mentioning.

Heavy metals

The EPA website states that the top three greatest environmental health concerns in terms of toxins are the heavy metals arsenic, lead, and mercury. Other toxic metals in the top ten include cadmium, exposure to which is on the increase in recent years. The EPA information describes the extensive array of symptoms exposure to each of these metals may cause, the numerous sources of exposure, and the scope of long-term disease that can result from chronic exposure. Unfortunately, the website then says, "If you think you may have a problem with this, go see your doctor," but unfortunately there is a 90–95 percent chance your doctor won't have a clue about this aspect of health and medicine.

Cadmium is commonly found in cigarette smoke, in many paints, batteries and household items. There was major concern about the lead-based paints used on children's toys made in China in 2009, so the following year the Chinese manufacturers switched out much of the lead for cadmium, but cadmium is, pound for pound, even more toxic than lead (based on the accepted cutoff for toxicity on urine excretion tests). Cadmium is present in significant amounts in some fish and seafood, but most of the total dietary exposure in American comes from vegetables, whole grains and potatoes collectively. It is more likely that industrial exposures or other, more concentrated, exposures may be dangerous.

Biochemically there is evidence that cadmium contributes to breast cancer formation, because it has estrogen-like activity on breast tissue, but a recent large epidemiological study in America did not show any relationship between dietary intake of cadmium (from grains, potatoes and vegetables) and risk of invasive breast cancer (Adams, 2012). A study from around the same time frame out of Sweden however, did suggest a relationship between dietary cadmium intake and overall breast cancer risk. The relative risk increase was around 25% for estrogen receptor (ER)-positive breast cancers, but there was no observed risk of increase in ER-negative tumors. This was a much larger, prospective study, and they looked primarily at other food sources than those evaluated in the American study. In fact, the Swedish study evaluated intake from vegetables and grains separately and found that those sources actually mitigated the risk somewhat, presumably because those foods contain healthy nutrients, which help the body eliminate the naturally occurring cadmium within them (Julin, 2012). The foods of concern are apparently the farmed seafoods and processed foods that have "ubiquitous contamination" with cadmium according to the Swedish study.

Heavy metals exposures are ubiquitous for all of us in every-day life. I find some amount of at least five different toxic metals in everyone I test, but generally at nontoxic levels. You are likely to encounter tin and aluminum in canned foods and beverages, and antimony is present in flame-retardant chemicals and certain industrial processes. There are many other less common metals to which you may be exposed, but lead and mercury are the ones I find most frequently in the people I test. Entire books are written on just one toxic metal, so I cannot go into detail about each of them, but I would like to elaborate on a few issues concerning these particular common metals and metals toxicology in general to help steer you in the right direction.

Lead and mercury are everywhere in our environment, thanks largely to the burning of fossil fuels. Automobile (diesel engines) and machine exhaust continues to spew lead into the environment, and hundreds of thousands of tons of mercury per year are released into our atmosphere from the burning of coal to produce electricity. There is also massive atmospheric mercury generated by forest fires, since trees absorb much of what is in the air from other sources. You get toxic metals with each breath. From there, the metals end up in our oceans, where they get into the food chain. They also end up in ground water and in plants grown in the soil.

Compact fluorescent light bulbs each contain a small amount of mercury, and gum wrappers, batteries and other common objects contain lead, as does that metallic-looking liner bag inside boxed wine. Those who work with metal, metal parts, machinery, oils, and other industrial solvents are often exposed to high amounts of lead and other metals. Almost all paint still contains toxic metals; even if the lead is now lower, cadmium has largely taken its place. Drinking water, from underground wells, is a major source of exposure to arsenic; it is important to know the trends in your region and have your own well water tested, because the levels vary tremendously from place to place.

Using solder (working with stained glass is particularly bad) or welding causes extensive exposure, and the largest lead levels I've seen have been in people who load their own ammunition or shoot guns frequently. In the commercial production of chicken in America the birds are given drugs containing arsenic (e.g. roxarsone) for the last six weeks or so because it causes them to fatten up dramatically. Dr. Oz got in big trouble with the apple juice industry for announcing that there were worrisome levels of arsenic found in apple juice samples; but the levels in chicken are more concerning in my opinion.

Arsenic interferes with cellular energy production and can cause acute toxicity leading to multi-system organ failure and rapid death from massive exposures. Chronic, lower level exposure to inorganic arsenic, most commonly from drinking water, has long been known to contribute to the formation of a wide array of cancers. Arsenic has also been shown to cause chronic toxicity and disease to various other tissues. We now know that inorganic arsenic contributes to obesity and type 2 diabetes in humans as well (Del Razo, 2011).

The argument with the chicken treatment is that the arsenic used is in an "organic" form (meaning it is combined with another molecule that is carbon based). There are many forms of arsenic in the environment and the organoarsenic forms are not thought to be toxic. Shrimp contains very high levels of organoarsenic for example, but more than 90% of that ingested arsenic can be measured coming right out in your urine the day after you eat the shrimp; it is therefore not accumulated in this form and is not harmful. A recent study showed that the arsenic given to chickens in those drugs converts at some rate to inorganic arsenic, which is toxic, and accumulates in their feathers and other tissues. This would not be a problem, except for the fact those chicken feathers and other parts are later ground up and fed to livestock animals that we also eat. The toxic arsenic may therefore become a problem in our food supply after all (Nachman, 2012). This type of contamination problem is one reason why I continually preach the consumption of only wild or pure organic animal foods in particular.

Wild animals are not completely safe to eat on this planet any more either however. I once did the math on a standard can of tuna (which is always wild), based on the typical mercury content and allowable daily levels of mercury intake posted by the EPA, and calculated that there is a toxic dose of mercury in one typical tuna can for anyone who weighs less than 190 pounds. Of course, let's not forget that dentists have been stuffing mercury, inarguably one of the most toxic substances on the planet, into our teeth for many decades now. Many dentists practicing today still use mercury amalgams and fervently deny any possible harm coming from them. Prior scientific studies have demonstrated very clearly that the mercury from amalgam fillings vaporizes on a constant basis, is swallowed and then conjugated into organic mercury compounds by gut organisms, and eventually deposits into tissues all over the body. Recent study has shown significantly lower thyroid hormone levels in women with greater numbers of mercury fillings (Ursinyova, 2012).

In short, everyone is at risk from toxic metals, some populations more than others. Whether you think you've been exposed or not, you have been exposed because you breathe, drink, and eat on this planet. I find elevated levels of toxic metals in people who have no identifiable significant exposure. Many of these people may have grown up in a house with lead pipes and/or lead paint, but it seems that most did not. The reasons for having an elevated heavy metals burden can be very specific to the individual, perhaps lying in their genetic ability to detoxify heavy metals. Lead, mercury, and other metals can stay in the body (especially the brain, because they tend to be fat-soluble) for several decades, and these toxins never decline significantly in some people because they continue to accumulate through ongoing low-level exposure. Your genetic or epigenetic potential for detoxification of metals may be an important factor.

Past studies of mercury levels in the hair found that autistic children had very low levels of mercury compared to "normal" control children; but more recent research has not shown this difference (Albizzati, 2012). Random urinary levels of mercury have also not been shown to be different between autistic children and control children without autistic disorders (Wright, 2012). Upon *provoked* urine metals testing, however, autistic children are often found to have significantly higher levels of mercury, lead and other toxic metals in their urine; and chelation therapy to remove toxic metals has been at least somewhat helpful in improving autistic symptoms for roughly 75% of children with autism spectrum disorders (unpublished Autism Research Institute survey of over 27,000 parents). This reflects an elevated body burden resulting from poor excretion and detoxification of heavy metals. Current research has correlated the elevated burden of toxic metals such as arsenic, mercury, copper and iron, with altered metabolism and biochemistry in autistic children with resulting oxidative stress, altered energy metabolism, autonomic nervous system dysfunction and other physiological derangements (Obrenovich, 2011).

These results suggest that poor heavy-metal detoxification physiology is a major risk factor for the development of autistic spectrum disorders and other conditions related to metal toxicity. While *exposure* may be similar for all children, there are vast differences in disease *susceptibility* related to that exposure. The vast majority of children today appear to handle the current environmental burden of heavy metals and other toxins without becoming autistic, but as the total load of molecular poisons mounts in our world more and more of our children are becoming affected in some way. As of spring 2012 the national news reported one in eighty-eight American children have autism. The number is even worse for boys as a subgroup, with their autism rate being one out of about fifty-four. The numbers are even worse in the United Kingdom, which industrialized a generation earlier than North America.

Autistic spectrum disorders seem to encompass a fairly broad array of problems, but there are many more developmental, neuropsychological, immunological and otherwise physiological problems increasing in our children as a result of, at least in part, these accumulating toxins. Some of these other conditions appear as low muscle tone, developmental delay, colic, constant irritability, reflux, apnea or SIDS, poor growth, frequent illness, learning disabilities, ADD/ADHD, visual integration issues, Asperger's syndrome (a form of autism), anger problems and oppositional behavior, and many other symptoms in infants and children, as well as some adults. The nervous system and immune system are particularly vulnerable to metals like lead, mercury and arsenic. The old expression "mad as a hatter" is a reference to mercury toxicity incurred by those who worked with felt making hats.

I usually test for heavy metals if an adult has any neurological problem at all, high blood pressure, psychiatric or psychological disturbance (even if it runs in the family since heavy metal retention problems may be genetic), hormonal deficiencies or imbalance without explanation, chronic fatigue syndrome, unexplained chronic pain problems, unusual vision problems (particularly common with mercury, as it has a predilection for the visual cortex of the brain), chronic rashes, multiple allergies, chemical sensitivities, cardiovascular disease, type 2 diabetes, lupus or rheumatoid arthritis and other complex autoimmune diseases, or some other conditions. In addition, if you have an unexplained condition, you should be tested for heavy metal toxicity.

Testing is a major area of contention between integrative and conventional practitioners. Conventional toxicology training still focuses on testing *blood* levels of metals like lead and mercury. Early investigations into metal toxicity used blood levels and found relevant results because the patients in question were being exposed all the time (e.g., children living in houses with lead pipes and paint at a time when automobiles spewed out tons of lead from leaded gasoline). Blood levels are certainly very useful for ongoing monitoring of those with known exposure, such as in mechanics, welders or mine workers, because blood levels rise for some time after exposure.

The problem is that blood levels of metals and many other toxins stay elevated only for a few weeks at best before the body stashes the toxic stuff away into tissues, rather than allow the poison to circulate around. Blood levels of lead the day after a child eats some paint chips will show high readings, but blood levels in the same child a month later may show no lead in the blood at all. However, just because metals leave the bloodstream doesn't mean they have left the body completely and are no longer a threat to health. Quite to the contrary, that lead will have been deposited in the brain, bones, kidneys and many other tissues.

We know now that toxic metals stick around for many decades; and with the ongoing exposure in the modern world, the body burden of heavy metals will continue to go up and up rather than down in susceptible individuals. To find out if chronic retention and toxicity of heavy metals is a problem, you have to "pull" some of the metals back into circulation and measure what comes out in the urine. I tell patients to avoid any sources of potential exposure to the common metals (e.g. tuna and other predatory fish, seafood, herbal medicines, boxed wine) for the week prior to doing their test. I just don't want the test results to be confounded by recent exposure; I want it to reflect long-term accumulation as much as possible. Hair analysis also only reflects fairly recent heavy metals exposure. Hair is also sort of an excretory tissue or substance, and there is great variability in how efficiently a given individual eliminates toxic metals through the hair; for those reasons, hair analysis is quite useless in my opinion and it can actually give you the completely wrong idea about one's toxic metals status.

As an aside, lead is of particular concern in women after menopause. Bone is a major source of "storage" for accumulate lead in the body, and most menopausal women will have some lead measurable even via blood testing as their bones are gradually breaking down. Lead toxicity is associated with increased risk of cardiovascular and neurological problems as well as other degenerative conditions. Risks of these conditions go up dramatically for women after menopause, and part of that increase could be related to this release of lead into the body once again. Also, lead is a very heavy and dense element; it is conceivable that this loss of lead from bone contributes to the loss of bone density seen after menopause. Since lead certainly doesn't make bone any stronger, this loss of density does not likely increase the risk for fractures as much as it would appear.

The standard among integrative practitioners is to give a patient some sort of chelation drug (e.g., DMSA, DMPS, EDTA) and then collect their urine for some length of time (usually about six hours). There are many different options for how to do this, and the choice of chelation substance depends upon which metals you are looking for. This whole field of medicine is its own subspecialty, so you need to find someone with modern training in this area. I repeatedly run into conflict with other providers who don't "believe in" provoked urine testing for heavy metals and claim that blood testing is the standard. However, any reasonable person to whom I explain the physiology seems to understand it right off. It's just another example of how those who are mired in medical dogma can't see past their blinders. The real problem with provoked testing is there are no published normal values or reference ranges in the literature. The reference ranges for urinary metals

Anyone with persistent medical complaints of almost any kind, psychological or psychiatric issues (including insomnia or extreme opposition in children), high blood pressure, recurrent infections, electromagnetic sensitivity, cardiovascular disease, metabolic syndrome or diabetes, allergies, or autoimmune disease of any kind should have his or her heavy metals tested. If done by blood testing, the results will be normal in the vast majority of cases and the diagnosis will be missed. However, it is nice to have a normal blood level in conjunction with provoked urine testing, because that normal blood level helps to rule-out recent exposure as the explanation for elevated urine collection levels. Many integrative practitioners do pre- and post-provocation urine testing in order to make this distinction as well. This is quite complicated, and I strongly suggest that one seek out a practitioner with modern understanding and practice in metals toxicology if they wish to explore this for themselves.

Toxic halides

The halides are one of the vertical columns in the periodic table of elements, and a couple of them—iodine and chloride—are essential nutrients. The larger ones are the essential elements, while the smaller ones (bromine and fluoride) bind to receptors for iodine and chlorine and obstruct normal physiology in various ways. Excessive exposure to fluoride has been proven to cause arthritis and sclerosis of the bone, severe damage to the enamel of teeth called "dental fluorosis", increased bone fractures, gastrointestinal bleeding (all noted as the "adverse effects" in my ePocrates drug database) and possibly neurological toxicity. Fluoride is pregnancy category "C", which means it has been shown to cause fetal harm in animal studies. Sounds like really great stuff, right? They should put it in the water!

A Harvard-based study showed a more than 540 percent increased rate of bone cancer (osteosarcoma) in boys exposed to fluoride through childhood (DeNoon, 2006), and fluoride is used in laboratory study to induce cancerous transformation in human cell cultures. One study of human populations in India showed that people living in regions with 2-3 times the usual amount of fluoride (typical for how our cities fluoridate their water) in their drinking water had correspondingly 2-3 times the rate of genetic mutation noted in their cellular DNA (Sheth, 1994). There is therefore a good possibility that fluoride contributes to other cancers, such as thyroid and breast cancers, since those tissues are somewhat dependent on iodine, but studies have not yet to my knowledge been done on this possibility.

Poison control centers receive thousands of calls every year about fluoride ingestion from toothpaste. It is a known cellular poison and toxic substance, and yet the authorities in the United States still want you to believe you need this poison for proper dental health. I encourage everyone interested in the dental health argument regarding fluoride to go the IAOMT (the International Academy of Oral Medicine and Toxicology) website and read their position paper on fluoride. It catalogs a great deal of the scientific research on fluoride and clearly states the argument against using fluoride in humans for any reason at all. You can also go to websites such www.fluoridealert.org and read the information posted by the Fluoride Action Network.

Toothpaste as a source is obvious, and you can easily find non-fluoridated toothpaste. Other common sources include fluoride-treated water supplies in many cities, under the argument that fluoride is good for your teeth. The reality is that aluminum and other mineral industries produce a waste product that is high in fluoride that is then sold to municipal water treatment centers for water treatment. This substance also contains mercury and other toxic metals, strong acids that have been known to leach lead from pipes, and who knows what else. This is the form of fluoridation used 90 percent of the time in our city water supplies, along with chlorine and other toxins. (Chloride in salt form is beneficial, but chlorine gas will kill you quickly.)

Most of Europe stopped fluoridating water a long time ago because they realized the toxicity and lack of benefit. They have gone largely to ozone systems, which is very clean and much safer for purifying water. I believe our country still uses water fluoridation because we tend to be controlled by the whims of industry; if the mining operations had to pay for proper disposal of fluoride rather than selling it to put into water, they would lose a great deal of money. All of this is of course my own opinion; while it is shared by many others, one could certainly write it off as conspiracy theory.

Our EPA set the upper limit in water at 4ppm in 1986, even against a great deal of uproar from the scientific community. A 2006 report of the US National Research Council suggested dramatically lowering the limit, but the EPA made no such change. In 2011 the Health and Human Services Department suggested lowering the limit to only 0.7ppm, but the EPA has not changed the enforceable standard. The EPA does have a lower "suggested" standard of only 2ppm, which is set so as to reduce rates of dental fluorosis in children. Widely published data suggests that one in six people will still suffer some dental fluorosis at this level (even posted on the EPA's own website!). I think the best current book on this topic is *The Case Against Fluoride*, by Paul Connett, PhD; anyone interested in fighting their local government on water fluoridation should acquire this book and use its references in their argument.

Hopefully fluoride will be completely removed from our water supplies at some point; I encourage you all to take whatever action you can on a local level to help achieve this goal. In the meantime, I contend that you should not drink fluoridated water or treated city water if you can avoid it. Get a good water purification system that utilizes reverse osmosis or a distillation system, and watch out for fluoride in manufactured beverages and processed foods. Every drink you buy in a bottle, can, or box is comprised mostly of water that had to come from somewhere, and that somewhere is often a city water supply.

Many store-bought drinks, including alcohol, have very high levels of fluoride. The main pesticide used to grow grapes for wine and grape juice is sodium fluoride. Baby foods with chicken have very high levels also because the bones of the chicken contain lots of fluoride, and the bones are partially pureed in the food. Tea, referring to the actual tea tree *Camellia sinensis*, has a major affinity for fluoride uptake into its trunk, limbs and leaves. Tea drinkers need to be aware there are significant levels of fluoride in nonorganic tea; the levels in black tea are quite a bit higher than in green tea, and as much as ten times greater than levels in white tea (the youngest leaves). There are far lower levels of fluoride in herbal teas made from other plants (until you brew it in city water that is fluoridated). Adults drinking five cups of nonorganic black tea daily may get up to three times the safe upper limit of fluoride consumption for the day (Malinowska, 2008). For these reasons it is very important to drink only organic tea.

The toxicity of fluoride is depends on body weight. Babies have an all-liquid diet, and babies on formula get a lot of tap water, much more than adults based on their body weight. In a typical city with fluoridated water, it is easy for an infant to get a harmful dose of fluoride every day when they're on formula. The current "enforceable" standard for fluoride in water supplies is a max of 4mg per liter of water. A liter is roughly 33.3 ounces of water; this amount if frequently consumed by infants on formula (four eight-ounce bottles in a day is 32 ounces). Many adults will get only two or three liters of water per day themselves, though they weigh easily six to ten times more than a typical infant. Therefore, the infant gets proportionally much more fluoride.

It is also important to note that fluoride is used in a number of prescription medications, from Prozac™ to asthma inhalers. My last comment on fluoride is regarding "perfluorinated compounds," or PFC's. These are the "non-stick" chemicals used in such household goods as nonstick cookware (e.g. Teflon©), carpets, furniture, and Scotch Guard™. These chemicals are highly toxic, causing reproductive toxicity, neurotoxicity and liver toxicity; some specific PFC's are considered likely carcinogens as well (Genuis, 2010). Unfortunately the body doesn't clear them well at all; they aren't even cleared effectively by sweating, one of our most common detoxification methods.

Less is known about the effects of bromine than those of fluoride because bromine hasn't been studied as much. We know bromine works in hot tubs to kill germs. (I for one can't breathe very well around the stuff.) Bromine binds in your cells where iodine should be and gets in the way, inhibiting normal iodine-mediated function. Some are concerned this may lead to increased rates of thyroid disease, thyroid and breast cancers and possibly other health problems; but there is no science to support these theories that I could find.

Bromine has been used in a number of inhaled and pill-form

medications and is present in significant amounts in some manufactured beverages. Bromine has been used in place of iodine as a dough conditioner in virtually all commercial flours (e.g., bread, crackers, cookies) since the 1970s, which may be responsible for the large amount of bromine exposure in our population as a whole. Apparently European countries removed bromine for their manufactured flours in the 1990's, but I am not aware of their publicized reasons for doing this. If you are concerned you can purchase non-brominated flour to bake your own products, but it is not always easy to find. One position would be to say that, like fluorine, bromine has no biological role in our bodies; and until there is proper proof of safety, perhaps we shouldn't be consuming either one.

Plant toxins

We likely consume many natural biological toxic compounds in plants regularly. They contribute to your *total load* of toxicity and can be reduced by general detoxification methods.

Some special cases I want to mention in this category are those that people inflict upon themselves. Caffeine is a powerful stimulant derived from plants that causes well-known signs of toxicity, including agitation, tremors, tachycardia, diarrhea, and sweating. Theophylline is a chemical found in tea that has similar properties to caffeine, it has been used for a long time as a prescription drug in the treatment of asthma or other chronic pulmonary disease; it has similar toxicity to caffeine and can cause seizures with overdose in some. Opium, morphine, and heroine are long-used substances derived from poppy seeds. They can be used therapeutically for pain control, but they also cause toxicity and death from overdose.

These are some obvious examples of plant-derived toxins. There is also cyanide in certain plant foods such as almonds, walnuts and cassava root (tapioca flour). There are many other naturally-occurring substances in plants that cause mild toxicity to the liver or other organs, have adverse effects on reproduction or other physiological processes. Eating healthy whole foods generally provides one with the healthy nutrients needed to aid detoxification of these plant toxins.

Mold and fungal toxins

Mold is a significant problem all over our country, especially in regions with a lot of humidity or cold winters. Mold grows primarily where it is wet or damp, such as in your bathroom and shower or along windowsills where the moisture from your indoor air condenses when it's cold outside. Any water leaks, from leaking roofs or plumbing or overflow accidents, may result in mold growth if not completely dried within 48 hours. Many houses and commercial or public buildings (like schools) have mold infestation, although often you can't see it because it's within the walls or crawl spaces. We refer to these places as "sick buildings" or "sick houses."

Even if you can't see the mold, the spores and toxins can spew into the air and make susceptible individuals sick. If someone in your home seems to be sick all the time with nasal congestion, coughing, sore throats, swollen glands, unusual fevers, headaches, strange red rashes that migrate, generalized fatigue, muscle or joint soreness, attention or thinking problems, irritability and moodiness, dark circles under their eyes, blotchy skin, or any combination of those symptoms, he or she may be afflicted by mold toxins or otherwise reacting to mold in the home or in his or her school or workplace. If the person gets better when he or she is somewhere else for several days or more—such as a child home for Christmas break (who is getting exposed at school) or an adult office worker who takes a two-week vacation and gets dramatically better after a week away from the toxic home or office—mold may be the culprit.

Infants can be particularly susceptible to mold toxins in their indoor air. Deaths from pulmonary hemorrhage can occur in babies who live in housing that has experienced water damage and has mold growth in the walls. It is thought that many cases of sudden infant death syndrome (SIDS) are related to indoor mold exposure (American Academy of Pediatrics Committee on Environmental Health Policy Statement, 1998). It has been postulated that molds may cause volatilization of toxic compounds derived from flame retardant chemicals in infant mattresses, thereby leading to SIDS, but research has not yet substantiated this (Warnock, 1995).

Because of the scope of this problem, some integrative practitioners are specializing primarily in the treatment of mold-related illness. Conferences are held nationally every year just to educate doctors about mold toxicity. It is a complex topic, and treatment and recovery can be difficult because it is often difficult for people to get out of the toxic environment or to repair it. The American Academy of Environmental Medicine is one organization frequently offering practitioners education regarding mold and its effects on human health.

People with mold issues often incur recurrent bacterial infections as well, beginning a cycle of antibiotic exposure, weakened immune system and constitution, intestinal yeast overgrowth, further worsened immune problems and increase inflammation, and increased susceptibility to more infections. If you suspect you have a mold-related illness, you should find someone who can recognize this cycle and help you break it, someone who can guide you gradually back to health. For some, the road back to health can take years.

A less well-known source of fungal toxins, also called *mycotoxins*, is the food supply. Fungi grow quickly on many fruits, nuts, and other plant foods, and they are added to a number of foods for fermentation or processing. Some foods and beverages very high in mycotoxins include red wine, apple juice, cherries, nut butters of all types (like the aflatoxins in peanut butter), most other berries, and many cheeses (particularly blue cheese). If you want to learn more about what these toxins do and which foods to be most concerned about, I suggest you look at the website for the UK Food Standards Agency, www.food.gov.uk/safereating/mycotoxins/about/ or the European Food Safety Authority at www.efsa.europa.eu/en/topics/topic/mycotoxins.htm and read their information. The U.S. EPA and FDA websites catalog lists of scientific articles regarding mycotoxins if you search their sites, but offer no user-friendly reference lists or information that I could find.

Another type of fungal toxicity is that which you may encounter out in the woods if you eat the wrong mushrooms; toxins from the amanita mushroom varieties (poisonous toadstools) can rot your liver out in a matter of hours. Then there are the "magic mushrooms" that produce psychedelic toxins that can take you on a bizarre ride through an alternate reality. These dangerous varieties are balanced in nature by a whole host of medicinal mushrooms that produce compounds that strengthen your immune system or improve adrenal function. Not all fungi are bad.

Most antibiotics and antifungal drugs are derivatives of fungal toxins that we use to our advantage, though they are not without direct toxicity and many people have allergic reactions to them. If you are sensitive to an array of antibiotics, you may be sensitive to environmental mycotoxins as well; you should avoid foods with high levels of mycotoxins and clear any molds from your environment. You may also have excessive amounts of fungi or yeast growing in your stomach and intestines and other places on your body (skin, nose, mouth). Some of these are harmless or even helpful to you, while others can produce a number of toxins that may contribute to chronic illness.

Bacterial toxins

Many bacteria produce toxins that can cause chronic illness. You may have experienced food poisoning from bacterial toxins in food that caused violent vomiting or diarrhea within twelve hours of ingestion. These effects are usually short-lived. There is a particularly nasty toxin called lipopolysaccharide, or LPS, derived from the cell wall of many common bacteria. It is not so much a direct toxin as it is a tremendous stimulus for immune system activation and inflammation. Your immune system sees this stuff and assumes you must have a serious infection; the resulting immune activation is designed to clear an acute infection and save your life. Unfortunately, there is often some unavoidable collateral damage as the dramatic immune response can cause high fever, blood vessel hemorrhage in various tissues, fluid accumulation in the lungs or other tissues, dangerous drops in blood pressure and even death (we call this process "sepsis").

Man-made chemicals and xenobiotics

Chemicals can cause tissue damage because they cause direct tissue injury or because they trigger an inflammatory response, create free radicals and oxidative stress, consume antioxidants, or affect nerve transmission or muscle contraction. Xenobiotic chemicals can cause problems through all these same mechanisms and by initiating inappropriate physiological activity. They can block or stimulate cellular receptors, affect enzyme activity, and alter other functions on a molecular level. When chemicals stimulate or influence hormonal activity it is now often called xenohormesis; we did not need a word for that fifty years ago, just like we did not need the word "organic" in relation to our food before the development of pesticides and synthetic fertilizers.

The third way chemicals can cause illness, which is quite controversial, occurs when the immune system becomes active against the chemical molecule in a way similar to an allergy. This problem is becoming a common occurrence in industrialized nations. I will discuss this problem in greater detail within the later chapter on allergy.

Xenobiotics are man-made or naturally occurring chemical substances that have biological activity of some sort. This term could be used to describe prescription drugs. Only a portion of synthetic chemicals behave in this manner; it is much more common for these toxic man-made substances to cause direct toxicity to human tissue because of their inherent chemical properties. Xenobiotics may cause some direct tissue injury or stimulate the immune and inflammatory response as well, but they also have some physiological effects on the body through molecular mimicry.

One could fill many books with all the different types of synthetic chemicals we have introduced into our work and home environments. I won't elaborate much on the different chemicals here but would like to make some general comments about synthetic chemicals and briefly enumerate some of the more prominent categories from industry.

These chemicals can cause illness in several ways. Of course, one is massive, sudden, direct toxicity, such as when you drink a bottle of drain cleaner or set off a bug bomb in your face. One of my patients set off a bug bomb in his garage to clear fleas that had infested a stray cat he had brought home. He left the house for the four hours the product label suggested to clear the area of the pesticide, but when he returned and went into his garage he had a grand mal seizure and nearly died; the cat seized as well and did die. I saw him ten years after this exposure, still having multiple seizures every day.

A second way these chemicals cause illness is through chronic low-level exposure, which is much harder to recognize. These patients repeatedly seek health care for chronic symptoms like headaches, fatigue, brain fog, sleep problems, neurological problems like numbness and tingling, pain, weakness or seizures, heart palpitations, and digestive complaints like trouble swallowing, heartburn, and diarrhea. I have another patient who worked in produce for grocery stores more than twenty years before developing seizures and electrical problems in his heart, both presumably due to long-term low-level pesticide exposure.

It is well understood that long-term exposures to organic pesticides leads to Parkinson's disease in some (searching "Parkinson's and pesticides" on the PubMed database yielded 1373 articles in May 2012). Agent Orange (an herbicide used heavily in Vietnam during the war) lead to lymphoma and other soft tissue cancers in some individuals; exposure has led to a greater than doubled risk of prostate cancer in exposed veterans, specifically more aggressive cancers in notably younger men on average (Chamie, 2008). Many other common chemicals, such as benzene and toluene, are known to contribute to cancer as well.

There are many widespread subtle symptoms of chronic chemical toxicity, such as those listed above, that often generate only symptomatic treatment or no treatment at all from conventional practitioners. Probably the most common treatments these poor people receive are psychotherapy or psychoactive drugs, which represents a significant failure of our healthcare system and medical education. The vast majority of medical practitioners never consider the possibility that chronic environmental chemical toxicity is causing a person's symptoms, but jump instead to psychiatric diagnoses.

In my opinion, pure psychiatric illness is uncommon; the vast majority of psychiatric symptoms are organic and physiologic in nature, but most providers don't know how to sort out the real causes.

A second way xenobiotics cause illness is through their potential for physiological and biological modulating effects. Biological effects of some well-known chemicals were fully intended by their creators. Artificial sweeteners were designed to trigger a response from your taste buds and trick the brain into thinking you've eaten sugar. You can also use artificial sweeteners to kill ants in your home; just sprinkle some in the corner of a room if you want to find a pile of dead ants there later. The suspected mechanism here is the conversion of these substances to formic acid and formaldehyde after consumption. Aspartame is known to convert to formaldehyde in our bodies, and has been suspected as a common cause of migraine (Abegaz, 2009) along with other artificial sweeteners like sucralose and acesulfame.

We now know that some chemicals act very much like hormones; this is an effect now called xenohormesis. Plasticizer chemicals act like estrogen in some cases; bisphenol A, for example, was originally *designed* as a synthetic estrogen by a drug company (Janssen, 2010). Some pesticides and solvents also appear to have hormone-like activity. These common environmental toxins don't always behave *like* a given hormone or neurotransmitter; instead, they may modify or block the function of those signal molecules in the body.

Type 2 diabetes is likely caused in some folks through this sort of mechanism; their bodies bio-accumulate solvents, pesticides, plasticizers, and other chemicals that block the insulin receptors or other pathways affecting blood sugar metabolism until they have serious insulin resistance problems. Certain PCB's (polychlorinated biphenyls – flame retardant chemicals banned in the 1970's because they were found to persist forever in the environment and cause a wide range of chronic human toxicity) have been found to increase the risk of type 2 diabetes in humans more than *one hundred fold* (Tanaka, 2011). Though these chemicals were banned well over thirty years ago now, there are still very high levels present in fish and seafood, dairy products and meats. This is of particular concern in *farmed* salmon, which may contain more than *thirteen times* as much total PCBs as wild Pacific salmon (Hites, 2004).

It shouldn't come as a surprise to anyone, especially medical doctors, that synthetic chemicals could have these sorts of biological effects on the body. After all, isn't that what the pharmaceutical companies have worked so hard to achieve all these years? Don't they manufacture synthetic chemicals that have profound biological and physiological effects? If Prozac™ can affect serotonin signaling, why can't yellow dye #5 do the same thing? If atenolol can slow your heart rate by blocking adrenaline receptors, why couldn't one of those chemicals in your hand lotion or toothpaste do the same? After all, many drug effects are discovered completely by accident; Viagra™, for example, was initially made to be a blood pressure drug.

Are drugs and pharmaceuticals a potential cause of illness and disease? You bet your astronomically high insurance premiums they are! What is the difference between a drug overdose reaction and toxic poisoning? What is the difference between a drug "side effect" and an illness condition? What is the difference between "medication discontinuation symptoms" and a drug withdrawal syndrome? The difference is that we are attempting to use medications to gain a therapeutic benefit, so any unintended consequences are accidental (though not unexpected; after all they run through the list of possible horrible side effects of a drug on every TV commercial).

Do drug companies ever study the potential toxicity of taking a given drug for many years on end? No.

Do they ever study the potential toxicity of taking five or six different drugs together every day? No.

How about the combined effects of taking a few prescription drugs, smoking cigarettes and having exposure to toxins like paint or solvents at work, household chemicals like fire retardants and formaldehyde, plus the diesel exhaust you are exposed to on the commute to work every day? Of course not; there's no way to study that directly. If pharmaceuticals can have toxic effects, they certainly add to your total toxicity load and certainly contribute to chronic illness. Even if there is no direct toxicity, they add to the burden of chemicals your liver and other organs must detoxify and excrete.

Acetaminophen (Tylenol™), one of the more toxic products in the grocery store, is responsible for many deaths from overdose, both accidental and intentional. Acetaminophen overdose is the leading cause for calls to Poison Control Centers every year, at >100,000 calls per year; it accounts for over fifty thousand emergency room visits and more than 450 deaths per year (Lee, 2004). Acetaminophen kills you by completely depleting your liver of glutathione, the most powerful antioxidant you have, and then destroying your liver through unchecked free radical damage. The only effective treatment is to load the victim with enormous amounts of the amino acid *N-acetyl cysteine*, which helps you produce enough glutathione to detoxify all the acetaminophen you consumed. The amount of acetaminophen, like any drug, it takes to kill someone is widely variable; one person could die from taking chronic doses within the recommended range, while others could take half a bottle every day and never suffer any consequences (but don't try it).

Pharmaceuticals, like other xenobiotics, must be detoxified and cleared by the body, and a body's ability to do that is highly variable. Some drugs are altered and detoxified by the body, some are exhaled through the lungs, and others may be excreted unchanged in the urine. Still others may accumulate in the body and stick around for years. For example, women are advised not to get pregnant for many months or even more than a year after taking drugs like ribavirin, Accutane™, or amiodarone. Doctors mean well when we use these products, but these substances are not without their risks. Prescribers and consumers must be aware of the potential harm incurred from exposure to a foreign chemical substance, especially when the exposure goes on for years.

Important principles involved in chemical toxicity include exposure, total load (every other stress on the body, illness, and chemical exposure encountered), and biological individuality. One of the most important factors in determining whether an individual will fall ill from an exposure or ongoing exposure over time is how well they detoxify the relevant substances. This ability is both genetic and nutritional because a number of genes are involved in detoxification, and you have to get the right nutrients in order to perform chemical detoxification (as in the Tylenol™ example). A number of gene mutations in detoxification-related enzymes have been identified; testing for some of them is currently available through specialty laboratories. These factors are also relevant to prescription drugs, which explains why people's responses to them can be so diverse.

Returning to the issue of chemicals in general, by some estimates, over a hundred thousand new chemicals have been introduced into our environment since World War II. There has been no testing for human safety on the vast majority of these chemicals, and testing for developmental effects has been done on only a fraction of one percent of all these chemicals (Janssen, 2010). The EPA was supposed to take a tougher stance regarding the safety of environmental chemicals after the passage of the Toxic Substances Control Act of 1976, but that debate has not manifested much at all. Sixty-two thousand substances were "grandfathered in" and not subject to review for health effects. The EPA has reported that eighty-five percent of the more than eighty thousand chemicals currently on the market lack chemical data regarding health effects, and sixty-seven percent have no health or environmental data at all (Janssen, 2010).

This situation has resulted because the burden of proof for safety or harm does not lie with the industry that produces the chemicals but with the EPA and its limited resources. As of early 2010, only five chemicals in production had been directly regulated by our government to any great extent (Janssen, 2010).

The FDA requires a great deal of short-term safety data on pharmaceuticals, but these chemical still sometimes cause severe, if unexpected, harmful effects, resulting in many drugs' being pulled from the market within a few years. Why doesn't any government agency require industrial chemical manufacturers to prove their substances don't cause any adverse health effects on humans before they can be spewed into the environment or distributed through our food or homes? It is probably because these substances are not *intended* for human consumption; but unfortunately they end up inside almost every one of us.

Legislation to control potentially harmful environmental chemicals has been proposed along these lines repeatedly in the United States and has been summarily shut down. Contrast this to the chemical and food safety policies of some European and other countries, and you start to feel that our government cares far more about the welfare of corporations than the health of its populace. The European Union filed The Water Framework Directive in December 2008, putting into place limits and measures to control surface water pollution with 41 priority chemicals. The directive also calls for ecological status measures, promoting the health of natural ecosystems as well as human health. This is further reinforcement of the prior Groundwater Directive filed in 2006, which provided specific measures to assess, monitor and control groundwater pollution.

Some of the effects of chemicals that cause the greatest concern are those that affect human development, especially prior to birth. A frightening study of infants born in 2004 found 287 industrial chemicals represented in the umbilical cord blood of ten infants at the time of birth (Crinnion, 2009). The truly frightening aspect of this study is that the researchers looked for only 413 different chemicals, a small fraction of the many thousands of chemicals around these days. Could that result have anything to do with the precipitous rise in autism, ADHD, learning disabilities, developmental problems, allergies, and other conditions in American children? You bet.

Numerous articles have been published that demonstrate the

relationship between low-level prenatal and infant chemical exposures and later developmental or cognitive problems. Occasionally, these studies make the national news, such as the press release in 2010 that described how organophosphate pesticides in chronic low amounts seem to contribute significantly to attention-deficit/hyperactivity (ADHD). The most commonly detected pesticide metabolite in one particular study was associated with a nearly doubled risk of ADHD in children (Bouchard, 2010). Every time you let your child eat non-organic fruits, vegetables, berries, milk, butter, ice cream, meat, eggs, or other foods, your child is exposed to these chemicals.

In my opinion, chronic chemical exposure plays at least some small role, if not a major one, in all chronic diseases of modern industrialized society. It has to be addressed in some way, even if it is just through self-directed measures like cleaning up the diet, protecting oneself from occupational or recreational exposure, and possibly taking some supplements that help the body detoxify. I personally believe our government should also take an interest in human health by doing something to stop the production and use of potentially toxic chemicals.

Electromagnetic radiation (EMR)

There is considerable concern about the potential harmful biological effects of electromagnetic radiation (EMR). Some sources suspect EMR from cell phones may contribute to increases in the incidence of brain cancers. Some European studies have suggested modest increased rates of gliomas, a malignant type of brain tumor, in people heavily using cell phones, particularly at younger ages. These findings have caused the World Health Organization to classify cell phone radiation now as a potential human carcinogen, category 2B. The WHO filed this publicly on May 31, 2011 in press release No. 208 from their International Agency for Research on Cancer (Grigor'ev, 2011).

There is, of course, an immense amount of money at stake in this issue, with many billions of dollars behind the desire to disprove the theory that cell phone radiation may cause harm. If you research this issue you will find a number of recent studies suggesting there is no such increased risk of tumors with cell phone use. These studies need to be evaluated very critically, because most of them do not evaluate long enough exposure times. It takes years to develop a clinically relevant size of tumor; therefore, looking at people with less than ten years of cell phone use shows no increase in brain tumor incidence. Review of the studies that do include long-time users shows a doubling of the incidence of malignant gliomas, and almost two and a half times the rate of a benign tumor called an acoustic neuroma appearing on the same side of the head as that where the individual holds their cell phone (Hardell, 2007).

It makes sense that children are at much greater risk than adults are because their skulls are thinner (anatomically, not figuratively–my kids are definitely "thick-skulled" at times). Authorities all tend to agree, and have stated so publicly on national news interviews, that children and teens have the greatest potential risk from cell phone radiation. The suggestion is to have them send text messages rather than talk on the phone (luckily, this seems to be their preferred method of communication anyway – which some authorities fear is making them a bit socially retarded, but at least they may have fewer brain tumors), and use the speaker phone feature rather than hold the phone against their head during a call. Those little wireless earpieces for cell phones emit radiation right into your skull and are probably not safer, but you can purchase earphones that have open tubes to transmit sound without any electrical device in the ear.

It has been suggested that large-scale EMR from power lines and cell phone towers contribute to immune illness, neurological symptoms, and cancer incidence. One study from Iran suggested a dramatic increase in the incidence of one particular childhood cancer in children living close to power lines. Children living within 600 meters (a bit more than one third of a mile) of high voltage power lines were found to have a ten-fold increased incidence of acute lymphoblastic leukemia (ALL) at 123KV or 230KV voltage, and a three-fold increase for ALL near 400KV lines. The risk for children dropped off by about 40% for every 600 meters they were away from the power lines (Sohrabi, 2010). This means that children living a mile away from such power lines would still be at some increased risk.

Much of the information about this issue is from large industry and government research here in the US; those reports provide very different statistics and greatly minimize the potential harms. European data and reports suggest that concern is in order, but the specifics of the relationship between electromagnetic fields and cancer risk are unclear. Some studies suggest there is potentially very high risk for increased childhood leukemias related to high voltage EMF exposure, but the statistical analysis is all over the place (Malagoli, 2010). Other studies from the UK suggest that there is a great deal of risk associated with electrical fields produced from within the home rather than the power lines outside (Maslanyj, 2007)). The relationships, direct causal factors involved and potential unrelated causes are still unclear; this means nothing is going to be done about this in the near future.

There is certainly a spectrum of sensitivity to electromagnetic radiation, and it may only adversely affect a minority of people. Significant EMF exposure is thought to cause other types of illness or bothersome symptoms in people who appear sensitive to this type of insult. A study was done in three schools in Minnesota, where they placed EMF "filters" in classrooms that previously had very high EMF readings caused by what is termed "dirty electricity" (usually resulting from old or faulty wiring). Teachers did not know which rooms had the real filters placed in them, and were asked to fill out health symptom questionnaires repeatedly over the course of the study before and after having the EMF-reducing filters in place. EMF was reduced by approximately 90% in the rooms with real filters; this corresponded to symptom improvement in 64% of the 44 teachers surveyed, but symptom worsening in 30% and no change in 6%. Symptoms that improved included headaches, general fatigue or weakness, dry eyes and mouth, facial flushing, asthma, skin irritations and overall mood measures (Havas, 2008).

I suspect there is probably some sort of biological harm when high exposure to EMF is present. I suggest you use cell phones or wireless in-home phones on speaker whenever possible, rather than holding them right by your head. (I get pain and heat in my ear when I use a cell phone for more than a few minutes.) Texting is likely to be much safer than talking on the phone, so your average teenage daughter is probably better off with the fifteen thousand text messages she sends and receives each month than if she were talking on the phone.

It is probably best not to live near high-voltage power lines or within a mile of a cell phone tower, if possible. I have used a small EMF detector in my office, and the fluorescent lights in my ceiling gave off an electromagnetic field many times larger than anything else in the building. I suggest you buy or borrow an EMF detector and scan your entire house for "hot spots." Sometimes things are just wired wrong, and those can potentially be fixed.

Some people who are sensitive to EMF experience fatigue, mental confusion, headaches, migraines, or body pains when in the presence of significant electromagnetic radiation (you can use one of them to detect the high-EMF zones in your house if you do not have access to an EMF detector device). Many people, especially medical personnel, consider these people to be irrational or of having psychiatric illness. Those who are sensitive in this way should be tested for heavy metals and appropriately detoxified. The modern bioenergetic machines (e.g. the Indigo™, SCIO™, QXCI™) have programs for desensitizing people to these frequencies as well.

Medical radiation

It should not be a surprise to anyone that medical radiation causes harm. We use radiation therapy in cancer treatment to destroy cancer cells directly, and many toxic side effects have been described. Some patients have significant burn-like dermatitis of their skin in the areas of their radiation treatments that continue to evolve and worsen many years after exposure. Others, years after their abdominal irradiation, still have evolving problems with intestinal adhesions, leaks, and fistula tract formations from bowel to bowel or bowel to the abdominal wall. We know from early study on ionizing radiation that it can destroy your bone marrow. (Madame Curie could tell you all about it if she hadn't died from radiation poisoning.)

We also know that the radiation used to kill one cancer can cause a new cancer to show up years down the line. A young woman I recently helped through her lymphoma treatment was told by the radiation tech that she should now expect to have breast cancer in twenty years or so because of the radiation treatments to her chest.

Cancer is not the only risk of radiation exposure. It is well described that radiation therapy to the head, to treat cancers and tumors within the head, can cause complete failure of the pituitary gland. The pituitary regulates many different hormone systems and this therefore affects all bodily processes. The effects of this are much worse if it begins in childhood or before full physical maturation, but may result in hypothyroidism, reproductive problems and life-threatening adrenal deficiency in people of any age. It has been shown that this "iatrogenic hypopituitarism" may manifest up to ten years following the therapeutic radiation exposure (Sathyapalan, 2012).

These are issues involving large amounts of exposure with the intention to cause genetic and cellular damage to tissues. What we don't know for sure is what toxic effects, if any, may be incurred by exposure to *diagnostic* radiation exposure from procedures like X-rays, CT scans, and nuclear imaging studies.

I was taught that the average X-ray has ionizing radiation equal to the background exposure (that which you get from the sun and the environment) of about two days. That doesn't sound like much, but that's modern X-ray technology. People from earlier generations involved in the early days of medical radiology, before they knew about the potential harm and when the radiation loads were far greater from a simple X-ray of the time, often developed some sort of cancer or other radiation-related illness. There is a reason that radiology techs wear those lead aprons and little radiation exposure trackers.

One related issue in the national news recently was the relationship between dental x-rays and the risk of benign intracranial tumors. The type of tumor found to increase with dental x-ray exposure is specifically *meningioma*, a benign tumor arising from the tough membrane sac around the brain rather than from brain tissue itself. These tumors cause problems simply due to the pressure they apply to the brain while they grow inside the skull. The most recent study done showed nearly a five-fold increase in meningiomas for those receiving panorex full-mouth x-rays prior to age ten, and twice the risk of these tumors for those ever having simple bitewing dental x-rays at any time in their life compared to those who never had dental x-rays (Claus, 2012).

If you can have increased tumor risk from a few mouth X-rays, what about CT scans? The modern multi-slice scanners generate a great deal of power and produce radiation equal to dozens or even hundreds of typical X-rays. If you have had a few CT scans, you may have more to worry about, though that concern has not yet been clearly elucidated by research. In fact, I'm not sure anyone is studying it at all. My attempts to search for relevant articles on PubMed using keywords including "cancer", "CT scan", "radiation" and similar things yield thousands of articles related to all sorts of cancer studies, with no studies relevant to my concern appearing near the top. Certainly the industry that produces these machines has not had to demonstrate long-term safety or toxicity levels applicable to patients (although they have had to do so for workers' exposure). It is difficult to know whether there is any harm because cancers and other illness usually develop many years after exposure, and they will likely never be linked to their cause.

The use of CT scans in medicine has been driven by legal concerns to some degree; if a doctor misses a diagnosis and didn't do every possible test, he or she is liable to be sued, especially if the doctor works in the emergency department. Before our local hospital got our own CT scanner, only about twenty patients per month were sent to Anchorage for an urgent CT scan (e.g., to rule-out an intracranial bleed or serious abdominal problem), but once the hospital got its own scanner, there were soon more than two hundred scans per month ordered within the facility.

CT scanners are expensive tools, and if you have one, the tendency is to use it to get your money's worth. Another major downside of the push to use CT scans is that our newer physicians don't often perform good thorough physical examination and clinical evaluation since it's much quicker and easier to order the CT scan and get your answers that way.

I'm not suggesting that you never have a CT scan or X-ray, as they can help save lives, but ask your provider if anything else may be useful in getting your diagnosis. Ultrasounds or MRIs may be acceptable alternatives and carry far less risk. Sometimes a stay in the ER for twelve hours or more for observation and repeated careful examination (which was the standard for abdominal pain prior to the scans) is sufficient. This approach leads to a higher rate of unnecessary surgery, such as in cases of suspected appendicitis that turn out to be something else following surgery, but at least unnecessary surgery doesn't increase your risk of cancer later in life.

This question needs more study, which it is unlikely to get as long as the burden of proof for human harm in our society lies with regulatory bodies rather than with industry. Until then, my advice is to limit your radiation exposure whenever it is feasible to do so, without depriving yourself of necessary medical care. One last important point is that radiation is an accumulative insult, and the risk drops off with prolonged time in between exposures. If you do have to have a CT scan or x-rays done, try to space out any future exposure as far as possible.

Ozone, carbon monoxide and radon: miscellaneous environmental toxins

Ozone is three oxygen atoms bonded together, O-3 rather than the O-2 we need to survive. That extra oxygen atom is very unstable and reactive because oxygen wants to bond together in couplets, not triplets. When ozone spontaneously reverts to the O-2 form, the extra oxygen atom becomes a powerful free radical until it finds another molecule with which to react. Ozone will thus react robustly with organic molecules in organisms and chemicals with which it comes into contact.

Ozone is generated as a byproduct from many electrical and combustion-based devices. Most people can smell it whenever standing near one of those ionic air purifiers—it's like the smell in the air after a lightning storm. Ozone is a double-edged sword because you can use it to sterilize water systems, hot tubs, or your entire home, but it is very toxic to your lung tissue because of the reactivity of that third oxygen atom when it separates from the others. I frequently recommend that environmentally ill patients get an ozone generator and use it to sterilize their homes because the ozone kills all the mold and bacteria and neutralizes and destroys most of the chemicals in the air and on surfaces. However, you should not be there while the generator is running or for several hours afterward. Be sure to carefully read all instructions that accompany an ozone generator used in this manner.

There are medical uses for ozone also; in Europe patients with serious systemic illness are often treated with ozone by drawing some blood out, infusing it with ozone, and injecting it back into the patient. This process has positive results for some with infectious or toxic illness, as well as in those with oxygen-deprivation conditions like stroke and other cardiovascular issues. This type of therapy is taught here in the U.S. as well, under the category of "oxidative therapies" that also includes blood UV irradiation and the use of intravenous hydrogen peroxide. It is a very controversial type of medicine here in this country, and few practitioners utilize these techniques because of fear they may have their licensure revoked by antagonistic and narrow-minded state medical boards.

Patients may administer their own ozone treatments at home by bubbling it into their bodies rectally or vaginally so you don't expose your fragile lung tissue, or by running it into an airtight suit that excludes their faces and heads. A few of my patients do this at home and get significant relief from various symptoms related to chronic toxicity or infection issues.

I put ozone here as a toxic substance, but I have spent considerable time describing its benefits. I reiterate that ozone is toxic if inhaled, and if you work around a lot of machinery or electronics, you may be over-exposed and at risk for lung problems, so be aware.

I put carbon monoxide in this short section because it is toxic, but it isn't exactly a complex chemical and it isn't man-made or plant-derived, but it doesn't occur frequently in nature under normal circumstances. Carbon monoxide has proven to be extremely toxic, and this one has no beneficial application at all.

Carbon monoxide (CO) is responsible for more than a handful of deaths in Alaska every year, usually in winter, and it is a potential hazard anywhere people have to heat their homes by burning carbon-based fuels. When wood, oil, gasoline, natural gas, or other fossil fuels are burned the process generates primarily water and carbon dioxide, and also a small amount of CO.

The CO can kill you by binding strongly to the hemoglobin proteins in your red blood cells and preventing oxygen from binding so you can't circulate oxygen to your cells. We can tell if someone has had significant CO exposure by measuring a carboxyhemoglobin level in the blood. Smokers always have some measurable carboxyhemoglobin in their blood, as do children who live with smokers. Chronic low-level exposure may not cause demonstrable harm, but it may lead to decreased mental and physical functioning.

High-level short-term exposure to CO can certainly kill. People occasionally commit suicide via carbon monoxide poisoning by running their cars within enclosed garages while they sit inside and breathe the exhaust. In Alaska, entire families die every winter because their home heating systems were not working properly and they did not have CO detectors in the home. This gas has no odor at all, so you usually do not know you are being exposed until it is too late. These tragedies are completely avoidable. If you use any kind of heating system other than electric, make sure your heating system is working properly and that your home has CO detectors on every floor. It is important to point out that your CO detectors should be replaced every three years, because they collect dust and lose sensitivity over time.

This brings me to the third orphan toxin. Radon is a naturally occurring gas from the ground that has no smell and can permeate your basement or cellar if your foundation happens to have been dug into a radon pocket. Cancer is the only consequence of which I am aware, but a major one. This problem is particularly frightening problem because you are unlikely to have any symptoms of exposure until you are diagnosed with lung cancer after years of exposure.

Radon is thought to be the second leading cause of lung cancer, after cigarette smoking. Ongoing exposure to radon leads to DNA damage and mutation in your lungs, but it doesn't seem to cause any chronic illness symptoms prior to the problems arising from a growing cancer. People who have never smoked a day in their life but are suddenly diagnosed with lung cancer in their forties or fifties may have had significant radon exposure years prior.

You are only at real risk of radon poisoning if you spend significant amounts of time in the poorly ventilated basement or cellar of a home. If you do have a below-ground space in your home, it is easy to go get a radon test kit at your local hardware store to check it out. You should certainly do this if a previous owner or someone on your street died of lung cancer, but it is a good idea in every home with an underground space. If there is detectable radon gas all you need is a simple ventilation pipe and fan set-up to keep it cleared out. If you have a good HVAC system running in your home (including the basement), you're probably fine, but test just in case. The test kits are cheap; chemotherapy and funerals are not.

There are other environmental chemical and elemental toxins I have not discussed. Don't be overly concerned and paranoid about all the deadly substances in your environment; but certainly take action within your home, workplace, community, country, and planet whenever possible.

Emotional and "energetic" toxicity

Emotional, psychological, or energetic toxicity is far too common in our society. It seems as though many people aren't happy unless they are making someone else unhappy, and too many people lash out at others when something is wrong in their own lives. Negativity abounds in the news, in magazines, and on television shows (especially the "reality" shows that are exploding on cable these days; the "real housewives" make me appreciate my wife, who must be "unreal," but I like her that way).

Cases of bullying in our schools that have led to homicide or suicide are now a regular topic on the national news. There seem to be kids shooting other students or teachers in schools every year. Employees show up at work with weapons and randomly (or specifically) murder their coworkers and bosses. Spouses, boyfriends, and girlfriends kill their significant others over minor spats or break-ups. The great State of Alaska holds top "honors" for incidents of domestic violence in the country, as well as incidents of physical and sexual abuse of children.

These dramatic examples, while uncommon, seem to be becoming more common, and I think they illustrate the point regarding toxic emotion leading to action. Far more common and much more subtle is the day-to-day adverse energy you can get from others. You may meet an angry driver on the road or upset irrational person in line for coffee in the morning. Your boss may be having a bad day and decide to take it out on you. You may have an unhappy marriage because your spouse has a substance abuse problem or hormonal issues so you must always watch what you say to avoid an explosion.

This onslaught of negative energy from other people is common in daily life for many in our culture. While most of us realize it has an effect on us, how it has that effect is more difficult to understand. In many cases, it translates eventually to physical illness, so it is important to learn to let the nonsense slide off you, rather than stick; maintain focused insight into your own feelings and dispel negativity your own positive emotion and energy. This is a life skill that comes easy for some, but for the rest it requires practice.

Very often *internal* negativity is the biggest problem. People who suffer from internal doubt, resentment, self-loathing, disbelief, guilt, and a sense of failure and worthlessness should consider counseling, stop eating processed foods, go off gluten, eat a whole-food diet, increase vitamin D level up, have their hormones and possibly heavy metals tested, get some exercise, and find something positive to do. Watch movies including *What the Bleep Do We Know?*, *Down the Rabbit Hole*, and *The Secret* to help improve your understanding and mastery of these issues. I encourage everyone to check out Masaru Emoto's book *The Hidden Messages in Water* (Emoto, 2005) for incredible visual images relating to this concept.

Routes of exposure

This section refers primarily to chemical substances. The exposure to radiation is by proximity, and I have mentioned that exposure to CO, radon, and ozone are by inhalation. My goal in this short section is to draw your attention to the scope of the problem from another perspective so you can make optimal choices regarding your surroundings, food, and drink. If what I have to say here scares you, that's good.

Airborne toxins

Airborne toxins are a major, global problem. (See section III regarding the need for clean air.) The exposure route for airborne toxins is, of course, primarily inhalation, but you are also at risk from precipitation that drops through the air, such as acid rain.

If you're behind a truck in traffic, you may become acutely aware that exhaust is spewing into your face, but you may not realize that you are exposed to a small amount of toxic air pollution every time one of these trucks passes through your city, even if you're not directly behind it. Before gasoline was "unleaded," high blood levels of lead in children (and adults, but they didn't get the attention) were the norm, and they weren't standing behind trucks all day; the lead was in the ambient air.

When those white streaks from jet planes are visible in the sky, some sensitive people tend to think they have more asthmatic attacks and headaches. The emissions from jet engines are of course the same every day, but the white trials appear when atmospheric conditions are of a certain type (Rossmann, 2011); perhaps that changes the toxin exposure in some way or causes symptoms in people directly. When the air quality is noted to be poor in an area, there is a significant increase in heart attacks in the local ER (Nuvolone, 2011).

There have been numerous cases of factories that produce lethal fogs when weather conditions and atmospheric inversions are just right. People who live near factories have a lesser but constant exposure even on other days and may be prone to chronic or latent illness. Some studies have reported chemical-induced illness even in spouses of those working at chemical plants (Cannon, 1978).

Burning coal for electricity spews hundreds of thousands of tons of mercury into the atmosphere every year, which is a major problem no matter where you live. The air currents are global and there is no longer a truly pure place on the planet. The circumpolar regions are particularly toxic now because air moves from the warm equator toward the cold poles where many toxins are "dumped." Studies of polar bear populations and water mercury concentrations have shown far greater levels of mercury in higher latitude polar regions (Beaufort Sea) versus sub-Arctic (Hudson Bay) waters, with an average of 79.8pg/L in the Arctic and less than half that (38.3pg/L) in the sub-Arctic region. The polar bears from the two regions had drastically different levels of hair mercury (14.8mcg/g versus 4.1mcg/g) as well (St. Louis, 2011).

Indoor air problems include fumes and pollutants from fossil fuels like natural gas (which those of us who are sensitive can smell instantly), fuel oil, and coal. Some people burn wood, which creates particulates in the air along with chemicals, depending upon the type and source of the wood. Modern houses are full of solvents, adhesives, formaldehyde, and flame-retardants, among other chemicals. This stuff doesn't dissipate and go away just because you open the window for a few hours either. New furniture, wood products, textiles, carpeting, and other household items will outgas formaldehyde for years after purchase. This chronic low level of exposure has been associated with adverse health consequences in those who are sensitive (Flueckiger, 2009).

Chemicals in the adhesive under your vinyl floor covering or countertops exude chemicals into your airspace for years also, as will VOCs (volatile organic compounds) from the paint on your walls. I am somewhat sensitive to these types of chemicals and still cannot stand to go into my wife's parents' house even three years after its construction, because they used lower quality paint, had formica countertops and vinyl floor covering placed throughout. They cannot smell anything, but it hits me like a fist when I walk through their front door. We had our house built just two years ago and I am completely fine in the entire house except the room above the garage where we had vinyl floor covering placed. The rest of our house has granite countertops, tile or hardwood floors, low-VOC paint and low-chemical nylon carpeting.

You can take measures to create a safer house in terms of chemicals by choosing less toxic building materials, no-VOC paints, hard flooring without adhesive (wood, tile, non-glued laminate), and granite countertops, and installing an air circulation and filtration system that constantly cleans your air. You can also use ozone from time to time to clean up airborne pollutants. The ozone treatment only lasts a few months in my experience, at least in that space above our garage.

Older houses often have mold buildup in the walls, even if you can't see any in the bathroom or around your windows. The molds can produce powerful biological toxins and spores that trigger your immune system and cause illness. This is a major problem especially in cold or damp climates. If there is mold in your home or place of work, and you are chronically sick, you should look for an environmental physician or practitioner who knows how to treat you properly since conventional physicians tend to just prescribe symptom-controlling drugs that may just make you sicker.

Most of us are exposed to toxins in the air now no matter how hard we try to avoid them. You can control your exposure only to a certain extent after which it is up to your body to detoxify these substances so your system isn't overwhelmed.

Do I even need to go into cigarette smoking? It baffles me that people still smoke, yet members of my own family and other people I care about still smoke or smoked for years in the past. The amount of self-poisoning involved in smoking is staggering; the fact that everyone knows it underscores the powerfully addictive nature of nicotine.

Water contamination

Water contamination is a major problem in developing nations in terms of infectious disease, but now the problem has extended to chemical toxins in water. Many factories have been built in third-world countries because of cheap land and labor and because these countries impose no or only very weak regulations on industrial safety standards and waste disposal. This lack of regulation leads to rapid contamination of ground water, even in the absence of large-scale spills like the one in Bhopal, India in late 1984 or the dioxin contamination of Times Beach, MO here in the United States in the 1980s.

Many companies have dumped toxic waste in various places around our own country over the years. Much of it was done decades ago, before it was obvious that was a bad idea, but the stuff is still there causing trouble. Many synthetic chemicals are called "persistent organic pollutants" (POPs) because they never biodegrade. Some of these substances are expected to last in our soils and groundwater for centuries (Weber, 2008). This means significant contamination of our water and food with chemicals like DDT and other pesticides, PCB's, dioxins and furans; all known to have devastating adverse health effects. By the time the toxicity and persistence of these chemicals was realized it was too late; what is more unfortunate is the continued development, production and use of new substances that have similar properties, without studying or regulating them any more appropriately.

Regions where there has been industrial waste dumping, mining or toxic substance manufacturing tend be over-represented in illnesses like cancers and neurological disease. Patients from several areas in Alaska, such as an area called Red Devil, have told me that their pets died after drinking water from puddles or even their own well water. These regions have typically hosted inordinately large numbers of cancer cases, autoimmune disease, and chronic neurological disease.

If you live in a city of any size here in the United States, you may be at risk of water contamination from modern water treatment, such as the addition of toxins like fluoride and chlorine, or from substances unintentionally re-circulated throughout the water supply, such as pharmaceuticals (many drugs are measurable in city water supplies all over this nation) and cleaning solvents. Many cities also have toxic levels of heavy metals because of such problems as older buildings with lead pipes.

Chlorine added to city water supplies as a disinfecting agent reacts with naturally occurring organic compounds in the water to create chemicals called *chlorates* and *chlorites*; it also reacts with certain common chemical compounds to create toxic chemicals called *trihalomethanes*. The most familiar substance in this class is the anesthetic drug *chloroform*, which has well-known toxic, carcinogenic, mutagenic and teratogenic effects. A recent study in Italy for the first time attempted to study the link between the presence of these substances in drinking water and the rate of certain birth defects in children whose mothers drank the city water. The researchers found that mothers drinking water with chlorite levels >700mcg/L had babies with more than tripled risk of kidney malformations, nearly seven-fold greater risk of abdominal wall defects and more than four times the risk of cleft palate. Moms drinking water with chlorate levels >200mcg/L were at risk of having babies with nearly triple the rate of urinary tract defects, almost ten times the risk of cleft palate and five times greater risk of spina bifida (Righi, 2012).

In light of the research above, I decided to look up the U.S. EPA drinking water standards. Trihalomethanes are actually regulated to very low level, only allowing 80mcg/L, presumably because it is such a well-known toxin. Chlorite levels are allowed by our EPA up to 800mcg/L. If you look back to the preceding paragraph you will see this is a full 100mcg/L more than the level found to create dramatic increases in certain birth defects in the Italian study. Chlorate is not listed as a regulated chemical at all, which is frightening in light of the Italian study results showing chlorates have even greater toxicity at less than one third the concentration. The 2012 presidential election cycle is underway as I write this, and some republican candidates have been running with a platform that includes defunding or complete eradication of our Environmental Protection Agency. I wonder what the standards will become like if that happens, since they already allow significant toxicity?

The vast majority of homes where I live have their own well water. While that sounds nice, many wells here are found to have high levels of arsenic. Other regions have problems with natural toxins likes fluoride (some areas of China and India, for example), and if you or your neighbors spray chemicals on your lawn or garden, those toxins will seep into your well water. Living next to a golf course often means you have an extremely large amount of fertilizer and weed killer in your well water. The common weed killer Roundup™, made by Monsanto, has been advertised as being "safe as table salt" by its manufacturer; but more recent research into some of its "inactive" constituents has shown incredible toxicity against human cells in laboratory tests. The research team discovering this suspects that even the residual amounts of these chemicals one would get from eating Roundup-treated crops such as soybeans, corn and alfalfa might cause problems with pregnancy and fetal development (Gammon, 2009).

There are also biological contaminants like bacteria and parasites in drinking water. The Department of Environmental Conservation (DEC) will usually test your water for "coliform" bacteria, which are commonly found in the colon, indicating that there is a little poop in your water. This isn't usually a problem for city water supplies in the US because of government regulation and enforcement, but it is a major one in developing nations and could be an issue for those with well water depending upon the sewage systems of your house and your neighbors' houses.

You should become aware of where your water comes from and the potential toxins in it. It is easy to find water filtration systems for your drinking water if you think there are contaminants in your water. Use a system that includes reverse osmosis, and also ozonation if possible. Europe has largely gone to ozonation to avoid toxins such as fluoride, chlorination byproducts and other chemicals in their water.

It is important to note that in addition to exposure through drinking water, organic chemical toxins in your city water can also absorb right through your skin. If you live in a city with a contaminated water supply (which is virtually all of them), you may want to get a filter for the shower and bathtub in addition to the one for your drinking water. You may get a far larger chemical exposure by lying in fifty gallons of contaminated water than you do from drinking a quart of it.

To make matters worse, once the toxic water is taken out of the ground or from your tap at home, people often place it into plastic bottles, cups, or containers that add more potentially harmful chemicals. The phthalates or plasticizers in plastic vessels can cause hormonal disruption and developmental problems and may contribute to increasing cancer incidence. Bisphenol A (BPA) is currently being heavily studied and has been associated with a wide array of hormonal and metabolic problems. BPA is being voluntarily removed from most plastic baby bottles and other items by conscientious manufacturers, yet still has not been formally restricted or banned by the US government. However, the removal of BPA from these containers does not mean any of the other commonly used phthalates are safe; they just haven't been studied to the degree needed to implicate them as harmful.

In spite of the mounting evidence proving the harms of BPA, you can find an argument to the contrary online at the *American Chemistry Council* website. They have links to "information" there from the *Polycarbonate/Bisphenol A (BPA) Global Group*, an organization that promotes the business interests and general welfare of the BPA and polycarbonate plastics industry around the world. They offer evidence suggesting BPA and other similar chemicals are safe. If you read their stuff, which I'm sure isn't biased in any way, I suggest you also read the posting by the *Environmental Working Group* chronicling the history of BPA in industry. They describe how it was intended for use as a pharmaceutical agent to mimic estrogen until diethylstilbestrol DES was found to be so toxic, and then it was later put into plastics from which people would eat and drink. You can also search PubMed for "BPA and toxicity"; I had 637 articles pop up in May 2012, and there are more every month.

Phthalates are common plasticizer chemicals used to make plastic containers for foods and beverages, also used in hydraulic fluid, dielectric fluid in capacitors and also as a solvent inside glowsticks. Mono-2-ethylhexyl phthalate (MEHP) has been shown to have significant toxic effects against human testicular cells even at very low concentrations (Muczynski, 2012). Another phthalate, di(2-ethylhexyl) phthalate (DEHP), has been proven to cause liver cancer in rodents and because of modern research has now been classified as a possible human carcinogen (Group 2B) as well (Rusyn, 2011). You may come in contact with DEHP from medical devices such as polyvinylchloride IV tubing, food, water and air contamination.

It is my opinion that all of the chemicals with similar properties that are in plastic, an organic (carbon-based molecules) substance, may have similar effects in your body to BPA and these phthalates mentioned—or at least they aren't worth the risk. I don't believe for a minute that "number 2" plastic is any safer than "number 7." Grading plastics in this way is right up there with "clean coal" technology on my list of industrial nonsense. In my opinion, buying water in any plastic bottle is a bad idea. You have no idea how long the water has sat in that plastic, to what kind of temperatures it has been exposed, or where the water came from. It is also important to point out that the commercial bottled water industry is largely unregulated; some of those companies simply bottle some city tap water and put a pretty label with a picture of mountains or something on it.

The plasticizer chemicals in the bottle just add to the toxicity. After the BPA and phthalate toxicity issue went mainstream, bottled water producers suggested that people should not refill their bottles but just drink the water and then discard the bottle. I don't understand how drinking out of it once is safe but drinking out of it twice is not. Does that sound as stupid to you as it does to me? The water that is in the bottle at the time of purchase is the most toxic water you're going to get from that bottle! It's been sitting in there for who knows how long while the phthalate concentration is at its highest.

If anything, you should buy the product, dump out the water that's been sitting in it for days, weeks, or months, and refill it with your own water that you do not allow to sit in the bottle for more than a few hours. The same goes for any other beverage you can buy at the store, even if it's a product advertised as healthful: if it's been sitting in plastic, it's probably toxic, especially if there is carbonation or some natural acidity to the contents. Don't forget that many tin cans are lined with plastic to prevent the food from tasting like metal, and most of that plastic lining is very high in BPA. In addition, many beverages in a box made of paper have a plastic lining. You're generally better off buying beverages in glass whenever possible—even aluminum cans—instead of plastic.

Start paying more attention to what you are putting in your body!

Toxins from cultivated or harvested foods

Food may be the biggest source of chemical exposure for the average person in the United States since most of us don't work with chemicals. Ingestion is a sure way to get chemicals into our bodies. Our food supply is contaminated in a variety of ways, from processes used in agriculture, to contamination of rainwater and groundwater, to chemicals used in food manufacturing, to those added in the final stages of preparation.

Chemical fertilizers have been the mainstay of agriculture for decades, and traces of these fertilizers are in your plant and animal foods if they are not certified organic. Chemical fertilizers often contain significant amounts of hazardous materials that are known to be toxic because the fertilizers are typically derived from the waste products of other industries. The only standard they are held to is that they must contain proper amounts and ratios of nitrogen and phosphorous; the frightening toxic compounds additionally within those products go unnoticed (Shaffer, 2001).

Pesticides are also certain to be in your food unless your food is an organic product. Studies have suggested links between consumption of pesticides and the development of neurological conditions such as ADHD in children (Bouchard, 2010), Parkinson's disease (Le Couteur, 1999) and epilepsy (Jett, 2011). This should not be a surprise to any chemist or health professional, since many pesticides are designed specifically to be neurotoxic agents, and those effects are not specific to insects. Even the prescription pesticides used on human children to kill lice have been known to carry the risk of inducing seizures; the drug lindane was taken off the market in the U.S. because of this, but the drug permethrin that is currently used has not yet been shown to induce seizures.

Industrial or occupational exposures and large toxic exposures to pesticides have been shown to clearly cause neurological damage and disease; it has not however been sufficiently proven whether chronic low-level consumption of pesticides from nonorganic foods may cause disease.

It is theoretically very likely, and the studies associating ADHD with levels of organophosphate pesticides in children certainly suggest this relationship. Pesticides and other chemicals have been shown to "sequester" in high concentrations within certain tissues of a given individual, and reach extremely toxic tissue-specific levels even when blood or urinary levels do not appear elevated. A colleague of mine has found a series of patients with head and neck cancers in patients without elevated blood or urine levels of pesticides, but extremely high concentrations of chlorinated pesticides within the tumor tissues themselves (Govett, 2011). This means that testing blood or urine levels of chemicals in no way accurately assesses your risk of chemical-related disease.

People will often buy organic fruits and vegetables preferentially in an attempt to avoid pesticides, but it is far more important to focus on organic animal-derived foods. The highest levels of pesticides are in animal products because of bio-accumulation up the food chain. Cheese, butter and ice cream, eggs, sausage, bacon, some meats, and other animal products are high in fat, so they contain higher levels of pesticides because they are fat-soluble chemicals. Human breast milk should be recognized as an animal-derived food as well (do vegans breastfeed?); elevated levels of pesticides and other toxic chemicals have been found in human milk (Bergkvist, 2012). I know organic foods are more expensive than the non-organic forms, but anti-seizure drugs and chemotherapy are quite expensive as well.

Herbicides are also common in the food supply. These toxic chemicals—which are designed to kill living things, so they are inherently poisonous—are sprayed onto crops during cultivation to keep weeds away. Roundup™ is very common, and since Monsanto Corporation has made "Roundup-ready" genetically-modified (GMO) crops, they can spray all the Roundup they want onto their food crops and not kill the plant. Of course, the higher level of herbicide residue in the food may poison whoever eats it in some way. Levels of herbicides and their chemical constituents are not found in foods in truly "toxic" doses, where cells in tissues would be directly damaged in a dramatic fashion. However, glyphosate levels (Roundup is a glyphosate-based herbicide) even at the low levels similar to those found in agricultural products and human urine, such as 1ppm, have been shown to cause dramatic decreases in testosterone production (35% decrease) by testicular tissue in vitro (Clair, 2012).

One very common herbicide, atrazine, affects the function of chloroplasts, the little energy-producing parts of plant cells that look and function a lot like our own mitochondria. Atrazine, the first or second most common herbicide in the world, is so commonly used on corn and others crops that it can now be measured in just about every water supply in the US, including our rainwater. (See the movie *Living Downstream* for some startling information about atrazine and other chemicals in our environment.) Laboratory studies have shown that atrazine can turn male frogs into females, and it is suspected to contribute to the development of obesity, metabolic syndrome, breast cancer and type 2 diabetes in humans, though the data is not conclusive. Atrazine is also thought to be linked to certain devastating birth defects with prenatal exposure (Lubinsky, 2012).

Fungicides are sprayed onto produce in order to protect your fruits and vegetables from mold; this will be the worst for berries and other produce sold fresh. You are better off buying frozen berries, especially organic ones, so you avoid both the fungus and the fungicide. Some fungicides have been clearly shown to interfere with the production of testosterone and other steroid hormones in rodent tissue studies in vitro (Manfo, 2011). Common fungicides have also been shown to have cancer-promoting effects on human ovarian cells (Paro, 2012).

Sprout inhibitors are biological poisons used to treat plant foods like potatoes and onions, which would otherwise start growing long sprouts or rootlets right there on the shelf if left too long. We don't know exactly what these chemicals do to humans, but a chemical designed to stop cellular growth and development can't be good for you, especially if you are a child or a developing fetus. The most common chemical sprout inhibitor, isopropyl-N-chlorophenylcarbamate (CIPC), has been identified as a xenoestrogen (Nakagawa, 2004) and has been demonstrated to cause direct liver toxicity in rats through mechanisms which would be expected to affect human cells as well (Nakagawa, 2004). CIPC has also been shown to cause impairment of sea urchin embryo development even at very small concentrations (Holy, 1998). The obvious criticism here is that humans are not the same as rats and sea urchins. If that's good enough for you, eat all the CIPC you want until some human data is published (which is most likely to be "never"); however, I suggest you make sure you buy organic potatoes and onions, which at this point certifies they are free of these chemicals.

Many other chemicals have been added to our non-organic produce with unknown effects on the people who consume them over long periods. Up to 80 percent of these chemicals are used simply to improve the color of the fruits and vegetables (Pollan, 2006), which is why organic varieties may not "look" as good; some organic producers use the slogan "Don't panic, it's organic!", to reassure consumers that looks aren't everything when it comes to food quality.

Heavy metals, primarily mercury, are a major problem in fish and other seafood. As discussed, the main sources are ultimately air pollution from forest fires, volcanoes or burning coal, which then gets into our oceans and up the food chain. The highest levels exist in the large predatory fishes or top fish-eating predators. The documentary movie *The Cove* (2009) explains the mercury problem incurred by the Japanese who eat dolphin in large numbers.

A typical can of tuna holds enough mercury to exceed the daily allowable mercury for anyone who weighs less than 190 pounds. What's more, recent studies have found that nearly half of high fructose corn syrup (HFCS) samples are contaminated with mercury because of the chemical processing used to create this artificial substance (Wallinga, 2009). The average American consumes gallons of HFCS every year. Don't let the television ads convince you that HFCS is just some "natural" product casually derived from squeezing the juices out of corn.

Plant foods are not necessarily free of heavy metals either. Irrigation using lead-based pipes still occurs in many parts of the world, so you have to watch out for this in foods and herbal supplements from places like China and India, even when the supplement tests within the US's allowable levels because the dose of bulk herbals is often large. There have been documented of cases of patients suffering anemia, liver toxicity and other adverse health effects from toxic amounts of lead or other heavy metals in herbal medications (Gunturu, 2011). I suggest buying herbal products only from manufacturers who test every single batch of bulk herb they purchase for heavy metals, pesticides, solvents and other toxins.

Don't forget about potential lead exposure from the liner in boxed wine, the metallic wrapper around your chewing gum, the aluminum from your beverage cans, and tin from food cans. All of these metals add up, especially in susceptible individuals.

PCBs and other POPs are prevalent in many seafoods and fish from the Great Lakes area and the circumpolar regions because of the movement of ocean currents from hot to cold climates. The Alaskan native diet was historically heathful when they consumed large amounts of marine life, but it is no longer so healthful because of this pollution problem. Farmed fish, such as salmon, have high levels of PCBs and other toxins (Hites, 2004); since 2009 or so the EPA has issued warnings that people should not consume more than one serving of farmed salmon per month because of the PCB content and the increased cancer risk that the PCB content carries. Why the heck would you eat any of it at all?

If you still think you probably aren't at risk, consider this: A study of almost six thousand people living in Texas found measurable levels of a metabolite of DDT in the blood samples of 99.5 percent more than a decade after DDT was banned in the United States (Stehr-Green, 1989). Imagine what amounts you are harboring in your body of the chemicals still actively produced and found within foods in this country.

Another important natural food contaminant class is the mycotoxins, which are produced by molds and other fungi growing on foods and produce. Most of the ill effects from these toxins take the form of unexplained systemic problems like fatigue, brain fog, recurrent illness or fever, rashes, digestive symptoms, neurological symptoms and other symptoms similar to those of chemical toxicity. Some of the foods highest in mycotoxins are figs, cherries, grapes, wine, apple juice, and peanut butter. Peanut butter usually contains some amount of a fungal toxin called aflatoxin b1, which is one of the most cancer-inducing compounds known. Aflatoxin b1 is still a major contributor to the development of liver cancers in humans living in developing nations (Kew, 2012), but the amounts allowed in peanut butter or other foods here in the U.S. are extremely low and not believed to pose direct risk to consumers. This is one solid argument in favor of the use of fungicides on peanuts; would you rather have the man-made toxin, or the fungal-made one?

Toxins from manufactured foods

In addition to all the chemicals that end up in our cultivated or gathered foods "incidentally" are a great many synthetic chemicals that are intentionally added to our manufactured and processed foods.

Nitrites, such as sodium nitrite, are added to almost all cured meats unless you seek out "naturally cured" or uncured items with no nitrites on the label. This includes all bacon, sausage, hot dogs, lunchmeat, jerky, salami, and pepperoni, as well as many smoked foods and other processed meat items. These simple chemicals are added to prevent spoiling by killing bacteria. A review of more than seven thousand studies by the World Cancer Research Fund suggested that these foods may be linked to pancreatic cancer and are possibly too dangerous for human consumption (Price-Pottenger Journal, summer 2008).

Artificial sweeteners are often converted to neurotoxins in our bodies;

for example, aspartame can convert to formaldehyde during metabolism (Patel, 2008). Many people get headaches from artificial sweeteners immediately. Some researchers believe there may be a link between artificial sweetener use and conditions such as lymphomas, leukemias, bladder or brain cancers, chronic fatigue syndrome, Parkinson's disease, Alzheimer's disease, multiple sclerosis, autism and autoimmune conditions like systemic lupus, although no solid evidence is yet available that would convince the conventional community and this is extremely controversial (Whitehouse, 2008).

Aspartame, the first of these sweeteners, took decades to earn FDA approval, and that was in a scandalous fashion according to some conspiracy theorists (see one account online at www.rense.com: "How Aspartame Became Legal – The Timeline"). The newer ones like Splenda™ (sucralose) appear to be no better. I suggest they be all be strictly avoided by avoiding most foods labeled "diet," "reduced calorie," or "sugar-free." You may be surprised to find them in most foods labeled "fat-free" as well, in almost every brand of chewing gum, and in many manufactured beverages, even if they contain sugar. You have to read labels carefully to successfully avoid these chemicals.

Artificial colors are all chemical agents with unknown biological properties. Most of these have been shown not to kill laboratory animals quickly when given in large doses in order to get approval as a food additive, but that doesn't mean they don't have developmental effects or don't add to your total load of toxins, taxing your liver's detoxification mechanisms. Some have been suspected as a trigger for asthma (i.e., yellow #5, aka tartrazine) and allergic-type reactions, but published scientific evidence supporting this claim has been lacking (Pestana, 2010).

I myself am sensitive to red #40 and yellow #5 and feel mentally and emotionally "off" for hours after ingestion. Many of my patients with ADHD or autism seem somewhat sensitive to these coloring chemicals, particularly blue #1 for some reason. This is an area where science has confirmed the association. A placebo-controlled, double-blind study performed in Australia did in fact dose-dependent adverse effects such as irritability, restlessness and sleep disturbance with the ingestion of tartrazine (yellow #5) by the majority of children suspected of being sensitive, and also ten percent of the "control" children (Rowe, 1994).

Some processed food preservatives, such as citric acid, are natural substances, but others, such as sodium benzoate, sodium bisulfite, and sodium metabisulfite, are chemicals. The "sulfites" are often used on lettuce at salad bars and added to wine and dried fruits to preserve texture and/or color. Preservatives are often chemicals that suppress or kill bacteria, so it is reasonable to conclude that a chemical that kills one type of organism can harm another.

Some people have sensitivity reactions to preservatives, especially the sulfites, that can manifest as wheezing, acid reflux, or other symptoms. One study attempting to evaluate the prevalence of sulfite sensitivity among asthmatics found that around 10% reacted upon initial challenge, though only 3.9% overall reacted after a double-blind rechallenge with a second dose (Bush, 1986). Criticisms of these findings, suggesting the prevalence they found may be artificially low, are that these patients were on active treatment for their asthma, they were looking for a fairly large effect (20% decrease in one-second forced expiratory volume by thirty minutes after ingestion), and the first dose could have induced a short-term adaptation or relative desensitization in some test subjects so that they did not react as badly upon repeat challenge. I myself can develop bloodshot eyes and mild airway constriction from consuming foods and beverages with high amounts of sulfites. Individual reactions may depend on recent intake of molybdenum and essential fats, as well as other recent chemical exposures and other factors.

Cooking and over-processing of food creates toxic substances derived from the food itself. Over-cooking foods creates advanced glycation end products (AGEs), chemicals that accelerate the aging process and appear to contribute to diseases like diabetes and cancer. Burning fats creates compounds that produce a high degree of oxidative stress in the body. We know that deep-frying fish takes away all the health benefits of eating fish, possibly making it harmful to you overall. One study found an association between consumption of fish cooked at high heat to a well-done state and the development of prostate cancer, but no such association for those who cooked their fish with lower heat methods or until it was just done rather than well done (Joshi, 2012).

One good example of the toxicity of processed foods was shown in a study done in which mice fed Cheerios™ cereal had a shortened life span compared to those fed mouse food. A third group of mice was fed only the cardboard box the cereal came in, and even those mice lived longer than the cereal group (Fallon, 1999). Other studies have shown similar rapid death in laboratory animals fed super-heated "puffed" grains and cereals (Stitt, 1981).

These results indicate there is potential harm incurred during the cultivation, storage, processing and preparation of foods. This is worse than just what risk results from stripping the nutrients from the foods. There are also plenty of toxins to worry about, even in some wild foods. There are health and safety concerns regarding food every step of the way.

Household items and personal care products

Flame-retardant chemicals are a major problem. PCBs (polychlorinated biphenyls) were commonly used chemicals until they were banned in the 1970. I have already discussed the association between PCBs and type 2 diabetes and other disease processes. These chemicals were replaced by PBDEs (polybrominated diphenyl ethers), which were not studied prior to their coming into our homes. Now, over thirty years later, we are realizing that PBDEs also cause adverse health effects. PBDE exposure has been associated with developmental neurotoxicity, hormonal dysfunction of various types, and reproductive disorders (Pellacani, 2012). PBDEs are also clearly implicated in what has been a huge surge in hyperthyroidism in cats seen by veterinarians across the country, a condition rarely seen in cats prior to the use of these chemicals. It is postulated that PBDEs may play some role in similar thyroid disease in humans (Mensching, 2012).

PBDEs and similar chemicals are common in carpeting, furniture, new clothing (especially children's clothing), and other potentially flammable household materials, so they are common in everyday house dust, such as that which collects on surfaces and behind your television set, where the air intake is. It is important that you clean dust from surfaces using a damp cloth, not a feather duster or other method that just stirs up the dust into the air. The chemicals aren't thought to get through your skin to any significant degree but to enter the body through the mouth when you passively ingest house dust.

Cats are at particular risk because they live very close to the floor and furniture. They also lick themselves, thereby ingesting large amounts of these chemicals relative to their body weight. Even if you don't own a cat, you may have an infant or toddler at home. Babies and small children also live very close to the floor and furniture and frequently put things into their mouths. They crawl around and put their faces on the floor and their mouths on the furniture, just as they frequently suck on their chemical-laden clothing.

Now this suddenly seems more important, doesn't it? Babies are trying to grow and develop, and their brains and other organs are more susceptible than adults' are to damage by these hormone-disrupting chemicals. It is important to be aware of the presence of flame-retardants, formaldehyde, and other chemicals in these household items. Wash new clothing several times perhaps before putting it on your kids—better yet, buy the clothing used—put your child on a clean blanket rather than directly on the floor or furniture, and dust with a damp cloth regularly.

If you have an outside wooden deck made with pressure-treated wood, don't let your child eat out there or crawl around too much. The pressure-treated wood used for outside decking often contains large amounts of arsenic, and other types of wood may be coated with paints and other chemicals. If your children drop food or other things onto this surface and then put the food or toys back in their mouths, toxic exposure can result. And don't forget about all the national news broadcasts regarding high levels of lead or cadmium being found within the paint on children's toys coming from China.

Many people in our society intentionally slather themselves with toxic chemicals. Those of us who are somewhat chemically sensitive or aware can't even get close to many people out there in public. Especially in closed areas like churches, many sensitive people have trouble with the perfumes and fragrances others wear. It isn't just perfumes and colognes that have fragrances in them; lotions, deodorants, soaps and other skin care items contain these as well.

Most artificial fragrances are chemicals derived from petroleum on some level and were never intended to be inhaled. There are people paid to take a whiff of these various toxic substances derived from rotten prehistoric plants and animals mixed with dirt, trying to decide which ones smell good to men versus women or what possible natural odor they resemble. That way they can get some consensus on which of these chemicals to use in the "vanilla" candles or a men's cologne for example. Bubble gum fragrance or flavor, for example, is a random petroleum-derived chemical with an interesting aroma and taste but no natural correlate.

Many chemicals are added to makeup, lotions, body sprays, soap, sunscreen, and other products we put on our skin. Most of these chemicals are lipid-soluble so they soak into the skin and into your body. Some phthalates, the same chemicals used to soften plastics as discussed above, are placed in skin care and cosmetic products to make them "smooth" and allow for more even application without plugging up the dispenser. Phthalates can now be measured in the bodies and body fluids if virtually everyone in modern society, and the suggested "safe" daily intake posted by the U.S. EPA is far more generous than the lower level tolerated by the European Food Safety Authority (Guo, 2011).

Parabens are common preservative chemicals placed in lotions and cosmetic skin products. Parabens have some xenoestrogen activity and have been suspected of playing a role in the development of breast cancers. A recent study from England analyzed breast tissue samples from women undergoing complete mastectomy for breast cancer and found phthalates present in 99% of the 160 tissue samples in the 40 women involved in the study. They also found much higher concentrations of the phthalates in the area closest to the armpit, which is where a disproportionate percentage of breast cancers tend to occur (Barr, 2012). These chemicals are easily avoided by choosing personal care products more carefully.

Some product lines have no phthalates or other potential toxins; many of these products can be found in health food stores or the "natural food" section of grocery stores. Skin Deep© cosmetics database, produced by the Environmental Working Group (EWG) is one resource for determining the safety of your personal care products. You can search their website at www.ewg.org/skindeep/ and see how scared you should be of you lotion, foundation or lip gloss for example.

Toothpaste, including kids' toothpaste, has many chemicals in it as well. At least kids' toothpaste doesn't usually contain fluoride because we know fluoride is a poison, and you wouldn't want kids to swallow it. One common chemical in toothpaste is sodium lauryl sulfate (SLS), which is added as a "detergent" to ensure your toothpaste foams up like you expect it to. Some people are sensitive to SLS and may develop mouth sores or a constant burning pain of the tongue or mouth due to daily brushing with SLS-containing toothpastes.

Non-stick cookware can expose you to perfluorinated compounds; they get into your foods during cooking and also vaporize to some extent so they can be inhaled. This could be seen as a food-borne exposure then, but these same compounds are also on carpets, furniture, and anything else with Scotch Guard™ or other stain-resistant treatment. These chemicals have been shown to cause immune system suppression, including significantly reduced antibody production in response to childhood vaccinations in kids even ages five to seven years of age (Grandjean, 2012). PFCs have been shown to induce mammary tumors in rats, and human epidemiological data has suggested an association between blood PFC levels and risk of breast cancers (Bonefeld-Jorgensen, 2011).

I have mentioned many different classes of chemicals, sources and routes of exposure, as well as some of the potential health risks posed by environmental chemicals. This has been a very small sampling, but hopefully enough to convince you the concept of environmental toxicity is an extremely important one as it relates to chronic human illness. I want to mention again that, though we have convincing data about individual substances causing disease in significant doses, we have no realistic way of determining what the risk is of someone being exposed to hundreds or thousands of chemicals at the same time in small amounts. That is the situation in which we all exist currently in industrialized society; in my opinion it has to be responsible for some portion of the current burden of chronic disease we are seeing.

Now that you are much more aware, perhaps frighteningly so, of the scope of chemical toxins in your environment, we'll further discuss the different potential health effects of these harmful chemicals and then explore what you can do about the problem.

Common symptoms and manifestations of toxicity in general

The potential symptoms and scope of disease caused by environmental chemicals and toxins is immense and includes just about everything. Environmental toxins are often involved in major killers like cardiovascular disease, cancer, diabetes, and autoimmune disease. Chemical toxicity is also involved when you are harmed by something your doctor prescribed you. Environmental toxins are frequently to blame on some level in mysterious chronic problems like fibromyalgia and other fatigue syndromes as well as in irritable bowel, migraine, epilepsy, Parkinson's, ALS, and other neurodegenerative problems.

It is important to point out that toxic substances can act much worse together than they do individually. This phenomenon is called synergy; it is very common among toxic substances with similar toxic effects. This concept makes it very difficult to accurately determine the risk of exposure, when we are always exposed to many substances in the world while research usually focuses on one at a time. Common PBDEs and PCBs together have been shown to have significant synergistic effects in terms of toxicity to human neurons in vitro (Pellacani, 2012). Enhanced neurological toxicity in a synergistic manner has been demonstrated with lead and arsenic, and more research is actively coming out showing synergistic effects between diverse types of toxins such as metals, alcohol, PCBs and pesticides (Pohl, 2011). This means that whatever you *know* you are exposed to is going to be made even worse by the stuff you don't realize you have already retained in your body.

The chronic symptoms of ongoing exposure to toxic chemicals or latent effects of a large short-term exposure may also manifest as chronic degenerative problems involving the immune system (frequent infections, allergies), nervous system, skin, cardiovascular system, digestive system, urinary system, or most other systems in the body. Headaches are common, as are heart palpitations or other types of cardiac electrical disturbance. Rashes may occur in some, but usually only if allergy or sensitivity develops to an internalized chemical. A chronic annoying cough may occur, or just a constant feeling of difficulty catching one's breath. Digestive system problems may manifest as heartburn or irregular bowel habits; the enteric nervous system can become improperly coordinated due to chemicals damaging those nerves.

Chronic toxicity problems may manifest as just annoying chronic symptoms, which don't meet criteria for any particular disease. People with chronic low-level toxicity issues are likely to have mild ongoing problems with fatigue, weight gain and eventually the development of insulin resistance, the metabolic syndrome and possibly type 2 diabetes. They may have primarily psychological or psychiatric manifestations such as problems with mood, sleep, thinking and memory. They may have random widespread pain problems of an aching, stabbing or burning nature, as well as numbness or tingling that moves around the body without any rhyme or reason.

Acute symptoms of chemical toxicity may include problems in almost any body system. Symptoms of effects on the nervous system include severe headaches, disorientation, confusion and possibly seizures. Symptoms of effects on the skin may include rashes, blisters, hives, or unusual itching. Symptoms of effect on the cardiovascular system include heart palpitations, full-blown cardiac arrhythmias, even sudden heart attacks or strokes in those without atherosclerosis. Gastrointestinal symptoms include nausea, vomiting, acid reflux, diarrhea, and abdominal pain from cramping. Respiratory symptoms are among the most common with acute exposure, especially with inhaled toxin exposure, and can include a runny nose, sinus irritation, cough, wheezing, and symptoms often diagnosed as bronchitis or pneumonitis.

I see many patients with toxicity issues, which are almost never recognized as such by practitioners without environmental medicine training. These patients come in with fatigue issues, mental complaints and many other symptoms as described above. The doctors they've seen have typically run some tests that were all essentially normal, have prescribed some symptomatic medications or nothing at all, and perhaps have referred them to psychiatry or offered a drug for anxiety or depression.

What's more disturbing is that you may not have any of these notable warning symptoms at all before you get your cancer diagnosis or have your first heart attack, diseases ultimately caused to some extent by the toxins you have accumulated. Therefore, it is the chemically "aware" among us who have a better chance of survival, because we avoid exposure. We may get annoying symptoms from small exposures, but that keeps us from wallowing in toxic chemicals like those without sensitivity are prone to do.

If you are the only guy working in the shop who always wears your respirator and goggles when working with solvents or other volatile chemicals, because they burn your eyes, nose or mouth, but they don't seem to bother the others, then you are the lucky one. If you are the only hairdresser in the salon who wears gloves when handling coloring agents because they burn your skin, but don't burn the others' hands, or you can't be in the room when someone is doing a perm because it makes you feel like you can't breathe, then you are the lucky one there. Those who feel a notable aversion reaction around chemicals, and are acutely aware of the chemicals that nobody else can seem to smell, are the bloodhounds of the chemically laden world in which we now live.

I reap considerable rewards from my colleagues' complete ignorance of environmental toxicity problems, though the general public does not; as this is a major area of discrepancy in modern medical education. As a patient, you can help fix this problem by politely requesting or demanding that your health care providers learn about these issues. Bring them resources, send them to websites, and suggest they go to environmental medicine conferences. (www.aaemonline.org, the environmental medicine website, lists upcoming teaching conferences and other useful information.)

With most environmental toxicity issues there isn't much you need a doctor for other than medications to help control symptoms while you detoxify, and guidance in devising an effective detoxification strategy. Hopefully you will learn most of what you need in that regard from the rest of this chapter. Some will need an integrative practitioner who performs chelation therapy in order to remove a toxic metals burden, others will need prescription medications to aid in the removal of other specific toxins.

The difference between "toxicity" and "sensitivity"

Many chemicals have direct harmful effects on your tissues and cellular biochemical function, which is the "toxic" effect. You can feel it when you drink a significant amount of alcohol or huff some type of volatile chemical that damages the brain (*not* a good idea). Virtually everyone sees these effects with enough exposure. There is a lethal dose of just about every chemical for every individual, over a very wide range within a given population.

"Sensitivity" to a chemical is different from toxicity or lethality and is much more like an allergy; I myself actually refer to these reactions as "allergy", but conventional allergists have a very strict definition of that word and would call these "sensitivity" issues. Some individuals become acutely ill upon very small exposure to a given chemical. They may have an instant headache around certain perfumes or fragrances, get a runny nose or wheezing around diesel exhaust fumes, or break out in a rash after wearing clothes washed in certain detergents. These types of reactions are not due to direct toxicity of the chemicals alone but are mediated in some fashion by the body's immune system, just like an allergy.

Therefore, in my view, a chemical sensitivity is an *allergy*, in that the person has an unusual adverse reaction to something in a non-dose-dependent manner. We have no problem understanding this when it comes to pollens, animals, or foods; we all know people who get a runny nose and watery eyes in the spring because of pollen allergies or "hay fever," and increasing numbers of people risk anaphylactic shock from eating certain foods, such as peanuts or shellfish.

However, for some reason, our population—and, unfortunately, our medical system and its practitioners for the most part—have trouble recognizing the same process as it relates to chemical substances, and doctors have a blind spot when it comes to realizing that patients with chronic headaches or recurring sinus infections may be reacting to common household or workplace chemicals. They don't believe patients who say they get brain fog or migraines around certain perfumes or candles or that they can't eat non-organic food without having diarrhea and abdominal pain.

This is bizarre because we readily accept the concept of medication allergy and write the drug name on someone's allergy list if the person develops a rash, vomiting or other symptom after taking it. Why don't we realize people can have life altering or life-threatening reactions to some of the thousands of chemicals our modern society swims in all day long? Ignorance of this problem is so bad in our medical system that the diagnosis of "multiple chemical sensitivity" is being considered a *psychiatric* illness! The medical professions wants us to put these patients on antidepressants or antipsychotics if they say they get sick around common chemicals because it just *couldn't* be a physical reality. Sometimes it seems to me that many of my colleagues haven't come far from performing frontal lobotomies or from ostracizing Semmelweiss for suggesting doctors should wash their hands!

I see these poor chemically sensitive folks in my office every week, if not every day. Other doctors all see them as well, but fail to understand what is happening to their patients and prescribe whatever relevant symptomatic drug they can think of, such as antihistamines, decongestants, acid-reducers, topical steroids, painkillers, sedatives, and psychiatric drugs. That approach means giving more chemicals to a person whose main problem involves chemicals! It is upsetting to me, and this sort of condition is becoming more and more common as we are exposed to greater numbers of chemicals over longer periods.

Treatment of chemical or biological toxicity

There is a difference in treatment approach between acute toxicity and chronic toxicity. Massive single exposures may be overwhelming and immediately fatal, with no effective treatment at all. Most emergency care in the hospital setting is purely supportive, cleaning any residual chemical from the body and helping to "flush" the substance from the body with hydration or perhaps alkalinizing the urine. If something was swallowed we may pump your stomach or make you swallow a bunch of charcoal in an attempt to bind it up to prevent absorption. There is the occasional actual "antidote," such as ethanol (that's the alcohol we can drink), for exposure to antifreeze or N-Acetyl Cysteine for acetaminophen overdose, but in most cases there is no specific treatment.

It is much more common that patients have ongoing lower-level exposures to toxins at their workplaces or homes, rather than large obvious exposures. People in certain professions have chronic toxic-level exposures to solvents, paints, pesticides, flame-retardants, heavy metals, petroleum, benzene, and a myriad of other chemicals. Some people may have recently remodeled their homes or moved into new homes and have excessive exposure to formaldehyde, paint, solvents, adhesives, and other chemicals. Some have hobbies, such as painting, making stained glass, or loading their own ammunition, that bring them into contact with heavy metals and other toxins.

Those patients who develop problems are likely to look for answers repeatedly in a primary care clinic or multiple specialty physicians' offices. They manifest all manner of symptoms in all the organ systems that are targets of environmental toxicity. If you have been to more than two practitioners trying to find answers to your persistent problems there is a good chance you have some component of chemical toxicity or sensitivity, but you could also have problems more related to hormonal imbalance, allergy, nutritional deficiency or one of the other chapters in this section. People with unexplained chronic problems are the main reason I wrote this book.

In the chronic situation, there are a few important components to treatment: avoidance, reduction of the "total load," detoxification, and support of normal physiology.

Avoidance, avoidance, avoidance!

Avoidance is the single most important aspect of successful detoxification. It's hard to get healthy when you are repeatedly exposed to what is making you ill. It is hard to rid your body of toxins if you keep putting them in. This all seems obvious and simple, but avoidance can be the most difficult part of the program to implement.

Avoidance essentially consists of identifying the sources of exposure and either getting away from the exposure, modifying the environment, or using proper protective gear. It is not always possible to quit a job but it may be possible to ventilate areas better, wear personal protective gear and use other precautions in the workplace. It may not be possible to move to a different house, but it may be possible to remove toxic materials from the home, abate mold completely, remodel with nontoxic alternatives, and use a good air cleaner system or ozone.

What makes avoidance most difficult is: *not knowing* what you need to avoid in the first place. Some people know exactly which chemical or other toxin is bothering them because they have immediate severe symptoms in its presence. Other people just have chronic, subtler symptoms and may only know that it is something at home or something at work. Some of my patients with environmental illness don't even know that, because they are never away from work for more than a few days, and that isn't long enough for symptoms to improve. Many environmentally ill people don't even realize their symptoms are environmental.

It is important to find a health practitioner with some degree of environmental training or understanding if you think you may have environmental illness. It is often not an easy thing to figure out and effectively treat, even for someone with training. Look for a conventional allergist or a good dermatologist if your symptoms seem like contact allergy reactions, because the standard methods for diagnosing chemical contact dermatitis are very effective; or seek out an environmentally trained physician or naturopath.

One of my patients was a laboratory tech at a hospital who had chronic severe dermatitis that caused her hands to be covered with hundreds of shallow cuts. They itched, the skin was thickened, and her hands burned constantly. She had been getting steroid shots every month or so for a year to keep the symptoms under control. The condition seemed to clear up when she was away from work, so I sent her to a dermatologist who did patch testing for common chemicals and found that she was highly sensitive to an agent common in many hand cleaners, including the one she used at work dozens of times per day. Once she started bringing her own soap to work, she was cured. Sometimes all you need is for someone to identify the substance involved, and the cure is simple: avoidance.

Reduction of total load

Reduction of total load involves reducing your total exposure to all potentially toxic substances in order to take as much burden off your immune system and detoxification systems as possible, thereby allowing your body to deal with the real problem more effectively. This clinically important concept requires a lot of education for most of my patients since most people are not aware of or don't believe in the adverse impact of all the potentially harmful substances in their environments. The preceding portions of this chapter were my attempt to convince the reader that you live in a toxic soup of harmful chemicals and substances.

You have to recognize and understand what sorts of things to avoid before you can avoid them, and this requires considerable convincing for some people, while avoidance can require some major lifestyle changes. Avoiding the initial major cause or causes of your symptoms may make you feel somewhat better, but many will still be chronically ill with symptoms like chronic fatigue, headaches, myalgias, brain fog, and neurological symptoms because their body has been taxed for too long. The body may be in such a deranged and depleted state that it begins to react badly to more chemicals (what we call "spreading" or "switching" phenomena) and can't keep up with detoxification of the usual low-level exposures that had been no problem in the past. In this case, it is imperative to reduce exposure to anything that puts additional burden on the body's detoxification system or that may be an immunologically reactive substance.

The individual in this situation benefits from avoiding all chemical fragrances, cleaners, detergents, cosmetic products, soaps, toothpastes, paints, petroleum products, inks, lubricants, and other common household or workplace chemicals. He or she should also avoid new clothing, new furniture, new carpet, and other newly manufactured goods that are treated with flame-retardant chemicals, formaldehyde, and other chemicals.

People with a toxic overload should eat only organic, whole foods, both for purposes of avoidance and for nutritional support. Even the small amounts of pesticides in foods like avocados and bananas can add up and tip the balance toward illness when your system is fragile and depleted. You must read labels and avoid anything with chemicals in it (ever read the ingredients in chewing gum?) and also avoid eating and drinking from plastic.

Patients who develop multiple chemical sensitivity problems often have to quarantine themselves inside their own homes and turn their homes into chemical-free sanctuaries. They become prisoners of sorts inside their own little bubbles or oases. Several thousand people in Anchorage, Alaska live like this, trapped in their homes unless they want to be ill and debilitated for several days from some minor exposure in the community. If they do venture out, it is usually to carefully selected destinations and they may wear charcoal masks to protect from automobile exhaust and other incidental exposures.

If you do need to create a safe haven for yourself, safe materials to choose include wood (but not cedar, because it has high levels of natural terpenes), concrete, granite, tile, metal, and glass. Most of the home interior finish materials we are used to, such as paint, carpet, vinyl, and adhesives for standard countertops, contain toxic chemicals that outgas into your air space for months or years. You may have to strip a room down to the studs and subfloor and start over from there.

Support of Physiology

Some vitamins, minerals, amino acids, and plant-based nutrients are very involved in detoxification. This is important for the environmentally ill patient because, even if you stop the exposure, your body still has to eliminate what is already inside. Internal detoxification is a very active process. Toxins don't passively come out in your urine or stool very quickly, if at all. Detoxification requires large amounts of energy and a great many cofactors for the physiological processes involved.

Many people think that fasting, going without food for days or even weeks, is going to help them detoxify. Fasting may be beneficial in that the person is avoiding toxins from foods and they are allowing their liver and digestive tract to focus on eliminating toxins and waste rather than digesting and processing foodstuffs. Fasting for more than a day is probably not a good idea for most people, and for the depleted, chronically ill patient, fasting even for a day is a bad idea in my opinion. When one starves for even a day they tend to start breaking down fat tissue, which is where many toxic chemicals are harbored. They are therefore exposing themselves to an increased load of toxins, while at the same time depriving themselves of the nutrients required to actively detoxify those substances and protect their tissues from the toxicity.

As I said, detoxification is an *active* process, requiring increased nutrients of certain types and a supply of cellular energy. It is important to get enough clean, healthy protein in the diet to supply the amino acids needed for conjugation and excretion of chemicals through the liver. Whey protein is probably the best if you are not allergic to it, but rice protein is a decent second choice, and both can be taken as a supplement if needed. Otherwise, eat wild meats, fish, beans, nuts, quinoa, and other healthful sources of protein. Certain individual amino acids are also heavily involved in promoting detoxification. I discuss them below as items to take additionally in supplement form.

Many vitamins are important in aiding detoxification and in protecting you from the harmful effects of toxins. Eating a broad whole-food diet provides most of these vitamins under typical circumstances, but supplementation can help your body get caught up. I suggest finding a good B-complex vitamin with high potency; you can usually find a B-100 or B-50 (two of the latter typically equal one of the former) to take daily. Many of the B vitamins are directly or indirectly involved in detoxification, and you will need to have them all in adequate supply.

Antioxidant vitamins like vitamin C are particularly helpful as well. Most people can only assimilate 5,000-10,000mg vitamin C per day orally before getting diarrhea; you therefore can't get your blood level very high at all with oral supplementation alone. We often give patients intravenous vitamin C, B vitamins, and other nutrients in the office for acute or chronic environmental illness. 400-800iu Vitamin E daily is helpful in protecting cell membranes, but remember to get a high-end product with mixed tocopherols. Vitamin B-12 is often depleted in the environmentally ill, because it is depleted when the body is actively trying to detoxify heavy metals and other toxins. It is very important to use *methyl*-B-12 in this setting, and I suggest doses of 2,000-5,000mcg per day.

Certain minerals are key in supporting the system against environmental toxins and in aiding detoxification. Magnesium should be taken in amounts as large as you can stand before getting diarrhea (though diarrhea helps clear out your colon, it depletes you of water and essential nutrients too). Zinc tends to be very low in people who are environmentally ill, so adults should get around 50mg daily. Selenium should be taken at 300-400mcg daily in the short term while you're catching up, and then at 200mcg per day for maintenance once the illness phase is past.

Molybdenum is very helpful in detoxifying sulfite-type chemicals and in some other aspects of detox; getting 2mg or so daily is usually sufficient. Manganese and some other trace minerals are also needed, so it is useful to find a good trace mineral supplement and cover all these bases because, if you're environmentally ill, you're likely to be generally depleted of most everything. Many people find products like "coral calcium," "glacial milk," and Cell Food™ helpful for getting the ultra-trace minerals. You can also start using liberal amounts of raw sea salt, which is loaded with necessary trace minerals and also helps to flush out your body if you hydrate well along with it.

Many plant-based nutrients are helpful in supporting detoxification because they act as antioxidants and otherwise protect your system from environmental toxins. I suggest eating lots of dark fruits and berries, vegetables in wide varieties, herbs and spices, and whatever other diverse plants you can get in your diet. Eat as much food as you can that increases glutathione levels, such as broccoli sprouts, blueberries, and watercress. An agent in prune skin helps improve liver and bowel detoxification; prunes also contain fiber that can bind toxins and speed bowel elimination. Organic, darkly colored plant foods are generally a good idea.

Finally, proper fats in the diet are important in protecting your tissue because your cell membranes are made mostly of fat, and they need improved integrity when they're under chemical or inflammatory attack. This is one reason why many Americans have high cholesterol levels: they are chronically inflamed and their bodies are trying to repair tissue. Getting enough omega-3 fats in the diet or supplementing with fish oil is also extremely important; they reduce inflammation and aid in cellular repair. A good short list includes salmon, walnuts, flax, purslane, and pumpkin seeds. I strongly suggest taking at least 1000mg of EPA (eicosapentanoic acid) in fish oil, krill oil or calamari oil supplements daily in this situation if possible.

Aside from all the nutritional elements that support physiology in a practical, physical sense, it is important to pay attention to the other aspects of health, such as emotional, energetic, and sleep issues. These stresses tax the system as badly as a low-level or moderate chemical exposure; it causes changes in hormones, the nervous system, and the cardiovascular system, and it drastically depletes B vitamins, magnesium, and other nutrients. Reducing emotional and situational stress is important for many with environmental illness (as it is in improving overall health for everyone).

Make sure you get adequate sleep, try to use only natural substances if you need assistance sleeping, and of course avoid caffeine and alcohol. It is also important to have physical activity every day because exercise ramps up your circulatory and respiratory systems and other systems involved in detoxification, and it signals your cells to perform all their processes more efficiently and robustly. I know when you are sick you do not feel like doing anything active, but it is critical. I tell people to act like they intend to *live* rather than lay down and die.

Pay attention to your body and don't overdo it, because many environmentally ill people have poor exercise capacity at first. Doing gentle energetic exercises like yoga, qi gong, and tai chi are particularly helpful in this case. They aren't physically taxing, and they promote energetic balance and flow. Having some sort of energy work done, such as acupuncture, craniosacral therapy, or Reiki, can improve your physiological ability to cope with your illness and help you detoxify.

Detoxification

As I've mentioned, detoxification is an *active* process, not a passive one. Toxins become "stuck" in your cells and tissues and don't usually leave the body passively. Detoxification is a diverse topic because heavy metals and chemicals require different approaches. Detoxification of chemicals has three general phases: *conversion, conjugation,* and *clearance.* Conversion means chemically changing the molecule through the action of certain enzymes we possess for this very purpose; conjugation means attaching the toxin to another molecule in order to facilitate excretion from the body. Clearance is the final act of actually getting the stuff out of the body.

Detoxification in the modern world is best viewed as a long term, ongoing practice. We are heavily laden with toxins now, and exposures are ubiquitous and continual. Many people like to do a short-term liver or colon "cleanse" now and then, subsequently returning to their usual routine. That really isn't effective, because there aren't just bundles of toxins sitting in your liver or colon waiting to be "dumped". The toxins are spread all over your body in every tissue; they are in your fat, your bones, your brain and your organs. I generally tell my patients who want to do the occasional "cleanse" strategy that "you can't expect to eliminate thirty years of accumulated toxins with three days of diarrhea."

Detoxification has to be seen as an ongoing process. It involves awareness and avoidance of toxins first and foremost, as discussed. It involves eating the right foods to provide what you need for the processes described below. It involves taking appropriate supplements to facilitate conversion and conjugation processes. It involves moving your body and exercising, so that your blood circulates readily to every tissue in your body. It involves making sure you sweat on a regular basis and that you bowels move easily every day. Next, I will review some key points to helping detoxify specific classes of toxins.

Heavy metals

Most conventional doctors cringe at heavy metals chelation, and it is often associated with "quackery" in medical practice. This is so ironic because of the widespread recognition that there are toxic levels of mercury in fish, lead in toys from China, arsenic in apple juice, and other such toxic metal exposure. The biggest problem with heavy metals toxicology is probably the belief that when you can't measure metals in the blood, they have left the body. Au contraire!

I have discussed testing before, but I repeat that you need to do provoked urine testing rather than hair analysis or blood testing if you want to a true reflection of your body's burden of metals. If you find a practitioner who knows how to do this test and interpret the results, you can target your therapy toward the metals that affect you. There are various chelation agents, each of which has it's own spectrum of coverage for the various toxic metals.

One chelation substance you can get over the counter, even though it is an FDA-approved "drug" for the removal of lead, is called EDTA. You can find it in capsules at many health food stores. It doesn't absorb well orally, but it helps remove lead from the GI tract if you take it multiple times per day by binding and extracting the lead your liver is excreting in your bile. Detoxamin™, is also available over the counter; a rectal EDTA product,

Detoxamin is supposed to have better absorption into the blood stream from that route. If you decide to take EDTA on your own, remember that it pulls out calcium, zinc and other minerals in addition to lead, so don't take it alongside a calcium or mineral supplement that will just bind it up. Take a good multimineral with zinc, selenium, copper and others on a regular basis at some other time of day, separated by a couple hours from the EDTA.

Other oral agents you can use on your own include DMSA, which covers most toxic metals and is very safe. DMSA is also available by prescription as Succimer™ or Chemet™, and it is the agent I use most of the time. DMSA is FDA approved even in children, for the removal of lead in particular; it also has an excellent affinity for mercury and many other toxic metals. I usually suggest patients take a dose of DMSA at bedtime three nights per week, on alternating nights. Doses range from 100mg for young children, to perhaps 750mg for large adults, depending upon how high their levels of toxic metals were and how well they seem to tolerate therapy.

Treatment often has to go on gradually like this for well over a year, whether you use EDTA or DMSA or any other oral agent. It is slower than intravenous chelation for sure, but gentler and far less expensive. Again, be sure to take a mineral replacement every morning if using DMSA or any other metal chelator.

Penicillamine another chelation drug that is available by prescription, may be taken orally to help clear certain metals, most notably copper (excess copper is toxic to the nervous system, and occurs particularly in certain genetic diseases such as Wilson's Disease). Practitioners can prescribe penicillamine for those with elevated metals, but it is not used as commonly as DMSA or EDTA.

DMPS is the most powerful agent for removing mercury, but it is generally given intravenously because oral absorption is poor. DMPS has more risk of adverse effects and toxicity, partly as a direct effect of the drug and partly due to the massive mobilization of mercury that can redistribute around the body and cause more damage if not readily eliminated. DMPS is probably the most risky and dangerous chelator to use; it is of tenuous legality in the United States, and many won't use it.

A mineral compound called zeolite may bind metals in the digestive tract and help pass them out in the stool, but it has not been shown to chelate metals effectively from the body's tissues, because it is too large to itself absorb into the blood stream. It is important to point out that facilitating elimination of metals from the body is extremely important. Chelation agents alone do not ensure the metals are removed from the body safely. Chelators find and bind metals from your cells, bringing them into circulation once again. Those metals then still need to be cleared from the body through the urine, stool, or possibly sweat.

It is important to stay well hydrated and make sure you are urinating large amounts when trying to clear metals. It is important to keep your bowels moving easily and regularly. It is important to take the amino acids, minerals, vitamins and other nutrients discussed in the following paragraphs to facilitate toxin clearance. This isn't as simple as taking some DMSA a few nights per week; detoxifying metals is a multi-step process, and can be dangerous if not done correctly.

I think it's best to undergo formal chelation under the supervision of an experienced practitioner. You can look at the ACAM (American College for Advancement in Medicine) website, www.acam.org, for providers trained in chelation and other means of detoxification through their courses. Environmental physicians can be found through the American Academy of Environmental Medicine at www.aaemonline.org.

Some natural elements help to remove toxic metals safely. These include all the foods that help promote glutathione as I discussed above, some other specific herbs and foods, amino acids and minerals. You can get oral glutathione itself, which works best in "liposomal" form, and you can get chlorella algae, which is very helpful in binding mercury and other metals, at health food stores or even in the grocery store and consume some a few times per day (about 500mg at a time). Cilantro also binds mercury well, and some of its relevant substances may even penetrate the blood-brain barrier to help remove mercury from the brain. Garlic and onions also contain substances that help remove toxic metals.

The amino acids I suggest people supplement with are N-acetyl cysteine (1200mg or more twice daily), glycine (2,000mg or more twice daily), taurine (500-1,000mg twice daily), and alpha-lipoic acid (300-600mg daily). The first two are key components of glutathione, and the last two help conjugate and remove metals. A B-complex vitamin is a good idea, and minerals like zinc, magnesium, and selenium are important as well in doses already discussed. Calcium is important if you are using EDTA, but I would only suggest about 500mg daily.

Avoid further exposure by reviewing the sources of metal exposure. Do the best you can, considering that you still have to breathe, drink, and eat. If you do have some noted ongoing exposure, take in whatever will aid in ongoing removal.

Chemicals

I lump "chemicals" all together here for the sake of brevity and simplicity. There are some general approaches that help your body eliminate many different substances efficiently and that cover most of the chemicals. Some chemicals are removed better by certain techniques, but I don't want to get too far into the specifics here. Even though there are thousands of chemicals, there are some fairly simple ways to remove them.

Remember that avoidance and reduction of total load are extremely important here, because you want to stop putting more stress on the system if you want to get ahead, rather than farther behind.

Sauna therapy or heat purification is the best overall means of chemical elimination (Genuis, 2011). Many indigenous cultures have had this figured out for thousands of years. They seem to have known that their health was improved through the regular use of sweat lodges or similar such heat purification. It is more than just the simple act of sweating, though that does help extrude chemicals out through your skin: heating up the body causes dramatically increased circulation especially to the skin, and there is something about heat that ramps up all of your body's detoxification systems.

You can use either an infrared sauna, which can be assembled easily inside your home with low energy costs, or any form of ambient heat sauna, but try not to expose yourself to fossil fuel exhaust or wood smoke. One does not seem to be better than the other overall. Taking supplements like niacin (200-500mg or more if tolerated), vitamin C (at least 2,000mg), and the amino acids mentioned above (N-acetyl cysteine, glycine, taurine, and alpha-lipoic acid) about thirty minutes before getting in the sauna to aid detoxification is a good idea.

I suggest you get the heat up to 140 degrees Fahrenheit or higher if you can stand it, though you may need to start at a lower temperature and work your way up, depending on your tolerance. Spend just ten minutes or so in the heat at first, and work up to thirty minutes or longer per session. Heat purification can be dangerous for those with heart problems or other serious medical issues, so you should consult a physician prior to starting a sauna program.

If you are very ill, try going into the sauna for five to ten minutes, then out for ten, back in for five to ten, and so on for several cycles. Work up gradually from there. Drink lots of clean, pure water with some sea salt in it (1/4-1/2 teaspoon per quart) to avoid dehydration and improve your detoxification. Shower off immediately after finishing your sauna, to avoid reabsorbing any toxins left sitting on your skin.

If you can't tolerate the sauna or if you're detoxifying a child, the second-best choice for overall chemical clearance is Epsom salt baths. Take the same supplements beforehand, get the water as hot as possible, and soak with at least two to three cups of salt per tub for as long as the water is hot. Sweating into the water is a key part of the process, so you have to get the body heated up.

Many people ask me about the ionic foot baths offered at spas, chiropractic offices, and other places. I think they may be useful for diagnosing toxicity issues, with the color of the water suggesting the presence of metals, chemicals, yeast, and other toxins, and they seem to make people feel better and to relieve a number of distinct symptoms as long as they are used regularly. I think that those benefits are due primarily to energetic effects, such as stimulation of the acupuncture meridians originating in the feet. However, I do not believe they aid in actual detoxification of the body, other than cleaning the feet well. I reviewed an excellent article on this subject for publication in a Canadian journal, which is not yet in print, and it was made clear that there is not any measurable amount of toxic metals coming out of the person into the water.

Intravenous therapy with high amounts of vitamin C, glutathione, B vitamins, magnesium, and other nutrients can be very helpful as well. This is particularly useful for those who are very ill and depleted, or those who for some reason do not absorb nutrients well through their digestive tract. This includes patients with Crohn's or other forms of inflammatory bowel disease, people taking stomach acid-reducing drugs, and those who have had gastric bypass surgery for weight loss. You must find a skilled practitioner to administer these kinds of therapy.

Some herbs are very helpful in detoxification, particularly through the liver. Milk thistle is the best studied, and I suggest that almost everyone take about 300mg twice daily, although there are some potential drug interactions, so have your doctor review your medication list if you aren't sure. Marshmallow, blessed thistle, dandelion, and some other herbs, which are commonly used for detoxification, can be found in various herbal mixture products. Essiac tea is one such classic mixture, but there are many others.

Chemicals are largely stored in fat tissue, therefore weight loss is helpful for those who are obese or overweight. Change your diet, decrease your calories to only what you really need, start or increase an exercise program, and lose some weight. Work with a provider who uses HCG if you can find one, or try some other supervised weight loss program. Make sure you do the chemical detoxification measures listed above (sauna, amino acids and nutrients) while you are losing weight because even more toxins will be released into your system as you break up fat tissue.

While breast-feeding or lactation is one of the best overall means of chemical detoxification for women, it is unfortunately potentially toxic for the child. Breast milk has a lot of fat in it, and many chemical toxins are excreted in milk at fairly high levels. I strongly suggest that women work hard on global detoxification *prior to pregnancy*, as I'm sure that toxins are a significant part of the surge in behavioral and developmental problems among America's youth, as well as allergic disease, metabolic disorders like obesity and type 2 diabetes in adolescence, autoimmune issues, and childhood cancers.

Of course, it is controversial to suggest that breastfeeding may not be a good idea, but it is without a doubt a potential exposure risk for infants to many toxic chemicals. It is possible to test breast milk for some chemicals, such as PBDEs. PBDEs have been found at high levels in women living in India and China, in regions near factories where the products made contain flame retardant chemicals; significant levels of PBDEs have also been found in human breast milk samples of women in Europe, the U.S. and Canada on a wide scale (Siddique, 2012). It remains unclear whether these levels are of serious concern to child health and development, but testing is becoming available to women, and if one had high levels of PBDEs or other potential chemical toxins in her breast milk she may opt to feed her baby formula instead.

Toxic halides, such as bromine and fluoride, are their own group of toxins. They are not "metals" and are not removed by chelation. They are single elements, rather than chemical molecules, so they are not removed by the same biotransformation processes as chemical and biological toxins are. They are so similar to the biological halides of chlorine and iodine that they become bound in your cells and require significant time to get out of the body, so avoidance is particularly important. It is theoretically possible that they may be removed more quickly from the body by taking iodine supplements. Iodine is what belongs where the toxic halides are usually stuck; iodine is larger and can't displace them very well directly, but if iodine is available, it will be able to bind where it is supposed to and help keep the bromine and fluorine from binding where they don't belong.

Estrogens and xenoestrogens—even the ones your body produces naturally—are certainly toxic. It is helpful that our bodies have mechanisms for detoxifying estrogen already because estrogen can have harmful effects. I suspect the natural means of eliminating real estrogens may not be effective in eliminating the estrogenic chemicals (xenoestrogens) as well, because their chemical structures are very different and diverse. Removal of xenoestrogens like bisphenol A, PCBs, phthalates and other chemicals is probably best achieved through the general chemical detox methods discussed above.

The primary route of clearance for our naturally occurring estrogens is conversion and conjugation in the liver, then passing out through the stool. Cruciferous vegetables have a compound called I3C (indole-3-carbinol) that facilitates the best liver transformation of estrogens. You can find I3C in supplements and its "activated" form, called DIM (diindolylmethane), to aid estrogen transformation. Eating plenty of broccoli, cauliflower, and Brussels sprouts or taking these supplements help detoxify the estrogens but do not necessarily clear them from the body.

To help clear estrogen from the body, you can take "calcium-D-glucarate," which helps ensure estrogens entering the GI tract from the liver remain in the stool to be passed from the body. The liver is supposed to attach glucuronic acid to the estrogen molecules (conjugation), and calcium-D-glucarate facilitates that process. If estrogens are not properly conjugated, they are reabsorbed by the intestines and put right back into circulation through your body. Certain intestinal bacteria interfere with this process by producing an enzyme that cleaves the glucuronic acid off the estrogen again, allowing the estrogen to be reabsorbed in the intestines once again. Taking calcium-D-glucarate helps override that interference, by tying up the enzyme to some extent.

Some substances, such as marijuana and a number of prescription drugs, impair your body's ability to transform and clear estrogens. These drugs impair the liver's ability to transform and detoxify estrogens because they are processed by the same enzymes.

Mold toxins are another special case in terms of detoxification. Your body is likely able to perform some degree of biotransformation or destruction of these toxins, but the major route of clearance is passage from the body through the stool. Like the estrogens, mold toxins tend to be reabsorbed in the intestines and re-circulated back into the body, so people can remain ill for months or years even after their exposure has ceased. An effective method for binding the mold toxins and helping to clear them from the body is to take a binding resin or compound that holds them in the stool so they pass out of the body.

The prescription substance cholestyramine is seemingly the best choice if you can find a practitioner to prescribe it for you. Dosing is in "scoops"zzz or partial scoops; usually ¼ to ½ scoop three or four times daily. It must be taken on an *empty stomach* so it doesn't become bound up in your food. People usually need to take it for only a month or two, unless they are being continually exposed. Alternative substances you can try if you can't get the prescription include activated charcoal and bentonite clay; these are widely available at health food stores.

The perfluorinated compounds used in non-stick cookware and stain-resistant textile products have proven particularly difficult to remove from the body. Studies of sauna and some other common detoxification methods showed no clearance at all. Cholestyramine is the only substance shown to help remove these toxins so far (Genuis, 2010), so it is worth adding this medication to a general detoxification regimen—possibly just a dose at bedtime nightly for general purposes.

There are many good books on environmental toxicity and detoxification with good reviews of available data and science. Of course, some books are somewhat far-fetched and extremist, which seems unnecessary, because the reality is scary enough. The EPA and CDC websites provide some mainstream data on the scope of the problem, which is on the conservative side, of course, but it will frighten you thoroughly nonetheless. Those agencies don't offer any advice regarding treatment of toxin-related illness or strategies for detoxification.

I want to end this discussion by saying that you *should* be frightened about this issue and that you *should* change your own habits, thereby helping to change the world and its environment for the better. The issue of environmental toxicity is one of the major upstream causes of all chronic illness we are experiencing today, and it's getting worse all the time. It will likely take several generations for the human species to recover, even if we completely halt all chemical production right now. There is much to do, but the first step is awareness. The best way to detoxify our future generations is to help detoxify the planet. Doing so will take everyone's cooperation.

Treatment of environmental sensitivity

A sensitivity problem is mediated by the immune system rather than a direct effect of the substances themselves; it is a form of allergy that can be caused by just about anything, even typically beneficial substances like foods and individual nutrients. Penicillin and peanut allergy are good examples, the symptoms of which can be severe from even very small exposures. The treatment of allergy to foods, inhalants, and other biological substances are discussed thoroughly in the following chapter on allergy and autoimmunity, so I will focus here on chemical sensitivity.

Conventional allergists and practitioners have no problem recognizing severe adverse reactions to drugs like antibiotics, painkillers, seizure medications, blood pressure drugs and others as allergies and no problem understanding skin dermatitis from nickel and other common metals, latex, detergents, and fabric softeners. However, the chronic, debilitating reactions many people have to common environmental chemicals are not viewed in the same way. That is tragic considering how common chemical sensitivities are becoming.

One study in Atlanta, GA found that 12.6% of a random sample of 1,582 adults reported having some sort of sensitivity reaction to at least one common chemical. Furthermore, 13.5% of that subset (1.8% of the entire population surveyed) reported having lost their jobs because of their chemical sensitivity (Caress, 2003). I have to wonder how many more people surveyed were ill due to chemicals and just didn't *know* it.

Respondents in the Atlanta survey mentioned above reported being initially sensitized by exposure to pesticides 27.5% of the time, exposure to solvents 27.5% of the time, and most others apparently did not know their inciting trigger. Only 1.4% of those with chemical sensitivity in this study had a history of prior emotional problems, suggesting there is a physiological cause to chemical sensitivity and not a psychological one (Caress, 2003). Most chemically sensitive people I know, including myself, tend to react to perfumes and other items with fragrance chemicals such as "air fresheners", body sprays, lotions, shampoos and other "personal care" products.

In reality these fragrant household chemicals aren't truly *safe* for anyone; and what's worse is that our government does nothing to protect us from them at this point. A study published in *Environmental Impact Review* evaluated just six common household products, three "air fresheners" and three laundry products, and isolate nearly one hundred different volatile organic compounds (VOCs) between them collectively. None of these chemicals appeared on any of the product labels, and only one had an MSDS (materials safety data sheet) listed for the product containing it. Ten of the VOCs isolated are supposed to be regulated as toxic or hazardous substances under federal law. Furthermore, three of the identified VOCs (acetaldehyde, chloromethane and 1,4-dioxane) are officially classified as Hazardous Air Pollutants (HAPs). The researchers looked into the legal aspects of this situation and found that there is no law in the U.S. currently requiring disclosure of all chemical ingredients in consumer products or fragrances (Steinemann, 2009).

Chemical sensitivity can usually be objectively demonstrated by skin testing or oral challenge techniques taught through the American Academy of Environmental Medicine. The biochemistry of these reactions has been worked out to some extent and can be understood in similar fashion to well-accepted chemical sensitivities, such as those to penicillin, other drugs, and biological allergens. Unfortunately, conventional medicine does not accept these sensitivities as legitimate; the biochemistry is ignored by the establishment and the skin injection testing is considered invalid. (In fact, many insurance companies consider it fraud to submit the costs of this testing for reimbursement.) Skin *patch* test kits for chemical allergies are considered acceptable mainstream testing, mainly used in diagnosing chemical dermatitis problems; these kits contain only a small number of chemicals to assess, and they may not detect milder reactions.

I think one difficulty in gaining acceptance of chemical sensitivity by providers is that the patients seem to be sick all the time, rather than to be sick in acute episodes. Those who are allergic to birch pollen are miserably ill the entire month of May where I live, and that is accepted. However, the chronic nature of the illness of those with chemical sensitivity occurs because they are chronically exposed to the chemicals to which they are sensitive in the modern world, and they carry small amounts of those chemicals inside their bodies at all times.

Another problem is the difficulty of believing that someone could be sick from something that seems harmless to everyone else. Again, this attitude is silly because we readily accept that a peanut might kill one child while every other child in his classroom can eat peanut butter all day long with no adverse effects.

The obvious reason that this attitude still holds is money (as with so many things that don't make sense). Imagine how much money in worker's compensation, personal injury claims, and retooling would be involved if it were widely accepted that normal exposure to everyday chemicals makes some people sick.

The number of chemically ill people is increasing dramatically, and it is only a matter of time before the whole thing blows up in the face of the chemical industry. But I worry that, by then, it will be too late for far too many of us. It is important to explore the possibility of chemical causes for your symptoms and to work hard to convince your providers of the importance of this issue. The best way to test this possibility on your own is to avoid the offending chemicals and see if you feel better; you can then confirm which chemicals are the triggers by challenge through intentional or accidental exposure later.

For those with skin rashes, formal diagnosis can be done through skin patch or injection techniques if you can find a good dermatologist who does patch testing for chemicals or an environmental physician who does intradermal testing. There are hundreds of environmental physicians across the country, but there may not be one within an easy drive or even your entire state depending on where you live. I recommend the Environmental Health Centers in Dallas, Texas, founded by Dr. William Rae, and Buffalo, New York, run by Dr. Kalpana Patel, to those who are extremely ill and may require inpatient treatment at first.

The mainstays of treatment with chemical sensitivity still include avoidance, reduction of total load, nutrient support and detoxification techniques. The unique aspects to treating chemical sensitivity, rather than toxicity, involve the immune system and techniques for immune desensitization.

You will need an environmentally trained physician or holistic practitioner who practices some of these nonconventional techniques to help you with immune therapy and desensitization. The treatments that may help include provocation/neutralization, low-dose allergy therapy (LDA), enzyme-potentiated desensitization (EPD), the Nambudripad's allergy elimination technique (NAET), electroacupuncture according to Voll (EAV) technology, and other energetic and homeopathic desensitization techniques (I myself have an Indigo Machine for this purpose). The next chapter focuses on allergy and offers a thorough discussion of these techniques.

Prevention on a population-wide scale

There is no real need for these toxic harmful chemical substances to be created and no need for us to keep digging up toxic, naturally occurring metals from the ground. The best way to prevent chemical toxicity is to stop producing chemicals, and the best way to reduce the amount of mercury in our food supply is to stop burning coal for energy. Another excellent way to reduce chemical and heavy metal pollution would be to stop pumping petroleum out of the ground.

These processes continue on a massive scale because corporations make billions of dollars in profits from the sale of toxic products. It's not just oil and gasoline; it's plastic bottles, non-recycled paper products, cheap household cleaners and detergents (the environmentally safe ones are more expensive), the practice of buying new items when old used ones could be restored, and other forms of waste.

The United States is clearly the worst about this on a relative scale; we consume and waste more than any other country by a staggering margin. The World Resources Institute, a subsidiary of the United Nations Development Program, found that in 2004 the U.S. accounted for 33% of global consumption though we accounted for less than 5% of the global population. The fact that our culture has been glamorized around the world has caused other populations to create far more toxic waste than they did before as well.

We have the power to change this situation by becoming more conscious of what we are purchasing and consuming and by using our voting power to swing our policies toward improved human health whenever possible. We can support recycling programs and the companies that produce cleaner, safer products or that are promoting truly clean energy. It will take resolve and strength of will for sure; many in our population do not care about "the environment" at all, and even ridicule those who try to make a difference in their own small ways.

You can't just wait for the situation to change on its own; the current situation is killing us, and our future generations. We may have only a hundred years before all of us are sterile, autistic, and chronically ill. I know that sounds dramatic and unlikely, but so have many other truths until they have become reality. Don't just sit back and wait for the world to change: watch for your opportunities to help change it. They occur every day.

CHAPTER 5 – ALLERGY
AND AUTOIMMUNITY

Introduction

I put allergy and autoimmunity together in this chapter because they both involve the immune system's attacking something it should not attack. That makes them similar processes even though conventional medicine wants to divide each type of allergy into a separate condition and each autoimmune disease into some useless specific "diagnosis". The common physiology of the two involves dysregulation of the immune system, causing a failure to recognize harmless environmental (or "self") antigens. That is a fundamental underlying problem with the immune system, the tendency toward which is somewhat genetic.

Autoimmunity refers to the immune system's attacking some aspect of the person's own body, including the skin (e.g., psoriasis), the brain (e.g., multiple sclerosis), the heart (e.g., rheumatic fever), the intestines (e.g., Crohn's disease and ulcerative colitis), the joints (e.g., rheumatoid arthritis), widespread connective tissues (e.g., systemic lupus), and any other organ or tissue type, or even blood cells (e.g., autoimmune hemolytic anemia and immune thrombocytopenia). This very diverse set of discrete diseases has common upstream causes.

As I've mentioned, the term *allergy* often engenders some disagreement. Modern conventional allergist decided around the 1920s or so, that a "true allergy" refers to an adverse response to an environmental (non-self) antigen (protein or other trigger molecule) involving a measurable antibody reaction of the IgE class or certain cell-mediated immune reactions demonstrable by skin testing. In *my* world, though, the word *allergy* refers to any adverse immune response to something that should be considered harmless. Physicians who practice conventional allergy care generally use the terms *sensitivity* or *intolerance* to describe a demonstrable illness reaction to something not involving IgE antibody or the typical skin test reactions. This distinction is just semantics, and is not helpful to anyone.

The immune system can react to a substance in many different ways in a molecular-biology sense; calling some of those reactions allergies and others something else is not helpful. It leads to failure to appropriately treat many people who are suffering. Therefore, when I use the term *allergy*, I am referring to any symptom or adverse reaction related to an environmental trigger like pollen, mold, pet dander, foods, and chemicals.

You may have noticed that people with one type of allergy frequently have other types as well and that these people sometimes evolve into having autoimmune disease. In addition, those with one type of autoimmune disease frequently have other autoimmune conditions because the immune dysfunction is the real issue, not the particular target causing a given symptom. Treatment should ideally involve correcting the aberrant immune response, rather than suppressing the entire immune system or merely treating symptoms.

These conditions are not all the way "upstream," meaning they are not typically the truly primary causes. Immune dysfunction problems are typically secondary to, or "downstream" from, various other underlying causes; they are usually due to nutritional deficiencies, hormonal imbalances, and environmental toxins mixed with genetic tendencies. I include these conditions in this section on underlying causes of illness because there is a point of intervention here that is sufficiently upstream to capture many of the downstream problems, and this immune response problem is a key treatable point for many people with chronic illness.

The scope of the problem

As a category, allergy-related complaints comprise the number-one reason for visits to primary care physicians in the US, and these problems are becoming more common all the time. Autoimmune diseases as a group are now thought to be the third leading cause of death overall in some studies, after cardiovascular diseases and cancers.

If you are over thirty, you may have a hard time recalling anyone in your elementary school classrooms who needed an Epi-Pen in the nurse's office because of life-threatening food allergies. But now it seems that there is at least one child in every class with severe allergies to one or more foods, and the nurse's office at every school likely has a dozen or more Epi-Pens. The prevalence of IgE-mediated food allergy in the UK is now around 5% (Holloway, 2011).

Asthma is usually an allergic disease related to inhalant or food allergies or both. Asthma and asthma-related death have become increasingly common in the past few decades, with higher incidence in cities than in rural areas, probably because of air pollution. The prevalence of asthma in the U.S. rose from 7.3% in 2001 to 8.4% in 2010, with notably higher rates in children and minorities than in adults and whites (Akinbami, 2012). How many children do you know now who have asthma versus how many you knew when you were young yourself? How many rescue inhalers does the school nurse have for students now?

Allergy problems are some of the most common problems I deal with every day in clinic, and the most severe cases are in children. Fortunately, there are ways to improve the immune response and function overall, to address the underlying factors to some degree, and to alter the immune response to help eliminate these problems.

Underlying causes of immune dysregulation

Allergies were far less common a hundred years ago, and virtually nonexistent before the late 1800s; they have blossomed as a problem particularly since the post-World War II industrialized era here and in other industrialized nations. Great Britain has had these problems the longest because of earlier industrialization and pollution (Waite, 1995). The Japanese had no problems with inhalant allergies to their cedar tree pollen until after World War II and the attendant industry-related pollution that occurred at that time, but it has since become a prevalent and increasing problem, along with many other inhalant allergies. Before the end of the twentieth century, one study revealed that more than one third of Japanese men had self-reported allergic rhinitis and 11% were found to have IgE antibodies against the cedar tree pollen specifically (Sakurai, 1998).

Air pollution, which is obviously part of the problem, is impossible to avoid in our modern society and in the modern world in general. A simple but elegant study proved a link between a common air pollutant and inhalant allergy. Healthy volunteers were exposed to an aerosolized protein derived from a deep-sea mollusk, with which no one had ever come in contact, and none of the subjects subsequently showed antibodies to the protein in their blood. A second group of volunteers was exposed to the same protein twenty-four hours after exposure to a small amount of aerosolized diesel exhaust, and *all* of those subjects developed a measurable antibody response to the mollusk protein (Meggs, 2008).

This test showed that an airborne irritant can trigger over-activation and dysregulation of the immune response, leading to allergy. We don't know exactly how much automobile exhaust, cigarette smoke, factory discharge, or other air pollution one must be exposed to for this sort of reaction to occur, but there is certain to be a wide spectrum of affect, depending upon the individual in question (like everything else in biology). Since everyone is exposed to these sorts of pollutants and irritants on some level, avoidance is currently impossible.

As for food allergies, our food here in the United States is now contaminated with so many chemicals that some of them may likely be irritating or toxic enough to trigger immune agitation in the gut, leading to food allergy. About seventy-five percent of your immune system resides in your GI tract because it is a major point of interaction with the outside world, including germs, food particles, and whatever else you might swallow. Of the thousands of chemicals the US government currently allows in our food, I suspect that none have been studied for their ability to induce allergy to other substances. I'm not even sure how one could go about doing that type of testing. Isn't that comforting?

Chemical allergies, which are increasingly common, are related directly to the presence of environmental chemicals in airborne, contact, or ingested routes of exposure. Other underlying causes may also contribute to chemical reactions, but the chemicals themselves are the key reaction point, as discussed in the preceding chapter. While there are ways to stop the immune response to the offending chemicals, avoidance, reduction of total load, nutrient support, and detoxification are also important.

Aside from the environmental poisons that cause immune system dysfunction, other causes include hormonal issues, stress and energetic problems, and nutritional deficiency issues. Weston Price, DDS found that allergy was nonexistent in indigenous populations that ate their traditional diets, while the newer generations that were beginning to eat processed foods were developing them (Price, 2006). Francis Pottenger, MD found that allergies began to arise in the cats fed devitalized food (cooked meat or pasteurized milk instead of raw forms), while the cats fed raw-food diets had none. He even described a case of asthma in one cat after a few generations of depleted food (Pottenger, 1983).

The hormonal issues involved primarily involve an adequate balance of thyroid, cortisol, progesterone, estrogen, testosterone, and DHEA. If you have problems with allergy or (especially) autoimmune disease, you should evaluate your status of these hormones. Many allergies arise right after a woman has a major swing in her hormones, such as puberty, pregnancy, the birth of a baby, or completing menopause. Many autoimmune conditions, which are much more common in women, are strongly influenced by pregnancy in one direction or the other (some improve during pregnancy and some worsen). The hormonal question is a stone you should not leave unturned.

Allergy to hormones themselves may sound like an outlandish concept, but it is not a rare occurrence. You can develop an adverse reaction to virtually anything, including sunlight, water, temperature changes, vitamins, minerals and your own tissues, so why not hormones? Some common conditions that may indicate this problem include PMS, endometriosis, depression, anxiety, and generalized fatigue or pain syndromes.

A person who is allergic to a hormone will note an adverse reaction to the administration of a hormone they seemed to clinically need; for example, a woman with PMS who has a low progesterone level may find that she becomes angry, gets migraines, or suffers worse PMS symptoms when she is given additional progesterone. She clearly seems to "need" it, but cannot tolerate it even in small doses. In this event, she needs to undergo neutralization for this hormonal sensitivity; some of these techniques will be discussed shortly.

The energetic/spiritual issues are hugely important as well. A good deal of modern research has demonstrated the effects of negative emotion on the function of your immune system. Negative emotion alters your resistance to infection and can cause abnormal shifts in your immune system, leading to increased allergy or autoimmune issues. One study demonstrated far greater increases of mediators of inflammation such as TNF and IL-6 in women than in men with chronic musculoskeletal pain conditions, and this was thought to be correlated with a greater tendency to display negative emotion during the experiment (Darnall, 2010).

Symptoms of inhalant allergy

Inhalant allergies—at least the most typical symptoms—are familiar to most people. Those with airborne allergies generally have symptoms involving the mucous membranes that are exposed to the air, such as the eyes, nasal passages, and lungs. Red, irritated, watery eyes, runny nose, sneezing, coughing, and wheezing are common and can progress to sinus infections, bronchitis, or pneumonia and to the chronic bronchial inflammation we call asthma. Though everyone is not bothered by the same triggers, we all understand the problem because it's common and the mechanisms have been worked out by medical science.

Some less common symptoms include headaches, mouth tingling, mild chest tightness, heartburn, generalized fatigue, body aches, and mental problems like attention deficit issues, trouble focusing, disorientation, memory problems, anxiety and irritability, sleep problems, and generalized unhappiness miserable. Some may have altered heart rates or palpitations, tremors or twitches, urinary urgency, or other strange and seemingly unrelated symptoms.

If the allergen is a chemical in the air, your only symptom may be a sudden desire to get away from the area (i.e., aversion). These symptoms can occur in the absence of the observable problems like runny nose or sneezing, and those around you may think you're making it up or just crazy if you have these reactions.

I get red eyes (often just my left eye for some reason), mild tightness in my chest, mild mental suppression, and a general sense that I'm in a bad place whenever I'm in most hotels and most second-hand stores. It has to be chemical and/or mold residues in the air or something similar, but I haven't been able to pinpoint it. I can barely stand to sleep on the sheets and pillowcases in most hotels because of the harsh laundry chemicals used to wash them. I don't let housekeeping come in to give me "fresh" linens on the bed for several days, so I can avoid the extra chemical poisoning every day.

Oral reactions to certain foods, or oral allergy syndrome, can be a cross-reactivity response from certain airborne plant allergies. Our best regional example in south-central Alaska is the itching, tingling, or burning in the mouths of those with significant birch tree pollen allergy when they eat thin-skinned fruits like peaches, apples, nectarines, and cherries or certain tree nuts like walnuts and almonds. This reaction occurs because of their tree pollen allergy, rather than specific reactions to those foods, and it will typically improve with just treatment of the pollen allergy.

Inhalant allergens typically include plants, molds, animals, and chemicals of all types. Some have such severe problems to foods that they can have "inhalant" or airborne reactions just by being in the same room with them. The most common example is peanut allergy, the most common cause of allergy-related death. Some individuals are so sensitive to peanuts that they go into anaphylactic shock if they just catch a whiff of a peanut butter cookie from twenty feet away. Children with a problem this severe usually have to be home-schooled because it is so difficult to get every other child in the class to keep foods containing peanuts out of the classroom, and it isn't worth the risk. Extremely careful desensitization is critical for those with allergies this severe.

Symptoms of food allergy

I diverge here from the mainstream view of allergy symptoms because the conventional view is so limiting that it fails a large number of children and adults. The typical concept of food allergy involves comparatively severe reactions, such as hives and anaphylactic types of reactions. Affected individuals may also have mild symptoms, such as itching in their mouths or throats or on their skin; they may develop a few hives that are mildly annoying or the reaction may progress quickly to swelling of the airway, respiratory failure, and death. In the absence of hives, mouth or throat itching or swelling, wheezing, or other severe respiratory symptoms, the reaction is not considered symptomatic of a "true allergy" by conventional allergists.

If a food makes you throw up or have stomach pain, it may be termed "intolerance" or "sensitivity," rather than an allergy. All these distinctions do is to prevent the patient from getting the advice and care they need. In *my* reality, food reactions can come in all forms and levels of severity. I call them all allergies for the sake of simplicity because human physiology is complicated enough, and doctors don't need to make it worse. If a patient has been to an allergist or done some reading on the subject, he or she is undoubtedly confused. Hopefully this chapter offers a relatively clear explanation.

The point I want to make is that food reactions can manifest as almost any acute or chronic symptom, anywhere in the body. If you come into my office with any persistent symptom, I'm likely to suggest food allergy investigation unless some other cause is evident. Following is a system-by-system abbreviated list of common food allergy symptoms and presentations.

General/Constitutional: Fatigue, weight gain/loss, poor growth in children, temperature regulation problems. It seems like almost everyone with "chronic fatigue syndrome" has food allergies, especially to gluten and dairy.

Neurological: Headaches or migraines, balance and coordination problems mimicking multiple sclerosis, seizures or epilepsy, numbness or tingling in various places, random shooting electrical pains.

Psychiatric: Depression or anxiety, panic attacks, irritability, attention or focus problems (most all those with ADD issues have food allergies), insomnia, nightmares, bipolar disorder symptoms, and even full-blown schizophrenia or psychosis (Randolph, 1987). These symptoms are the most difficult to accept as being related to food allergy, but they are very common.

Skin/Integument: Rashes, eczema, psoriasis, hives, acne (especially in an adult), folliculitis, random sores, papules or pustules, itching without visible rash, brittle or abnormal nails, persistent toenail fungus or warts.

Musculoskeletal: Muscle tension or spasms, soreness in the muscles or joints for no apparent reason, joint swelling and pain, joint stiffness. Many rheumatoid arthritis and other autoimmune arthritis syndrome symptoms are triggered by food allergies, especially gluten. Many patients with "fibromyalgia" diagnoses have food allergies.

Respiratory tract: Runny nose, recurrent sinus infections, recurrent ear infections, mouth tingling or itching or sores in the mouth, coughing, wheezing, recurrent bronchitis in a nonsmoker, asthma. These reactions are very common, and most people with asthma have food allergies in addition to inhalant allergies. Almost all children with frequent ear infections are allergic to milk and should eliminate dairy.

Cardiovascular: Heart racing or palpitations, irregular heart rhythms, chest pain or vasospastic angina, high blood pressure (especially if your BP is highly variable throughout the day), unusual bruising.

Gastrointestinal: Heartburn or GERD (the vast majority of people with these symptoms have a food allergy), nausea or vomiting, stomach pains or cramps, trouble swallowing, gallbladder pains or attacks in the absence of gallstones, constipation or diarrhea or both, rectal bleeding, recurrent anal fissures, anal itching. Virtually all patients diagnosed with "irritable bowel syndrome" have food allergies, as do many with inflammatory bowel diseases like Crohn's or ulcerative colitis. Anyone who has had endoscopy with the pathology showing "eosinophilic" inflammation (e.g., esophagitis, gastritis duodenitis, colitis) certainly has food allergies.

Urinary: Persistent bedwetting past age four, chronic urinary urgency or frequency, recurring urinary infection (most common in girls), interstitial cystitis, recurrent bloody urine without explanation (typically *milk* allergy).

Reproductive system: Infertility in women or men, endometriosis, PMS, painful intercourse, chronic vaginitis, recurrent yeast infections.

Blood-related: Chronic unexplained anemia, chronically low or high platelets, elevated eosinophils (a type of white blood cell that responds only to allergy, fungus, worms and parasites).

Nutritional deficiencies such as low iron, calcium, magnesium, protein levels (e.g. albumin) or amino acids, and low vitamin B-12 may result from food allergies. This is because the intestinal tract becomes inflamed to the point where it doesn't work properly in its absorptive function. Proteins and minerals are the most difficult nutrients to digest and absorb. Vitamin B-12 has a very complex absorption process and is easily disturbed as well. Therefore, symptoms related to any of these deficiencies themselves may ultimately be the result of food allergy as well.

You see why any persistent problem eventually gets a food allergy evaluation if I can't figure out another cause. There are still other possible manifestations of food allergies, but this list should suffice to indicate the wide variety of possible symptoms.

If you have more than a couple of the symptoms listed above, you most likely have more than one food allergy. One allergic food can cause twenty symptoms, and twenty different allergic foods can all cause the same symptom. For example, a person with an egg allergy may have eczema, nausea, diarrhea, headaches, and insomnia; while a person with allergy to egg, milk and soy may have diarrhea as their only symptoms for each. If multiple foods are causing the same symptoms, you have to eliminate all of the foods before the symptoms will go away.

Specific foods worth mentioning

Some foods are more commonly allergens than others. I want to address a few of them here in detail because they are relevant to a significant portion of the population and especially to children. Those who are chronically or recurrently ill, who have an autistic spectrum disorder or severe behavioral problems, or who "don't seem right" otherwise should first remove these most common allergic foods from the diet to see if their health improves. The foods listed below constitute what are probably the five most common food allergens.

Milk

Milk allergy is arguably the most common food allergen in children, especially infants and newborns. We are supposed to have *human* milk, not milk from other animals. Our culture has been effectively brainwashed by the dairy industry and poorly trained pediatricians and nutritionists to believe we need to give our kids cows' milk for them to grow properly and have a skeleton. That is totally ridiculous considering the vast majority of humans naturally become milk intolerant by the age of four! I like to ask people to imagine suckling on a cow's udder and tell me if that feels natural to them – there is no reason we should be drinking out of cows!

Common symptoms of milk allergy in an infant include spitting up or reflux, fussiness or crying during feeding, irritability, colic, recurring ear infections, constipation or diarrhea, chronic diaper rash, and poor growth. Kids and adults may have chronic rashes like eczema or what looks like acne, chronic nasal congestion, or even wheezing. Some children with allergy may grow very rapidly, while more often they will fail to thrive. No single symptom is the only one to watch for, so be vigilant. My milk-allergic son was colicky and had numerous ear infections, but I didn't understand this until he was about ten years old; I wish I had known when he was a baby.

As we get older, the most common symptoms often change to eczema and asthma problems, severe acne, headaches or migraine, persistent heartburn, stomachache, bloating, diarrhea or constipation. A strange one is excessive earwax production or chronic ear itching; excessive nasal mucous is also common.

Most who are allergic to cow's milk will also react badly to goat's milk as well, contrary to what many believe. Goat milk may be closer to human milk in protein composition, but it is still from a barnyard animal. Goats don't look any more like a drinking fountain than cows do in my opinion. Soymilk and other plant-based milk substitutes (which of course are not "milks" at all because they come from plants) are acceptable alternatives to mammalian milk.

How the animal was fed has a lot to do with whether you will react to its milk. If you buy the typical milk available at a grocery store, it likely came from a relatively unhealthy cow that was kept in a little pen with no room to exercise, fed corn and other grains, treated with antibiotics so its stomach wouldn't explode, pumped full of hormones to keep it producing milk in quantities many times greater than it was ever supposed to produce, and victimized by chronic infections of its udder that require antibiotics and generate traces of pus in the milk.

Since this kind of milk is not organic, it will also have significant levels of pesticides in it. (Shouldn't organic milk be *cheaper*, since it doesn't have antibiotics, hormones or pesticides in it?) Yogurt, butter, ice cream, cheese, and other dairy products obtained as cheaply as possible (not organic bargain brands) are equally toxic and also offer suboptimal nutrition. The dairy products that have been processed and contain traces of these harsh chemicals seem much more likely to trigger adverse symptoms. I have seen many patients who tell me they tolerate organic milk or especially *raw* organic milk just fine, but can't drink the regular stuff from the store.

If you react badly to the standard mass-produced type of dairy, you may not react badly to organic milk from the same store. You are even less likely to react badly to milk from a grass-fed, free-range cow that lives a happy, normal life free of stress and is milked only when appropriate. Granted, this type of milk is much more expensive, and difficult to find (look for local milk co-ops) but that brings me to an extremely important point: you don't have to drink any milk at all. Let me just plead with you to take any child who is chronically sick off milk products for a few weeks, and see if they improve.

It is possible that you or your child won't react to goat's milk, so it is worth a try if you have an infant who can't breast feed and won't tolerate cow's milk or an older child or adult with high nutritional needs (e.g., cystic fibrosis, cerebral palsy). Just make sure it's privately produced raw milk from an animal fed grass and natural fodder, not the toxic goat milk at the store that is produced similarly to cow's milk.

An individual who is allergic to liquid milk may not be reactive to dairy products that have been fermented or cultured, such as yogurt or kefir, and he or she is usually not going to be reactive to butter. Butter is made from just the fat portion of milk, and allergies are usually responses to the *proteins* in a food. If you are severely milk allergic, you may react to the traces of protein in butter and should try using *ghee,* which is "clarified" butter, as a substitute. Many of us (I'm mildly milk-allergic myself) can have cheese without restriction, as it has been altered quite a bit through the culturing process; different types of cheese can affect folks differently. I'm sorry to say that ice cream is not usually going to work.

That brings me back to dairy substitutes. The dairy substitutes most people think of are probably soymilk and related products like soy cheese, soy yogurt, and soy ice cream. Since soy is one of the top five most common food allergens, try other alternatives first. Also, about eighty percent of soy is genetically modified now, so if you do use it, make sure it's organic. There are also some concerns about the hormonal effects of soy, but I believe they are blown out of proportion, so don't let those concerns stop you from eating it.

Other dairy substitutes include rice milk, oat milk, coconut milk, hazelnut milk, almond milk, and hemp milk. Coconut milk is my favorite. You can find "fake" cheese made from almonds or soy, but they really don't taste like cheese at all and make very poor substitutes in my opinion. Yogurt substitutes are mostly soy or coconut-based. You can get ice cream substitutes made from soy, rice, or coconut milk. Nutritionally speaking, any of these that you can get from coconut are probably the best for you because it has the best type of fat. Unfortunately, coconut seems to be an increasing allergen in our culture, so watch out for that. Rice products may be the least allergenic for now, because soy allergy is very common and coconut allergy has been increasing dramatically, but rice allergy is also on the rise.

One final point to make here is that lactose intolerance and milk allergy are not the same thing. If you have lactose intolerance, then you are a "normal" human because humans are phylogenetically supposed to stop drinking milk around age two. Lactose intolerance means you don't have the enzyme in your small intestine that digests the sugar (lactose) in milk. The symptoms of the resulting sugar malabsorption include increased gas formation in the intestines, since the bacteria there get to digest the sugar through fermentation, leading to belching, bloating, and lots of farting, as well as watery diarrhea, accompanied in many cases by cramping and discomfort.

An allergy is an immune reaction to a protein in a food, not a sugar digestion problem. If you get any symptoms from milk other than those associated with the GI tract, then you have an allergy and not just lactose intolerance. (Vomiting and heartburn are not symptoms of lactose intolerance either.) Some of my patients experience fatigue, headaches, and rashes from milk, as well as the diarrhea and stomach pain, and they think they just have lactose intolerance, but they're wrong. If you do just have lactose intolerance and not milk allergy, then you can have milk products with lactase enzyme support, or take lactase enzymes with foods as a supplement.

Gluten and grains

Gluten probably adversely affects more than a third of us to some degree. Gluten is a protein complex common to many grains. Grains are grass seeds, and grass apparently doesn't want us to eat its seeds because we tend to chew them up and ruin them, so these seeds often contain compounds that may be harmful to us (at least this is the anthropomorphic way in which I choose to look at it). The grains that contain gluten include wheat, rye, barley, malt, spelt, kamut, and amaranth. It is worth doing your own research on this because the topic is extensive and complex. There are numerous books and cookbooks out there now about gluten-free living.

Gluten-free alternatives include rice, corn, quinoa (pronounced "keen-wa"), millet and sorghum, arrowroot, buckwheat (which is not related to wheat at all), flax, and chia seeds. Oats may contain gluten because they are often processed in the same facilities as gluten, but you can get certified gluten-free oats. Other products used to replace wheat flour include flours made from potato, garbanzo beans, buckwheat, almonds, tapioca (cassava root), and peas.

Many of my patients buy their own wheat or other grains, grind it themselves, and make their own baked goods. That is certainly a healthier option in terms of nutrition and chemical avoidance, but does not save you from the allergy problem. Soaking your grains first won't help either, although *sprouting* your grains may be useful. Once the seeds are sprouted, they drop their defenses, so to speak, so the potentially toxic compounds and gluten are metabolized and broken down rapidly. I believe wheat grass juice has no gluten, for example.

I don't know how long you have to let grains sprout or whether you can count on every little kernel's sprouting like it should or at the same time. Therefore, don't rely on the sprouting of grains if you are truly sensitive to gluten. What's more, many of the sprouted grain breads for sale at stores include regular flour or even added gluten (even Ezekiel bread contains added gluten; read the labels).

Those with gluten allergy or sensitivity may commonly experience fatigue, depression, headaches, attention problems, stomach pains, chronic diarrhea, random joint and muscle pains, and chronic rash. Neurological symptoms like brain fog, numbness or tingling, limb weakness or coordination problems are also very common. Conventional physicians almost always diagnose a well-described syndrome called *gluten ataxia* as "multiple sclerosis", because the symptoms are largely the same. It often takes years to be properly diagnosed with gluten sensitivity, even in the most severe cases. Many of the patients I diagnose with this affliction have seen five other doctors or more prior to coming to me.

Almost all symptoms can be caused by gluten, and gluten is the most common food problem we deal with in adults. It is present in most of our processed foods, and it requires some serious attention and discipline to avoid. Gluten-related problems too often just end up being misdiagnosed as separate symptoms or problems that conventional doctors treat with a fistful of drugs that may make the patient sicker.

Most patients I see with chronic fatigue syndrome, fibromyalgia, rheumatoid arthritis, Crohn's disease and various other autoimmune disease issues have gluten sensitivity as part of their problems. The only way to be certain you don't have a problem with gluten is to eliminate it from your diet, and people just don't seem to want to do that. I struggle with this issue with patients every day in my office because it is difficult to eliminate gluten from your diet, but it is one of the most important actions many people can do for their health.

The difficulty is that you have to avoid all the grains I mentioned, but is even worse because you also should avoid processed foods of all sorts, including sauces, soups, mixes, and seasonings. You have to avoid some raisins and other dried fruits because they may have flour sprinkled on them to prevent them from sticking together, and these kinds of sources are often unlabeled. Gluten may also be listed on a label as "modified food starch," "hydrolyzed protein," "TVP," or in other ways.

While going gluten-free entails a major life change, that's exactly what many people have to do to achieve optimal health. Most chronic illness relates to lifestyle issues in various ways. I can't stress enough that it is important to give this a real try for at least a month, although very ill people have to be off gluten for three months to recover fully. Many websites, books, and other resources explain how to avoid gluten (e.g., *Gluten-Free for Dummies*), and I urge you to check them out if you have any chronic health issues at all.

People often tell me that they saw no difference after going off gluten, but when I ask whether they read every label and avoided soy sauce, chewing gum, raisins and so forth, the answer is always "no." They usually admit they ate a bit of a cracker or some pasta once in a while, "but just a tiny amount." It is likely that they don't want to believe they have a gluten problem because it's so difficult to avoid; therefore they try in some manner to "reduce" their gluten intake, rather than eliminate it completely, and then convince themselves it was never an issue for them. Unfortunately, lying to yourself won't change the fact that your gluten problem is killing you.

A growing number of my patients have finally taken my advice to get off gluten after months or years of my telling them about it. They almost all tell me afterward that they wish they had listened to me at the beginning and saved themselves a great deal of suffering. You have an opportunity now to spend a month of your life seeing if you can stop a lifetime of suffering for you or your child. It's worth it.

Tangent on "Celiac Disease"

Celiac disease (or celiac sprue, nontropical sprue, gluten enteropathy, or whatever you want to call it) is a term used to describe the most severe gastrointestinal manifestations of gluten sensitivity. It is a clinical syndrome that presents many diverse types of symptoms, but it usually involves chronic diarrhea and malabsorption, resulting in malnutrition, nutrient deficiencies, weight loss, and various non-GI symptoms like rashes, depression, and neurological symptoms. Many will have issues related to nutrient deficiencies like easy bruising from low vitamin K, low bone density from low vitamin D, anemia from low iron, and so on.

Celiac disease has a nice, neat clinical description that technically involves having a biopsy of your small intestine that shows damage to the villi, the small, fingerlike projections that line the small intestine. We call this biopsy finding "villous atrophy," and it comes in several grades of severity. The most eminent, strict interpretation of celiac disease requires that the patient have *total* villous atrophy on a biopsy; otherwise, he or she is told they do not have celiac disease and therefore no problem with gluten either.

This approach is inadequate, and it leaves more than ninety-five percent of people with a gluten problem out in the cold. Doctors like to make the definition of disease very narrow, perhaps because it makes us feel important, when diseases almost always present with a wide range of possible forms and symptoms—none more so than gluten allergy.

Some blood-based antibody tests are anti-gliadin, anti-endomysial and, anti-tissue transglutaminase IgG and IgA levels. These tests can cost more than $600 of your hard-earned money, and they are not worth it. They are supposedly "95 percent specific," but that is the case only in patients who demonstrate total villous atrophy on an intestinal biopsy. These tests are negative in the vast majority of patients who do, in fact, have significant problems from gluten, so they may leave the neediest patients untreated yet again; even worse, the ordering clinician may now convince the patient they "definitely don't" have a problem with gluten.

Genetic testing can tell you whether you are *at risk for* celiac disease by looking at the HLA-DQ2 and DQ8 markers, although those tests will not tell you whether you are at risk for gluten *allergy*. Celiac disease is not really an allergy but an autoimmune reaction to gluten in which the immune system of people who are susceptible (about a third of us, based on the epidemiology of the HLA-DQ2 and –DQ8 markers) attacks their own tissue in response to gluten ingestion. Allergy is different; like any other food allergy, it is mediated through antibody reactions to the food proteins. Antibody types can include IgE, IgA or IgG (IgG has four described subtypes also, and there is controversy about which is the most relevant).

Anyone can develop an allergy to gluten, wheat, rye, or any of the other relevant grains because allergy is not a genetic disease. It may be worth determining whether you have the genetic susceptibility or not because, if you do, you should consider avoiding gluten forever even if you don't have allergic symptoms. A corollary to this discussion is that the treatments for *allergy* are not likely to cure *celiac disease*. The only real solution for those with celiac is complete gluten avoidange.

The only valid test for gluten allergy is the total elimination of gluten from the diet for at least a month. If we were talking face to face, I might be yelling right now because I've had the discussion hundreds of times, and people seem so resistant to hearing it. If you want to waste your money on laboratory tests, endure the risks and expense of undergoing intestinal endoscopy and biopsy, feel free to do so, but they won't tell you whether you have a problem with gluten.

If you do have a gluten problem, no intervention other than getting off gluten will fix you! Some may not see truly good symptom resolution until they have eliminated gluten for three months, so this takes a lot of patience and discipline (two things that far too many of us lack). You have to get the adverse influence out of your life to achieve health; there are no medications, vitamins, or herbs that will overcome it. The best part is that it costs you much less to do the "test" of dietary elimination than to do other kinds of tests that tell you nothing useful.

One of the most common questions my patients ask when I tell them to avoid gluten is "Well then, what am I supposed to eat?" About 99 percent of foods *don't* contain gluten; it just takes some determination to change how you eat because our culture is so heavily into bread or flour-based products and processed foods. There are hundreds of foods that don't contain gluten. Beginning with the letter A, there are apples, apricots, almonds, arrowroot, anchovies, artichokes, anise, agave nectar, asparagus, avocados, arugula, alfalfa, antelope, aardvark, abalone . This really isn't that hard, unless you choose to make it hard. I have dozens of patients who have done this successfully and state that it is quite easy once you make the change and figure out how to shop and prepare foods differently. Once you're there, your perspective will change.

Corn

Corn allergy is very common, probably because it is present in so many foods, and we are more likely to develop allergies to the things to which we are exposed more often. Of course, some foods are much more inherently allergenic than others, for reasons we don't understand. The most common allergens in the diet tend to meet both of these criteria: They are common in our typical diet, and they are inherently allergenic. Corn is a grain, and therefore a grass seed, though not a gluten-containing grain. Rice is also a grass seed and a type of grain, but it remains relatively hypoallergenic in our society.

Corn, corn starch, corn syrup, and other corn constituents are present in a large majority of processed foods in the United States, so avoiding corn poses just about as big a problem as avoiding gluten does. Corn may be present under other names like "vegetable protein," "gluten" (because the pulp inside corn is sometimes called gluten even though this meaning is completely different from the meaning of the word that it refers to in wheat), and "vegetable oil." Aside from what is on the label of a processed food, many packaged foods in plastic wrappers have cornstarch lightly sprinkled on the inside to prevent the food from sticking to the wrapper.

The vast majority of livestock in this country is fed lots of corn, so these animals are essentially *made of corn* to some extent. As a result, many corn-sensitive people cannot eat standard beef from the grocery store because of allergy reactions but can eat all the grass-fed beef they want without consequence. Some infants break out in bad rashes when their mothers (who are breastfeeding the babies) eat corn-fed beef but not if the mothers eat grass-fed organic beef. I have seen these scenarios repeatedly in clinical practice, though I have not seen published "scientific proof" of the phenomenon.

It is not completely clear how the allergen travels through one animal into another, but it probably has something to do with the energetic signature of the offending substance. Corn is particularly bad in this sense perhaps because of a specific change that occurs in the carbon atoms themselves when they become part of corn. Books like *The Omnivore's Dilemma* describe this phenomenon very well. With a particular analysis of the carbon in your cheeseburger, for example, you can determine how much of that ground beef was "made" from corn.

The majority of corn is now genetically modified (GMO) in our society, which may affect how allergenic it is and whether it poses other illness risks. One common GMO corn product is called "*Bt corn.*" The initials "Bt" stand for a strain of bacteria called *Bacillus thuringiensis* that produces a toxin that kills insects by causing their stomach or elsewhere in their GI tract to hemorrhage or deteriorate. In other words, if bugs try to eat the Bt corn, they will die.

It would be great if we could be sure that the toxin did not cause similar problems in humans, but that question was not studied so we can't be sure. However, several reports have been made of cattle dying from gastrointestinal bleeding or other distress after eating this type of corn (Smith, 2007). Do you know anyone with irritable bowel syndrome, chronic colitis, or inflammatory bowel disease? Perhaps he or she should try going off corn to see if those problems go away. They could try eating organic corn to see if it affects them similarly. Organic products are still not allowed to be GMO, but that could change at any time as our government continues to sell out our health to big business.

This is as good a place as any to discuss GMO or GE (genetically engineered) foods a bit further. There are many ways to genetically alter plants and animals to improve food production and even human health. Bt corn, for example, has been shown to have greatly decreased rates of crop loss from the primary corn-eating insect predators and also from certain fungi. These fungi produce toxins that are certainly harmful to humans, and Bt corn contains significantly lower amounts of these mycotoxins (Wu, 2006). Unfortunately, there is a very dark side to GMO/GE foods that seems to be widely suppressed by immense political and economic forces.

There is a great deal to discuss within this topic, but not space enough for an adequate discussion here. For now, I would simply advise people to avoid GMO/GE foods as much as possible; this means eating only organic corn and soy in particular. I would urge everyone to vote for legislation that forces the labeling of GM foods as such also, so people at least know what they are eating. Before you decide this whole thing is some silly conspiracy theory and choose to ignore my warning, I suggest reading Jeffrey Smith's book *Genetic Roulette: The Documented Health Risks of Genetically Engineered Foods* and William Engdahl's *Seeds of Destruction: The Hidden Agenda of Genetic Manipulation.*

Soy

Soy became a huge cash crop in the United States in the last hundred years or so. It was primarily used first as a rotational crop for nitrogen fixation in the soil to improve corn production. Since soy is edible, the agricultural industry, needing a market for this huge crop, began putting soy products into all sorts of foods as filler and making margarine and other artificial foods out of soy. Unfortunately, soy is not necessarily a good food to eat in such large amounts (Fallon, 1995).

Because of all this soy exposure, soy has become one of the five most common allergens in our diets. If you start reading labels, you will find soy in the majority of processed foods. What makes the soy allergy issue worse is that GMO soy now makes up more than 80 percent of the soy market. Some people believe that GMO soy is more allergenic than other soy because the genetic modifications increase the content of the allergenic proteins, and this is currently under study. In addition, there are often genes from the Brazil nut spliced into GMO soy, so those with nut allergies may cross-react.

Eggs and Peanuts

Egg allergies seem to me to be more common than peanut allergies, though no other food seems as dangerous as the peanut. Still, I love eggs and think they are a wonderful food nutritionally, as long as they're from naturally fed free-range hens. I have much less love for peanuts, and peanut allergies are the worst in terms of the severity of anaphylactic response and risk of death.

One of the reasons that eggs are a common allergen is that we use eggs often, either as ingredients in our various foods or just as themselves in our diets. We feed commercial hens a lot of corn and grain, which probably increases the allergic potential of their eggs. It is unfortunate that eggs are so commonly allergenic, but you shouldn't eat most eggs from the grocery store anyway because of how they are produced. The one good thing about having an egg allergy is that it will excuse you from the influenza and some other vaccines without a fight from your doctor or your child's pediatrician.

Egg allergies are linked to gallbladder problems. In my experience most patients with non-gallstone-related gallbladder disease and inflammation have egg allergy, and most people with problems this sort do much better if they go off eggs. They may have acquired diagnoses like "acalculous cholecystitis" or "biliary dyskinesia", but the problem is often egg allergy.

The other most common food triggers for gallbladder problems seem to be garlic and onions.

As for peanuts, they don't offer anything special to the diet other than allowing vegetarians to falsely believe they have a decent protein source. Peanut butter is almost always contaminated with aflatoxin, the most potent cancer-causing natural substance on the planet, and it's often adulterated with sugar.

Peanuts are far easier to avoid in the diet than the other items on this list, but peanuts are ubiquitous, and the severity of the allergy can be extreme. Faculty physicians in the American Academy of Environmental Medicine have emphatically recommended against even having peanut antigen in the office because the reactions can be so bad.

Alcohol and Food Allergy -

Alcohol found in beverages is always derived from some plant source—you never see "beef beer" or "venison vodka"—that has been fermented by yeast organisms and has had its sugar converted into ethyl alcohol. Two considerations related to alcohol are relevant to the allergy discussion here: the ubiquitous presence of yeast, and the plant source as a potential allergen.

Many people are allergic or sensitive to yeast organisms in some way, and the yeast residue left in alcohol may be a trigger for those who are most sensitive. The issue of the food of origin is important in terms of allergy. Even though the grain or other plant from which the alcohol was made was fermented thoroughly, traces of its antigens or its energetic signature remain. If you are allergic to wheat or barley, you will probably react to beer; if you are allergic to corn, you will likely have issues with whiskey; and so on.

Dr. Theron Randolph demonstrated that most alcoholics have an allergic sensitivity to the food from which their drink of choice is derived (Randolph, 1987). Most people who fall into this category become "different" or seem intoxicated immediately after having the first drink, way before they should have been technically intoxicated from it. Randolph's explanation is that this represents a neurological manifestation of their allergy.

Those with alcoholism of this nature must eliminate the food of origin for their alcohol of choice—and the alcohol—completely from their diets. For example, if a person is hooked on vodka, he or she must eliminate potatoes from the diet if he or she wishes to kick the vodka habit (of course, vodka can be made from other foods than potato, so you need to know the food source of the person's favorite brand). If the person becomes clean and sober but then eats some potato (or whatever plant source), he or she may suddenly feel the same intoxication felt from vodka and begin a downward spiral back into alcoholism. I know it sounds crazy, but this is a very real phenomenon.

People with allergies get allergies

Some underlying factors that cause allergies are present in those with allergies and promote the advent of even more allergies. Some have a genetic predisposition, some have become toxic with environmental chemicals or heavy metals, some are very deficient in vitamin D or essential fatty acids, and others have chronic inflammation in their respiratory tract or gut that causes the immune system to react against certain inhalants or foods.

This is what makes the food allergy problem particularly bad. Once you develop a food allergy in the GI tract, it causes an inflammatory response and over-activation of the gut's immune system (gut-associated lymphoid tissue, or "GALT"), which comprises roughly 70-75 percent of your total immune system. This reaction causes two issues that promote allergies to other types of foods: the hyper-vigilance of the immune system itself and the fact that the damaged intestinal lining allows food proteins to leak into the bloodstream before being properly digested, exposing them to the systemic immune system as well.

Because of this process, eating foods that cause inflammation, even if you do not feel the inflammation or have noticeable GI symptoms inevitably makes the problem worse, leading to becoming allergic to more and more foods. This effect may also pertain to some extent in inhalant allergies because patients often develop new and more numerous allergies in that area. It is very important to remove allergens from the diet, to avoid exposure to known environmental allergens or irritants, and to control inflammation if you want to avoid making these problems worse.

People with one type of allergy are very likely to have others. If you have airborne allergies, you are much more likely also to have food allergies and/or chemical sensitivities than is someone who does not have any known allergies. When people come in with complaints of hay fever symptoms or cat allergies, I often find they have food or chemical issues as well. For example, I commonly find that they get migraines, acid reflux, eczema, or chronic constipation or IBS issues or that they have some sort of aversion symptoms to perfumes or cleaning agents.

It is important to treat all your forms of allergy if you want to make your whole allergy problem better and improve your overall health. Identifying what foods and chemicals to avoid will make your asthma much better even if you just thought you reacted to cats and dust. Discovering and treating all of your allergies is a form of "total load" reduction for the immune system.

Testing for allergies

As in all of medicine, the most important way to determine a person's allergies is through logical deduction and elimination of exposures. If you have nasal allergy symptoms only in the spring, think about tree pollens and weeds. If you have symptoms all year, it is more likely an indoor allergen problem like molds, dust mites, or animals. If you have issues only in certain places like work or school, then think about molds, animals, chemicals, or other things to which you are exposed only at that location. In this last case, you may find that you improve over the weekend or when you go on vacation.

Making deductions about food allergies is more difficult. It's easy enough to pinpoint "classic" food allergy problems involving IgE (immunoglobulin, or antibody, of the "E" class) reactions and anaphylactic symptoms because the person generally experiences severe problems within minutes of exposure. However, since we tend to eat many different foods at one time or eat processed foods with many ingredients, the puzzle may not be so simple. If you break out in hives after eating a candy bar, you are just as likely to have reacted to one of the many chemicals in that "food" as to one of the actual food constituents.

The toughest thing to figure out by deduction is non-anaphylactic food allergy or "delayed" food allergy, which are far more common than the immediate IgE reactions. These reactions involve lower-grade, chronic, smoldering inflammatory responses, rather than the dramatic and immediate ones. These kinds of allergies cause persistent or episodic symptoms like fatigue, depression, joint pains, eczema, psoriasis, headaches, migraines, and chronic constipation that the patient may not experience until twenty-four or even forty-eight hours after ingestion. If they eat their triggering allergic food every day, the symptoms will just be there all the time or ebb and flow, having no apparent association with eating.

It is certainly possible for those with IgG-related and IgA-antibody-related delayed reactions to have immediate symptoms also, rather than delayed. Those with IgA reactions will only have gastrointestinal symptoms because that antibody class only acts across mucous membranes such as in the eyes, mouth and GI tract. IgG reactions can be the most diverse, causing symptoms like stomach pain, vomiting, skin itching, muscle or joint pain, headache, mental suppression, or emotional problems shortly after eating the allergic food. In the event that symptoms occur right away it is easier to convince people that their symptoms are related to those foods, and easier to test them via dietary challenge. That leads us to testing methods other than deduction or patient history.

For all types of allergy, "challenge testing" or "elimination-rechallenge" are the best ways to discover or confirm the foods or other allergens to which you're sensitive. For example, if you think you may be allergic to dogs, you can rub your face on a dog or let it lick you and find out very accurately. If you wonder whether a certain perfume or lotion causes a skin reaction, you can just put some on your skin and see if the rash forms. Of course, if you have dangerous symptoms, such as trouble breathing, I don't advise this kind of challenge testing. If you ate a candy bar with peanuts in it and aren't sure whether it was the peanut or something else that caused your throat to swell shut and nearly killed you, I am not going to suggest you eat some peanuts to find out.

If you get a stomach ache or a headache after eating or have some relevant chronic symptoms of delayed food allergy, the gold standard for identifying your triggers is to go on an "elimination diet" and then "challenge" by adding one thing at a time to see if you react to it.

I can't stress enough how important the elimination test is; it is the *only* accurate test for delayed or chronic food allergy because there are so many different ways in which the immune system may be reacting biochemically, and we don't know how to measure all of them in terms of laboratory testing. It sounds like a lot of work, and it is. In my practice I would say fewer than 20 percent of people agree to try an elimination test, and many of those still won't do it right. In order to do a good elimination trial, you have to *totally* eliminate the food in question, not just cut down on how much of it you eat.

Of course, if you just significantly reduce a certain food in your diet and you feel notably better, that is a positive test too, but you got lucky. In most cases, you have to eliminate the food completely for several days before you challenge yourself with some of it. For example, if you think milk may be causing your child's eczema, you must take the child off all milk products for about five days and then give him or her a glass of milk. You then watch closely for any symptoms to develop over the following

24-48 hours, although symptoms often occur within the first few hours in this setting. The resulting symptoms may not have anything to do with their initial problem of eczema; the child in this example may instead get a headache, a stomachache, or cramping and diarrhea the next day. Any adverse symptom that develops after ingestion could be a positive test.

What makes elimination-challenge testing difficult is: not knowing what foods to test. We all eat hundreds of foods, and it is difficult to avoid them all, but that's exactly what some people have to do in order to figure this out. I may suggest that more severely ill patients eat some extreme diet like: only rice, lamb or wild game, pears, and steamed broccoli for several days and then start reintroducing one new food each day. The five or six foods I discussed previously in this chapter are the most common dietary allergens, so I often suggest people start by eliminating just those foods first. Doing so will identify the major problems for most of those with delayed food allergy.

Unfortunately, one of the problems with our ability to undertake this kind of test is our lack of imagination when it comes to food. Most of us don't want to cook or plan ahead for meals; we think anything other than the foods we like is too expensive or too complicated, or we just lack the necessary motivation and discipline.

If you can't do a proper elimination trial for some reason, or just *won't* do one, there are some laboratory tests and other forms of testing that may help you sort things out. Identification of inhalant allergies is best done by skin prick testing, which involves poking tiny lancets dipped into various airborne antigen mixtures into the outer layer of the skin. You can test dozens of antigens at a sitting and then watch for redness, swelling and itching at any of the test sites. This works great for inhalant allergens because the skin and respiratory tract are continuous tissues and share the same immune system cells and signaling pathways.

Unfortunately the skin prick technique does not work well for identifying *food allergy* reactions, because the gastrointestinal tract really has its own separate immune subsystem that does not communicate directly with the skin. Studies showed poor accuracy and utility of skin prick testing for food allergies more than sixty years ago, and this poor success has been confirmed with more recent studies (Marco, 2006). IgE antibody levels to foods have been shown to correlate poorly with food reactions as well; oral challenge testing is still the most proven method, but is dangerous if anaphylactic reactions are suspected. Skin *patch* testing, leaving food antigens in contact with the outer layer of skin for a prolonged period of time in order to catch the more delayed type of reactions, is still only about eighty percent accurate, but is better than skin prick or serum IgE (Cudowska, 2005).

Many allergists now use a combination of skin prick and skin patch tests for foods, which does increase the accuracy of skin testing overall, but is still very poor in my opinion. Another huge problem with this type of testing is that individuals are usually only tested for up to a couple dozen different foods; this is because there are not that many commercially available food antigens for this type of testing, and also because there is only so much space on a kid's skin. Considering people tend to eat more than a hundred different foods, this is not likely to cut it.

If there is no or is only a weak reaction to the skin-prick test, it may be possible to inject antigens into the outer skin layers ("intradermal" testing) in order to see positive tests. This form of testing is more painful, takes much longer, and may not be covered by insurance because it is still considered a controversial method. Training in intradermal testing for food, inhalant and chemical reactions is taught by the American Academy of Environmental Medicine (AAEM), and it has been validated as a testing method in at least one independent, placebo-controlled trial (Fox, 1999).

If you do have positive test results on skin-prick testing and want to do specific desensitization therapy, it is helpful to then do intradermal injection testing with those positive antigens at various sequential concentrations to determine your "end point," the dose or concentration at which you first begin to react to an antigen. Practitioners can then formulate a more effecting starting treatment concentration based on the end point.

Inhalant allergies may also be tested through blood laboratory tests that look for IgE antibodies to various airborne antigens. Every region has different plants, and IgE tests for these are often offered in panels based on your area of the country. However, these tests are expensive (thousands of dollars rather than a few hundred for skin testing), they are not as accurate as skin testing for inhalant allergies, and they are often not covered by insurance as a result.

In my opinion, the only reason to test for airborne allergens is if you want specific desensitization treatment or want to know what you should try to avoid. The only allergens you can possibly avoid are molds, animals, and dust mites, so if you just have mild seasonal outdoor allergies, you may not want to bother with testing at all. Most people know if they react to dust or animals, therefore those with chronic indoor allergies all year are most likely reacting to mold. The form of treatment I use most often doesn't require knowledge of your specific allergens so it doesn't require any testing. Therefore I personally do very little skin testing for allergies of any sort in my practice.

Chemical testing can be done by skin patch testing, where a small amount of each chemical is applied to an area of skin and then covered with a non-absorbent patch for a day or more. If you develop itching, redness, or other skin changes in a tested area it is a positive test for that chemical. There are serious problems with this type of testing because you may have systemic problems with chemicals, reacting in tissues other than the skin; therefore, your test may be "negative" even though you have bad reactions to the chemical elsewhere than the skin. However, skin patch testing can certainly be useful for those with skin problems from contact with chemicals; as long as the kit contains the chemical or chemicals to which you react (and most only have a couple dozen chemicals to test).

To my knowledge skin prick testing is not performed for chemicals. Practitioners trained in environmental medicine may do intradermal injection testing with dilutions of various chemicals to determine the chemicals to which you react. This is the only good, objective test for chemical sensitivity, and it can lead to some very effective treatments, such as the "provocation-neutralization" technique taught by the AAEM. It may be difficult to find a practitioner who does this kind of testing because it is expensive to obtain all the chemical antigens needed, because environmental physicians who do this kind of testing are often attacked by their state medical boards for doing something so far outside the conventional medical arena, and because the tests are unlikely to be covered by insurance. You can find an environmental practitioner on the AAEM website at www.aaemonline.org.

Some companies are working on blood tests for various chemical sensitivities and allergies, but the tests are not yet very good in my experience. In any case, there are so many relevant chemicals that you are still not likely to have all the right ones tested, no matter what type of objective testing you do. Chemical allergy identification often requires upon careful detective work and observation on the part of the patient, so it's important to pay attention to your exposures and experiment with different household products.

The treatments for chemical toxicity discussed in the previous chapter can also be very helpful in decreasing chemical allergy or sensitivity. It is important to get the offending substances out of the body. The problem of build-up in the body is not an issue for inhalant allergies at all, and likely of no consequence for most food allergies. I do have a suspicion that the reason it takes so long for patients to improve when avoiding gluten is that the protein incorporates into the body tissues of the sensitive individual to a meaningful extent, and must therefore be "washed out" by protein metabolism and turnover before things will fully improve. Mycotoxins are biological allergens that also share the bioaccumulation problem with chemicals, since they usually do not clear from the body passively.

In terms of actually testing for specific allergies, the type I deal with most often is food allergy. If the food that caused a person's anaphylactic reaction is not evident from the patient's history, blood IgE tests are available for the more common allergic foods, such as milk, wheat, eggs, and peanuts. Blood IgE tests are a much safer option than challenge testing, and they are usually acceptable to insurance companies, in contrast to IgE testing for inhalants. However, as discussed previously, serum IgE antibody testing is not very accurate for foods. It is in testing for delayed-type or chronic food allergies that the controversies really lie.

As I discussed previously in this chapter, conventional allergists still prefer skin prick and patch testing even though those methods have been shown to have fairly poor accuracy and utility. While it's fine to perform a substandard test, doctors should take the results for what they are really worth and be honest about its limitations. Skin testing is usually meaningful if there is a positive result, but a negative result does not at all sufficiently rule out a food allergy. You must have a particularly bad problem with a food for it to react on your skin, and there are certain types of reactions that cross-react on the skin while other types do not.

In any case, in my experience skin testing fails to identify most food allergies. I tell people who have had skin testing done to pay attention to anything it showed as positive but not to believe anything it said was negative or safe to eat. Even if skin tests are positive, there is a significant documented false-positive rate as well (Cudowski, 2005). I therefore advise my patients that even a positive result for a food through skin testing methods needs to be validated through food elimination and subsequent oral challenge.

While the immune system can produce several types of antibodies against any given immune target, conventional allergists believe that IgE is the only one involved in "true allergy." Most delayed or chronic food reactions, in my experience, are mediated by IgG or possible IgA antibodies rather than IgE. IgA is secreted onto mucous membranes like those of the eye, the mouth, and the GI tract, to act as your first line of defense against

653

outside organisms and antigens. IgG circulates in your bloodstream, "remembers" what has bothered you in the past, and provides long-term immunity like that created by vaccines and natural infections.

If you have only gastrointestinal reactions to a food, you may have manifested only the IgA antibody reaction against it. Gastrointestinal reactions are the earliest food reactions to develop in some cases, and a small number of foods can be tested for by stool IgA testing from certain labs. Only a few labs in the country do this type of testing, it is still expensive, and it has some bugs to work out in terms of quality and accuracy, but it should soon be a useful tool. IgA antibody in the stool is not at all helpful in determining what foods may be causing symptoms not involving the mouth and GI tract however.

The testing I do most often for patients is blood IgG testing. Maybe a dozen companies in the United States now do this type of testing, but it is not yet standardized, and each company has had to make its own testing materials with their own antigens. Therefore, there is a wide range of testing quality and cost among these labs. I currently use a company called *Alletess Medical Laboratory*, which is based in Massachusetts. Their test has been shown to be reliable by independent third-party testing, and they are also the cheapest in the country currently. A couple of other reliable labs include *Immunolabs* and *Genova Diagnostics*

The IgG test panels have the opposite general problem from that of the skin tests because IgG testing is overly sensitive, meaning you will get numerous false positives or test results that suggest you are allergic to a particular food when in fact you are not. This is the main criticism allergists have regarding IgG testing, and it is a valid one. These types of tests generally give scoring categories of varying severity, so the results in the highest category are usually the real problem foods, while the ones that barely make the cut into the abnormal range won't tend to bother you in a clinically evident manner (meaning: no observed symptoms after eliminating and then challenging with the foods in question).

The way to sort this out and validate or confirm the IgG test results is to eliminate everything from your diet that the test says is positive, see if your symptoms improve, and then re-introduce the allergic foods one at a time at the rate of one new food each day. In this way, you can tell which ones bother you and in what manner. I know this is what I told you to do in the first place without any testing, so you may be wondering why you should bother with the blood testing at all. The benefit of the test is that it narrows your foods of concern down from "every food imaginable" to just those indicated by the test. This makes the elimination phase much easier.

If you have many positives on the test, you can try first eliminating only the foods that react at a high level and not the ones that react at lower levels. That makes the process easier in practice; but it is important to note that people can have very bad reactions to foods showing only lower-level positive responses on an IgG test. Additionally, if someone is allergic to several foods they will have to eliminate them all in order to see symptom resolution; this process is often not easy. If your symptoms are severe you can usually tell when you have eliminated the right foods within several days to a week; if they are very intermittent or not as severe it may take quite a bit longer to tell for certain.

The blood IgG tests are useful teaching tools for patients because they most often reveal at least one food to which the patient reacts badly, and after dietary modification the patient is likely to better believe in the idea that food can cause illness. I run these tests on people every week in my office, and they work well as long as you understand their limitations.

One other limitation of the IgG test is that it may not identify foods to which you have severe anaphylactic reactions because those reactions are usually mediated by IgE antibody rather than IgG. As a result, even if you have had hives, mouth or throat itching or swelling from a food in the past, the IgG test may show up negative for that food, possibly tempting you to try eating it again. No! Those are IgE reactions, and would not necessarily be expected to show up on an IgG test. Misunderstanding the nature of these tests can be deadly.

Because not all food reactions involve IgG antibody, because "true allergy" reactions are IgE-mediated, and because the IgG panels have a high rate of false positives, most conventional allergists think IgG testing is useless. However, in my experience, these tests are far more useful than skin testing, though it may be ideal to do both. I would rather use a test that shows you more foods than you really need to avoid than a test that misses the causes of some serious problems. You can always determine the false positives on the IgG panel after several days of elimination with no harm done, while the skin testing may lead you to keep eating a food that is harmful to you because you think the food has been "proven" to be safe.

Before we leave the subject of allergy testing, I want to mention some of the more unconventional "energetic" methods of testing for allergies of all types. These methods all involve the attempt to measure some sort of energetic disturbance in the body upon exposure to a vial of antigen (e.g., a little bottle of milk solution, formaldehyde, or cat dander) or even just the idea or essence of the antigen. These methods are often tough for westerners to comprehend and will seem very strange when a practitioner uses them.

One common example of this type of testing is muscle strength testing (MST), where the patient holds a little bottle of a food antigen while the practitioner presses down on the patient's outstretched arm or finger. (The patient's strength is tested first without holding anything in order to establish a baseline.) Some practitioners don't use physical samples of potential allergens because it can be expensive to buy a set of hundreds of possible allergen samples in little vials; instead, they just speak the name of the item or substance while pressing down on the patient's outstretched arm. If the patient retains his or her level of strength at about the same as at baseline, then the potential allergen being tested is not considered an allergen for that patient.

If the patient appears to become weaker, and it is notably easier for the practitioner to press the patient's arm or finger down, the item in question is considered to have tested positive as an allergen. You can test many potential allergens in a short period of time in this manner, but I have some serious issues with this type of testing. The most obvious issue is that it seems like nonsense unless someone explains the science behind it. It isn't nonsense. There is a certain body of science behind the concept that even the idea or "intention" of an allergen can disturb your body's electromagnetic field or function, and since your muscles work with electrical and electromagnetic processes, that disturbance can be measured by muscular function. Machines have been developed that can measure this process much more precisely than a human can.

The main problem with muscle testing by a practitioner is the human variable. The patient isn't going to resist with exactly the same strength each time, and he or she gets progressively weaker as his or her muscles fatigue with repeated testing. The practitioner is not going to apply exactly the same amount of force each time, and he or she may subconsciously press a little harder when testing the allergens he or she *believes* are going to be positive. You can't eliminate the human bias with this testing, although many MST practitioners are extremely confident in and certain of their testing ability.

Unfortunately, a number of my patients who have had MST by experienced providers got sick eating foods for which they tested negative; even more have found no apparent reaction to foods tested positive through

MST when they did elimination and subsequent challenge trials. I think there is some use for this type of testing, but people have to acknowledge the obvious limitations. The most useful application of this test is when the patients learn to do their own testing on themselves. You can hold something new in your lap, link your fingers together (make circles with the index finger and thumb of each hand and interlock them), and pull them against each other as a means of MST.

If your fingers break through one another without having to exert much force with the pulling, then whatever you are testing is presumably bad for you. You can get the feel for this quickly, especially if you test some things you know to be safe and some you know to be harmful for you. When you get the feel for it, you may even be able to hold something up close to your chest and simply "sense" whether it is good or bad for you. I have a number of patients who use this type of self-testing to determine what foods, supplements, medications or personal care products will be safe for them.

I have tried using a digital handgrip strength analyzer to do muscle testing in an attempt to be more objective, but you have to exert maximal effort each time in order to be consistent, and this effort causes the score to drop notably over time because of muscle fatigue unless you allow for a significant rest between tests. It's best to practice this on yourself and develop your own feel for it.

One of the original machines to objectively measure this type of energetic disturbance in the body was referred to as electro-acupuncture according to Voll, or EAV. Dr. Reinhold Voll was a German medical doctor, who in the 1950s developed the technology whereby you can measure a person's electromagnetic field using wires at the ends of the fingers where the acupuncture meridians start. You get a baseline reading and then place samples of different substances in vials on a metal tray attached to the machine, not on the patient or practitioner. If the antigen being tested is harmful for the patient, there will be a significant alteration in his or her electromagnetic field profile.

This type of technology has been around for many decades and has been used to help identify disturbances in organs or systems, sort of like running a diagnostic check on the computer in your car. It is very objective and its results seem to be reasonably reproducible, suggesting its results are valid at least in terms of their consistency. There were later versions of the EAV machine like the Vega© and the Mora©, which could administer the corrective frequencies as a form of treatment for medical problems, rather than simply diagnose what was causing a disturbance. Later improvements have included the QXCI© and SCIO© devices; the newest one, and the model I myself use, is called the Indigo© Machine.

The machines can also tell practitioners how to treat the patient using homeopathic remedies to correct their organ disease or sensitivity problems. They can test for foods, airborne items, chemicals, internal tissue structures, and basic nutrients. There are a myriad of problems that can be helped with this type of technology.

The Indigo is the only FDA-approved bio-energetic device of this type in the United States at this time, and is technically approved as a biofeedback device. It has more than eleven thousand vibrational frequencies programmed into it, as well as the capacity to test specific items on a tray like the original EAV. It can both receive signals diagnostically and send back corrective frequencies to treat allergies and sensitivities directly, and it may help to correct many physiological imbalances. It is an exciting piece of technology with a wide range of potential applications.

The last sort of testing discussed here is the Nambudripad Allergy Elimination Technique (NAET), which was developed by Devi Nambudripad, a chiropractor/acupuncturist/PhD/RN. You can learn more about it in her book, *Say Goodbye To Illness* and *Freedom From Allergy*. NAET operates on the principle that allergens cause an energetic disturbance in the body and approaches the problem diagnostically and therapeutically through the acupuncture meridians. This method is particularly good with "internal" antigens or nutritional items like your own saliva or blood, vitamins, minerals and other things.

In summary, there are many ways to test for allergies or sensitivities. Don't believe wholly in any one thing, and don't throw anything out either. If you have significant problems with many illnesses, it may be difficult to identify everything to which you are allergic or sensitive. Find a practitioner who will help you attack the problem from several angles.

Dr. Vincent's "chaos theory" of allergies

The "why" of allergies in terms of what you are allergic to and the types of reactions you may have frequently comes up. People want to know why they react to something they have eaten for many years or were around without problems in the past, or why they react to something they have never eaten or had contact with. Some people assume they are allergic to something just because their mothers were or others in the house are allergic to it. These are all valid questions, but are useless intellectual exercises because the answers are not there, and in my view can only be explained by *chaos theory.*

Exposure to a potential allergen when your immune system is agitated by a toxin or irritant likely often triggers an allergy. Many allergies originate coincident with significant hormonal changes, such as puberty, menopause, pregnancy, and initiation of a hormonal therapy. Some substances are more highly allergenic than others, so they are much more common allergens due to their nature. Despite these potential contributing factors, however, there is most often no rhyme or reason to why or when an allergy or sensitivity develops, nor how it manifests for that individual. Why does corn cause diarrhea for one person, joint pains for another, and migraine headaches in yet another person? And how can corn cause all those same symptoms within a single individual at different times in their life?

The substances to which you are most often exposed are statistically more likely to become allergens for you. Periods of stress or illness may agitate the immune system and generate an allergic response pattern, and certain infections may trigger the allergic type of immune response. Circumstances involving significant hormonal changes (e.g., pregnancy or menopause) may correspond to the development of new allergies, such that whatever potential allergens you are exposed to around the time of these events may become targets for your immune system. While you can point to all these explanations for why you develop a given sensitivity, in many cases the cause is a *group* of underlying and triggering factors, making it unclear why an allergy developed when it did.

In addition to the allergies that seem to make sense in terms of the issues mentioned above, people often have other sensitivities that don't fall neatly into these categories of explanation. Your child may have different allergies than you do, even though you eat the same diet and live in the same environment. Your allergies can also change at random. All of this points to chaos theory as the guiding "principle" of allergy development. When someone with imbalances that may lead to allergic tendency steps into a world with thousands of potential immune targets, you cannot predict what will happen or what his or her immune system will decide to attack. If a person works with a certain individual food or chemical all day at high exposure it makes sense they will become sensitized to it, such as the emergence of widespread latex allergy in health care workers or wheat allergy in bakers and bread makers. Most allergies will seem far more random or sporadic than that.

The second part of the chaos theory concerns how your allergies manifest, and this relates more to foods and chemicals than to environmental inhalants. The symptoms of food allergy range from headaches and rashes to arthritis and diarrhea and can involve every organ system in the body. Why a particular allergen may manifest a particular symptom is a question that has not been answered. However, what I have observed in practice is that a person with a dozen foods allergies may have completely different symptoms for each of them or the same symptom from all of them. The person may get headaches from eating wheat, stomach pains and diarrhea from milk, and pain isolate to the right index finger from eating corn. The symptoms may be specific for a given food or chemical, such as a rash in one particular spot or pain in one particular joint.

This range of symptoms is confusing to both patients and providers, and it is a major part of why practitioners have a hard time figuring out these types of sensitivities. Since we are trained to understand allergy in terms of the more global IgE allergy responses (e.g., anaphylactic shock or widespread hives), these discrete diverse reaction patterns don't make sense. Patients get extremely frustrated with their health practitioners who don't believe them when they explain how a certain strange thing happens when they eat or are exposed to a certain food or chemical. Those concepts just don't fit into the conventional medical dogma related to "allergy".

The types and patterns of reactions range so widely from individual to individual that they seem to be ruled only by chaos. There may be some "reason" why eating corn make a certain person's index finger hurt—perhaps the person jammed that finger the day their corn allergy developed, and the immune system focused the corn-related inflammation where there was inflammation already—but we may never know that reason.

The third issue with allergies seemingly driven by chaos is the *fluidity* of an individual's allergies. A person's reactions can get better and worse and even disappear for a while. A given allergen, especially a food, can trigger one type of symptom at first and then switch to causing completely different symptoms at some point for no clear reason. The reasons for these changes may be similar to those listed that contribute to the onset of allergies (e.g., hormonal changes and stress), but it often makes no sense at all. It seems to me that there are no hard and fast rules here, and it makes it much easier to understand the stories and symptoms people tell me if I keep an open mind and don't have some rigid cause-and-effect pattern in my head.

Nutritional and natural remedies for allergy (and autoimmunity)

A number of nutritional, herbal, hormonal and homeopathic things help reduce allergy reactions by improving the function of the immune system. Vitamin D is probably the most critical one; the widespread problem of vitamin D deficiency in modern society certainly has something to do with the rise of allergic and autoimmune diseases. One recent study out of Iran found severe vitamin D deficiency was six times more prevalent in those with allergic rhinitis as compared to the general population (Arshi, 2012). Vitamin C and Vitamin E can often help also. Vitamin B-12 is important for some, and it is important to get adequate amounts of all the other B vitamins just for general metabolic function.

Minerals like zinc and selenium are important to immune function and worth supplementing. Manganese and molybdenum are important to prevent chemical sensitivity issues and aid in detoxification. MSM is a useful supplement for allergy (Barrager, 2002), likely acting as a sulfur donor.

Fish oil and other sources of omega-3 fatty acids are likely important in allergy and autoimmune disease because they help modulate the inflammatory process. Studies have shown very high doses of fish oil are very safe, but studies to date have not shown convincing benefits in the treatment or prevention of allergy (Anandan, 2009). The reasons for this in my opinion are that the allergic triggers have not been identified nor dealt with, and the individual's diet likely still contains far greater levels of inflammatory components (sugar, trans fats, omega-6 or omega-9 oils). Taking fish oils may be a helpful part of a comprehensive overall program for improving allergic disease, but certainly don't cut it as a stand-alone therapy.

Fish oil supplementation *has* been shown to improve autoimmune disease to some degree. Studies have demonstrated reduced severity and progression of joint disease in people with rheumatoid arthritis (Miles, 2012). Fish oil supplementation has shown mixed results in patients with inflammatory bowel disease (IBD) such as ulcerative colitis or Crohn's disease; positive studies suggest that it is the ratio of omega-3 to omega-6 fats that is the critical factor. Patients maintaining remission of their IBD using fish oil or other omega-3 supplements generally had to maintain a much better fatty acid ratio (Uchiyama, 2010).

As I discussed in the chapter on fats within section III, it is the ratio of polyunsaturated fatty acids that is critical. The typical American diet is crammed full of unhealthy fats and is far too high in omega-6 and omega-9 fats from plant sources like safflower, sunflower, corn and other vegetable oils. Therefore, in order to achieve proper balance and correct the 3/6 ratio, one has to both reduce their intake of the bad oils and supplement with fish oil, krill or calamari oils. No intervention study I've seen had patients change their diet in this manner as part of the intervention; they just gave them extremely high doses of fish oil or other omega-3 fats to override the ratio.

For those eating the "SAD" (standard American diet) this often means taking more than ten typical over-the-counter fish oil capsules per day for a couple of months before you'll see a change—not just one capsule here and there. I strongly advise getting the sugar and unhealthy oils out of the diet, and also supplementing with fish oil. Find a molecularly distilled (purified, free of toxins like mercury and PCBs) product, preferably one that is highly concentrated so you don't have to take so many capsules. I always dose fish oils based on the amount of EPA (eicosapentaenoic acid). I suggest people with allergies or autoimmune disease try to ensure a total of 1,000 to 2,000mg of EPA daily.

Don't forget you need to get the sugar, bad fats, processed foods, and probably grains in general out of your diet if you want to reduce your inflammation.

Eating locally produced honey (preferably raw honey) is a potentially effective treatment for outdoor inhalant allergies because the bees have incidentally gathered up tiny amounts of local pollens into their honey, which can act as a kind of oral allergy desensitization.

Some food constituents and herbal items that may help with allergy include plant enzymes like quercetin (found in apples) and bromelain (found in pineapple), which are frequently found in natural allergy remedies and can help relieve inhalant allergy symptoms. Digestive enzyme complexes can reduce food allergies by improving how well the food proteins are broken down before they reach your small intestine; these must be taken while eating.

Boswellia (frankincense) can improve airborne allergies by blocking the inflammatory cascade in a way similar to the action of the prescription drug Singulair™. One product containing boswellia, licorice root and turmeric showed a pronounced beneficial effect in asthma patients compared with placebo (Houssen, 2010). Turmeric presumably helps because of its generally anti-inflammatory effects, and licorice root increases internal cortisol levels. Boswellia has also been shown to potentially offer help for some types of cancer including prostate, breast, pancreatic and colorectal varieties (Shen, 2012); and I personally know someone who seemed to have their leukemia go into remission with the addition of boswellia to their regimen, when they had not fully responded to the drug Gleevec™.

I use a Chinese herbal formula called *Bi Yan Pian* in my office that works surprisingly well for nasal allergy symptoms in many people, even when none of the antihistamine medications worked for them. Milk thistle, and the other herbs and nutrients I listed previously for aiding detoxification are useful for those with chemical allergy or sensitivity problems.

Conventional medical treatments

Conventional medicine offers those suffering from airborne allergens a number of medications that help control symptoms for many people. These include antihistamines like Benadryl™ and Claritin™; nasal steroids like Flonase™ and Rhinocort™; eye drops like Patanol™; leukotriene inhibitors like Singulair™ and Accolate™; inhaled steroids for asthma like Flovent™ and Pulmicort™; and rescue inhaler medicines like Albuterol™. These drugs are indeed effective and important tools, but they only serve to control symptoms and do nothing to treat the actual underlying *causes* of allergies and asthma.

Treating causes involves providing better nutrition to decrease inflammation and improve immune functioning; supplementing with vitamin D and some of the other nutrients or hormones discussed; identifying and avoiding allergic triggers; and utilizing treatments that directly influence the immune system in such a way as to reduce or eliminate the allergic reactions themselves. Therapies that alter the immune response in this manner include forms of antigen-based immunotherapy and some of the energetically based therapies mentioned for use in allergy diagnosis.

The conventional style of immunotherapy uses diluted samples of the antigens to which you are allergic as an injected treatment to counter your symptoms. Escalating concentrations and doses or given over time, and this works presumably by flooding or overwhelming the immune response to those particular allergens. Mixtures are made specifically for every given patient, based on their particular allergies, and solutions at the various concentrations are injected under the skin at the back of the upper arm beginning at two doses per week usually. The doses go up every week or two depending upon individual response, and over time the shot frequency can be spaced out further and further if things go well. A portion of patients will be able to stop therapy after a few years or so, and be essentially cured.

This type of specific immune therapy requires first doing skin-prick or some other valid form of testing to find out what you're allergic to, then diluting those substances down to the proper starting concentration based on the individual's level of sensitivity. The concentrations of the mixtures are steadily increased as you go along in order to keep challenging the immune system at higher levels, right around the threshold where they would have symptoms triggered.

This type of injection therapy has significant risks because you are using sizeable doses of substances to which you are allergic. Injection site reactions like pain, redness, and swelling are very common, and it is not rare for people to have mild anaphylactic reactions in the office, requiring emergency medications. Deaths can occur, though very rarely, in allergists' offices from this type of treatment, although proper treatment is usually quite safe works well for most people.

Sublingual immunotherapy (SLIT) for inhalant allergies is taught by the AAEM and some other nonconventional allergy organizations. The concept is the same as with conventional subcutaneous injection immunotherapy (SCIT), but the treatments have some distinct differences that serve to improve both effectiveness and safety. The test concentrations for finding treatment doses are made in 5:1 serial dilutions rather than the 10:1 dilutions used in conventional therapy, which means there is greater precision in determining the treatment threshold.

In the experience of environmental physicians, the sublingual route seems to be both more effective and safer, presumably because the mouth is a "natural" site of inhalant allergen interaction with our immune system, while the immune system contingent lying beneath the skin is not. Published clinical research has demonstrated the superior safety of SLIT over SCIT (Bahceciler, 2011) and suggested similar effectiveness of the two styles of therapy (Bahceciler, 2011 and Saporta, 2012). Major problems with either if these styles of *specific* immunotherapy lie in the facts that testing methods may miss some of the individual's allergens, meaning they never end up included in the treatment; and an allergic individual is likely to develop new allergies at any time, which would require repeat testing all over again.

The primary conventional treatment for food allergies is simply avoidance, although even this simple treatment is problematic when the testing done is of poor sensitivity, and some allergic foods are not accurately identified. The conventional style of allergy shots used for inhalant allergies doesn't work nearly as well for food allergies, so they are not often used. The drug Gastrocrom™ helps block certain aspects of the immune reaction within the gastrointestinal tract only, but it isn't used much. Taking digestive enzymes with meals may help degrade tiny amounts of allergenic food proteins, but don't really offer that much protection. Therefore, desensitization to food allergies is a very appealing option, especially for those who have so many sensitivities that it is difficult to find may safe foods to eat.

An oral desensitization process in sublingual form that uses highly diluted doses of antigens every day with slowly increasing strength over time can serve to "turn off" severe immune reactivity safely and effectively. The SLIT technique used by environmental physicians for inhalant allergies can work for foods and even chemicals or other types of allergens as well.

Researchers at Duke University made national news in 2008 or 2009 when they showed that they could safely desensitize children with even life-threatening peanut allergy by giving them oral doses of highly diluted peanut solutions and very slowly increasing the strength of the doses over time. They gave their test subjects doses of liquid solutions with a spoon, and it looked like a very crude version of what environmental physicians have done successfully for decades in a much more precise and clean fashion using carefully titrated drops in a glycerin mixture. This therapy was presented on the news as a totally new idea and an important medical breakthrough, I suppose because Duke was doing it, though it was not truly new or innovative at all. I spent several minutes yelling at the television when I saw this.

In 2011 the Duke researchers published that they had successfully desensitized a whopping fifty peanut-allergic patients using their technique (Kulis, 2011). I would guess that those successfully treated by environmental physicians over the years number into the thousands. But, it is wonderful that a prominent institution such as Duke is making this concept mainstream; this should make this safe and effective treatment available to far more people with life threatening food allergies.

Nonconventional/Integrative medical treatments
Environmental medicine has been training practitioners to do immunotherapy for decades. These techniques should not be considered "nonconventional" because they use the same stock antigens and involve

the same a process of dilution and administration back to the patient that conventional treatments use. The differences lie in the route or style of administration.

Another treatment process taught to environmental practitioners is called provocation/neutralization, or P/N. This technique involves performing skin injections with sequential concentrations of various antigens to assess specific reactivity. A fairly high dose is used first as a test; if the initial injection site reacts (gets larger), sequentially weaker doses are then injected until a concentration is found that *does not* react. This concentration, called the "neutralizing" dose for the given item, will generally take away the person's symptoms. A vial of the corrective dose can be given to the patient for use at home; they simply inject themselves with the neutralizing dose whenever symptoms are triggered by exposure, or perhaps on a daily basis for preventive therapy.

P/N can be used to test and treat outdoor inhalant allergens, molds, foods, chemicals, vitamins, neurotransmitters, and whatever else you can possibly get into a solution for injection. If you have a chronic allergy issue, you may need to use the shots on a daily basis, or it may be possible to use a sublingual route. The major problems with this treatment are related to time, financial issues, and legal concerns. P/N takes considerable time because you test just one potential allergen at a time and must wait ten minutes after each concentration is injected. It takes days to thoroughly test patients for all the possible substances.

Conventional medicine does not accept this process as valid, for reasons that are not clear to me (at least no valid *scientific* reasons). Therefore, this type of treatment is not covered by insurance, and the practitioner risks being sued for fraud if he or she tries to bill insurance companies for the procedure. State medical boards sometimes even try to revoke the licenses of practitioners who use this method.

I rarely use the P/N method, not because it doesn't work or I'm afraid of the legal issue but because the treatment I use is so much simpler and usually works very well. I use an injection technique called "low-dose allergy therapy", or LDA. It is derived from a treatment called "enzyme-potentiated desensitization", or EPD, that has been used in the United Kingdom for many decades with good results and acceptance.

LDA involves injections just once every seven to eight weeks, rather than daily or twice per week, using antigens that are diluted down near the homeopathic range—one part per trillion (1:1,000,000,000,000) or farther in most cases. In contrast, conventional allergy shots are often given in the 1:1000 range and stronger (1:10 eventually); therefore the risk of severe reaction to LDA shots is virtually zero and anaphylactic reactions have not been reported.

LDA involves using a few standardized mixtures of antigens made at a compounding pharmacy; one mixture of inhalant allergens contains more than three hundred different inhalants, another mixture contains a large number of common chemicals, and two mixtures contain hundreds of different foods. The food mixtures both contain the same foods—more than three hundred individual food items—but one is diluted even farther than the regular mixture, to use in those patients with very severe reactions. The treatment is very simple because, if you have airborne allergies, you get the inhalant mixture; if you have food reactions, you get a food mixture; and if you react to chemicals, you get the chemical mixture. If you have all different types of allergy you may receive all three mixtures at once with no problems.

With LDA, you don't have to do any preliminary testing because it doesn't matter what your specific allergens are. Most practitioners do some form of food testing at first so patients know which foods to avoid until the treatment kicks in effectively. Children usually see improvement in their symptoms with the first few doses, but adults often take longer—several shots and up to a year (essentially six doses) for some people.

This treatment is so easy, safe, and user-friendly that I rarely do SLIT or any skin testing any more. We no longer even make patients wait for thirty minutes after their shots to ensure they don't have a dangerous reaction because there are no dangerous reactions. LDA is also much cheaper than other styles of immunotherapy, because the doses are so infrequent. Dosing starts at seven to eight week intervals, but then spaces out further over time as patients respond better and better. A significant proportion of patients no longer need therapy after a few years.

So why doesn't everyone use LDA? Again, it is an issue of acceptance and cost. Conventional allergists generally think LDA is "homeopathic nonsense" because the concentrations used are so small, so it is not accepted as valid therapy and not covered by insurance at this point. There are currently only about ninety of us in the country who use LDA, so you may have trouble finding a provider near you. Also, most providers in the country insist on cash-only payment for the therapy; I am the only one I know of who bills insurance for these visits, and I charge only ten dollars cash for the cost of the antigens themselves each round. It is so profoundly helpful and safe I wanted to make it more "available" to my patients.

There was an effort years ago to get the FDA to approve the treatment, but the FDA wouldn't even consider it because the mixtures are pre-made at a pharmacy rather than mixed by the practitioners themselves in their offices as in conventional immunotherapy. This objection seems inappropriate to me because we use compounded medications all the time. LDA may seem like "homeopathic nonsense" to some, but it takes only a few molecules of pollen, cat dander, or peanut protein for a violent allergic reaction to occur, so there's no reason you need a big concentration to get a big therapeutic effect. Moreover, homeopathic remedies have been proven to work for all sorts of conditions, even by modern evidence-based research standards (Kim, 2005).

LDA works by administering very small doses of antigen in conjunction with a special enzyme (beta-glucuronidase) that signals the specific lymphocytes you are trying to "retrain" with the therapy. Those T-lymphocytes come to the injection site, which must be within the skin layer itself, not under it, and "see" tiny amounts of all these antigens. The effect is that those lymphocytes are directed to view all these antigens as "normal" or "harmless"; they then "spread the word" to the rest of the body's immune system through systemic chemical signals. This is the job of those particular lymphocytes; they are there to experience the world and tell the body what is "normal" out there.

The relevant concept here is *tolerance*. This is what our immune systems do right from birth, when we are exposed to tiny amounts of myriad substances in the environment through the air, breast milk, other foods, and contact with objects. All along the way, our immune system has to learn what it can tolerate before it can learn what it must defend against. Even before birth, our immune systems must effectively learn to recognize "self", taking note of every single protein comprising our own tissues.

Allergy and autoimmunity are, in essence, a failure of that tolerance process, and LDA works to restore tolerance to environmental antigens. Since early 2010 I have experimented with using various extracts from patients themselves, diluted to similar concentrations and combined with the beta-glucuronidase enzyme, to desensitize them to "self" antigens and correct autoimmune diseases of various types in similar fashion to using standard LDA therapy for allergies. I have had truly amazing success with this in patients with autoimmune conditions including Crohn's disease, ulcerative colitis, rheumatoid arthritis and other inflammatory arthritis, polymyalgia rheumatica, certain types of psoriasis and other autoimmune skin conditions such as discoid lupus. I intend to publish cases in the near future, and later on publish a book on the topic of autoimmune disease and the utilization of this simple technique.

That brings me to another category of allergy treatment entirely, treatments that involve energetic systems like those addressed in the testing discussion. Bio-energetic diagnostic and therapeutic machines like the SCIO and Indigo can sometimes be used to treat the patient by administering an energetic treatment or "re-balancing" their energy frequencies regarding specific substances. NAET is another potentially effective means of treating allergy for some, and a number of my patients have benefitted from that as well.

Acupuncture is frequently used for asthma and allergy issues. It works in a general way to tone down the allergy response and to help achieve normal energetic and physiological balance in the immune system. Acupuncture is in my opinion a general, nonspecific therapy for allergies; it would make a useful adjunctive treatment to be used with any of the other techniques.

There are many other energetic treatments now, as well devices to reduce allergy issues. One I know of involves coins or medallions that are "charged" and then placed on the allergy-sufferer to keep him or her "balanced" and free of allergy symptoms. Some people also use crystals, flower essences, or energy healing. These types of remedies should be completely safe, even if you doubt their effectiveness or don't understand how they could possibly work. If you suffer from allergies you don't have much to lose, other than a little money, in trying some of these things.

Autoimmunity

Autoimmune disease is a major topic, as autoimmune diseases (AID) as a category are by some reports the third leading cause of death in the United States. Autoimmune reactions can be the main diagnosis, or it may be an underlying factor in many seemingly unrelated chronic conditions, such as thyroid imbalance, infertility, gastrointestinal problems, and nutritional deficiencies.

You can look at autoimmunity the same way you look at allergy. Allergy is a failure to tolerate things in the world, and autoimmunity is a failure to tolerate proteins within the body itself. Autoimmunity is arguably is a much bigger failure on the part of the immune system than is allergy, but the concepts are similar.

The nutrients I suggested for reducing allergy problems all help with autoimmunity as well, especially vitamin D. Many autoimmune diseases are far more common in vitamin D-deficient regions, and some have shown clinical improvement with the therapeutic administration of vitamin D. This seems related to vitamin D effects on the immune system itself, as well as hormonal actions, influences on gene expression, and also interactions and effects involving the gut microflora (Hewison, 2012).

Detoxification seems even more important for AID than for allergy because AID involves a more significant derangement of the immune system to lead to its attacking the body. I often test patients with AID for heavy metals and seem to more commonly find elevated mercury or lead. Those with lupus often seem to have issues with chemicals and food additives, particularly formaldehyde and artificial sweeteners, as well.

The great majority of autoimmune diseases spring from immune reactions to substances outside the body first. A well-known classic example is rheumatic fever, which every doctor knows is an immune reaction to certain strains of *Streptococcus pyogenes*, the bacterium that causes strep throat. The immune reaction cross-reacts and spreads to the person's own tissues because a protein in the bacterium's cell wall looks like one of our own proteins; this is a phenomenon called "molecular mimicry." This process is widely accepted in modern medicine, and we know it can lead to progressive permanent changes in heart valves and other tissues in the instance of rheumatic fever.

This same bacterium, *S. pyogenes*, is known to cause an immune reaction in the kidney called poststreptococcal glomerulonephritis, which looks in some cases like an autoimmune disease; and it is clearly linked to a certain type of psoriasis called *guttate* psoriasis. We also know strep can cause a chronic inflammatory problem in the brain, which manifests as psychological and behavioral problems. This condition, which is called "pediatric autoimmune neuropsychiatric disorder associated with streptococcus" (PANDAS), can occur in both adults and children in my opinion. It typically manifests as obsessive-compulsive behaviors, irritability, sleep problems, and other neurological issues, including seizure-like episodes in some.

Though these four immune or autoimmune conditions are known to spring from just one particular bacterial species, conventional medicine still does not understand other AIDs as being related to bacterial pathogens or other outside triggers. There is considerable data showing other associations, such as ankylosing spondylitis's association with the common bacterial organism *Klebsiella* colonizing the gut of genetically predisposed people with the HLA-B27 genotype (Jones, 2005). Following similar mechanisms, conditions like rheumatoid arthritis and autoimmune thyroiditis have been suggested as related to *Mycoplasma* bacterial infection or colonization (Brownstein, 2001). The antibiotic minocycline is even FDA-approved for the treatment of rheumatoid arthritis (RA), suggesting there has been some prior understanding of that disease as being triggered by a bacterial organism. I have seen this work in some of my patients with RA and also other forms of inflammatory arthritis.

Many of my patients with persistent inflammatory or autoimmune conditions are afflicted by food or environmental allergens. I routinely test patients with rheumatoid arthritis and many other types of AID for food allergies using IgG food testing. In many cases when people eliminate the indicated foods their arthritis and other symptoms improve. These same people may also have relevant bacterial infections, chemical or heavy metals issues, thyroid or adrenal deficiency, or vitamin D deficiency as well. Most chronic complex illness conditions are going to be multifactorial, and require multiple forms of intervention for complete resolution.

Autoimmunity's underlying triggers are similar to those of allergy, but autoimmunity's triggers are more complex on certain levels. I firmly believe we can get most AID under control by addressing nutritional, hormonal, allergic, toxic, psychological, and energetic factors, but the immune inflammation and self-attack is so ingrained in some people that more drastic measures must be taken. The conventional approach is to suppress the immune system using powerful drugs like steroids (e.g., prednisone), chemotherapy and other immunosuppressants (e.g., methotrexate and cyclosporine), immune modulators (e.g., tacrolimus), or monoclonal antibodies against various immune signal molecules (e.g., Remicade™ and Enbrel™).

As I mentioned previously, I believe we can use the concepts of immunotherapy from allergy treatments in cases of autoimmunity also, deriving suitable antigens from the patient or other relevant sources and help turn off the relevant immune response. Some practitioners have had some success using dilutions of the patients' own blood serum or urine to do general neutralization treatments for a wide range of autoimmune and other conditions. Enzyme potentiated desensitization, EPD, as used in the United Kingdom, contains some bacterial antigens known to trigger autoimmune problems in some cases. This therapy has had success against conditions like rheumatoid arthritis, ankylosing spondylitis, and nonspecific inflammatory arthritis.

The mixtures they use with EPD contain only a few bacterial types such as *Bacteroides*, *Proteus* and *Klebsiella*; and I am certain there are many people who are reacting to other types. Most often the source of immune inflammation arises from the intestinal tract, where the majority of the immune system resides, so my technique as I mentioned above involves simply using a stool sample and desensitizing patients to all of their gut organisms at once. Using self-derived samples likely also works for autoimmune diseases because they contain the immune targets, whatever they may be, on a molecular level. Following this principle I have cured conditions such as discoid lupus by making antigens from a patient's skin biopsy.

I again think it is best to remove whatever is "afflicting" a person with AID and to provide what they need to improve normal functioning, balance hormones, detoxify, and adjust their diet as necessary. If that doesn't work, there are many other treatments short of derailing the entire immune system with potent and toxic drugs that dramatically increase their risk of cancer and life-threatening infections. Just look for a good integrative or environmental practitioner to help guide you through this process.

CHAPTER 6 — INFECTION, IMMUNE DEFICIENCY AND IMBALANCE

Introduction

I lumped three potentially very different issues—infection, immune deficiency, and immune imbalance—together into one chapter because they often present as the same sorts of symptoms and they encompass one broad area of thinking. The complaints of patients with these types of problems, which include chronic or recurring infections and strange and diverse symptoms that suggest an underlying or occult infection, often indicate something is wrong with their immune systems in terms of defending against infectious organisms. In many cases, the key to solving these problems is to focus on the immune system itself, helping the body achieve balance, control, or clearance of a chronic infection.

Of course, achieving balance, control, or clearance of an infection is often not a primary issue for the patient, who just wants to feel better. Infection usually has more to do with the *host* than with the infectious agent. A patient may keep having sore throats or ear infections because something else is bothering his or her immune system, such as a food allergy or chemical toxin. A patient who appears to have generalized immune deficiency may have a genetic basis for it or may have had environmental exposures that damaged his or her immune system.

Hormonal deficiencies, such as hypothyroidism and adrenal insufficiency, can adversely impact the immune system, as can broad influences such as nutrient deficiency or stress. The relative immune system suppression caused by these problems can lead to persistent or recurring infections. Similarly, immune system suppression can lead to increased risk for cancers as well.

Chronic infection and immune defense in general is a complicated area of medicine that requires an understanding of everything we have discussed to this point. These immune system issues are often "symptoms" themselves, and not the upstream cause, so the real root issues will still need to be addressed. However, the infectious or other immune problems that develop and become chronic must be treated in order to return people to health, and that's what we're going to discuss here.

Recurring or chronic infections

Many patients complain explicitly of recurring infections of some sort while others don't realize that their various problems are caused by infection at all. Infections that aren't obvious to the patient are "occult" infections. The following discussion addresses some common recurrent infection problems and what may need to be done to resolve them.

Bacterial infections

Bacterial infections are the types of infections people commonly think of when you mention "infection." Bacterial infections can include bulging red eardrums that burst and leak pus, recurring sinus infections with thick green snot and pain in the face, urinary tract infections, and recurring skin boils. Most people who know about these have had repeated courses of antibiotics and may have developed infectious organisms resistant to some of the drugs over time.

Let's take each area of infection and discuss what you can do to prevent recurrent infections or help reduce the need for antibiotics. You want to avoid antibiotics because overuse of antibiotics leads to drug-resistant bacteria, which can become increasingly nasty and lethal. In addition, using antibiotics orally can derange the normal microbial population of the gut. Finally, antibiotics are potentially toxic to humans. Those first two issues are well known to most people, but I should elaborate on the statement about toxicity.

I'm not referring to the idea of drug "allergy" though antibiotics do commonly cause allergic reactions, possibly because most of them are derived from fungus. Antibiotics are, by definition, designed to kill or inhibit the cellular function of living things, and thinking that they do not have adverse effects on our own cells is naïve.

We know that many antibiotics offer some diverse side effects like nausea and tooth discoloration that are annoying enough, but some antibiotics have unusual and specific toxicities, such as the aminoglycosides (e.g., gentamicin), that cause damage to the auditory nerve. A more consistent problem is that antibiotics can kill the energy-producing organelles called *mitochondria* that are inside all of your cells; mitochondria are like little bacteria with which virtually all multi-cellular organisms developed a symbiotic relationship billions of years ago (according to the scientific view of evolution).

An important goal of any prescribed antibiotic drug is to have *selective* toxicity for bacterial cells over human or animal cells. It is easy to find those differences for the uniquely human parts of our cells, but mitochondria are usually still susceptible. The membranes, DNA, and proteins of your mitochondria are similar to those of bacteria, therefore your mitochondria may be inadvertently damaged by antibiotics. Since mitochondria are responsible for producing the vast majority of energy used by your cells, common symptoms of antibiotic use include generalized fatigue, decreased mental function, muscle weakness, neurological deficiencies, and other specific organ dysfunction.

I try to avoid the frequent use of conventional antibiotics, and use them only when it really seems necessary. For those with recurrent infections of certain types, alternatives include addressing any allergies that are affecting the particular body region or compartment. For example, treat inhalant allergies in those with recurrent bronchitis or sinusitis and food allergies in those with recurrent urinary, ear, skin, sinus, or other types of infection.

Colloidal silver is often used as a "natural" antibiotic for the treatment of acute minor infections and for prevention purposes in those with recurring infections. Colloidal silver has been used for a long time to treat infections of all types; it does not have any known human toxicity, other than to turn the skin a bluish gray color (argyria). Silver susceptibility among bacteria is genetically determined and very broad spectrum. There may be some activity against fungi as well (Lansdown, 2006). I found one published case report of a boy with cystic fibrosis who was doing very poorly and then showed dramatic improvements with the institution of daily colloidal silver. He had dramatically reduced lung infections and more than doubled his pulmonary function (FEV1 up from 24% to 60%) while using the silver, then had his only infection leading to hospitalization when he had a temporary lapse in the colloidal silver therapy several months later (Baral, 2008).

Silver products for use as antibiotics are available over the counter. Look for a product that is in "colloidal" form or "nano" form rather than "ionic" form. Many products will say they are colloids, but if you do some research you may find they are ionic. The colloidal and ionic forms can accumulate in the body, while the manufacturers of nano silver forms claim it does not accumulate. Some practitioners, usually in other countries, will administer silver intravenously for severe infections.

I would caution anyone with serious infection symptoms that they should not rely upon only silver products for treatment, as I have seen many cases where silver alone failed to cure infections. If things seem to be getting worse in spite of using silver, seek conventional medical attention right away. It is certainly safer to try using silver as a daily preventive therapy for those who seem to be susceptible to recurring infections.

There are other interventions for specific regional infections. For those with recurring ear or sinus infections, it is often helpful to avoid dairy products and to take daily doses of N-acetyl cysteine (NAC), which boosts glutathione levels and helps thin and clear mucous from the sinus and middle ear compartments. NAC is also helpful for those with chronic or recurring lung infections (especially smokers) and those with chronic liver infections. Children should take 600mg daily and adults up to 1200mg twice daily for prevention, with greatly escalated doses during any actual infection. There is no toxicity whatsoever of NAC, and it is good for a wide range of illnesses.

Garlic and mullein in warmed olive oil placed in the ear is a common folk remedy that works well for most ear infections. Rinsing the nasal passages with salt water—perhaps with the addition of a little silver or peroxide—using a neti pot also works well for many people who suffer from recurrent or chronic sinus problems. Saline nasal sprays can be helpful for those with recurrent sinus or ear infections. Afrin and similar nasal sprays should be used for only a few days at a time, to prevent dependence. Some with recurrent ear infections may benefit from having their tonsils and/or adenoids removed.

Some people get recurring infections of the tonsils, most frequently from streptococcal bacteria. After the tonsils have been repeatedly infected, they can become chronically inflamed, and their immune activation sometimes can't be calmed down (tonsils are primarily immune tissue). Sometimes removing the tonsils is the best option, after which the person's overall health will frequently rebound. Of course, some people just keep getting sicker or get sick in a new way. Probiotics specific for oral flora, which usually contain *Streptococcus salivarius*, are useful for those who have recurrent sore throats.

Chronic bronchitis is seen most often in smokers, many of whom have persistent bacterial colonization in their airways because of the damage to their normal mucosal defenses. NAC and colloidal silver on a daily basis may be helpful, and a good herbalist can often find a helpful combination of herbs, although occasionally conventional antibiotics may be needed to treat exacerbations. Intravenous vitamin C infusions, sometimes including glutathione, can be useful for those with lingering viral or bacterial lung infections, including bronchitis, viral illnesses like influenza, or even mold and other inhaled exposures.

Recurring deep skin infections are often caused by nasty, drug-resistant species of staphylococcus bacteria (e.g., the dreaded "MRSA" so prevalent today). Acne doesn't count so much as a chronic infection in my opinion, because it's usually related to food allergies and hormonal imbalances, but it is often treated with chronic antibiotics by conventional practitioners who don't realize there may be other causative factors. For the recurring boils or other more severe infections, it may be helpful to shower with chlorhexidine (Hibiclens™) every day and to place mupirocin (Bactroban™) or bacitracin ointment inside your nose every day to reduce the bacterial burden. It's best to avoid repeated courses of oral antibiotics for skin and other common infections for reasons I'll discuss shortly; colloidal silver is a good alternative to try daily as a preventive measure.

Urinary infections are common in women and young girls. An isolated urinary tract infection (UTI) here and there is not unusual, but some girls and women get them frequently. This condition always leads me to test for food allergies, which I find present in most of these cases—most commonly dairy. Patients with any type of recurrent infections should be tested for food allergies in my opinion. The antibiotics used for UTIs, and any other bacterial infection for that matter, frequently cause problems later on and are best avoided if possible, so I want to give you some strategies for prevention and natural treatment of recurrent UTIs.

One simple tactic is to drink more water, but that doesn't help much unless the individual was taking in too little water in the first place. It is helpful for sexually active women to urinate right after intercourse if they notice that is a contributing factor. Drinking cranberry juice is helpful, but you should choose a juice with no added sugar because the sugar feeds bacteria; for that reason you're better off with cranberry capsules. Vitamin C taken at 500-1000mg several times per day can be helpful. The herb *uva ursi* has been shown to help, but it is canceled out by cranberry, so don't take them together.

Taking colloidal silver every day at a low dose and then increasing to treatment strength when UTI symptoms first begin is sometimes a useful strategy. It is also very helpful to use an over-the-counter product called *mannose*, an inert sugar. The sugar is almost totally eliminated into your urine, and any *E. coli* bacteria will let go of your bladder and be flushed out while they go after the sugar. (*E. coli* love mannose like it's their "crack".) The down side of mannose is it won't work on other types of bacteria, but since about eighty percent of UTI's are caused by E. coli, it helps most of the time and doesn't disturb the gut flora at all. I suggest using mannose at about ¼ to ½ tsp daily for prevention in those prone to recurrent E. coli infections.

Chronic gastrointestinal problems caused by bacterial organisms are more common than conventional medicine would have you believe. We are trained to identify the bacterial causes of diarrhea, such as salmonella, campylobacter, *E. coli*, shigella, and *Clostridia difficile*. Those first four are generally self-limited and don't usually require antibiotics at all; they are usually the cause of infectious food poisoning. Certain *E. coli* infections can be life threatening and severe, but still aren't supposed to be treated with antibiotics in most cases because that just makes it worse in the short term.

Infections with *C. diff* can be life threatening even in otherwise healthy individuals and do require rapid institution of appropriate antibiotic therapy (and there are only a couple antibiotics that are typically effective). People often pick up the *C. diff* organism in the hospital, and the bacterium is carried asymptomatically in a significant proportion of health care workers. The organism usually does not cause any trouble, until something happens to disturb the overall balance of the intestinal flora. Taking most antibiotics, targeting other bacterial infections, tends to kill of the competition and allow dangerous overgrowth of Clostridia bacteria. It has also now been noted that chronic use of acid reducing medications such as Prilosec™, Aciphex™, Nexium™, Prevacid™, Protonix™ and Dexilant™ can allow overgrowth of C. diff as well and potentially lead to this life threatening infection.

If a patient has chronic diarrhea, bloating, discomfort, and other symptoms in the bowels, the doctor will often order a stool culture, looking for just these particular pathogenic bacteria mentioned above. If they aren't found, the doctor often assumes that you don't have a bacterial infection. Giardia and other parasites are usually ruled out too, with a cursory stool examination that tends to miss real parasites a significant percentage of the time at conventional labs. When these tests are normal, and perhaps a colonoscopy appears normal as well, conventional doctors often diagnose the patient with "irritable bowel syndrome" even though there are many other types of bacteria that could be present and explain the symptoms.

Some providers, including me at times, will presume the patient has "small bowel bacterial overgrowth", and treat them with broad-spectrum antibiotics that kill most types of bacteria. The one used most often currently—and I have good success with it myself for this type of issue—is rifaximin (Xifaxan™). Rifaximin tends to kill Clostridia organisms as well, and will relieve symptoms in most who have a bacterial cause of their problem (even when the stool tests were all normal—which is why I often skip the stool tests).

Many people with chronic diarrhea problems developed them after having had antibiotics for some other infection or during a medical procedure. The typical antibiotics prescribed for respiratory, urinary, and skin infections usually do not kill the anaerobic (meaning they can't live in oxygen) bacteria that populate the GI tract, but they do kill most of your "good" bacteria that normally keep the other bacterial populations under control. Sometimes taking antibiotics leaves a major overgrowth of the wrong types of bacteria such as other species of Clostridia, not just the *difficile* variety, which aren't tested for (there are dozens of Clostridia species and many cause human disease), or other anaerobes. It is often helpful for those with chronic diarrhea after antibiotics to use a course of metronidazole (Flagyl™), rifaximin, or possibly neomycin, in order to kill the offending germs.

Some people with inflammatory bowel disease (IBD) problems have chronic bacterial infection with an atypical organism class, which are called *mycobacteria* because they have components in their cell walls that are similar to those of fungi. These organisms are often acquired through milk and other dairy products. In many people, there is a small, quiet population of these bacteria; but in some people the immune system mounts a full-scale attack on them. One particular organism likely associated with Crohn's and ulcerative colitis is *Mycobacterium avium paratuberculosis* (MAP). The MAP organism has been identified through various techniques in a significant percentage of IBD patients and is known to cause chronic intestinal inflammatory disease in dairy cows, nonhuman primates and other animal species (Pierce, 2010).

There is a very real risk of acquiring the MAP organism from store-bought dairy because the infection spreads readily through dairy herds and is known to survive extreme conditions such as the heat of pasteurization, the acidic environment of fermentation into products such as kefir and yogurt, and the low temperatures during refrigeration (Klanicova, 2012). The organism has been cultured from a small but significant percentage of dairy and beef products sold at grocery stores (Eltholth, 2009). Again, it is dangerous to assume the food at the store is safe.

Some harsh antibiotics target these types of bacteria specifically (e.g., ethambutol, rifabutin) but common drugs like azithromycin and ciprofloxacin are often effective as well. Similar to the treatment of active tuberculosis, antibiotic therapy for MAP infection typically must include three or four different drugs to be very effective. This leads to a high rate of adverse effects. Treatment frequently has to continue for a year or more for complete resolution, and many of those patients will relapse again later because their infection was not fully cleared or because they were re-infected. For this reason, my autologous immunotherapy technique using stool-derived antigens to turn off the adverse immune response to these organisms becomes an attractive option and seems to be quite effective.

The last group of bacterial infections to be discussed here is chronic systemic infections, though I of course have only mentioned a few focused infections thus far and there are certainly many more that are relevant to chronic disease. Some strains of bacteria can hide from your immune system inside your own cells, some cause diverse and widespread symptoms, and others can trigger autoimmune reactions that seem to be completely unrelated to bacterial infection. Syphilis, a disease caused by the spirochete bacterium *Treponema pallidum*, is a classic example of one such bacterial infection. Many people died from syphilis prior to the discovery of antibiotics, and it was known to cause an incredible scope of disease depending upon where the infection was focused. Luckily the antibiotic penicillin still kills this bacterium easily, so syphilis is rarely seen these days.

Other spirochete infections are still prevalent today, and like syphilis, they can spread to almost any tissue and cause almost any type of symptom. Lyme disease, a well-known example, is caused by a spirochete bacterium in the genus *Borrelia*. Lyme disease can be treated with antibiotics if it is caught early, but if the infection is not treated aggressively in the first week, the bacterium gets into tissues from which it is difficult, even impossible, to extract. It can cause long-term and progressive problems with the nervous system, the heart, and other vital organs.

There are many *Borrelia* organisms other than the one that causes classic Lyme disease, and they are all difficult to test for. Most are carried by ticks, but they can potentially also be carried by other biting insects and arthropods, such as mosquitoes. The classic initial rash called erythema migrans indicates the initiation of such an infection, but most people with Lyme-like disease have no memory of such a rash. These germs can burrow inside own cells and hide from your immune system for as long as they need to in between exacerbations; they also evade your immune system by changing their surface antigens and preventing effective antibody formation.

Patients with chronic spirochete infections often see numerous doctors and have many chronic symptoms like fatigue, mental focus problems, headaches, body aches, depression, insomnia, strange neurological symptoms, and heart palpitations or arrhythmias. Conventional practitioners rarely consider spirochete infection, and it is unfortunately very difficult to verify infection by lab testing even if it is suspected. Recovery from these infection problems often requires long-term intermittent antibiotics as well as other complementary and integrative therapies. It is common for other co-infecting organisms to be present along with a borrelia infection; the most common organisms include *Bartonella* and *Babesia*. These agents must be identified and addressed as well in order to achieve remission of illness.

A small number of integrative practitioners around the country specialize in these sorts of chronic problems, often calling themselves "Lyme" doctors or stating a specialty in tick-borne infections. These practitioners can be difficult to find, because they are often persecuted by dogmatic conventional physicians and state medical boards. You won't likely find them advertised in the phone book as "Lyme doctors". Call offices that seem to be holistic or integrative and ask specifically about this area of treatment, or check out the International Lyme and Associated Diseases Society (ILADS) website at www.ilads.org for information and a list of trained practitioners near you.

Chronic Lyme-like illness should be considered in anyone with chronic fatigue, widespread pain, brain fog, neurological symptoms and other associated complaints that don't seem to make sense and don't appear to be associated with other identifiable causes. I often test these folks for hormonal deficiencies such as thyroid, cortisol, DHEA and testosterone first; put them on vitamin D and appropriate nutritional therapy; test them for food allergies; screen for carbon monoxide exposure and maybe test them for heavy metals first. If all that stuff is unhelpful I may give them a course of antibiotics (usually doxycycline plus azithromycin for a full month) to see if they respond. I usually run a western blot antibody profile test for Lyme, but it is frequently all normal/negative even in those with rampant infection, so I generally treat folks based on suspicion anyway.

It is important to mention that if you do in fact have a Lyme-related infection problem you will likely feel absolutely horrible for the first several days to one week on antibiotic therapy. This is because your immune system will be seeing all the pieces of dying spirochete, with exposed antigens that cause profound inflammatory responses. This is called the Jarisch-Herxheimer reaction in the medical arena, or a "die-off" reaction in lay terms. Steroids may be helpful through this period of several days, but you just have to tough it out to some extent as well and come out better off on the other side.

Other types of chronic intracellular infections include certain *Mycobacteria* and some atypical bacteria, such as *Mycoplasma* and *Chlamydia*. The classic systemic mycobacterial infection is tuberculosis (TB), caused by *Mycobacterium tuberculosis*, which used to kill people every day in this country. We now have antibiotics against this organism and widely screen our population for occult infection so it no longer a major problem here except in certain regions, such as rural Alaska. (It's still the Dark Ages up here in some ways.) Vitamin D and natural sunlight were the most effective treatments for TB prior to antibiotics.

Another classical mycobacterial infection is leprosy, caused by the organisms *Mycobacterium leprae* or *lepromatosis*. Leprosy is of course very rare these days, but still plays an important role in human history as a chronic systemic infection. (I wrote a term paper on the subject in my undergaduate microbiology class.) There are other types of Mycobacteria, some of which are common in your own everyday environment. I mentioned those in milk products that cause GI infection, most commonly *Mycobacterium avium paratuberculosis* (MAP). Others in the *Mycobacterium avium* group include MAI (I = "*intracellulare*"), which are literally everywhere in your environment; for example, they roost in your showerhead, and you inhale them during every shower.

Mycobacterium avium complex (MAC) organisms are usually a problem only for those who have immune system or chronic lung problems. Kids with cystic fibrosis get chronic MAC infections, as do smokers and those with chronic obstructive pulmonary disease (COPD). Patients on immunosuppressive drug treatments for cancer, transplant, or autoimmune disease are susceptible as well. These infections are tough to treat because few antibiotics kill these organisms and repeated exposure is likely to occur, leading to recurrent infection. Your best bet is to improve your immune system. You can also take NAC and colloidal silver or some other appropriate preventive treatments as I have discussed.

The last specific bacterial organisms I want to discuss here are *Mycoplasma* and *Chlamydia* species. These bacteria are smaller than most and don't have a cell wall. They get inside your own cells—even your white blood cells—and hide from your immune system. They don't usually cause problems directly, but most people know about the sexually transmitted disease Chlamydia causes (*C. trachomatis* species specifically). This organism is also a major cause of blindness worldwide because it will damage your eyes if it gets into them. This is one reason we put antibiotic ointment in babies' eyes at birth. (And perhaps it is the root of mother's telling their adolescent sons they will go blind if they keep masturbating.)

The bigger problem with these organisms is the chronic colonization some species can achieve and the immune system inflammation they generate. Cardiovascular disease leading to heart attacks or strokes is in some cases thought related to *C. pneumoniae* infection in the body and the resulting inflammation in the arterial walls (Luque, 2012). Numerous other chronic infectious agents, including various bacteria and viruses, are thought to contribute to the intravascular inflammation that leads to atherosclerosis and cardiovascular disease (Tufano, 2012).

As discussed earlier, rheumatoid arthritis and autoimmune thyroiditis and other autoimmune diseases have been suspected related to chronic *Mycoplasma* or other bacterial infection. One reason for this is possibly the fact that these bacteria are inside our own cells, and our immune system is forced to attack our own tissue to get at them. That problem is both related to infection and the chronic inappropriate immune response that cross-reacts with our own tissues.

Only certain types of antibiotics will kill these types of intracellular bacteria that have no cell wall. The antibiotics must be the kind of agents that penetrate into cells and effect intracellular function rather than cell wall synthesis (which rules out the penicillins, cephalosporins, vancomycin, and others). Erythromycin and tetracycline derivatives usually work, but it may take months of treatment to clear up these infections because of where they hide. One possible regimen involves taking a weekly dose of azithromycin for several months, and I usually prescribe it daily for the first week or two.

This is an example of what we call "empiric therapy", meaning we don't really know there is infection there and are treating based on clinical suspicion rather than verified test results. There is the risk of adverse effects, yeast infections and gut organism derangement from the antibiotics, but it is worth trying for many patients with chronic inflammatory arthritis and other problems. I advise taking a good probiotics, and prescription or natural items to control yeast, while on antibiotics and for a time afterward. I am not sure whether using colloidal silver works as well here, but it's worth a try perhaps because it is safer and available without a prescription.

The most common types of chronic bacterial infections are gum disease (gingivitis and periodontitis), cavities and other dental infections. Gingivitis is to some extent present in more than 90 percent of adults in the United States (Li, 2010), making it the most prevalent infectious disease problem we have by far. Dental cavities represent a very common infectious disease as well; and this condition effects the poor and certain ethnic groups to a greater extent than white middle class folks. One recent Indian Health Services (IHS) study found that 75% of American Indian and Alaskan Native kids have dental cavities by age five (Phipps, 2012). Many don't realize that cavities are the result of infection but they are caused by acid produced from certain types of bacteria (*Streptococcus mutans* specifically) acquired in the mouth, usually from your mother (don't forget to thank her on mother's day).

The effects of these infections are not confined to the mouth since they release variable amounts of bacteria and biological toxins into the bloodstream every time you eat, chew gum, or brush your teeth. Gum disease has been associated with cardiac death and chronic disease since ancient Greek times. The association between periodontal infection and inflammation and coronary artery disease has been confirmed by modern research (Bazile, 2002). Periodontal disease and poor oral hygiene have shown some association with stomach cancer (Salazar, 2012). There is also some evidence to suggest that control of periodontal disease improve blood sugar control in diabetics (Taylor, 1999). This is why simply using a waterpik after brushing twice per day may extend your life!

The keys to keeping infection out of your mouth are simple: Eat a healthy diet with no refined sugars or starches. Don't smoke or use drugs that may cause dry mouth. Brush your teeth twice daily with fluoride-free toothpaste. (You do not need fluoride!) After brushing, irrigate your gum line thoroughly with a water pik, and consider putting a little iodine and/or colloidal silver in the tank. If a tooth is broken or decayed past the point of repair or otherwise disease such that it causes chronic pain, it is best to simply remove it. You should not have a root canal done, because all that does is kill the nerve to the tooth so that it no longer hurts; and it leaves the tooth "dead" and relatively defenseless against the oral bacteria. Performing a root canal on a diseased tooth would be like severing the nerves to your finger when it has gangrene at the tip, rather than amputating the end of the finger.

The dead teeth left after root canals are completely infected, loaded with dozens of different species and millions of bacteria (Rocas, 2008). Again, I advised people to *never have a root canal performed*, and if you have already done so, my opinion is that you should have those teeth pulled straight away. The chronic infection left behind after root canal can trigger systemic inflammatory responses throughout the body. I've noted this phenomenon in diabetic patients; when some have had their blood sugars running persistently high without any explanation, I have had them go to the dentist and remove old root canal teeth, to see their blood sugars drop immediately back down afterward. Pulling a tooth is much cheaper than having a root canal done anyway.

Yeast and fungal infections

Chronic fungal problems well known to conventional medicine include histoplasmosis and coccidiomycosis. These and other fungal infections like them are contracted through the lungs by exposure to the fungal spores in certain environments, such as caves, dense brush, and areas with lots of bird droppings. Just living in certain regions, like the San Joaquin Valley, is enough to become infected to some degree. Severely infected people may have an acute respiratory illness with fever that can become severe. Alternatively, they may not have any acute symptoms at all. Most will just have nodules or enlarged lymph nodes inside their chest that may be visible incidentally on later X-rays and CT scans.

These fungal organisms may live dormant in these nodules and reactivate if the immune system weakens. If a patient is going to have an organ transplant and go on immunosuppressive drugs to prevent rejection, develops AIDS or is going on an immunosuppressive drug for autoimmune disease (Enbrel™, Humira™, Remicade™, etc.) he or she is often tested for these fungal infections, especially if he or she has spent time in certain regions. If the patient has suggestive radiological findings or a positive antibody test for past exposure, he or she is usually put on chronic antifungal medication, such as fluconazole, along with their immunosuppression. Problems with fungal reactivation are not common at all in the general public.

However, what *is* common in the general American population is chronic mild fungal or yeast infection/infestation/overgrowth. This problem usually relates to the "environment" in your body's being too conducive to the growth of fungi, and has a lot to do with the level of sugar consumption in our culture. Less often, the problem is due to your having contracted a particularly nasty, atypical strain of fungus somewhere. Everyone has fungus living on their skin and yeast in their bowels, vaginal area, and oral area. We have many bacteria and parasites in these areas too. These microorganisms are part of the ecosystem living in and upon us that is not human.

Under normal conditions, if you have a well-functioning immune system and aren't feeding your little "pets" sugar all day, the fungi are kept at low or moderate levels in terms of population, and all your microbes live in harmony. Less than ideal conditions can allow the overgrowth of fungi or yeast, and various symptoms may result. Athletes' foot is one well-known condition that results when feet are allowed to remain hot and sweaty for too long at a time, and they pick up some new strain of fungus from the locker room. This same type of skin infestation can occur in the groin, under the breasts, in the armpits, and between rolls of flesh (if one is obese).

These local skin infections with fungi relate to there being a dark, warm, damp area of skin in which the organisms can frolic—they love it! In these situations, the skin being kept *dry* is more important than it being clean; washing with soap and water will not help if you don't dry the area thoroughly afterward. You should even dry your toes, groin, and other such areas with a hairdryer after bathing. Water is the only essential item needed in common by all forms of life; you must deprive the fungi of their water.

The skin can become deeply and chronically infested with fungal organisms and require the use of oral antifungal drugs or topical agents. This commonly happens in the scalp (tinea capitis) or around the eyebrows and nose (called seborrheic dermatitis, but it's really a yeast infection on your face), on the feet (tinea pedis), and in the toenails too (tinea unguium). You can try over-the-counter topical antifungal agents for each of these conditions. Use Selsun Blue shampoo (soak your feet in it, put some on your face or wherever your infection resides), tea tree oil products, oil of oregano, and some other natural antifungals. These attempts don't usually work because the agents aren't strong enough and they don't penetrate into your tissue deeply enough.

Toenails are particularly hard to clear, probably because they have no blood flow except at the very base. Having a toenail infection with fungus isn't harmful by itself, but it can be spread to the rest of the foot and lead to cracks in the skin that can become secondarily infected with dangerous bacteria. This is of particular concern for those with diabetes. Fungal infection in the feet is often the inciting event that leads eventually to amputations. Of course, diabetics maintain high levels of sugar in their tissues, making this very tough for them to treat.

Chronic toenail fungus is best cleared by improving overall health and immune function and possibly using a course of oral antifungals like Lamisil™ for three months or longer. Chronic toenail fungus is usually not a serious problem and is just cosmetically annoying, but it may be of concern primarily because it indicates something may be wrong with your immune system on a broader scale. If you have tried repeatedly to eradicate toenail fungus or foot fungus without success, you must attend to your overall health in other ways.

The most important factor when it comes to fungal problems in the body environment is the availability of sugar to the organism. Yeast and fungi feed almost exclusively on sugars, so they love when you eat the typical American diet, and they especially love people with diabetes because their blood and tissue sugar levels run high. Diabetics often develop yeast and fungus problems in the mouth, intestinal tract and on their skin, and diabetic women are much more prone to vaginal yeast problems than non-diabetic women are.

Anyone who eats "excessive" amounts of sugar (which means the majority of Americans) may develop overgrowth problems with yeast, at least in the gut. It is critical for those with diabetes or pre-diabetes to avoid all simple sugars and starches and to be on the lookout for fungal overgrowth problems. The infestation causes a stress response in the body, which raises sugar levels and creates a vicious cycle that promotes more fungal growth and increases inflammation, thereby increasing blood sugar levels again as part of the inflammatory response.

It is very important to reduce or eliminate sugar from the diet if you want to clear up any type of yeast or fungal problem. This means avoiding corn syrup and added sugars, any type of bread products and other processed carbohydrate products including pastas, crackers; corn; excessive amounts of potato or rice, and other starches. Of course avoiding things like ice cream, candy, cookies and cake should be obvious. If that sounds impossible to you, you may just need to get used to having problems with yeast.

You may never truly win your battle with fungi and yeast unless you eliminate the sugar and simple carbs. This also means avoiding grapes, melon, fresh berries, and some other high-sugar fruits for some. There are entire books written about how to eliminate yeast from your body naturally, including these dietary suggestions and some natural items that kill yeast, so I won't spend too much time on it here. Just think about what food items tend to mold quickly, and don't eat those foods. The *Paleo diet* is a particularly good strategy, and excellent for long-term health as well.

Herbal items that act against yeast and fungi include pau d'arco, black walnut, caprylic acid (present in coconut oil), oregano, berberine, Oregon grape root, and tea tree oil. You can take these herbs internally or put them on the skin as appropriate. People with bad yeast or fungal problems usually require prescription antifungals, at least initially, to get the problems under control. You can try to starve your yeast out with a strict diet and help eradicate it with the herbals and some probiotics, but it may take months.

I frequently prescribe nystatin and fluconazole together for people I suspect of having significant chronic intestinal yeast issues. If someone has visible focused fungal infection problems, such as ringworm on the skin, fungus on the scalp, or toenail infection, he or she probably needs oral antifungals (fluconazole is safest) for a month or longer. Toenails frequently require six months or more of treatment, and Lamisil (terbinafine) is the most effective for this specific problem. However, if you don't eliminate sugar from your diet, you will probably fail regardless of how long you take the medications.

Other chronic fungal issues include those in the sinuses and vaginal areas. Mucous membranes are all naturally colonized with yeast organisms; they are in the air, and every time you take a breath or eat, you ingest some yeast and fungi, so "total eradication" of fungi is a fantasy.

Anyone who has had several courses of antibiotics may end up with excessive fungus in the body cavities, including the sinuses, the vagina, and the GI tract. Most women know about this, and it is well accepted by physicians that if you have irritation, itching, and thick, white discharge from the vagina, you probably have a yeast infection. We treat it with vaginal antifungal creams or oral fluconazole, and the infection symptoms usually go away readily. For tough cases, have a doctor prescribe compounded vaginal suppositories of boric acid (600mg, one nightly for a week), which will acidify the area (lower the pH) and make it unlivable for the yeast.

Babies with angry red diaper rashes often have a yeast infection issue that can be treated with topical antifungal creams, oral nystatin, or fluconazole. Probiotics are important in this instance as well. Older children and adults may incur similar problems, but usually just isolated itching and redness right at the anus area, because we usually don't wear diapers.

For some reason, if a patient has chronic irritation, itching, pain, and thick, whitish discharge from the *sinuses* instead of the vagina, physicians never seem to suspect the problem is related to fungus. Physicians are taught about a particularly severe fungal infection of the sinuses caused by organisms in the genus *Rhizopus*, which infects those with immune deficiency or poorly controlled diabetes and virtually eats away the middle of your face. Most conventional doctors see that as the only "real" fungal infection in the sinuses, and don't believe there are other fungal infections in the sinuses of milder varieties.

However, anyone who has had a number of bacterial sinus infections treated with antibiotics, especially if nasal steroids are used too, is likely to end up with some chronic fungal colonization and infection there afterward. If the patient has some anatomical problem obstructing sinus drainage, like a deviated septum, chronic fungal infection is even more likely. After a while, these patients often notice that they need longer and different courses of antibiotics to clear their infections, or antibiotics no longer seem to help at all. If this scenario fits you I suggest you stop using antibiotics completely unless you develop a high fever and greenish nasal discharge, and try to address the fungal element.

The chronic symptoms and those repeated flares of pressure and increased mucous without fever are mostly related to fungus and related inflammation, rather than bacteria, in folks treated repeatedly with antibiotics. In this setting one should take N-Acetyl Cysteine (NAC) at least 1,200mg twice daily, take lots of vitamin C (just short of causing diarrhea), and avoid eating any sugar or dairy. Consider doing rinses with saline and colloidal silver using a Neti pot. If that doesn't clear things up, find a practitioner who will prescribe a nasal antifungal spray to use every day in both nostrils. I prescribe a compounded itraconazole spray in 0.5-1% strength with a little EDTA (0.1%) to help break up biofilms. This spray has to be made at a compounding pharmacy because there are no currently mass-produced nasal antifungal sprays. It often has to be used for six months to a year for complete resolution of tough cases.

Viral infections

There are a great many chronic viral infections we have described in humans, and certainly many more we still have not identified. Warts are caused by HPV (human papillomavirus), and some strains are associated with cervical cancer, anal cancer, laryngeal cancers and vocal cord lesions. We know the cancer Kaposi's sarcoma seen almost exclusively in AIDS patients is caused by a human herpes virus (HHV-8), a virus which usually causes no apparent symptoms. Around 7% of healthy adults in the U.S. have antibodies against this virus, suggesting prior exposure (Qu, 2010). It is likely that other cancers are related to other types of viruses yet unrecognized.

Chronic viral hepatitis caused by hepatitis B or C is well understood, and the donated blood supply is screened for these, as well as HIV and some other known viruses. It wasn't until the 1980s that hepatitis C was identified, and donated blood screening started in 1992. Prior to that time, it was all too common for a patient to develop hepatitis after a blood transfusion and to contract what was then termed "transfusion hepatitis" or "non-A, non-B viral hepatitis." Many Vietnam veterans who were injured and required blood transfusion became infected accidentally.

Many people also contracted HIV from blood transfusions before that virus was identified and the blood supply was screened appropriately starting in 1985. This situation was especially bad for hemophiliacs, who receive blood factors from hundreds of pooled donors. More than one third of all hemophiliacs became infected with HIV from the years the virus came on the scene until 1985, and then new infection virtually stopped (Cowan, 1999). It probably wasn't a good idea to pay for blood donations since many drug addicts, whose blood was likely to be infected with hepatitis and HIV and other blood-borne diseases, were eager to sell their blood for money so they could buy more drugs.

I have to wonder what yet-undiscovered viruses are still in the blood supply, wreaking havoc in some transfusion recipients. It would be foolish to think we had identified all the viruses by now.

We know that most viruses in the *herpes* family can set up chronic infections, partly because they incorporate themselves into your DNA. Some viruses are composed of DNA, and others of RNA strands. Other than their "genome" (the DNA or RNA), these viruses are made of proteins and cell membranes that our human cells make for them. The only thing unique to the virus is its genetic material. Some RNA viruses set up persistent infections inside us as well. Hepatitis C is an RNA virus and can be eradicated completely from the body with medical therapy, whereas hepatitis B is a DNA virus and can never be completely cleared because it can lie dormant within your own tissue, incorporated into the nuclear DNA of liver cells.

The herpes viruses, which are well known, include herpes simplex virus type 1 (HSV-1), which causes mostly cold sores, and HSV-2, which causes mostly genital herpes. By the time we reach adulthood, the vast majority of us have HSV-1, but only a few people experience recurrent cold sores. The rest of us have immune systems strong enough to keep the virus locked away and dormant. People can experience severe neurological problems from HSV-1 including meningitis or encephalitis leading to death if not treated. There is also some evidence that high HSV-1 activity is be linked to Alzheimer's disease. Other chronic infections with spirochetes like those causing Lyme or syphilis and atypical bacteria such as *Chlamydia pneumoniae* show significant association with the development of dementia as well (Miklossy, 2011).

About a fifth of adults have HSV-2, but the genital sores only show up occasionally or not at all. Stress and immune suppression can trigger reactivations of viruses, as can direct sun exposure in the case of cold sores. Some people have frequent severe eruptions of the painful genital lesions and require ongoing suppressive therapy. Again, the specific functioning of an individual's immune system has everything to do with how well one handles these infectious agents. Taking the amino acid lysine every day, usually in doses of 1,000 to 2,000mg, seems to reduce the frequency of herpes flares in both oral and genital regions. One study found that getting the serum lysine concentration above 165nmlo/mL was the threshold for effect, significantly reducing the occurrence of cold sores in a group of volunteers with a history of recurrent lesions (Thein, 1984).

Chicken pox, which is also a herpes virus, can reactivate later on to cause a dreaded "shingles" outbreak, at times leading to chronic pain in the area. Other common herpes viruses include the Epstein-Barr virus (EBV), the most frequent cause of mononucleosis, and cytomegalovirus (CMV), which also causes some mononucleosis cases. Both EBV and CMV tend to stay in the body forever after initial infection, because their genomes are both comprised of double-stranded DNA and they can incorporate into our genes. The great majority of adults are infected with one or both of these viruses within their lifetime. EBV has been implicated in some cancers, such as Hodgkin's and Burkitt's lymphomas, nasopharyngeal cancer and cancer involving the muscle of the uterus. These cancers are all rare, but EBV infects more than ninety percent of the world's population.

A number of viruses, like HPV, EBV and HHV-8, have been shown to cause cancers. Infection with hepatitis B dramatically increases the rate of liver cancers, and hepatitis C increases that risk as well. How many other cancers may be caused by viruses? How many viruses lie within adults, just waiting for us to drop our guard and have some degree of immune dysfunction? Cancer is our second greatest cause of death; I think that makes chronic infection a very important potential cause of chronic disease and death as well.

Some people with chronic fatigue syndrome (CFS) symptoms who are tested for EBV activity show elevated viral counts in their blood; their practitioners may point to these elevated levels as the cause of their symptoms. However, since ninety percent of people are going to have this virus, some are going to have elevated viral levels without it meaning anything. If their viral activity levels are high and you treat them with an appropriate antiviral drug, they should get better—but it doesn't work that way; therefore there is not cause-and-effect relationship with EBV and chronic fatigue.

Similarly, in recent years there has been a suspicion that CFS may be caused by a relatively new virus called XMRV (xenotropic murine leukemia virus-related virus), a gammaretrovirus identified in 2006. This virus was thought possibly related to prostate cancer, and then later thought to be a common cause of CFS. These theories have since been disproven (Mendoza, 2012). Repeated studies have demonstrated no XMRV in humans sampled, and there is suspicion that the studies finding the virus in some subjects may have been the result of contamination (Hong, 2012). Some clinicians have attempted to treat CFS patients with antiretroviral drugs (like those used to treat HIV, which is also a retrovirus) and found no improvement in their symptoms, further demonstrating that the virus is not a likely cause of the condition.

The real issue with chronic viral problems, in my opinion, is the immune system; it is impossible to avoid contracting dozens—more likely hundreds—of chronic viruses in your body. That is just the nature of the world in which we have evolved and adapted. We should be used to having various viruses and other infectious agents colonizing us. If you are healthy and have a functioning immune system, you should be fine; otherwise, you may have chronic symptoms. Living in harmony with these agents is the key.

The JC and BK viruses are two other examples of this concept. They are *polyomaviruses*; a name which reflects an association with multiple types of tumors. There has been suspicion that the BK virus may be involved in certain cancers (though not yet proven), and the JC virus is known to cause a devastating neurological condition called progressive multifocal leukoencephalopathy (PML). These viruses are present in the great majority of people, 60% having the JC virus and more than 95% having the BK virus by middle age adulthood (Antonsson, 2010), but the viruses seem to lie dormant and asymptomatic in those with a functioning immune system. These viral problems generally only crop up only when a person's immune system is taken out by HIV or another virus or immunosuppressant drugs. I suspect that for some all it takes is severe vitamin D or nutritional deficiencies, or perhaps chronic severe illness, to leave them susceptible.

We don't have effective medical treatments for most viruses. There are a few antiviral drugs for influenza (amantadine, oseltamivir, and zanamivir) and herpes viruses (acyclovir, valacyclovir, and famciclovir) but not many other options. Influenza is generally cleared by the body on its own; and the antivirals aren't often further helpful. Herpes viruses cannot be totally cleared from the body because they incorporate into the DNA, but the drugs can be taken regularly to suppress symptoms. Don't forget to try daily lysine supplementation for this as well.

Some common natural and herbal antiviral items used by integrative and alternative practitioners include colloidal silver, olive leaf extract, grapefruit seed extract, pau d'arco, and lauric acid. One of the most helpful vitamins to take is vitamin D in large doses since vitamin D is very helpful with viral problems (Gal-Tanamy, 2011). There are likely homeopathic remedies, other herbals, and energy-based treatments that help directly combat viral pathogens as well.

Parasitic infections

Parasites are another category of invading organisms. When Americans think of parasites, they often think of giardia, flukes, tapeworms, and other intestinal parasites. They are also likely to think the whole topic is disgusting and rare in people who are "clean." Granted, having parasites is far more common in developing nations where people live close together without clean water; but these types of organisms are common in our industrialized society as well.

Malaria, which is caused by parasites in the genus *Plasmodium*, remains one of the leading causes of death worldwide, even in so-called civilized regions where the parasite is endemic. We have drugs to prevent and treat most infections, but those without access to these medications either die or have recurring problems from the parasite throughout their lifetimes. Recall that those carrying a single genetic mutation for sickle cell anemia are immune.

It is estimated that well over one billion people worldwide have worms of one or another species. One study even found that nearly a third of school children in Turkey (not a third world country at all) had intestinal parasites (Okyay, 2004). It is possible that half of the world population has one or more parasites in them at all times, as disgusting as that may sound. Just think about how often you are supposed to de-worm your dogs because they keep picking up worms from the environment. We live in that same environment, and while we don't intentionally eat poop like our dogs do, we likely come into contact with parasites all the time.

A "good" parasite doesn't kill or even harm the host because that would be counterproductive (if the parasite doesn't want to end up homeless). Many of us are walking around with little protozoans in our GI tracts and worms and other larval forms as cysts in our brains, muscles or other tissues. The *Taenia solium* tapeworm from undercooked pork, or the toxoplasmosis parasite (*Toxoplasma gondii*) from cat feces are common examples.

As long as our immune systems are functional, the toxoplasmosis parasite is not often a problem. It can however cause problematic lesions in the brain when people develop AIDS or are on immunosuppressive drugs; it can also get into the fetus and cause devastating neurological damage if a pregnant woman becomes exposed or infected for the first time. Cysticercosis is the term for the pork tapeworm larva forming cysts within our tissues, and neurocysticercosis is the term for this occurrence in the brain. The latter condition is unfortunately common in certain regions of Mexico and other developing nations, leading to recurring seizures in many of those affected (Correa, 1999). There are many other creepy and disgusting parasitic conditions seen in third world country, with various worms and parasites traveling through or bodies in various ways. It all serves as a reminder that we are not truly at the top of the food chain.

Diarrhea is a more common parasitic condition in our culture; and when most people say they think they may have "parasites", they are usually referring to their GI tract. Some well-known examples that cause symptoms like diarrhea in people include *giardia, cryptosporidium*, and *cyclospora*. Drinking water from a natural source while out hiking in the wilderness is the common way of contracting giarda, but the parasite can also be found in daycares and occasionally local water supplies. Cruise ships seem to be a favorite home of some of the other causative agents of parasitic diarrhea.

Parasites survive only in particular hosts, so many environmental parasites that are a problem for some animal species are not problems for us. For some of these, we are an occasional, "accidental" host, and we may get temporary symptoms when we encounter them. My favorite example of this is "swimmers' itch," which is caused by a type of fluke that burrows into your flesh if you swim in a contaminated lake. Your immune system finds and destroys the fluke larvae in your skin, preventing true infection but causing an itchy rash in the process.

Some worms and flukes are important examples of how dangerous parasites can be. The pork tapeworm is an important cause of epilepsy in Mexico and other places because the worm larva encysts in the brain, causing seizures to develop. Some flatworms, or "flukes," take up residence in the liver, lungs, or bladder and cause chronic inflammation and progressive destruction of those tissues. Alaska has a couple endemic tapeworm species of the genus *Echinococcus* that can create cysts in the liver, with risk of sudden anaphylactic shock if they are ruptured by accidental trauma. Those parasites cannot use us as a normal host to complete their life cycles, but they can kill us anyway.

Parasites are generally very good at evading the immune system, and most do not cause trouble directly. Intestinal worms can cause chronic microscopic bleeding and iron deficiency anemia however, which could eventually kill someone. The "fish tapeworm" *Diphyllobothrium latum*, which can grow to almost thirty feet long in your intestines, can steal the vitamin B-12 from your food, leaving you with symptomatic B-12 deficiency. Parasites are a diverse and fascinating area of medicine, but significant parasitic problems are fortunately uncommon in America.

Many practitioners in complementary and alternative medicine circles believe that practically everyone has parasites and that clearing them solves all sorts of health problems. According to these practitioners, if you're tired, you must have parasites; if you have headaches, it's parasites; and if you have an itchy anus, you most certainly have parasites! However, in my opnion there are causes of all these issues much more common than parasites in our society.

The best way to know whether your symptoms are from a parasite is to take things that should kill parasites and see if you get better. There are a number of herbal and natural remedies to clear your parasites; many companies produce "parasite cleanse" products, and there are a number of prescription antimicrobials that kill various parasites.

If you think you may have some sort of GI parasite, try wormwood (*Artemisia absinthium*), which is the origin of the alcoholic spirit absinthe and which has antimicrobial activity against most parasitic worms, or neem (from the tree *Azadirachta indica*), which is an important East Indian herb used in various health conditions (especially skin-related) and environmental pest control. Be aware that excessive internal use of herbal antimicrobials like wormwood, neem and pau d'arco (which also has anti-parasitic activity) can potentially lead to toxicity problems (a substance that kills other living things should always be handled with care). In addition, neem is probably the worst tasting medicinal item I have ever tried, and that's saying something!

In summary, parasites are probably very common, although they are not likely a common cause of illness here in the United States. If you think you may have parasites, there are some relatively safe over-the-counter remedies you can try first, but don't wait too long before seeing an experienced practitioner if you think you have significant problems. Doing stool testing for parasites through conventional laboratories is usually a waste of time and money, though some specialty labs that integrative practitioners use do a much better job.

Miscellaneous infectious agents and oddballs

There is always a "miscellaneous" category because we can't possibly know everything. Before moving on, here is some information about mites, insects, and prions.

Mites, which are arachnids, not insects, can come in very tiny, microscopic varieties like dust mites. Certain mite species can burrow into your skin and cause the itchy, infectious rash called "scabies." Other mite species live in your skin more harmoniously but can cause a milder rash that looks like little red dots, usually at the hair follicles. Insects are much less common parasites, but certain varieties, notably the botfly, lay eggs in your skin.

Other little arthropods (mosquitoes, ticks, and other biting bugs) play a much bigger role in infection by carrying parasites, viruses, and bacterial agents, such as malaria, leishmaniasis, various encephalitis viruses, Rocky Mountain spotted fever, and Lyme disease.

Prions, which rarely cause illness, are single mutated protein molecules that trigger the infected person's cells to manufacture the same mutant protein in mass quantities. The prion then accumulates in the person's tissues, most notably the brain, leading to tissue destruction and eventual nervous system shutdown. Mad cow disease, or "bovine spongiform encephalopathy" (BSE), is currently the most widely known prion condition; when people eat affected meat, they can develop the same disease problem. We call that "variant" Creutzfeldt-Jacob disease (vCJD), but it is caused by the same prion as BSE.

Another uncommon condition seen in sheep and goats is called scrapie, but it is not transmissible to humans as far as we know (but who knows when we will end up with a "mad sheep disease" scare). Kuru, a known human-to-human prion disease, was spread among certain tribes in Papua New Guinea through cannibalism. There is no known treatment for it, so just try not to eat other people, especially their brains. Prion diseases are not common at this time, but you never know when something new will pop up.

Chronic occult infections

The term "occult" refers to infections hidden below the surface so they are not overtly evident. I have already discussed many of these, including bacterial infections like Lyme disease and TB, viral illnesses like hepatitis C, and chronic intestinal colonization with yeast or *Clostridia* bacteria. Here I want to mention a few important indicators of infection's being the cause for chronic illness and some of the more common signs to look for.

Chronic systemic complaints like fatigue, random aches and pains, depression, and mental suppression are very common with infections. Fever without an obvious cause is possible, but fevers seem relatively rare in this setting. Recurring neurological symptoms like burning or electrical pains, tingling, numbness, and other symptoms without an apparent cause may occur, although these symptoms are also common with environmental toxicity problems. Many chronic digestive system problems are the result of chronic undiagnosed infection, as are inflammatory arthritis problems and other autoimmune phenomena.

Persistently high or spiking blood sugars in a diabetic that cannot seem to be controlled may be a sign of an occult infection. The presence of infection in the body may not manifest typical localized signs and symptoms of infection but may activate the body's systemic inflammatory or stress response. One of the effects of this stress response is to release extra sugar from the liver into the blood stream, which causes a diabetic person's blood sugar to go out of control. It may also be the final trigger to tip someone over into an initial diabetic state; many childhood diabetics manifest the disease right after having some sort of acute infection.

If you are a diabetic or you care for a diabetic with unruly, high, or spiking blood sugars without any apparent cause, there are a few common infections to look for. One is dental abscess, which may not be painful at all but will cause major systemic inflammation. A trip to the dentist for X-rays is one of the first things I suggest; any suspicious teeth must usually be pulled out. Chronic sinus disease is also common; there can be significant inflammation in the sinuses without notable symptoms if the sinus drainage has not been blocked to create pressure and pain. Skin infections like small boils or toenail infections can go unnoticed, especially on the feet of someone with peripheral nerve damage related to their diabetes.

You don't always see the typical signs of infection in the very young or the very old. Babies with fever often get broad evaluations that include chest x-rays, blood cultures, spinal taps, and urinary sampling with a catheter because they often don't exhibit focal signs of infection such as a cough and they can't complain about localized pain. Urinary tract infections in elderly women are common, but they may not have typical symptoms of urinary frequency, urgency, or burning. Often the first signs of UTI in an elderly woman are mental confusion, elevated blood sugars, or urinary incontinence.

The modern medical literature has confirmed the long-known fact that oral disease, such as chronic gum disease or periodontal disease, is linked to heart attacks, our number-one killer. The best way to keep your gums healthy is to use a water pick twice each day after brushing; I can't over-emphasize the importance of this simple habit. Don't let dental staff do "gum scraping" on you; just get a decent water pick and use it.

Root canals are very common, but you are far better off just having the tooth pulled. A tooth after root canal has no feeling because the nerve has been removed, and many of these teeth become a site of permanent chronic infection down at the jawbone that can't be kept clear through oral hygiene. If you have root canals in your mouth and signs of chronic infection, you may want to have advanced imaging done to look for infection and have the relevant teeth pulled.

Osteomyelitis is a chronic infection of bone or bone marrow. It is not a common type of infection unless you have a deep skin wound that reaches all the way down to the bone or a puncture wound like an animal (or human) bite. Cats bites are particularly dangerous because of the dangerous bacteria in their mouths (i.e., *Pasteurella multocida*). Children occasionally develop spontaneous osteomyelitis without any skin wound, possibly because their bones are so metabolically active and have tremendous blood flow.

Chronic undiagnosed viral infections like hepatitis and HIV are occult infections. Undiagnosed patients can complain of the general systemic symptoms mentioned above for years before being diagnosed. Those with a history of injection drug use or other high-risk behaviors are likely to be tested right away, so be honest with your doctor about your history. Even shooting up just one time twenty years ago could have infected you. Having had a blood transfusion is a major risk factor as well, especially before 1985, as is having received any other blood-derived product (e.g., platelets, plasma, clotting factors).

It is ridiculous to think we know about all the possible viruses and other infectious agents out there. We didn't even know about hepatitis C until about twenty-five years ago, and we didn't know about HIV much before that. The blood supply cannot be totally safe when we don't even know everything to look for. I'm not suggesting you turn down a blood transfusion when you need one to save your life, but blood transfusions can be over-utilized in those with gradual causes of blood loss. There are exceptions, of course, such as for those with heart or lung disease, but you should ask your doctors very directly about the risks and benefits of blood infusion. If possible, donate some blood to yourself prior to surgery in case a transfusion is necessary or look for donors in your family or close personal contacts.

If you think you may have some sort of chronic occult infection like Lyme or other spirochetes, other bacteria, or viruses, look for an appropriate integrative practitioner who specializes in these sorts of chronic infections. Consider therapies like blood ozone therapy, hyperbaric oxygen, or blood UV irradiation; take your vitamin D; try some colloidal silver; make your nutrition as perfect as possible; and try to detoxify your body.

Immune deficiency problems

In many cases of chronic or recurring infection, the real problem may be some deficiency of the immune system itself. These problems can be genetic, such as in severe combined immunodeficiency syndrome and X-linked immune deficiency, but those genetic conditions are rare. Some have a mutation in the vitamin D receptor or in the genes that are involved in antibody formation or utilization.

Some people seem to have problems defending against particular types of agents, such as certain viruses. For example, those who are prone to cold sores or shingles may have some such specific problem with herpes strains, and those prone to warts may have trouble with HPV strains, but they could also have problems with immune defense in general. Those who have lost their spleens tend to have trouble with certain types of bacteria (particularly encapsulated bacteria) and may have some general immune problems as well because they have lost a major breeding ground for antibody-producing lymphocytes.

Some seem to have trouble keeping fungi under control, which involves a different arm of the immune system. Some people have various types of mutations, usually affecting T-lymphocyte function, which lead to poor immune defense against Candida and other yeast organisms. These people end up with persistent yeast infection problems involving the mouth, GI tract, skin, nails and vagina. The condition is called chronic mucocutaneous candidiasis, and is probably more common than doctors suspect (Plantinga, 2012). These people will generally be experiencing recurrent yeast problems requiring medical intervention, especially if they eat sugar and starches to any degree at all.

Generalized immune deficiency is more often an acquired problem than a genetic one. Everything I've discussed in this book can play a causative role here. Those with poor nutrition in general tend to have weak immune systems. Those with vitamin D deficiency, thyroid, or adrenal problems may be prone to recurring infections. Those with environmental toxicity issues frequently have immune system problems. Heavy metals like lead and mercury are particularly bad for the immune system. Sleep deprivation impairs immune function. Chronic psychological or emotional stress can suppress the immune system, as can general unhappiness or sadness.

Cancers, especially leukemia and other blood-related cancers, can weaken the immune system. Leukemia in children is often eventually diagnosed because of work-ups to find the cause of recurring infection problems. Many drugs cause suppression of the immune system as well. Numerous drugs designed just for this purpose are used to treat autoimmune disease or to prevent rejection of transplanted organs, but many other types of drugs impair the immune response to some degree and leave you susceptible to prolonged or severe infection problems.

Acetaminophen, aspirin, ibuprofen, naproxen, and all other non-steroidal anti-inflammatory drugs (NSAIDs) may weaken the immune response and can cause an infection to go on significantly longer or evolve into something much worse than it would otherwise. Severe life threatening skin infections with common bacteria, termed necrotizing fasciitis or necrotizing soft-tissue infection (NSTI) have been shown to be strongly linked to giving otherwise healthy individuals NSAIDs during certain viral infections such as chicken pox (Souyri, 2008). These drugs block a critical aspect of the immune response, which results in a double-edged sword.

Blocking the fever response with these drugs is part of the problem because fever helps kill viruses, bacteria and invading organisms. Acetaminophen dramatically weakens your general defenses by depleting glutathione reserves; the other drugs mentioned here deplete it as well, although to a much lesser degree. I personally advise against ever using acetaminophen, unless someone has a very high fever (>104 F) and cannot take the other NSAIDs for some reason. Fever itself can be damaging and trigger seizures or brain injury, so there are cases where it must be treated aggressively. Using cool baths is a better option if possible.

Reye's syndrome is a devastating reaction to aspirin by children when they have certain infectious illnesses. The syndrome could be caused by altering the immune response with the drug, although this is still a mystery. The recommendation is to avoid giving aspirin to children under the age of 19 in the presence of viral illness, and not to use aspirin at all in those under age 16 unless they have one of a few rare conditions where aspirin is the treatment of choice (e.g. Kawasaki syndrome).

My advice is to let your children's fevers go up to 104–105 degrees to help them kill infection. If you want to bring it down, try a tepid bath, using fans and cold drinks, keeping their hair wet, or giving them sponge baths with some eucalyptus oil in the water. It may helpful, if you can tolerate it, to bundle up and sweat when you have an infection; just watch your body temperature if you try this and make sure it doesn't go too high (above 105 degrees for children, 104 degrees for adults). Febrile seizures can occur in children, but that is generally from the temperature's rising quickly, rather than from its staying high; therefore, seizures may be more likely when you drop a child's temperature rapidly with drugs, with a subsequent rapid rebound spike back up in temperature.

Other drugs that can affect the immune system are used for respiratory allergy. Antihistamines can impair the normal immune response to respiratory infection and thicken your mucous, potentially leading to increased and more severe sinus infections and bronchitis. The drug Singulair™, which is frequently used for respiratory allergy, has been shown to increase the rate of respiratory infections, as noted in the package insert. (It increases suicides as well, which is a strange effect.) Nasal steroids suppress local immune response in the nose and increase the presence of fungal organisms, probably contributing to chronic sinusitis related to yeast and fungi.

Certain infections can themselves impair the immune system. The most obvious is HIV. Those who have had HIV infection progressing to AIDS have shown us in gruesome detail just how many maladies a normal immune system protects us from. These "opportunistic infections" include oral and throat infections with fungi (e.g., thrush, or esophageal candidiasis), pneumonia with a typical bacteria, skin infections with fungus or bacteria, or possibly atypical organisms like what we used to call "PCP" (*Pneumocystis carinii* pneumonia), although the name has been changed because the organism appears to be a yeast rather than a bacterium.

Certain types of infections or tumors are considered "AIDS-defining conditions" because they appear only when the HIV virus is present and has substantially impaired the immune system. Kaposi's sarcoma is a cancer caused by a common virus that fits this category. Other common indicators include herpes simplex infection in the esophagus, shingles that flare up and cross multiple skin regions (dermatomes), and PCP.

Chronic or recurring infections themselves can cause a relative immune suppression simply due to wearing down our defenses or distracting our immune system away from other potential duties. There is a limit to what your body can cope with, so a persistently taxed immune system will eventually reach a breaking point. Sometimes the key is to break the cycle of recurrent or persistent infection by treating with relevant drugs (e.g., antibiotics, antivirals, antifungals), but it is also important to support the immune system nutritionally, hormonally, and energetically.

Whatever may be the cause of the immune deficiency, it is important to feed the individual as well as possible. When someone is ill, he or she needs healthy high-quality food even more than when they are well.

Homemade chicken soup is a standard, but I suggest using organic chicken and other ingredients and rice rather than gluten-containing noodles. All the foods I've discussed as having antioxidants and beneficial nutrients are important; examples include dark berries and fruits, green tea, and organic vegetables.

In my opinion, vitamin D is one of the most important supports for the immune system. Those who aren't already supplementing can take a massive dose to help clear an acute or prolonged infection, especially viral infections. Up to 200,000iu for adults (roughly 1,000iu per pound) as a single dose is good for the first day; then take suggested maintenance dosing as discussed earlier. Supporting with other relevant hormones like thyroid or cortisol can be important as well, so I advise having appropriate testing or evaluation for these.

Vitamins C and A and zinc are helpful in clearing infections, and selenium may be needed if there is deficiency. Herbs like astragulus and possibly good-quality *Echinacea* can be very helpful as well. Colloidal silver may be used on a long-term basis. There are many folk remedies and other nutrients, but it is helpful to seek the help of a good herbalist or acupuncturist rather than just flail about with various things you find on the internet.

Adequate rest is vital for the immune system, which is why it is common to advise people to spend time in bed when they are ill. I'm not sure this is always good, and it should be kept in moderation, because we know that lying down too much makes you more prone to developing pneumonia. Clinical research has demonstrated improved recovery in patients with pneumonia when they are encouraged to get up and walk, with gradually increasing activity (Pashikanti, 2012). I suggest you make sure to get up and move around several times per day no matter how bad you feel. Get your blood pumping and your lungs moving now and then so nothing stagnates and your immune system cells and signals are sent coursing around the body.

They way I explain it is that "germs don't have calendars." The infectious agents are cleared based on how rapidly your body's immune system can functionally clear them, which is based more on how many times your blood circulates rather than days on the calendar; therefore, staying active and keeping your circulation up should shorten your illness—it tends to work well for me.

Immune imbalance problems

Imbalance or "distraction" of the immune system may be a common factor in chronic infectious problems. In this case, the immune system is being taxed or steered in an abnormal direction by other factors, allowing persistent infection problems to develop. Allergy is certainly the most common such immune influence. For example, many of my patients with persistent warts, acne, or toenail fungus clear those problems when we get the allergic foods out of their diet. This imbalance, where the immune system is distracted by something and does a poor job handling certain infections, may also theoretically allow cancer cells to grow unchecked. Autoimmune disease is another type of immune imbalance, where one type of immune response is favored over another. We call these two general categories of immune response "TH1" and "TH2".

TH refers to "T-Helper" cells, a class of lymphocyte involved in regulating the immune system. TH1 responses involve immune system cells directly attacking invading pathogens (or your own tissue in the case of autoimmunity), while TH2 type reactions involve antibody production against pathogens or self antigens; the former is termed "cell-mediated" immunity and the latter is what we call "humoral" immunity. Psoriasis and multiple sclerosis are common examples of TH1 reactions, while lupus and autoimmune thyroiditis are TH2 reactions.

Hormones have a definite effect on TH reactions. Cortisol and other mediators seem important in shifting from TH1 to TH2, and DHEA (another adrenal steroid) seems to be important in shifting from TH2 to TH1, but these relationships are more complex than we currently understand. Progesterone appears to generally push the immune system toward TH1 and away from TH2 inflammation. In many instances, progesterone supplementation decreases allergy issues, and pregnancy has a significant effect on the activity of many different autoimmune conditions. There are likely other hormonal and non-hormonal regulators of inflammation that can be used as therapeutic tools.

A third type of T helper cell, called the T-regulatory cell, regulates and tones down both TH1 and TH2 forms of inflammation. The T-regulatory cell is involved in immune tolerance and in decreasing allergy, autoimmunity, and other types of excessive immune activity. I mention it because vitamin D (my favorite) increases your T-regulatory cells and thereby decreases inflammation of every sort.

There is much more immunology that is known and certainly even more that is not yet understood, but the key points I want to stress here are the benefits of vitamin D and the idea that rebalancing the immune response with the right hormonal influences, nutritional support, and other interventions may be helpful. Homeopathic remedies and herbals (e.g., turmeric and boswellia) can play helpful roles here as well by regulating the inflammatory response in broadly beneficial ways. Quercetin decreases hitamine release and is helpful in allergic conditions. As usual, you should find an experienced and competent practitioner to help guide you.

Addressing upstream causes

The point of this chapter is to point out how chronic infections can be the cause of many illnesses, to provide you with some strategies for dealing with them, and to discuss the immune system in general and ways to deal with deficiency or imbalance. Before moving on, I want to reinforce once again the importance of looking upstream and correcting the problems that lead to the development or persistence of infection or immune problems in the first place.

Of course, genetic causes of immune deficiency, irreversible upstream problems like spleen removal, and difficult primary infections like Lyme disease don't involve prior deficiency problems. If possible, though, it is important to address the factors that may have caused or perpetuated the problem.

Nutrition is the foundation of health, and it is vital to eat a healthy diet full of nutrients and helpful phytochemicals that are devoid of poisons and toxins. Environmental toxicity plays a major role in modern health, so it is helpful to avoid exposure as much as possible and to pursue relevant methods of detoxification. Hormones, which are essential to the immune system, can make a major difference in the treatment or management of chronic immune problems and recurrent infections even though they don't seem on the surface to be directly related.

It is well documented that stress and sadness have a very negative impact on the immune system through various mechanisms (Prossin, 2011). These influences can cause a very real sort of immunosuppression, making one much more susceptible to infection or cancer. On the other side of that coin, happiness and social support can be highly therapeutic. Perceived happiness has been shown to significantly decrease inflammatory cytokine chemicals and improve overall immune balance (Matsunaga, 2011).

I would be best if the repeated treatment of infections with antibiotics were replaced by attention to upstream issues that could solve the problem definitively. It would be ideal to avoid the unrelenting use of drugs that block the immune system when the disease could be modified by nutritional or hormonal interventions; symptomatic drugs for allergy when it is possible to retrain the immune system. And other sorts of conventional downstream approaches that cause as much or even more harm than good cannot realistically be as good as treating the cause of the problem in the first place.

Of course, it is appropriate to use antibiotics when they are necessary to save your life or to prevent significant tissue damage, take antihistamines for your allergies, and use chemotherapy for your cancer when it has been proven effective. However, you should also attend to all the other factors that can promote your overall health and prevent future or persistent problems, in addition to treating the downstream disease state.

Vaccines and the immune system

One last thing I want to discuss again is vaccine reaction and vaccination in general, which is an admittedly controversial and potentially dangerous topic to discuss. I have brought it up previously in the book but it bears mentioning again in this chapter. There is major debate in this country about whether vaccines can cause or contribute to chronic illness. It has been established that vaccine reactions do occur and that they can have catastrophic effects, such as the triggering of permanent seizure disorders or irreversible and profound brain damage.

The CDC data lists about a 1 in 14,000 to 1 in 16,000 chance of severe neurological injury in children receiving the pertussis or measles vaccines; but for some reason they don't acknowledge the possibility of milder, chronic neurological conditions being caused by these vaccines. The current questions concern whether they can cause problems with the immune system or trigger conditions like the autistic spectrum disorders. The current evidence does not adequately demonstrate these associations, so the idea is summarily dismissed by the government and vaccine manufacturers. This is the area of debate that gets people's ire up for sure.

On the positive side, some vaccines have made major contributions to our public health. Smallpox was eradicated from the planet by the vaccine, childhood meningitis caused by *H. influenza* was dramatically reduced by the Hib vaccine, and polio is no longer seen in this country today, although it still exists elsewhere. Chicken pox has decreased dramatically in incidence since the use of that vaccine as well. Some people claim that vaccines don't work and that these diseases were all going away anyway, but that claim is clearly false and ridiculous in my opinion.

One annoying issue to me is the tendency for people to talk about "vaccines this" or "vaccines that," when each vaccine is really its own separate issue. Each vaccine, and the disease it is meant to prevent, are unique, and warrant their own discussion. You cannot make global comments about vaccines in either the positive or the negative context.

I am not a big fan of many vaccines, but the concept is sound and some vaccines have made major impacts on our life expectancy and public health. However, some vaccines do not accomplish much or aren't worth the effort and expense. The measles vaccine may be one such because the incidence of measles infection was dropping dramatically on its own in this country before the vaccine was developed, and that vaccine (MMR) causes a lot of immune inflammation because it is a combination live-virus vaccine. There is also evidence that in some children the live vaccine virus is not killed by the body, and continues to replicate in the brain and other tissues (Jepson, 2007).

The pertussis vaccine wears off within ten years, and the bacterium is still spread widely by adults, so it is now suggested that adults get pertussis boosters with their tetanus every ten years. This is a much better strategy in my opinion, because it will more effectively reduce exposure for those who are susceptible and cannot get the vaccine themselves (infants under 8 weeks of age, and immuno-compromised individuals), and older teens and adults have more fully developed brains without the risk of neurological injury seen in children as a result of the vaccine.

One problem is that new strains of pertussis have been identified that are not covered by the existing vaccine. What's more, the pertussis vaccine has been one of the worst in terms of causing catastrophic brain injury, though this reaction is rare. However, despite these problems, the pertussis vaccine is one of the few I suggest parents consider giving their kids in the first year of life because outbreaks of whooping cough (the common name for pertussis) continue to kill small numbers of children and infants every year in this country. Infants under two months of age are at greatest risk, but are too young for the vaccine.

When my last child was born I made sure everyone in the house, including my wife and I, received necessary booster doses for pertussis. I still have not immunized my youngest two children, born since I started researching this issue so heavily, for pertussis or measles, and will likely not do so until they are around twelve years old.

The first pneumococcal vaccine (Prevnar) hadn't decreased the already rare cases of meningitis in kids by much at all. I declined this vaccine for my fourth child in 2006, although I accepted all the others at that time, and I caught a huge amount of grief from the nurses at the public health office. In 2010 a new formulation of this vaccine came out, the 13-valent version instead of the prior 7-valent vaccine, because the data continued to show a lack of benefit for the version I turned down. I encourage parents to do their homework on each vaccine and make the best choice they can for their own kids. Don't use just one source for your information, as you can't believe everything you read. And, don't let health professionals, who may well know *less* about the vaccines than you do, pressure you into doing something you don't think is right for *your* child.

Vaccines can certainly be an upstream cause of illness. We know that children can suffer fevers, irritability, and pain after their vaccines, and some cases of seizures occur after immunization that sometimes evolve into persistent epilepsy or catastrophic brain damage. Several of these individuals are in my own practice, and it is tragic indeed. There is a federal vaccine injury fund to pay victims of vaccine-related harm, so the fact that vaccines can be dangerous should really not be disputed by anyone, as unpopular as the idea may be. Parents really need to be informed of the real statistical risks for both the vaccines and the diseases they are meant to prevent, and be allowed to make appropriate *choices* for their child's health.

What is much less commonly known is that live-virus vaccines can cause direct infection with an atypical strain of virus in those who have weak immune systems at the time of administration. This effect occurs in those who develop atypical chicken pox or shingles even after having the varicella vaccine and those on the autism spectrum who clearly regressed right after having their MMR vaccine and have living atypical measles virus in their bloodstream, brain and spinal fluid, and gastrointestinal tract. A good source of information on this issue is *Changing the Course of Autism* (Jepson, 2007). It is not currently possible to test kids for this phenomenon, outside the research arena, and it is nearly impossible to get a medical provider to believe it happened to your child.

I am not trying to scare everyone away from vaccination in general, but I believe that people should educate themselves about vaccines to the degree possible and that the medical community should let them make informed decisions about the benefits versus the real risks. We should then respect the decisions made and try to tailor vaccination to the desires of individual parents. I have compiled a manual of the relevant information on each childhood vaccine and the disease it prevents in my office for parents to read. I encourage parents to vaccinate their children fully if that's what they decide to do, with some cautions and suggestions, and I gladly sign vaccine waivers for those who conscientiously decide to forego vaccinations.

The other side of this discussion includes the idea of "herd immunity" and the "free rider" phenomenon. This is where those who cannot vaccinate their children for some reason (certain genetic immune dysfunction syndromes for example) or their children are immune suppressed and at greater risk of severe infection (due to cystic fibrosis, immunosuppressive drugs or other causes) rely heavily upon the entire population being immunized and the overall incidence of disease being low. This is an unfortunate circumstance for sure, but in my opinion does not mean that thousands of children should receive unnecessary or unwanted vaccinations to protect that one child. These children are usually susceptible to most every type of infection, and general infection control measures like avoiding public places and hygiene are of paramount importance; after all, the vast majority of the infectious threats to these kids have no vaccine to prevent them.

Those who *can* vaccinate their own children have no argument here at all in my opinion, because they can just go ahead and immunize their kids if they want the potential protective benefit; it shouldn't matter if they are exposed through unvaccinated children in that case.

My general advice with vaccines is the following:

- Accept only preservative-free vaccines (no mercury, aluminum or chemicals) whenever possible. Vaccines such as the polio vaccine do not come in a preservative-free form unfortunately.
- Give vaccines only to completely healthy, well-nourished children who are already on a good dose of vitamin D. This reduces the risk of adverse immune response and inflammation, and improves their odds of mounting good immune response to the vaccine.
- Give infants probiotics. Research has shown improved immune function and even potentially improved

response to vaccines if the infants are given good probiotics around the time of vaccination (Youngster, 2011).

- Take only those vaccines that have been shown to be important in our population, or are relevant for expected travel.

- -Avoid vaccines that are unnecessary in our population or that have been shown to be unhelpful (e.g., Gardasil/HPV, Rotavirus, HepA) first, if you are trying to reduce the overall number of vaccines. The Gardasil vaccine is of little benefit in the U.S. because our pap smear screening programs have already greatly reduced deaths from cervical cancer; and, as of September 15, 2011, the Vaccine Adverse Events Reporting System in the U.S. included nearly 21,000 total reports including 71 reported *deaths*. I would suggest seriously weighing the potential risks and benefits of each vaccine.

- Take vaccines only one or two at a time to avoid excessive stress on the immune system and to improve the immune response to the administered vaccine. This is a highly theoretical concern, as our immune systems are geared to react against thousands of things at once; but one study in "healthy" two-month-old infants showed a small reduction in immune response (to only the rubella virus) when they were given vaccination to nine viruses and bacteria at once (West, 2001).

- Give vaccines at ages that make sense rather than cramming them into the first couple years of life when the immune system is still developing. For example, it would make sense to delay the hepatitis B vaccine until the late teen years or adulthood when there may be risk of exposure, delay polio until age two when there begins risk of neurological damage from the infection, delay Varicella until age twelve or so when the infection becomes potentially deadly, delay mumps and rubella until shortly before puberty when the relevant effects on fetal health and male fertility become an issue. The only vaccines I advocate giving in the first year are Hib, DTaP and maybe pneumococcal, because the respective diseases are problems for infants.

- If you prefer, take just one or two installments of the various vaccines, rather than the three or four in the series recommended for the population. One or two doses will cover the vast majority of people just fine. Three or four are suggested because of the 5 percent or so who don't respond well to one or two.)

Vaccines are an important topic. If you are a parent, I suggest you do extensive research on each vaccine before you decide what you want to do with your children. Don't just take *my* word on any of this, and certainly don't let the conventional medical providers bully you into hammering your child's immature immune system with several toxin-laden vaccines at a time. This can be done quite safely if circumstances are taken into proper consideration. There is a great deal to be gained from vaccinations, but my opinion is that the current conventional approach is potentially unsafe in its scope and methodology.

If you don't want to vaccinate your child at all, that should be your right. It is still legal to have a religious exemption or medical vaccine waiver in all fifty states, though some states no longer honor a "philosophical" exemption. (Though I'm not at all sure how that differs from a religious exemption.) If you want a medical waiver to keep your child from having vaccines, look for a pediatrician or family practitioner who will respect your decision and sign one for you after appropriate discussion.

In my view, it is not correct to say that vaccines "cause" autism because the condition involves so many complex underlying mechanisms; it is just not that simple. The vast majority of children can receive all the suggested vaccines without developing autism, which is why the establishment points to mass research as an argument against blaming vaccines for the condition. Unfortunately, many children today are *susceptible* to developing autism because of genetic factors, environmental toxins, chronic infections, nutrient deficiency, and immune system abnormalities, and a vaccination episode can be the final straw that triggers a regression into autism for some of them.

CHAPTER 7 – INTESTINAL DYSBIOSIS

Introduction

The concept of _dysbiosis_ may be new to many of you, but it is likely to have affected almost everyone reading this book. The term refers to a state in which the wrong population of microorganisms is present in the GI tract. This state is different from the concept of infection, where there is typically a single dominant organism wreaking havoc on your tissues. It is also different from immune inflammation or "die-off" reaction, with resulting symptoms from enzymes and toxins produced by the infectious agent or collateral damage from your own immune response.

In order to make dysbiosis clear, I should first explain the normal or optimal state of affairs in the human intestinal tract. Then I will discuss what can happen when that environment is not optimal. I will discuss the nature of our gut flora in general, what those commensal or symbiotic organisms do for us, the negative consequences of not having the right organisms there, and the consequences of having too many of the wrong organisms.

Probiotic species

The term "probiotic" here refers to favorable (pro) life forms (biotics). In the context of dysbiosis, it refers to an organism that is supposed to live in your body and that promotes normal or optimal health. All the probiotic organisms taken collectively represent our "normal flora," "microbiota," or "microbiome," all fairly synonymous terms here. Probiotics constitute an important area of nutritional and medical products, and research on this topic is currently exploding in every direction.

Probiotic organisms include not just bacterial species but also certain types of yeast or fungi, protozoa, and possibly even some multi-cellular critters. There is certainly far more we *don't* know in this area than what we do know. I focus on bacteria and yeast here because they are the groups about which we know the most.

The bacterial species or strains that inhabit the human gut under optimal circumstances likely number in the hundreds, or maybe even the thousands. Certain genera like *Lactobacillus* and *Bifidus* are well known to the public because some brands of yogurt advertise them in their products and tout their health benefits. *Streptococcus* species are also important all through the GI tract, from the mouth to the anus, though the name recalls a particular species of streptococcal bacteria that causes strep throat. There is another streptococcal species that is the most common cause of pneumonia, but there are also many species in this genus that are good for us.

Certain strains of *E. coli* and *Enterococcus* are also important in the GI tract, even though they are common causes of urinary tract infections. It is obviously important to keep your bowel organisms out of your bladder, but that doesn't mean that they are inherently bad. If you get germs in an area where they don't belong (e.g., the urinary tract, the blood stream, the lungs, or the brain fluid), then you will have a problem. For our purposes here, we'll assume these "good" bacteria and other germs are good only as long as they stay where they belong. We also know about toxic strains of *E. coli* that cause occasional outbreaks of fatal diarrhea combined with red blood cell destruction and renal failure (enterohemorrhagic *E. coli*), or others that cause travelers' diarrhea (enterotoxigenic *E. coli*); these exceptions are not normal flora.

Many other bacterial species have been shown to have positive health effects in our GI tract. This field of study is still evolving, and subspecies or specific strains of bacteria are being proven beneficial in very specific ways in terms of health promotion and altering discrete disease states. Inflammatory bowel disease is an obvious target for probiotic therapies (Veerappan, 2012). Some specific bacterial strains are even being patented as medical therapies and used for issues such obesity and resulting metabolic diseases such as type 2 diabetes (Cani, 2009).

The particular species and strain are very important; for example, study of various species of *Lactobacillus* has shown that administering *L. acidophilus* results in significant weight gain in humans, while the administration of *L. gasseri* is associated with weight loss in obese humans and in animals (Million, 2012). Giving probiotics to older children and adults is not nearly as useful as starting with the right organisms in the neonatal period, because immune system signaling becomes important immediately after birth (Ly, 2011). Additionally, vitamin D appears to be very important in this early gut-microbe communication and immune system "tuning" (Ly, 2011); so make sure your newborns get their vitamin D!

Yeast and fungi are the other major category of probiotic organisms. While there are many different types and species of them as well, in contrast to bacteria, not many fungi have yet been shown to be useful therapeutically. The best-known yeast genus is probably *Candida*, and the best-known species is *C. albicans*. Everyone has *Candida* in them, but it is not a probiotic or beneficial yeast. *Candida* yeast species are always pathogenic (or bad), but they are ubiquitous and impossible to avoid. Everyone with a functioning immune system has a positive skin injection test reaction to Candida antigen, and this used to be used as a "positive control" when testing people for exposure to TB.

These fungi, along with many other species that live in your gut and all over your skin are just waiting for you to die so they can consume your body, as nature intended. Fungi are the major force behind decomposition of organic materials. It's all part of the "circle of life," so in a real sense we aren't at the top of the food chain after all, and neither is anything else (because it's a circle, right?). It's not so much a food chain as a food wheel, and we're just one of the spokes.

We have used yeast species in cooking and beverage fermentation for thousands of years. Baker's yeast and brewer's yeast are both subspecies of the yeast *Saccharomyces cerevisiae*, and we have all consumed lots of those fungi. Though they have practical benefits for us in terms of food production, they don't have biological benefits to my knowledge. Allergies to these yeast species are common; and severe immune reaction against this yeast can play a role in the development of inflammatory disease it seems, most often the version we call ulcerative colitis (Takaishi, 2012). The IgG food antibody panel I run at my office includes testing for these two types of yeast, and I would say the majority of people I've tested have elevated reactions to them.

A related probiotic species of yeast in the same genus, called *S. boulardii*, is a cousin of sorts to baker's and brewer's yeast that has proven to be medically useful. This strain of yeast has considerable research evidence that it helps prevent or treat colitis colon inflammation or infection of autoimmune origin, such as Crohn's disease or ulcerative colitis (Cain,

2011), or that is caused by overgrowth of *Clostridia* bacteria specifically used to prevent diarrhea caused by *C. difficile*. The evidence that it helps with C. difficile diarrhea is mixed (Na, 2011), and some of it slightly negative in fact (Pozzoni, 2012). *S. boulardii* is available at pharmacies under the name Florastor™.

Other types of organisms, aside from bacteria and fungi, may promote health. Some protozoan species are frequently seen in stool samples of healthy people, so they are typically considered "normal flora." However, these organisms may or may not do anything beneficial for you, so they may or may not be "probiotic." It is also possible that certain viruses, worms, and parasites trigger some sort of benefit. There is an emerging area of research and therapy that uses certain worm eggs to alter the immune response in some conditions therapeutically. They are enrolling patients for clinical trial right now in the U.S. to study the possible benefits of ingesting eggs of the pork whipworm to treat autoimmune or allergic disease, and this practice has shown some promise in early phase trials (Bager, 2011).

More on the benefits of probiotics

Probiotics have two major categories of benefits: those that these organisms do for you on a daily, ongoing basis to promote normal health, and those that deal with the therapeutic properties of some of these organisms in particular disease states.

The day-to-day benefits gained from your intestinal organisms include production of vitamins and other nutrients, production of neurotransmitters and other signaling molecules, digestion of food components, exclusion of pathogenic organisms through environmental competition, "attunement" of the immune system, and strengthening of the intestinal lining. I will go into a bit more detail on each of these issues so you can more fully appreciate the trillions of germs you're toting around. And I do mean "trillions"; you have about one trillion human cells comprising your body's tissues, but about 9 trillion "non-human" cells inside you from mouth to anus and on your skin.

Two vitamins we derive in large proportion from production by our intestinal flora are biotin and vitamin K. You may recall that biotin is in the category of B vitamins and is involved in cellular energy production, fetus maturation (a deficiency of biotin has been linked to cleft lip or palate), and maintenance of head hair, among other functions. If you have experienced some ongoing hair loss sometime after having had antibiotics, you may need to supplement with biotin until you can replace your intestinal flora with probiotics.

Vitamin K is necessary for functions like normal blood clotting and bone matrix formation, and who knows what else. The average American derives the majority of his or her vitamin K from intestinal bacteria for sure because we don't eat many fruits, vegetables, or other foods high in vitamin K (e.g., seaweed, grass-fed dairy products and fermented soy products). People can experience easy bruising or bleeding after having antibiotics if they depleted their intestinal organisms, which can be a particular problem for patients who are taking the blood thinner Coumadin™, which works by blocking the effects of vitamin K. I always advise those getting broad-spectrum antibiotics to hold their Coumadin while taking the antibiotics and to monitor their blood tests closely.

Other nutrients provided by intestinal bacteria include short chain fatty acids (SCFAs), which are important sources of energy and nutrition for the cells that line your intestine, especially in the colon. These nutrients are made primarily through fermentation of certain types of fiber in food; we don't have the enzymes needed to do this ourselves, so we rely heavily on our intestinal bacteria to do it for us. Having the right bacteria is therefore very important for normal intestinal health and the integrity of its lining.

Our intestinal florae also help perform some processes of digestion. Some bacteria help digest sugars and fibers we don't handle well on our own, and without enough of these bacteria, we may develop diarrhea because of relative malabsorption. Many people experience this effect after taking antibiotics. The digestive function of bacteria doesn't always work in our favor; a good example occurs in those with lactose intolerance since, if you can't digest the lactose yourself, the bacteria will do it for you, and the fermentation processes they use create gas and intestinal cramping from the resulting distention.

The digestion of nutrients by bacteria is much more important for certain other animal species than it is for us. Cows given corn instead of grass develop significant imbalance in their intestinal flora and severe problems with their stomachs and digestive tracts, which leads to frequent need for antibiotics (Pollan, 2006). Rabbits keep a population of bacteria and other organisms in their appendix (which is far more developed than the human appendix) and produce a stool pellet from that organ they pass every morning and then eat again, because those organisms further digested the fibers in their foodstuffs and liberated many more calories for the rabbit to assimilate.

Of course, termites are probably the best example of reliance on gut bacteria, as they rely entirely upon their bacteria to digest wood pulp for them. Termites actually feed each other these bacteria in the form of a droplet from the rear end of an adult termite consumed by the newborn termite. (Aren't you glad we don't have to do that?) The assistance we get from our gut organisms in terms of digestion is not nearly this dramatic, nor this disgusting, but is still very important to our health nonetheless.

The gastrointestinal tract has its own nervous system, which functions independently from the brain, so your food will be churned up and moved along without your having to think about it. This enteric nervous system, or ENS, uses the neurotransmitter *serotonin* as the primary signal to perform peristalsis, the progressive mouth-to-anus movement of the GI tract. This is the same neurotransmitter in the brain that, when it is deficient, seems to be involved in depression and anxiety states. In fact, more than 90 percent of your body's serotonin is in the GI tract, while less than 5 percent resides in the brain.

Other strains of bacteria in the gut produce, or help to produce, serotonin to promote normal smooth muscle motility in the wall of the stomach and intestine. People deficient in these particular bugs may experience problems with constipation and have problems with anxiety or depression. Replacement of flora with appropriate probiotics can improve all these problems to some degree. This kind of deficiency may be involved in many cases of "irritable bowel syndrome," which is frequently accompanied by symptoms of mood disorders, and seems to be greatly improved by certain types of probiotics (Bixquert,-Jimenez, 2009)

Some of the normal residents of our gut produce signaling molecules that promote integrity of the intestinal lining, make growth signals for the cells lining the intestines, and promote the production of the proteins that link the intestinal cells together. This process directly influences the barrier function of the intestine, so intestinal flora are important in preventing the intestinal leakage that could promote allergy, toxicity, and infection (Koninkx, 2008).

Our complex and vital symbiotic relationship with our gut flora has developed over millennia. Some organisms inside us promote our health in various ways, and many organisms could be damaging if allowed to overpopulate. We are supposed to be colonized at birth with germs from our mother's birth canal that should colonize our guts at the same time our immune systems are trying to learn about the world. We also obtain common organisms from our parents' skin, from the soil, and from the environment starting immediately after birth.

It is very important for our immune system development that we have the right organisms present right away. They help our immune system learn to tolerate the "normal" germs in our environment and to recognize enemy organisms. The right organisms are also likely to be important to our immune systems' ability to recognize the "self." We know that those born by cesarean section have significantly higher rates of asthma, other allergy problems, infections, and autoimmune disease. Evidence shows that babies born vaginally at home have lower rates of asthma and allergic disease than babies born vaginally in the hospital as well (Van Nimwegen, 2011). There is likely increased risk of these problems if the mother receives antibiotics during labor, because one major difference appears to be whether the infant is colonized with *C. difficile* shortly after birth (Van Nimwegen, 2011).

There is very good evidence that giving newborn babies probiotics reduces their chances of developing allergic diseases, and I encourage parents to do that. In fact, given that our food supply is so "clean" and that our livestock are given antibiotics given that end up in our food, I suggest everyone take a good probiotic regularly or find some other way to ensure proper gut flora because we probably don't have enough healthy bacteria intake.

Many therapeutic applications of probiotics are now available for various medical and health complaints or established disease states. There is new knowledge coming out of this field all the time, and this area of medical practice will be actively evolving for a while yet, so I don't want to offer too many specifics because the current "truths" will probably change. My general advice is to do lots of research on probiotics if you want to figure out what's best for you in this regard, just search Pubmed for your condition "and probiotics," and to find a knowledgeable practitioner if needed (i.e., not a doctor who tells you to "just eat some yogurt").

Where probiotics come from

All of these beneficial germs can be found in the environment; you should be able to get many of the organisms you need in a handful of good quality soil. However, in modern society people tend to eat exclusively from grocery stores and restaurants where all the food is as clean as possible, and we live our lives far removed from the dirt in every sense. In fact, most people live in cities where they may not ever encounter biologically normal soil. This state of affairs contributes to the "hygiene hypothesis" as a proposed cause of some of our immune and infectious problems in the modern world.

The hygiene hypothesis suggests that some of our chronic disease problems arise from the fact that our lifestyles are now too clean, and we do not get all the germs we need or exposure to enough microorganisms. You can still obtain the proper organisms if you seek them out. You can eat locally grown organic produce, which often still has a little dirt on it that is not contaminated with pesticides. Organic fertilizers contain composted animal feces and plant materials mixed with soil; those are the germs we evolved with as long as the animals lived on a normal diet (like grass).

You can also eat fermented foods made with good probiotic organisms, such as yogurt and kefir (if you aren't allergic to dairy), coconut milk kefir, kimchi, sauerkraut, miso, and kombucha. Cultures for traditional fermented foods are obtained from natural sources, and some have very specific strains of bacteria native to the regions where those foods originated. Wine was traditionally made using bacteria and yeast from the feet of the grape stompers, and other traditional foods were made with the help of germs from the body or soil without people's even knowing that bacteria existed.

Our first intake of probiotics is supposed to occur at the moment of birth, through vaginal delivery. This is likely an extremely important occurrence in regards to our long-term health, since evidence has suggested that early exposure to the right organisms is vital. There is evidence of this as it relates to allergic disease in research finding that being born by cesarean delivery increases the risk of asthma in the child by 15-20% (Magnus, 2011).

Of course, you can instead take manufactured probiotic supplements, but even the best commercial probiotics contain maybe twenty different strains of bacteria, a drop in the bucket when it comes to the number of different species we are supposed to have. We cannot hope to make a probiotic that recreates nature, and we will probably never catalog all the beneficial bacteria in the human gut. However, in today's society, probiotic supplements are often the best we can do.

Where the "bad" germs come from

Pathogenic (bad) bacteria can be found in nature right alongside the good bacteria. For example, the bacteria that cause tetanus, gangrene and botulism, which are all *Clostridia* species (those guys are usually nasty), are common organisms in the soil in most parts of the world. Other opportunistic bacteria that cause human illness can propagate in any water supply; some of these cause infections acquired in hospitals or chronic problems for people at home. Modern ranching techniques in this country have increased the exposure to potentially harmful bacteria because the animals are crowded together, living in filth and excrement, and fed loads of antibiotics. It has also been shown that feeding cows corn rather than grass or hay dramatically increases the levels of bad bacteria in their guts (Pollan, 2006).

Every time you inhale or eat something that has been exposed to the air, you are colonized with more yeast organisms because they release spores into the air. If you don't believe this, just leave your freshly baked bread out for a few days and see if it starts to grow mold on it. The yeast you put in the dough was killed by the heat of cooking, as were any other organisms in it prior to cooking. That new mold found your bread through the air. You can also demonstrate this by making sourdough starter with regional wild yeast; all you have to do is leave a little flour and water out on the counter for an hour or so, and you will have your own wild yeast population.

This fact is important when we talk about ongoing fungal infections of the respiratory tract or gut, fungal infections in immunosuppressed patients, and regional fungal infections like valley fever and histoplasmosis; it's also important in terms of beneficial yeast and fungi. We have to intentionally ingest the right things to get the bacteria we need, but all we have to do to get some of our fungi is breathe. Those who are immunologically sensitive to yeast organisms have no chance of completely eradicating or avoiding yeast and fungi because of their presence in the air, just like they can't completely avoid tree pollen in the spring. The solution for these people lies in immune desensitization.

Probiotic products

Although probiotic products are inadequate compared to natural sources of bacteria, they are therapeutically useful for many people. Those who have taken antibiotics would do well to take a good probiotic for at least a month after their infection has been treated. Those with chronic gastrointestinal issues of any sort would do well to try one also, although patients with inflammatory bowel disease may well flare up against even purely beneficial flora because their guts are so deranged in terms of immune response. I have also seen patients with rosacea and irritable bowel problems flare up when taking beneficial probiotics at times. These problems generally do improve on probiotics however, so they are certainly worth a try. It is very helpful to me if someone flares up in response to a probiotic product, because I can then use that product itself to help desensitize them, just as with immunotherapy for allergy.

Anyone with an allergic disease, such as asthma or eczema, those on the autistic spectrum, and those with rheumatologic disease should take a probiotic in my opinion. There is ample data to show that probiotics help to prevent allergies and asthma in children and actually therapeutically improve some children with eczema (Ozdemir, 2010). Giving the probiotic organism Lactobacillus GG to pregnant mothers in one study was shown to decrease the risk of eczema (which is almost always related to food allergies) in their children by half, but did not appear to reduce the risk of asthma or inhalant allergies (Kalliomaki, 2001). Several more recent studies have not been able to replicate this result, so this topic remains controversial; but probiotics are harmless, so it is worth a try in my opinion.

As I mentioned above, the microbiota of the gut interact with our gastrointestinal nervous system as well as the central nervous system, and they influence neurotransmitter regulation. There is mounting evidence that the organisms of the intestinal tract play an important role in early "wiring" of our stress response systems. Animals raised in a germ-free environment have been shown to have exaggerated stress reactions involving the hypothalamic-pituitary-adrenal axis; and treating these animals with probiotics blunts this exaggerated response back toward "normal" (Dinan, 2012). This means that certain probiotics may well be helpful for people with anxiety, panic, depression, or even issues in addition to all the other things they seem to improve. I feel that, when supplementing with probiotics for some therapeutic indication, one should see a benefit in a month or less; if you don't, then it may not be worth continuing that particular product.

Regarding probiotic products, I suggest you use a powdered product in bulk or capsule form that is kept in the refrigerator. The liquid products are usually all dead (the live bacteria eat up their food supply and then die off), as are the hard tablets, and the hard tablets may not even dissolve properly. I suggest you find a probiotic with many species of bacteria; the more the merrier. Make sure it has a high colony count ("colony forming units," or "CFU" number) with at least 25 billion organisms per capsule or dose; I usually suggest getting 100 billion CFUs or more per day for therapeutic purposes, and studies of inflammatory bowel patients have often used more than 200 billion per day.

Many probiotic products are on the market, and they vary in terms of quality. There is very little regulatory control to speak of, so some products have been found to have mostly dead organisms or even some pathogenic strains included in them by accident. Consumer quality assurance websites like www.consumerlabs.com are useful for determining which products are worth buying. When in doubt, you can purchase VSL#3 from most pharmacies; it has about 225 billion organisms per capsule in more than a dozen varieties and is a prescription-quality product. The double-strength form, VSL3-DS, is even covered by some insurance companies as a prescription drug.

Dysbiosis

In addition to the bacteria, yeast, and other organisms that are health-promoting, there are numerous germs living in your gut that don't do "good" things for you but also don't cause problems under normal or ideal conditions. These are termed "commensal" flora. It is conceivable that under certain circumstances, such as an immunosuppressed state, some of these organisms could take the opportunity to invade your tissues and cause infection or disease; the organisms that do this are termed "opportunistic" in terms of disease. Under normal healthy conditions there are far more beneficial bacteria and other beneficial organisms living in your gut than there are potentially harmful organisms, so the potential bad guys are kept quiescent and everything goes along fine. If something happens to disturb this balance, however, you may develop various problems manifesting within the GI tract or perhaps with cascading symptoms throughout the body.

We call this condition "dysbiosis" because it is not usually associated with an infection-level overgrowth of any dominant organism but simply with an imbalance. Unfortunately, conventional medical teaching has as yet made no place for this concept, so those with GI dysbiosis problems are usually labeled with irritable bowel syndrome, told there is actually nothing wrong, or placed on various symptomatic drugs or antidepressant medications. Inadequate treatment of dysbiosis is a very common problem in our culture, and I think a majority of Americans have GI dysbiosis on some level because of several factors, but antibiotics use is the most common reason. We don't always know the effects antibiotics will have on the gut flora since there are so many different species.

Antibiotics may be necessary to save lives in many instances, but they are clearly overprescribed in our culture and others around the world. Overprescription of antibiotics and other drugs is an even bigger problem in China, where doctors have direct income and financial incentives from prescribing medications (Li, 2012). At least the U.S. does not allow doctors to make money directly prescribing drugs! Antibiotics are also present in our food, since they are fed in mass quantities to our livestock and therefore end up in the meat and milk of the animals. The practice of broadly giving our livestock antibiotics to promote faster growth has led to a serious problem with drug-resistant pathogenic bacteria (Price, 2005). The U.S. should consider stopping this practice as an act of government, as was done in the European Union in 2006 (Bywater, 2005).

The other big factor in promoting GI dysbiosis is the typical diet in our culture. The consumption of processed foods with various foreign chemicals and high amounts of the wrong sort of carbohydrates promotes the growth of the wrong sorts of bacteria and yeasts we don't need. Eating more whole foods with the right type of natural fiber promotes the growth of bacteria in our gut that in turn reduces our risk of developing obesity, metabolic syndrome and diabetes (Parnell, 2012); whereas eating processed foods high in starches and sugar clearly worsens those conditions. There is also evidence suggesting that our diet influences risk for cancer in part because of how it alters the population of bacteria in our intestinal tract (Rooks, 2011).

Symptoms of dysbiosis can include acid reflux, excessive belching and gas, chronic nausea, stomach cramps or pains, diarrhea or constipation, and other symptoms that range from mild and occasional to chronic and debilitating. There can also be many diverse symptoms outside the GI tract, such as fatigue, weight gain, mental fog, headaches, mood changes, insomnia, rashes, joint or muscle pains. These types of complaints are common, but primary care practitioners usually treat them symptomatically and rarely consider whether the body's microbiome plays a role.

Diagnosis of dysbiosis generally relies upon the patient's history alone, not laboratory testing. The typical stool tests that are run for diarrhea-related problems through conventional labs are usually unhelpful in these cases unless you're "lucky" enough to have giardia, some other parasite, or possibly *Clostridium difficile* because they test for those agents. Some specialty labs do more comprehensive stool testing, which can be helpful, but the results can also be misleading in my experience. There are just too many different types of organisms there to really be able to figure out what is going on through the stool cultures or DNA tests available today in my opinion.

I hope that the information in the rest of this chapter will enable you to prevent or fix the problem on your own most of the time. If you can't resolve your issues, be sure to track down a practitioner with appropriate experience and skill in this department.

Preventing and correcting dysbiosis

Dybiosis was probably not an issue for early humans at all, and probably not even a minor issue in our country as recently as a hundred years ago. The problem likely began when we started growing grain and eating a lot of flour-based foods like bread. The issue was made much worse I'm sure when we developed foods with processed white sugar. When we stopped eating more fibrous natural foods we stopped feeding the healthy bacteria what they needed and slowed our bowel transit. When we eat higher amounts of simple sugars, we drastically over-promote the growth of yeast and fermenting bacteria, with all the negative health consequences that brings.

The real key to preventing gut dysbiosis is to go back to a natural, whole-food diet with no processed carbohydrates. We should eat things "closer to the soil" with healthy organisms on them and no chemical agents. Of course, avoiding antibiotic exposure would important as well for many reasons.

As a momentary aside, the paid editor from my publishing company left repeated comments through here (obviously personal comments and not professional editorial type comments about grammar and such) about "animal feces" being on organic produce. I will assume perhaps there are some readers out there thinking the same thing, so let's address it head-on. When an organic "fertilizer" such as compost is made, it isn't just pure cow poop dumped on the ground. Organic fertilizer is a very complex mixture of good soil, broken down plant and vegetable matter, and yes, some feces from animals fed on a natural diet. As I've mentioned, herbivores such as cows eating grass or their otherwise natural diet will breed the proper organisms in their gut, just as we do when we eat the proper foods. Therefore, the bacteria in these foods are actually many of the same ones we need—and how exactly do you expect them to get into your intestines if not through your mouth? Modern "civilized" humans such as "Word Queen" (which I assume is an alias, and not the editor's real name) are so far removed from nature they don't realize how badly we need germs and where germs come from; they tend to try to keep things too sterile and fail to realize that all the germs in their own poop initially got in through their mouths. I hope for their sake that they never have babies either, because they are likely to get "animal feces" all over them, like I have many times from my own six little humans.

Don't kill the good guys

Avoid unnecessary use of antibiotics, take shorter courses of antibiotics when you do need them, and avoid eating nonorganic meat products to avoid antibiotics in your food. If your doctor or your child's doctor prescribes antibiotics for a simple urinary infection, you can usually stop after just three days, perhaps five days if you still have symptoms. If your child has an ear infection, antibiotics are not usually needed longer than five days, and you can generally stop them when the child's fever and pain have subsided for more than a full day. Antibiotics for skin infections may usually be stopped when the redness is completely gone for at least a full day. Basically, antibiotic treatment for infection can usually be stopped once it seems like you or your child are "all better now". You can always start them up again if symptoms seem to resume; no harm done in trying to stop them sooner and then restarting.

Eradicating or decreasing the bad guys

While I realize this seems to be contradicting what I just said, sometimes specific antibiotics are needed to correct bacterial imbalance. This is obvious in the case of typical "infections." Many cases of dysbiosis are caused by common antibiotics, which are good for killing the aerobic bacteria common in respiratory or urinary tract infections but poor or ineffective against the anaerobic bacteria that heavily populate the gut. The result can be overgrowth of *Clostridia* or other anaerobes.

Antibiotics like Metronidazole (Flagyl™) and Rifaximin (Xifaxan™) can be helpful in eradicating the leftover "bad" bugs; then you can start over by replenishing your gut flora with good probiotic products and fermented foods. Some natural or herbal products that can also help clear the gut of pathogens include colloidal silver, pau d'arco, turmeric, and wasabi.

The benefits of stomach acid

The acid in your stomach is supposed to help prevent infection or colonization of the gut by pathogenic bacteria and other organisms. There is significant overuse of antacid drugs in our culture, from TUMS™ to

Pepcid™ to Prilosec™ and related drugs in those classes. Chronic use of these medications disables the normal disinfectant function of the stomach by reducing the acid. The real keys to resolving acid reflux are to identify and address food allergy and GI dysbiosis. Taking apple cider vinegar (2 teaspoons) or betaine HCl (one to five capsules depending upon the amount of food) with meals can help replace and support stomach acid, improving digestion, helping to kill pathogens, and often improving acid reflux symptoms themselves. Digestive enzyme supplements can sometimes complement these effects well.

Probiotic replacement

It is frequently necessary to supplement with beneficial flora for at least a month or two when you have GI dysbiosis. Don't forget about using yeast probiotics like *S. boulardii*, especially after taking antibiotics that promote *C. difficile* diarrhea. Some people will feel better from taking a probiotic long-term, and never stop using them. This is generally fine, since there is no toxicity or realistic risk of harm in people with functioning immune systems. Autistic kids are one group that tends to benefit from continued intake of probiotics. My guess is that there is something preventing successful gut colonization by and persistence of certain beneficial bacteria in these situations; it could be that the right "pre-biotic" fibers and nutrients are lacking (as discussed below), or it could be that the individual's immune system is targeting normal flora inappropriately.

Feeding the troops, selectively

It is important to limit or eliminate sugar and processed carbohydrates in order to avoid feeding the wrong organisms too well. Eating foods rich in natural fibers such as fruits, vegetables, and whole grains, can promote the preferential growth of healthy bacteria over unhealthy ones. Certain foods contain particularly good fibers and nutrients to support the preferential growth of beneficial oorganisms; we call these substances *prebiotics*. Some of these nutrients are fructooligosaccharides (FOS), which are added to some probiotic supplements to improve their benefits. Foods with particularly high amounts of these nutrients include Jerusalem artichokes, chicory root, bananas, asparagus, onions, jicama, and tomatoes.

Normal bowel elimination

Continuously moving the bowel contents through and out helps ensure that only those organisms most appropriate to inhabit your intestines will persist. Constipation allows overgrowth of all sorts of bad bacteria and other organisms and increases the absorption of too many toxins from the stagnant GI tract. In my opinion, the best ways to promote proper bowel elimination are to eat abundant high-fiber foods, drink plenty of water, get daily exercise, and take magnesium and vitamin C regularly as needed. People rarely need to do more than that. Some people recommend frequent enemas or "colonics," but that should be necessary only in extreme situations.

Intestinal Candida or "yeast dysbiosis"

The Candida issue, which I believe is the most common form of dysbiosis, is an important topic in alternative medicine. The organism is present in everyone and is impossible to eradicate, as I mentioned earlier in this chapter. It overgrows quickly and dramatically with most any type of antibiotic use, and it's growth is promoted dramatically by sugar and starch consumption. Yeast dysbiosis and yeast-related inflammation are common in my patient population and are frequent underlying conditions that must be addressed in order for most people to achieve optimal health.

Symptoms of yeast overgrowth or "intestinal candidiasis" (which is an actual medical diagnosis, with its own billing code) frequently include constipation, excessive gas, and bloating; common non-GI symptoms include fatigue, weight gain, mental fog, memory problems, depression or anxiety, muscle or joint pains, random numbness or tingling, elevated blood sugars, and unusual rashes. It is important to separate yeast "hypersensitivity" problems from yeast overgrowth or infection. I think that this difference constitutes the biggest reason for the rift in the appreciation of chronic yeast problems between conventional and alternative practitioners.

Infection with yeast or fungi manifests in discrete ways, such as vaginal itching and discharge, localized skin rashes, yellow flaky toenails, and urinary tract infection, all of which are widely accepted types of true infection with yeast. It is also possible to have yeast or fungi invade other body cavities or the bloodstream. If the organism does get into the blood, it is an extremely severe problem that may lead rapidly to death. Many alternative medical practitioners promote the idea that some people have yeast growing in their blood and other tissues, which is how they attempt to explain the distant and diverse symptoms seen in some people with yeast problems. Most practitioners know that this idea is incorrect and seems absurd, because yeast in the blood is not very compatible with life.

I resolve this rift by thinking about it in terms of allergy or immune hypersensitivity. It is entirely possible to mount an excessive inflammatory response against yeast or any other potentially infectious agent, or even for the body to react against the presence of yeast in the gut, the same way it would in the case of food allergy, and with all those diverse consequences. It is this immune reaction that I believe generates all the myriad distant symptoms frequently associated with Candida problems in susceptible individuals. Symptoms may occur in dramatic fashion without any GI, skin, or vaginal symptoms being present, which tends to cause major confusion and misunderstanding for alternative and conventional medical providers alike.

Testing for Candida in the conventional sense is useless, unfortunately, which serves to further the disbelief of conventional providers. Stool testing for Candida reveals that it is in just about everyone, as does skin testing, so both are virtually useless. Candida is a pathogenic organism to which everyone has been exposed, so you should manifest a positive skin test if you have a functioning immune system.

You can get a better sense of yeast overgrowth by doing urine organic acids testing, which looks for common yeast byproducts like arabinose and can indicate whether you have more yeast than the average person, although it does not tie that yeast to your symptoms. In my opinion, treatment itself—a trial of therapy—is the best "test." If I suspect yeast is the problem, I prescribe antifungal drugs for a couple of weeks or longer, depending on the patient's circumstances, and watch for response. If the patient's relevant symptoms all improve, then they were probably related to the presence of yeast; if nothing improves, then they may have some other problem or they may have a very tough yeast infestation involving a biofilm, or perhaps drug-resistant organisms.

When I prescribe antifungals in response to a suspicion about yeast, I strongly suggest the patient strictly limit sugar and starches, and also take a good probiotic. I usually prescribe two antifungal medications, typically Nystatin and Diflucan together, because there is a significant possibility of drug resistance to one or the other alone. It is also a good idea to treat for possible biofilms by giving oral EDTA (ethylenediaminetetraacetic acid) and digestive enzymes an hour before the antifungals. The EDTA pulls out the mineral ions that link together and solidify a mat of fibrous material and mucous that comprises the bulk of the biofilm. The complex of digestive enzymes breaks up the biofilm matrix material, leaving the yeast organisms (or certain bacterial organisms that do the same thing and form colonies within protective biofilms) exposed to the medications we use to kill them.

Those with just bowel yeast *overgrowth* issues usually improve quickly with antifungal medications and stay improved even after stopping them. Those with a *hypersensitivity* problem do well while on the medications but then relapse fairly quickly after stopping their antifungal medications, usually experiencing symptoms again in about three days. When this happens, an immune sensitivity is likely because there hasn't been enough time for the patient to have accumulated a large yeast burden and have problems with overgrowth so quickly. Some of these people can maintain improvement long term by strictly avoiding sugar and all grain products, taking a good probiotic, and perhaps using various herbs that work against Candida and other yeasts.

Common herbals I suggest in such cases include pau d'arco, caprylic acid (present in coconut oil), black walnut, olive leaf, berberine, and Oregon grape root. I suggest switching herbs every week or two to reduce the chances of toxicity from any one agent and to keep resistance from developing in your yeast organisms.

Summary

- The most important points in this chapter follow:
- The germs in your gut are important to your health.
- Most of these germs can be obtained by eating organic produce with traces of healthy dirt or by consuming healthy fermented foods.
- Don't eat sugar.
- Don't eat any grain products or starches at all if possible. This includes bread, cake, cookies, crackers, noodles, rice, corn, tortillas, tortilla or potato chips, mashed potatoes and other related products.
- Having the wrong population of microorganisms in your gut can create many diverse health problems.
- Avoid antibiotics whenever possible, and use the shortest courses necessary to clear relevant infections.
- Don't be afraid to *use* antibiotics when they are truly needed, but take probiotics for a while afterward.
- Taking a daily probiotic is a good preventive health measure for most people.
- Keep your bowels moving easily by eating lots of high-

fiber foods, drinking water, and exercising. Take daily doses of magnesium and vitamin C as needed.

- Eat foods that promote the growth of the right organisms. Recall that fructooligosaccharides can be found in tomatoes, bananas, asparagus, Jerusalem artichokes, onions, and chicory root.
- Identify yeast overgrowth problems early and correct them in order to prevent the development of hypersensitivity.
- Memorize the following poem I composed on the subject, to help remember the importance of your gut microbiota (just for fun):

Probiotics, probiotics,

What would I do without you?
I'd cough and I'd wheeze,
In the spring I might sneeze,
and have all sorts of trouble with poo.
In addition to this, I have a confession:
Without you, I suffer from mild depression.
My joints may all hurt, without the right dirt.
I may suffer from rashes,
Or lose my eyelashes.
I see clearly now in no uncertain terms
that my health depends in part upon germs.
I'll have and I'll hold you,
With my diet embold you,
Else I shall go feed the worms.

CHAPTER 8 – STRUCTURAL AND ANATOMICAL ABNORMALITIES

Introduction

Structural and anatomical abnormalities are a common, and often obvious, cause of chronic health problems. I include a chapter on the subject both for the sake of completeness and also to point out some of the more subtle ways by which structural problems can cause symptoms, so you can seek appropriate care rather than being mired in confusion or just stuck using symptomatic medications.

I spend most of the time discussing structural and anatomical problems related to the skeleton and related structures because those are the most common issues that afflict us here. I also point out structural issues in other organs and tissues that can sometimes cause confusing symptoms.

Symptoms of spinal misalignment

Spinal misalignment is a good place to start because it's probably the most common type of structural issue that causes chronic problems in our society today. Much of this has to do with our poor ergonomics. We are meant to lay around all day or casually roam about, changing positions regularly and putting our bodies through a complete range of motion regularly. We are not suited to sitting in a car or chair for prolonged periods, leaning our heads forward to look at a computer screen for hours at a time or staring straight ahead in class all day. These protracted positions are not good for our spines.

We are also not supposed to be exposed to the tremendous traumatic forces some of us encounter accidentally or repeatedly, including automobile and bicycle accidents, falling down stairs, being tackled on the football field, smashing into the boards in a hockey game, wiping out on the ski slopes, bucking on a horse or bull, slamming onto the pavement when skateboarding, being crushed in the surf, and many of the other various physical traumas to which we willfully expose our bodies.

In the process of either gently or violently abusing our spines, we can incur some serious alignment problems, such as herniated disks, torn or stretched ligaments, sprained or chronically tense muscles, misaligned vertebrae, and altered curvatures of the spine. These issues can lead to chronic pain problems in the area of the spine itself or within the distribution of impinged nerves coming from the spine. They can also lead to more diverse symptoms that conventional physicians often fail to recognize as being related to the spine.

Gradual degeneration of the spine or disks can cause altered curvature, as seen quite obviously in people with bad osteoporosis. Altered curvature and mobility of the thoracic (chest region) spine can even begin to interfere with breathing past a certain point. Osteoporosis and age-related spinal degeneration are preventable—or at least "delayable" to a large degree—with proper diet, regular exercise, mobility exercise, vitamin D, correction of the causes of chronic inflammation, avoidance of smoking and excess alcohol as well as many medications, and appropriate hormone replacement therapy (progesterone, testosterone, DHEA).

Aside from pain and restriction of movement, spinal misalignment may cause symptoms like poor ability to nurse, colic, or general fussiness in newborns; and headaches, swallowing problems, chest pain, heart palpitations, breathing difficulty, problems with digestion, constipation, bladder control issues, sexual dysfunction, and other problems in older children and adults. These internal organ issues are most often thought to arise from altered autonomic nerve functioning, because the sympathetic nerve roots all emerge from the thoracic spine; but there are potentially other mechanisms as well, and these issues are the basis for the development of osteopathic and chiropractic medicine as primary care professions (Bolton, 2012). The philosophy of these fields includes the idea that your nervous system controls many of the body's functions; since those nerves often pass through the spine at some point, many different health problems can be related to spinal or other musculoskeletal system alignment issues.

Low Back Pain

Lumbar or low back pain problems are among the most common reasons for visits to doctors and certainly chiropractors in this country. The explosion of chiropractic clinics is indicative of the scope of the problem. Some studies have suggested that as many as 90 percent of us will experience at least a short period of debilitating back pain in our lives, and one recent statistical review reported more than two million emergency room visits for low back pain across the U.S. from 2004 to 2008 (Waterman, 2012). The majority of these acute pain issues will resolve on their own within six weeks, but if the problem persists beyond that, it may become chronic.

The most common reasons for low back pain are chronic positioning problems and repeated or incidental trauma, but the obesity problem certainly exacerbates or directly causes this problem for many. Therefore, some obvious things to do for prevention include avoiding activities which may cause trauma to your body, staying at a healthy body weight, eating an optimal diet (so you can make bones, ligaments and disks properly), and getting plenty of exercise with some focus on spinal mobility and strengthening (with yoga being the most obvious).

Vitamin D deficiency is also a common underlying factor, and androgenic hormone (testosterone, DHEA) deficiencies are common problems leading to back pain in my practice as well. Research has shown vitamin D deficiency to be strongly related to widespread muscle and joint pains, which of course includes the back and spinal areas, but not so much to isolated back pain (Heidari, 2010). Male testosterone deficiency has been associated with osteoporosis and back pain for a long time (Bain, 2010); in my experience it is also associated with widespread muscle, joint, and skeletal pain in both men and women.

Checking your vitamin D status and keeping your level in the optimal range is very helpful for spinal and musculoskeletal health. Evaluating testosterone and DHEA status and using appropriate HRT is vital for some as well, including both men and women. I personally developed significant chronic low back pain (likely originating initially from a severe auto accident at age seventeen, followed by many years of heavy weightlifting) when I came off my testosterone replacement to have child number six in 2010. It did not improve until I had been back on my hormone replacement therapy (HRT) for about six months.

I see many men with chronic back pain who improve tremendously on HRT, which is an important tool in my view even when testosterone levels aren't in the deficient range. I use this therapeutic tool on people who need to heal other musculoskeletal injuries as well. The anabolic steroid helps strengthen all the stabilizing muscles and ligaments around the spine, improving function and relieving pain. It is critical to do proper exercises to stretch and strengthen the spine as well because those tissues will get stronger only if you give them the signals to do so.

The best advice I can give most folks with chronic low back pain is to use an inversion table for spinal traction. Many people with disks that are shrunken or out of place can restore disk space or normal alignment if they utilize traction to pull the spine apart a bit instead of always having gravity pushing down on their axis. For those with intervetebral disk disease, spinal alignment problems or even facet joint arthritis, this type of spinal traction is one of the most helpful things.

Most people with low back pain see rapid and significant improvement when they use an inversion table just ten to fifteen minutes per day. It not only unloads pressure from the disks and returns space to the spine, it also takes a load off all the little joints we have between the spinous processes coming off the back of the vertebrae. Traction in this manner also allows spasmed muscles to relax and resume their full length. This works only if you can hang and relax on an inversion table or in a similar manner, not if you hang from your arms or are forcibly stretched with a machine. Many chiropractic offices have traction machines like DRS, VAX-D, and IDD, which are useful alternatives if you cannot tolerate hanging upside down.

If traction doesn't offer some relief, the pain is likely to be coming from ligaments, small joint degeneration, and other more permanent tissue damage. In that event, you should focus on nutrition, exercise, and hormone replacement (which includes vitamin D) as needed. Some therapeutic interventions can help heal damaged tissues in the back, block inflammation on a local level, scar down and secure the torn ligaments or muscles, or just fry the nerves that carry the pain signals. These sorts of interventions include steroid injections, prolotherapy, and radiofrequency ablation.

I strongly recommend against using opiate pain medications (e.g., hydrocodone, oxycodone, methadone, morphine, codeine) on any sort of ongoing basis. Using narcotic or opiate painkillers does nothing to improve your problem and gives you a host of other issues to deal with. Anti-inflammatories may theoretically impair the healing process and perpetuate your problem as well, so I don't suggest using them even for acute injuries if you can help it; though the NSAIDs are a much better choice for chronic use than are opiates. Natural options for treating back pain include heating pads, arnica, Zeel™ or Traumeel™ (homeopathics), turmeric, Zyflamend™, and other herbal anti-inflammatories. Meditation and positive visualization are helpful also. The safest and therefore best prescription option in my opinion is lidocaine patches, which send local anesthetic directly into the area of pain without the risk of systemic side effects seen using oral medications.

Chiropractors and osteopaths who perform manipulation can get the majority of people out of pain without undue risk or expense. An inversion table replaces a chiropractor in many cases, but some people cannot use one or cannot get access to one for various reasons. My advice is to try chiropractic or osteopathic manipulation for a couple of weeks to see if helps you. If you have had six treatments without obvious sustained improvement, try something else instead or in addition. If a chiropractor can't get you straightened out in short order, you may have other factors perpetuating the problem that must be addressed in some other way.

For chronic problems related to soft tissue damage, I suggest you try acupuncture, magnetic therapy, microcurrent therapy, prolotherapy (injections of a strong sugar solution to cause focal areas of tissue scarring), or neural therapy (superficial injection of anesthetics). Massage, stretching, and exercise are helpful also. If the small joints are arthritic, you can try acupuncture, magnetic or electrical therapies, or possibly steroid injection into the joints, nerve roots, or the epidural space. Injections are very expensive, have a high failure rate, and don't last very long in many cases; however, they can work well for some folks and are worth a try if more conservative treatments have failed.

For severe back pain that is not responsive to these methods or that involves nerve root impingement to the point of risking serious nerve damage, it is reasonable to consider surgery. However, spinal surgery has a high failure rate so you may want to try everything else before moving to surgery unless you have an emergency or severe risk to a nerve. Research your surgeons carefully; look into their success, failure, and infection rates, and make sure you completely understand what sort of surgery options you have (e.g., artificial disk replacement versus spinal fusion).

<u>Non-spinal skeletal problems</u>

The spine is highly susceptible to alignment problems because it has so many joints, easily losing stability as a result. It is also possible to have alignment problems elsewhere in the skeleton. Most of these problems, such as joint dislocations, are obvious and do not need to be discussed here. Others are subtler and may be missed.

Starting at the top, the skull and its associated bones are an important area of focus. Conventional allopathic practitioners are taught to believe that the bones of the skull are fused together and have no movement relative to one another, but other practitioners, such as those who perform cranial-sacral therapy (CST), believe that the separate bones of the skull do have movement and that problems with that articulation can cause impaired flow of cerebrospinal fluid and brain dysfunction.

Therapists who perform CST can often help with headaches, insomnia, mood or cognitive disorders, ringing in the ears, and other problems involving the head, brain, and the rest of the spine or axial skeleton. Behavioral problems in children, mood disorders like anxiety and depression, and issues like insomnia can often be improved with cranial therapy. One recent study reviewing the use of CST in 157 patients found a 74% success rate in improving their primary problem, particularly helpful for headaches or migraine, neck and back pain, anxiety, depression, or fussy and colicky babies (Harrison, 2011). Serious limitations to this published outcome are that this was a retrospective review of patient charts, there was no control group, and no comparison to placebo.

The jaw is part of the skull, and various problems with the way your jaw articulates with the skull can cause issues ranging from problems with feeding in infants to temporomandibular joint (TMJ) pain and headaches in adults. Many chiropractors and CST practitioners are good at adjusting the jaw to improve alignment and reduce these symptoms. One recent randomized trial involving thirty patients with TMJ pain associated with myofascial pain and dysfunction of the jaw muscles found myofascial manipulation therapy (like having aggressive massage of the jaw muscles and surrounding muscles of the face and head) to be slightly superior in reducing pain compared to botulinum toxin injections; though it was noted that those receiving the botulinum toxin injections had slightly better jaw range of motion following treatment (Guarda-Nardini, 2012). Studies evaluating the use of acupuncture in TMJ pain-dysfunction syndrome showed it has similar efficacy to the use of decompression splints (Vicente-Barrero, 2012).

Moving down the skeleton, you can have alignment problems with the shoulder bones, collarbones, and ribs that generate pain from the chest area out to the shoulders. Some people also experience some difficulty breathing or the feeling that they can't quite catch their breath. These symptoms can often be improved with manipulation as well. Bony problems responsive to manipulation in the elbow, wrist, or hand are less common, but they do occur.

Alignment problems with the pelvis are much more common. The pelvis is a large ring comprised of four bones (the sacrum in the back and two pelvic halves comprised of the ilium, ischium, and pubis fused together) with a joint in the center-front of your pubic area (the pubic symphysis) and on both sides of the sacrum in the back (the sacro-iliac joints). These joints, which are more or less at the center of your body from top to bottom, is subject to many forces from different directions through the normal movements and positions of the body.

It is possible for the pelvis to be torqued out of line with some unusual forces, especially in those who are not in good muscular condition. This misalignment can cause the pelvis to twist a bit and functionally tilt to one side, which causes one leg to ride higher than the other and forces compensatory sideway curves in the spine. Significant pain in the spine or elsewhere and visceral dysfunction problems with abdominal or pelvic organs can result due to nerve impingement on the concave side of these curves. I have had an osteopath adjust my pelvis, which was still out of alignment nearly ten years after an auto accident; it was a strange feeling, but it made a noticeable difference even after only one treatment.

Hip, knee, ankle, and foot alignment problems seem much more common than upper extremity issues. This is most likely because we bear our weight on the lower extremities. I see few people who need adjustments in these extremity joints, but I think a good osteopath is your best bet if you suspect your leg or arm joints might be out of alignment or moving wrong. Some chiropractors and certain well-trained physical therapists can work wonders here too. These issues usually manifest as pain, and the pain may even be some distance away from the actual alignment problem.

People who have real leg-length discrepancies (not just a twisted pelvis or curved spine) or foot deformities may experience pain anywhere along their spine. This is because of the lateral bending and curving it requires to keep your head on straight when your leg length discrepancy would have you leaning to one side. Those with pain problems and other symptoms related to this alignment issue require a lift or shoe insert on one side to achieve proper alignment. Seeing a podiatrist or orthotic specialist is best if you suspect this problem. Some physical therapists, osteopaths, and chiropractors have this expertise as well.

Musculoskeletal manipulation

In general, there are two types of manipulation: fast and slow. Most people are familiar with the fast sort, which is what the chiropractor does when he or she suddenly twists your neck to one side and makes it crack all along the vertebrae, or shoves down fast and hard on your lower spine and creates the same sort of noises. This type of manipulation, which is often called "high-velocity" manipulation, can get your spine back into alignment, although there is a small potential risk of damage to cartilage, ligaments, and tendon attachments. Chiropractors and osteopaths are highly trained in doing this sort of thing, and they can perform high-velocity, low-amplitude adjustments with no problems the vast majority of the time. However, I have seen a number of patients who experience worsened or new pain after having manipulation of this sort. I am not suggesting that you avoid chiropractors or avoid this type of manipulation, just discuss it with your practitioner if you are concerned and ask about other options.

The slow type of manipulation is practiced by some chiropractors who use machines like the "pro-adjuster," which act like little jackhammers to shift your vertebrae gradually back into line in an arguably safer fashion. Osteopaths often use their hands to peform more subtle, slower manipulation techniques with the spine and other joints. In some cases, the manipulation techniques may even focus on the muscles and other soft tissues rather than the bones and joints. This approach makes more sense to me than fast manipulation does in many cases because the abnormal pull of muscles in spasm is the reason for the persistently altered skeletal alignment, and jerking the bones back into place in the setting of improper muscle mechanics does not yield long-term relief much of the time.

Techniques such as strain-counterstrain, fascial manipulation, the Berry method, rolfing, and even deep tissue massage can help release the muscles that are pulling the spine out of line. Craniosacral therapy is very gentle and in many cases the patient feels like nothing is happening at all. The next day, however, the patient may feel significant relief or even deep aching or new pain. This effect often surprises them because they didn't think anything had been done to them. The point is you don't have to be rough on the body to make big things happen.

With manipulation, I believe you should notice some improvement within the first three or four treatments; otherwise, you may want to consider a different type of treatment or a different provider. I'm sure many chiropractors and other practitioners would argue with this point of view and suggest you have six to ten sessions perhaps, but I think an effective therapy should work more quickly and that, if you have to keep coming back for manipulation every week for more than a couple of months, you should look for another or an additional form of treatment.

For example, if your spine keeps going back out of alignment a week after being manipulated, then you probably have a leg-length discrepancy or some chronic muscle tension problem, and just having your spine repeatedly straightened under force may not be the best approach. You may want to see someone who works with muscles as well, such as a rolfer or other specific physical therapists with advanced training of this sort; you may also want to see about the need for a lift in one shoe or do particular strengthening exercises to achieve more permanent improvement. Yoga is my favorite form of exercise for correcting spinal and muscular issues of the upper and lower back; neck and limb problems may not do as well with yoga.

Other structural problems

Aside from the muscles and bones, structural problems can occur in other organ systems and tissues. These problems manifest as pain, altered function of an organ, obstruction to the flow of a fluid, pressure or mass effects, tissue death, and general physiological problems. These issues can be congenital and cause problems of varying severity right at birth, or they can develop over time from tissue injury or chronic dysfunction. These problems usually require surgery for ultimate correction.

Sometimes it takes a long time and multiple providers to figure out that a problem is structural. Most alternative practitioners first attempt functional and physiologic remedies, while many conventional physicians and other providers first treat the symptoms with drugs if the symptoms are mild. A surgeon often looks for a structural or surgical problem preferentially, but it is unusual to see a surgeon first for a problem that does not seem obviously surgical in nature. If you yourself are aware of the possibility of a structural issue causing your symptoms, you can help guide your provider to look for it.

There are many such structural problems that are possible in the body. Starting at the top, some babies are born with malformations in the back of their brain stems (e.g., Chiari malformations) that interfere with the normal flow of cerebrospinal fluid and can cause pressure inside the skull; these are often not identified until the child is several years old and manifesting various developmental difficulties. Adults can develop tumors or cysts in the brain or neighboring structures that cause severe headaches, seizures, vision disturbance, hearing loss, or focal neurological problems.

As for the mouth and neck area, babies can be born with cleft palates and be unable to nurse properly. Some may be born with abnormal connections between the throat and the esophagus or with the throat draining into the lungs. Older children or adults can have enlargement of the tonsils, which obstructs swallowing or breathing, particularly during sleep. A deviated nasal septum, with possible obstruction of one nostril, is quite common.

Structural heart problems are of particular concern; some may be present at birth and others may develop or worsen with age. Severe congenital heart problems may not be compatible with life, but newborns with milder malformations can undergo surgery and live a normal life expectancy. These more notable defects are usually not a mystery in the way they manifest, and in the age of prenatal ultrasound they are often identified prior to delivery. Some subtle issues like abnormal valves or holes in the septum dividing the atria or ventricles may not cause overt problems early in life but may result in altered physiology later on—even first becoming apparent in adulthood.

With heart issues, the main symptoms to worry about are exercise intolerance, chest pain, dizziness, and fainting. A particularly tragic heart deformity is called "hypertophic cardiomyopathy" (HCM) (formerly termed "idiopathic hypertrophic subaortic stenosis", or IHSS; it is a genetic condition that leads to abnormal thickening of the muscular wall between the ventricles. HCM can cause blood flow obstruction specifically during exercise, and occasionally causes sudden death in young athletes during exercise of sports competition. HCM is a major reason that sports physicals are required for school athletic participation, but the abnormal heart sounds are often not present or are difficult to elicit during physical examination. If your child has any unusual sound in their heart, the doctor should order an ultrasound (echocardiogram) just to make sure.

Digestive organs can have structural problems of a wide variety, with most problematic issues causing some sort of obstruction. Achalasia is a disorder involving tightness at the bottom of the esophagus with resulting trouble swallowing and extreme dilation of the esophagus just above the tight spot. Pyloric stenosis is a common problem in which there is tightness on the way out of the stomach into the small intestine; it usually presents as *projectile* vomiting in a newborn or recurrent vomiting with poor growth. There can be problems with the structure of the pancreas, the liver and bile ducts, the colon, and the rectum. It is also possible for the intestinal tract to rotate abnormally during development such that the sigmoid colon is easily twisted. Each of these issues is most likely to present with extreme abdominal pain.

Structural problems with the urinary tract can lead to kidneys being placed incorrectly, joined together into a single kidney, or absent a ureter connection and not functioning at all. Children can have recurring urinary tract infections that are due to improper connection where the ureters meet the bladder. The genital and reproductive structures can also be altered, leading to visible malformations and reproductive or menstrual problems.

Blood vessels can have abnormal structural development, or they can develop blockages over time because of atherosclerosis. The process of atherosclerosis is of metabolic origin, but the end result is obstruction to flow, and that is a structural problem of sorts. Some people have unusual kinks in coronary arteries, or arteries to other parts of the body, causing plaque to build up in these places much more readily than normal. Aneurysms are abnormal dilations in arteries; when they occur in the brain and suddenly rupture, they often kill people who were otherwise very healthy and young. Aneurysms in the abdominal portion of the aorta are more often acquired rather than congenital; they occur primarily in smokers. Dilated veins can develop anywhere in the body through various mechanisms and can lead to bleeding from internal organs or deep, aching leg pain.

The nervous system can experience structural problems as well. Nerve sheath tissue can enlarge, causing "neuromas," which may be painful if they occur in tight places, such as between the bones of the feet. The most common structural problems that affect nerves are spinal problems, when herniated discs or spinal degeneration put pressure on nerve roots.

Many of these soft tissue structural problems require surgery as the ultimate and sometimes urgent solution. I went through this select list of issues just to make you aware of the potential scope of structural problems and to suggest that you and your provider consider this possibility if other explanations aren't making sense or yielding results. This is one area in which a *conventional* medical practitioner is usually superior to naturopaths and other alternative medicine providers. Our allopathic training is heavily weighted toward severe problems like these, while alternative medical training focuses on physiological function and metabolism.

Chapter 9 – Psychology, Energetics, and Spirituality

I want to emphasize the aspect of your "being" one more time and give the idea due respect with its own chapter. I also want to provide some scientific evidence for the connections between psychology and physiology and mention an amazing example of the power of belief–even someone else's belief.

Aside from the active daily thoughts that affect your energy and physiology, you may also be persistently affected by past negative events. I'm not talking about how your mother didn't love you enough; I'm talking about real abuse, traumatic events, intense fear episodes, perceived serious neglect, and other experiences that may have had a lasting impact on you in a tangible sense. This impact is not just psychological; it becomes intertwined with the energy in every cell of your body, and it causes dysfunction on multiple levels. We all know acute stress can cause short-term increases in heart rate and blood pressure and change digestive functions and blood sugar levels, but I contend that there are other effects not visible on the surface.

Aside from the known effects that stress and trauma have on measurable chemicals and physiology in the body, there are lingering energetic signals or abnormalities within your cells and tissues. You cannot separate matter from energy, as they are one within a living system. A crystalline matrix connects all our cells to one another, with conduits that carry signals throughout the body, such as the "meridians" of acupuncture theory (Gerber, 2001). The effects of this matrix are diverse and are usually

742

impossible to explain through modern conventional medical approaches with our typical process of interview, examination, and testing.

Unfortunately, many of my adult patients, including a majority of the women it seems, has been abused in some manner during their lives. Some people have persistent awareness or psychological reliving of their traumatic experiences that lead to named disorders like PTSD, and others have stuffed it away psychologically or "dissociated" from their traumatic experiences. We use terms like "repressed" and "suppressed" to describe how the bad stuff is still there even when you choose to ignore or deny it.

I think we've all experienced how we can physically feel much worse when we are in a low mood or state of relative depression. The obvious symptoms of psychological illness include sadness, lack of pleasure, and sleep disturbance. They exacerbate pain problems, digestive symptoms, and other physical or physiological issues. These symptoms are all more obviously associated when we are mentally aware of our psychological or energetic issues, but they also occur when we ignore or deny those issues and don't readily see the connection.

On the other hand, we have all experienced how being genuinely happy can seem to make physical problems and illness symptoms much less important or even objectively better. The old expression "laughter is the best medicine" has some real truth to it, and this seems true even if you are basically "faking it" by making yourself laugh intentionally (Mora-Ripoll, 2010). The converse of that could be that sadness, fear and anger may cause disease. Research has shown that those with chronic pain issues and negative emotional attitudes do significantly worse than those maintaining positive personality traits such as optimism, hardiness and internal locus of control (Radat, 2011).

These psychological and emotional states can translate to physiological changes in the nervous and hormonal systems involving chemicals like serotonin and cortisol, either toward positive or negative outcomes. That is still a *physical* aspect of who we are, and not the topic of this chapter. There are also less "physiological" processes going on in these situations. We all have an energetic aspect—call it your spirit, your qi, your essence, or whatever you like. Dr. Emoto's work showed that water crystallization is dramatically affected even by artificially imposed ideas of emotional states (Emoto, 2005). These concepts form the bridges between psychological or spiritual disharmony and physical illness and symptoms.

In traditional Chinese medicine (TCM) these ideas about linking

743

emotion and health are explicit and accepted as fact. Each sphere of influence, labeled with a particular organ name, has corresponding positive or negative emotions that promote either health or disease within that sphere of influence. The emotion of fear is damaging to the "Kidney," affecting not only the urinary tract but also adrenal function, the sense of hearing, low back pain, bone issues, decreased overall vitality, and strength in every sense. The emotion of anger is damaging to the "Liver"; this sphere of influence involves the liver itself, movement of blood, the eyes and sense of vision, and several other functions. The emotion of grief is hard on the "Large Intestine" and can lead to issues like constipation or even colon cancer.

These negative relationships go both ways in TCM philosophy; real disease in an organ will tend to trigger certain emotional states or perseverations. Kidney disease therefore tends to create fear, liver disease tends to promote anger, and so on. This relationship can be beneficial as well as detrimental; for example, the emotions of elation or extreme happiness, is very healing and good for the heart; and acceptance and positive regard are good for the liver and its sphere of influence. "Acceptance" is an extremely important concept in Buddhist philosophy and practice in general, and reaching a state of acceptance is key to being at peace and in balance with the world.

This ancient system of healing (TCM) is based on centuries of careful observation, not laboratory tests. Similar concepts involving relationships between emotional or spiritual disturbance and physical illness or health can also be seen in other traditional systems of healing, such as Ayurveda, although our culture has mostly lost touch with this connection in the same sense. While on some level we acknowledge that extremes of emotion can influence your health in one way or another, it is said more as a superstition than with real conviction. We readily observe that acute anxiety can increase one's heart rate and blood pressure, but we are not taught that chronic anxiety, fear, or worry can cause lasting *physical* illness.

Similarly, we are not taught how positive emotion can heal. We tell people to "think positive" when they are experiencing bad things, though it is more of a cliché than a prescription. We now have scientific evidence for the beneficial health effects of positive emotion and visualization (McCraty, 2010). This connection should be taught throughout all medical training as a first-line therapy in my opinion because there are proven benefits, absolutely no risk of harm, and the price tag is very reasonable.

The science here refers to what is called "coherence." Coherence is a term in physical science and harmonics that describes how electromagnetic fields can become entrained with one another into a cohesive concordant rhythm, thereby creating a signal much greater in focus and intensity than the sum of the individual fields. For example, coherence can be achieved with artificially generated light and sound waves to create laser beams and shock waves. It can also be observed in association with human beings, as the separate electromagnetic field generators can come in line with one another in such a way that a focused summated signal is generated that is far stronger than their sum.

You can measure the energetic rhythms of physiological parameters like heart rate variability (HRV), respiratory rate and rhythm, blood pressure, the wave pattern through the vascular system, and brain waves. Since these energetic rhythms each generate their own electromagnetic fields and harmonics, they can generate individual, discordant rhythms or they can harmonize with one another and generate a compound signal.

HRV has been shown to be the best measurable predictor of heart disease and cardiac events like heart attack—far better than traditional risk factors such as cholesterol, blood pressure, or CRP (Kotecha, 2012). HRV, which represents the beat-to-beat variability in heart rate, is affected by blood flow through the coronary arteries, neurological inputs from the brain and autonomic nervous system, and much more. The greater the level of the HRV pattern, meaning the *more* irregular it is, within the individual, the lower the chance for heart disease. A low five-minute HRV correlates with risk of coronary artery disease in a linear fashion (which reflects a very strong association, rarely seen in medical research), and those with HRV below 250ms(2) have about two and a half times the risk of obstructive coronary disease compared to those above 250 for example (Kotecha, 2012).

It is simple to measure HRV; all it takes is a fingertip pulse sensor and some computer software. You can get your own setup for this at home with a biofeedback trainer called Heartmath™, which has a pile of clinical and scientific data in support of its benefits. This program trains people to coordinate their brain, focus, and autonomic nervous system. It is useful not only for cardiovascular health, but neurocognitive issues and perhaps other problems. One study found that children with ADHD showed significant improvements in behavior, learning and cognitive function using this biofeedback program (Lloyd, 2010).

Studies of the factors that influence biorhythms such as HRV have found that emotional and mental states have profound impact on coherence. Anger and frustration wreck your coherence pattern, while appreciation, love, and positive emotional focus generate good coherence. Relaxation exercises don't promote more improvement in coherence than does performing a simple mental task, although relaxation shows a better peak frequency. Meditation performed by a very experienced person can achieve very good sustained coherence that is much better than a novice can achieve. Focusing on the concept of "acceptance" was shown to generate a dramatic spike in coherence (McCraty, 2010).

The most important message here is that positive emotion has a significant effect on this important physiological parameter. Anyone off the street can profoundly influence their level of bioenergetic coherence as well as a highly trained meditating Zen Buddhist monk by just visualizing something very positive that elicits a feeling of intense love or happiness.

This means that one of the best ways to heal yourself of all ills is to focus on positive emotion whenever possible. If you take some time here and there to focus your attention and thoughts on beautiful things, love, gratitude, joy, hope, dreams, and experiences that brought you great happiness, you will create the brightest of lights inside and spread wellness to all your cells. You will likely feel this effect immediately, and others around you may sense it as well, even if only subconsciously. The more you practice this, the easier it will become.

An entire issue of *Alternative Therapies in Health and Medicine* (Jul/Aug 2010) is dedicated to the concepts of physiological and energetic coherence and how it relates to psychological and physical health and wellness. Coherence is grounded in measurable science, with studies showing the short- and long-term consequences and benefits of having discordant or positive coherence in your biorhythms.

An important new field of mind-body practice and healing, termed "mindfulness," has arisen that is very much in line with Buddhist philosophy and teaching, albeit with a more western scientific approach. Research has shown that the brain's function and connectedness can be dramatically affected through mindfulness. Current research has even demonstrated significant improvements in mood, quality of life, sense of wellbeing, and even the adverse physical affects of treatment in women undergoing therapy for breast cancer (Hoffman, 2012). These concepts can easily be applied to any type of chronic illness. Self-help systems in mindfulness training are available to the public now on CDs and digital audio, and I encouraged anyone who wants to improve psychological balance to try it out.

A 1985 scientific study now called the Gracely Study clearly demonstrated the power that the belief and intention of one person may have on another physically. (You can certainly extrapolate this to the conclusion that the effect you can have on yourself is almost certainly even greater.) This simple study used postoperative dental pain after wisdom tooth extraction to examine the power of feelings, emotion, and intention.

The oral surgeon was told that some of his patients would be given the narcotic drug Fentanyl for pain during and after the procedure and that another group would be given a placebo. The surgeon was not "blinded," so he knew which patients were supposedly getting the Fentanyl and which were getting the placebo, but the patients themselves did not know anything about the study, so all expected to receive the typical treatment for pain (Fentanyl). The results showed a dramatic difference in perceived pain by the patients following the procedure, with those in the placebo group reporting far more pain than those in the Fentanyl group.

The most interesting part of this was that all the patients received only placebo. Nobody got the real drug. Think about that for a minute.

What happened was that the surgeon's expectations influenced the patients' experiences. If he thought they were going to be in pain, they were; if he expected them to have comfort and relief, they did. This was no small difference either: the placebo group had a perceived pain level increase of 6.5 on their scale, while the Fentanyl group experienced a decrease in their pain to the level of -3. This difference was measured one hour after the procedure (Gracely, 1985).

This result ties in with Dr. Emoto's research into the effects of feelings, emotions, and intention on water crystallization and shows that the beliefs of your medical provider are important to how well you do. It suggests that both negative and positive emotions from yourself and others can have a very real impact on your health and wellbeing.

I have no doubt that some of my patients get better simply because I "expect" them to, sometimes in spite of what therapy I've prescribed for them, rather than because of it. I go to work every day knowing that my intention to heal and belief in the human body's capacity for wellness generates positive outcomes. Frankly, it makes my job that much easier. If I tell you in a convincing manner that your symptoms will improve, and I know you have the ability to stick with whatever difficult program I've suggested for you, you are very likely to improve just as I have predicted. I have no earthly clue why so many of my colleagues wish to tell patients the complete opposite: that their prognosis is very poor, there is no cure for their condition, they are going to die in six months or less, or some other horrendously negative and pessimistic thing. By telling people those things, they are making the negative outcomes far more likely to occur.

Similar mechanisms could lie behind positive benefits of faith healing, Reiki, therapeutic touch, intercessory prayer, and other practices of that nature. The positive effect of expectation helps explain why those with loving, supportive families and social networks do so much better with their medical conditions than do those with the opposite situation, who tend to struggle with many more complaints. It could also explain any real effect of negative practices like voodoo, curses, and black magic. It is therefore very important that we hold each other in positive regard and engender good feelings for each other and ourselves. Sometimes all that keeps a person sick is negative emotion—from themselves or others.

Before I end this short chapter, I want to mention some things you can do to help heal this aspect of your being or your physical ailments. These suggestions can be important not only for the recent or obvious issues but also for the long-standing, consciously forgotten issues that still have an ingrained physical presence. You can use positive emotional expression and visualization, exercise, mindfulness meditation, prayer, and other types of self-care; exercises like yoga, tai chi, qi gong, and others that blend the physical with the energetic; biofeedback training programs and devices like *Heartmath* to train yourself; and other people by spending quality time with loved ones and friends, seeing a good counselor, or doing uplifting group activities.

Some external healing therapies to help correct problems in this realm can be performed by others. Homeopathy is one way for a practitioner to prescribe an energetic input for you, but it is very complex, and practitioners must have extensive training to be proficient. Reiki and other forms of energy healing are very effective for some, and craniosacral and "cellular energy retraining" techniques (CERT) may also be practiced by someone in your area. There may be excellent healers around you who can help you make these connections and reestablish energetic and physical harmony. If you open yourself up to these therapies, they work far better—remember the power of positive thinking and expectation.

Acupuncture is a very effective means of correcting disease states involving these types of problems; it is particularly good for releasing old, stuck energetic problems you don't even remember. I know a number of people who have experienced surprisingly intense emotional reactions from acupuncture treatments that were not even targeting those problems. I was taught a particular treatment protocol to help release blocked energy related to past trauma or negative experiences that seems to work very well for what we would call PTSD, dissociative disorder, or repressed memories. I performed this treatment on my father and he swears it helped him significantly regarding his prior traumatic experiences in Vietnam.

One of the most exciting treatments in my opinion is the use of bioelectric machines like the Indigo, Vega, Mora, SCIO, and QXCI. These machines have traditionally been used to assess your energetic imbalances, disturbances, or "sensitivity" to potential environmental or internal substances in a diagnostic sense so appropriate homeopathic remedies can be prescribed to correct the problem. The newer machines, like those I listed, also have some capacity to deliver a *corrective* energetic signal back to the patient. As I mentioned previously, I have begun using an Indigo machine, in early 2012, and I have been very impressed with its benefits.

These machines and their effects on our biorhythms represent what I feel is the future of medicine. This type of technology has the potential to help correct chronic imbalance or dysfunction on an energetic or physiologic level. Indigo's applications for treatment include problems with the nervous system (including psychiatric issues), neuromuscular system, the immune system (allergies, autoimmune disease), the cardiovascular system, digestive system, and many others. There are also programs related to addiction such as smoking cessation. There are programs that delve into the metaphysical as well, designed to help you reconcile issues with past lives or better align yourself with your "higher purpose." These aspects of the technology risk alienating a relatively conservative-minded subset of our population, in which case just the more "physical" aspects of the machine can be utilized.

This is one of the shortest chapters in the book, but it is very important. I urge you to take charge of this part of your being and focus just as much effort on it as you do your diet or exercise program to promote your own health. Your psychology, energetics, and spirituality should not be ignored. This could be the most difficult, but most important, part of your personal health management.

Chapter 10 – Specific
Medical Problems

I have covered what I believe are some of the most common upstream causes of most chronic illnesses. However, I want to discuss some specific examples of common disease conditions in terms of what the real causes may be and what sort of treatment approaches one can take. By using an integrative perspective, I hope to help you think a bit differently from the mainstream view about them.

In the final section of this book that follows this chapter, I recap the essential aspects of health in what I hope is a succinct and useful summary of the book.

Cancer

When people develop certain symptoms, such as weight loss, headaches, abdominal pain, and palpable lumps, they may worry about having cancer. Cancer is a potential "cause" of illness symptoms that must be investigated and ruled out. Cancers as a group are a major leading "cause" of death in our society, so they are a very important topic. Many organizations raise money toward finding a cure for "cancer;" however, the many different types of cancer that are each their own unique disease in many respects.

Each type of cancer shares certain characteristics metabolically, such as altered energy production and oxygen utilization, increased cell division rates and metabolic activity, the loss of normal programmed cell death mechanisms, and the breakdown of normal growth boundaries that leads to cancer cells invading neighboring tissues inappropriately. In spite of those general similarities, cancers that arise in different primary tissues have very different growth patterns, spreading habits, responses to conventional therapies, symptoms, and survival rates.

Each type of cancer, designated by its tissue of origin and its cell type or characteristics, is a unique disease with its own ideal treatment protocol in terms of conventional medicine. The field of oncology is highly complex and diverse as a result; oncologists must keep current on all the available forms of chemotherapy and methods of radiation therapy and know which combinations have most recently been shown to be the most effective. While there is a constant flow of research coming out of this field, for some types of cancer, none of it works very well.

For certain other types of cancer, the conventional approach works very well. For example, Hodgkin's lymphoma responds very well to the conventional chemo and radiation treatments, and the great majority of patients survive. Unfortunately, many of these survivors will develop a new cancer decades later because of the toxicity of the therapy they received (Demoor-Goldschmidt, 2012). Other cancers, such as pancreatic cancer and many forms of lung cancer, have low survival rates in spite of our best efforts with conventional therapies. For those cancers, researchers get excited if they find a new therapy that seems to offer even just one month of added survival, although that month may be fraught with serious side effects.

It is important to note that cancer is always part of "you," and there are underlying reasons why you developed it. Those reasons include most of the underlying causes of disease discussed earlier in this section, including genetic factors, nutrient deficiencies, environmental and internal toxins, hormonal imbalances, and psychological or energetic factors. I discussed evidence linking many of these issues to cancer in one form or another. If you want to prevent cancer, you should work hard in all of those areas and try to make your overall health as optimal as possible. Remember that having a genetic predisposition (i.e., family members with cancer) means you have to *behave* even better; it does not mean cancer is *certain* in your future.

Keep in mind that screening for cancer with tests like mammograms and blood PSA levels is not "prevention" of cancer but methods of early detection that may help you get treatment much sooner, when it can be most effective. They do nothing to decrease the initial development of cancer. Real prevention lies mainly with lifestyle factors. Cancer usually takes a decade or more after your cells have initially transformed to manifest clinically.

We spontaneously generate dozens or even hundreds of cancerous cells every day, even under good health conditions, but mechanisms in the immune system constantly kill these small numbers of cancer cells. The key to avoiding death from cancer, whether you have it now or not, is to live as healthfully as possible, eat well, detoxify, exercise regularly, and promote peace and happiness in your life. It is NOT about taking drugs like aspirin, which shows a possible reduction of colon cancer in some epidemiological studies.

The media gives lots of attention to studies suggesting aspirin reduces colorectal cancer, even though results from studies have been very mixed, and two out of the four best randomized controlled trials actually showed a negative impact of aspirin on colorectal cancer (Rostom, 2007). On the other hand, the media makes no mention at all of studies like the one showing a 78% *increase* in small cell lung cancer risk (a much worse cancer than colorectal) taking a regular aspirin per day (Brasky, 2012). This is not to even mention that aspirin use as much as triples the risk of developing stomach ulcers (Rostom, 2007) or other adverse complications. I searched "aspirin increases cancer risk" on Google, and all that came up was a long list of media articles about aspirin reducing colon cancer. We really like to promote drugs as being the solution in our society.

I give a twelve-page handout (written by myself) on natural interventions for beating cancer to my patients, which includes advice regarding diet, supplements, exercise, stress reduction, energetic and spiritual wellness, and herbal and intravenous therapies. I stress that research shows you have to get regular vigorous exercise if you want to beat cancer; diet alone is not enough, no matter how strict you are. Physical exercise is associated with all-cause mortality, and also death from breast and colon cancers specifically (Ballard-Barbash, 2012). Physical activity greatly improves pain, constipation, fatigue, breathing, insomnia and emotional disturbances associated with having even late-stage cancers (Albrecht, 2012). Apparently, you have to tell your body you want to live by *using* it.

Dietary factors need to stress non-toxic foods, strictly wild and organic whole foods. My suggestion is to avoid grains completely and of course eat no processed sugars at all. I suggest people consume large quantities of dark berries and fruits such as blueberry, pomegranate, acai and others. There is a system termed *Gerson therapy*, developed by a German physician named Max Gerson many decades ago, which has a strong following and good track record in helping people fight cancer. The Gerson protocol includes consuming large quantities of organic fruit and vegetable juices (juicing allows you to get the nutrients from twenty pounds of produce each day without having to swallow all that fiber and bulk), taking iodine and doing coffee enemas. I usually skip the coffee enemas unless people have a lot of pain, as they seem mainly helpful for the pain.

Green tea has been associated with decreased cancer risk and has also been shown to work synergistically with conventional anticancer drugs and chemotherapy (Fujiki, 2012), and I suggest having a few cups or more per day (organic only, of course). I mentioned before that melatonin has been shown to have anticancer properties (Margheri, 2012), and I suggest up to 20mg nightly if tolerated. I suggest people consider many other supplements as well including turmeric (liposomal form preferably), mushroom extracts (reishi, shitake, maitake, cordyceps), boswellia and Zyflamend™.

I of course strongly encourage those with cancer to take vitamin D, and get their 25-OH levels up as close to 150ng/mL as possible. The only direct intervention we offer at my office is intravenous vitamin C, which as I discussed in section III is even proving to be a very useful adjunctive anticancer therapy in the conventional medical literature (Monti, 2012) and has virtually no toxicity. If you can find a practitioner who performs insulin-potentiated chemotherapy (IPT) I encourage you to consult with them as well. Look for a practitioner through the International Organization of Integrative Cancer Physicians (IOICP) at www.ioicp.com. Despite this type of therapy and its practitioners being targeted by "Quackwatch", there is evidence in favor of IPT coming out in the conventional literature (Damyanov, 2012).

The psychological, energetic and spiritual aspects of health are probably more important in cancer than in any other chronic disease condition. This condition instills tremendous fear, dread and helplessness in people; and those very thoughts and emotions are themselves barriers to success. It is very important to address the psycho-spiritual stuff utilizing whatever modalities you have interest in and access to. Find a counselor, clergyman, energy healer, hypnotist, or practitioner who uses a bio-energetic device such as the Indigo or SCIO. Perform regular yoga, tai chi, qi gong, mindfulness meditation, positive visualization, journaling, prayer or whatever else helps *you* feel centered and balanced.

Those who survive their initial cancer are often at much greater risk for a recurrence or even a new cancer than is the general population because they had factors that once led to cancer, because their cancer may not have been totally cleared, or because they had treatments that promoted the development of new cancers. Therefore, it is even more important for cancer survivors to live an ideal lifestyle after their cancer is beaten than it was prior to their cancer diagnosis.

This is one type of illness where almost everyone will seek medical care, often medical care of various types. I urge everyone with cancer to work with alternative or integrative providers as well as their oncologists, even if those practitioners don't get along with each other.

Cardiovascular Disease

I bring up cardiovascular disease here because it is our leading cause of death and therefore warrants a bit of synthesis. Cardiovascular disease can be the cause of symptoms like leg pain, erectile dysfunction, chest pains, dizziness, and mild cognitive problems. However, the first "symptom" of up to half of those with coronary artery disease is a heart attack, and half of those folks will die from that first event. Clearly, prevention is very important, as is adequate screening for the disease.

Our modern understanding of vascular disease—at least our understanding of atherosclerosis—suggests that it begins with inflammation and ends with plaque buildup inside arteries at the site of that initial injury to the vessel lining. Prevention therefore lies in reducing the chances of chronic inflammation in the blood vessels, and this is a key component of treating established disease as well. Prevention of cardiovascular disease involves diet, exercise, hormone balance, environmental toxicity concerns, emotional wellbeing, and everything else discussed in this book.

Some people have a genetic predisposition to getting vascular disease, but even a genetic predisposition leaves the chances of getting vascular disease far from a certainty. It just means those folks must live a very healthy and optimal lifestyle if they want to live longer. Vascular disease that can kill takes many years to develop to the point of illness or symptoms, so we tend to disregard proper preventive lifestyle habits when we're young because we don't suffer enough immediate consequences for bad behaviors. With the terrible food they consume and the serious lack of exercise among our young people today, we are now even seeing evidence of early atherosclerosis changes in the arteries of teenagers at autopsy (McGill, 2000).

We have to start taking this issue seriously beginning in early childhood. That does not mean we should be putting children on cholesterol drugs, although the American Academy of Pediatrics is now suggesting we consider doing so with kids as young as eight years old. It means we need to relearn what real food is and get the junk out of our children's diets, make them shut off their electronic devices and get off the couch for a couple hours per day, promote love and happiness in our households, ban the manufacture of cigarettes (why hasn't that been done already?!), and somehow make them *want* to be healthy. I know, it seems unlikely.

It is also important to avoid sugar, processed foods of all sorts, and all unhealthful mass-produced animal products. Exercise is a must in this case. Supplements such as vitamin D, iodine, fish oil, magnesium, vitamin C, garlic, niacin and some others have been shown to be important. Importantly, you should start all this at least twenty years *before* you might expect a heart attack if you want to be successful, so don't wait. It is easier to prevent cardiovascular disease than to treat it.

Testing for the presence of coronary artery disease in conventional medicine often involves tests that are often not helpful in reality, but are quite expensive. A standard EKG can be performed in a physician's office, but rarely tells you anything about the presence or absence of plaque in the arteries and can even look normal in a startling percentage of folks who are actually having a heart attack. Treadmill stress tests have quite poor sensitivity and accuracy, particularly in women; adding nuclear imaging (as in a "cardiolite" study) to the stress test in order to see blood flow to the heart muscle improves its sensitivity but costs thousands of dollars more and exposes you to radiation. The cardiolite still doesn't tell you for certain that you don't have plaque in your arteries either, because one can grow substantial collateral vessels around the site of a blockage over time; this makes it appear that the area of heart muscle still gets adequate blood flow, without showing the presence of a lesion that may kill the person suddenly at any time if the plaque were to rupture.

The "gold standard" in testing in allopathic medicine is intravascular angiography, where they enter your arterial system through the groin or arm and inject dye right into the coronary arteries to look for any visible blockages. This is quite accurate and tells us what we really want to know, but typically costs in excess of $10,000 in our country and subjects the patient to substantial risks. Angiography is typically reserved for those having acute symptoms that are strongly suspected to be cardiac in origin. This is not a test you perform on an asymptomatic individual for screening purposes; therefore that 50% of people who have a heart attack as their first symptom are not going to be helped by this.

My preferred *screening* test for coronary disease is called a coronary calcium score. This test can be done by CT scan, which exposes one to radiation, or in some places by electron beam scanning, which does not involve radiation (therefore the latter is preferable). The coronary calcium scores look anatomically at the heart and quantify any visible calcified plaque present. This tells you the presence and extent of established disease, but does not adequately visualize any early soft plaque that is still made strictly of lipids. The test is non-invasive and only costs a couple hundred dollars in my area. It is the best way, in my opinion, to get an early warning about this condition and reasonable assessment of disease severity without an expensive invasive procedure.

Medical treatment of coronary atherosclerosis in conventional medicine includes a handful of drugs like statins to reduce cholesterol, beta blockers to reduce the workload of heart muscle, angiotensin-converting enzyme inhibitors to reduce heart muscle remodeling, aspirin to reduce blood clotting and others as needed to control arrhythmias or otherwise improve blood pressure; perhaps some nitrates to reduce angina symptoms. This approach has been shown to extend life expectancy, and is potentially an important part of an integrative approach to the condition.

Coronary bypass grafting surgery is fairly common in our society as well, but has only been shown to be superior to medical treatment (as described above) in those who have more severe coronary disease to the point it is causing deficient heart pumping (McGee, 2007). Therefore, bypass surgery should not be recommended for those who are stable (i.e., not having ongoing chest pain or heart failure symptoms) on medical management. Also, bypass surgery does nothing to prevent the development of new disease like diet, exercise, certain supplements and medications do. People who have had bypass surgery will just plug up again in short order if the real causes of the disease are not addressed.

Intravenous chelation therapy with EDTA is a popular option among integrative practitioners in this country and is a common therapy in mainstream medicine in Japan and much of Europe. A patient of mine had intravenous EDTA chelation as part of his overall treatment in Japan. Chelation was readily advised there by his cardiologists, though my search of PubMed for "EDTA chelation and Japan" yielded no studies from that country. There are very few published studies on the topic, and results most often show no clear effect; there are a couple small studies suggesting a positive effect (Villarruz, 2002). There is a large trial going on in the U.S. right now, funded through the NIH, called the TACT trial to try and answer the question of using EDTA for coronary disease more clearly.

There is also a rectal form of EDTA on the market, and there is at least one published case series showing success of its use combined with antibiotic therapy. I discussed in the chapter on infection how there has been suspicion of various bacteria being involved with the development of atherosclerosis. One study of just 19 patients having significant coronary artery disease showed improvement, or even complete resolution, of coronary atherosclerosis at four months using oral tetracycline (500mg) and rectal EDTA (1500mg) nightly, for an overall 84% success rate (Maniscalco, 2004). If this effect is real it would certainly be an inexpensive and low-risk option; I would encourage people to try it.

Other important interventions include strict attention to the dietary recommendations I've repeatedly lined out in this book; high intake of dark fruit and berry juices; taking supplemental vitamin D, magnesium, fish oil, iodine, niacin, garlic, turmeric, and nattokinase or serrapeptase (the latter two are enzymes that help degrade the plaque). Exercise is critical as well, and should be undertaken in a slow, gradual manner if you do have some coronary disease. One comprehensive approach to diet and lifestyle management for those with heart disease can be found at www.heartfixer. com. Many experts advocate a vegetarian or vegan diet when trying to combat heart disease, but I would strongly disagree with that. What I would stress is that any animal products eaten have to be wild, organic, grass fed or otherwise completely clean and eating the diet nature intended the animal to eat.

Detoxification is going to very important, especially in terms of heavy metals. I suggest reviewing the chapter on toxins and avoid sources of heavy metals; consider having provoked urine testing to see if chelation treatment may be indicated. Sauna therapy or Epsom salt baths would be strongly recommended as well. Taking NAC in large amounts, as well as supplemental zinc and selenium would help with this as well. Paying attention to oral health is extremely important for cardiovascular disease. Be sure to clear up any gum disease by using a water pick twice a day after brushing.

For those who have symptomatic chest pain or limb pain due to vascular disease, hyperbaric oxygen can be very helpful. I advise working with both a cardiologist and an integrative practitioner or naturopath if you have vascular disease; just be prepared to get very conflicting views and information on your problem, which you will then have to reconcile.

Inflammation

Inflammation is the initial metabolic disturbance in cardiovascular disease, and it is also a key underlying process behind diverse diseases like cancer, osteoporosis, some fatigue syndromes and psychiatric conditions. Inflammation is clearly present in allergy, chronic pain conditions, arthritis, and autoimmune conditions. It has become a bit of a buzzword in modern self-help books that contain advice about anti-inflammatory diets, supplements, and herbs.

While inflammation causes many diverse symptoms, it is not really an *upstream cause* of disease. Inflammation is always triggered by something else; if you want to be successful, you have to figure out what is causing the inflammation rather than just trying to keep it under control with such treatments as anti-inflammatory or immunosuppressive drugs. Those treatments are important while you are searching for the true causes, but don't rely on downstream remedies alone.

Extremely important in combating inflammation is avoiding sugar, gluten, corn, dairy (for many), trans fats, overcooked meats or fats, and food chemicals of all sorts. They keys to an anti-inflammatory diet are avoidance of the aforementioned foods and liberal consumption of organic fruits and vegetables, the dark fruits and berries I repeatedly mention, wild fish and sea foods, olives and olive oil, nuts and seeds. Be cautious not to overcook foods, as that creates inflammatory byproducts.

You should try to avoid chemical exposures and smoke, whether from cigarettes, machines, or automobile exhaust. Get regular moderate exercise and try to keep your emotional stress level low. Use supplements and herbals like vitamin D, fish oil and turmeric. Pay attention to toxin avoidance in general and consider taking NAC to improve general detoxification. Perform moderate exercise but be careful not to over-exercise, as that can increase oxidative stress and inflammation.

Failing to look for the *source* of inflammation and only treating the symptom is like continually wiping up the water overflowing from the sink without simply turning off the faucet. Look for dietary factors, chronic infections, gut dysbiosis, food and other types of allergies, heavy metals and other environmental toxins, hormonal deficiencies (adrenal and thyroid most prominently), abdominal obesity, emotional disturbances, and energetic imbalances.

Excessive body fat directly contributes to systemic inflammation, and weight management is a very frequent concern in our population. Following the dietary and exercise principles mentioned in this book should help most people achieve a healthy body weight. Others will need to attend to hormonal deficiencies or imbalances, possibly undergo aggressive detoxification. Some may benefit from the HCG weight loss protocol at first for one or two rounds, but this should not be relied upon as a means of long-term weight control. Losing the excess body fat can be an important part of reducing systemic inflammation.

It can be difficult to sort through all the possibilities, but my advice is to think back to when problems began and try to identify the triggers or predisposing factors. It is also helpful to consider seemingly unrelated symptoms or problems that originated at around the same time. This is one chronic disease issue where identifying the triggers is of paramount importance.

Depression

I mention depression here largely because conventional practitioners too often consider it a "cause" of illness symptoms. I quickly abandoned this way of thinking after completing my conventional medical training. Depression is almost always a *symptom* of something going on and is not a primary cause of illness.

I admit that depression itself can go on to *cause* a long list of more downstream symptoms like insomnia, fatigue, weight changes, digestive problems, and pain issues. Many illnesses can themselves become causes of other problems. However, it is more likely that the associated symptoms depressed patients experience are caused by the same upstream factors that led to their depression. It is the pattern and timing of associated symptoms that generally help me determine an underlying problem.

In my opinion, practitioners should always look for upstream organic or physiologic causes of depression symptoms, rather than just putting people on antidepressant drugs. When I was trained the standard of care was to treat depression with medications for up to one year only, then try to withdraw the medication; this is because the medications may cause undesirable alterations of brain chemistry (and depression resolves on its own within a year the vast majority of the time). If you never identify and correct the underlying processes it will be very hard to get off the medications when the time comes. It's okay if they treat serious depression and emotional problems with symptomatic drugs while you search for the upstream cause, but we shouldn't leave it at that!

Common upstream causes you should consider if you experience symptoms of depression include hormonal deficiencies (thyroid, adrenal, testosterone, estrogen, progesterone, vitamin D); food, environmental or chemical allergies; poor diet and nutrient deficiencies (B vitamins and folate, omega-3 fatty acids, magnesium and trace minerals, and phytonutrients); heavy metals and other toxins; gut dysbiosis; and psychological and energetic factors. You can also consider lack of exercise as a cause since exercise has been shown to be one of the most effective treatments for depression. Depression is *not* a Prozac™ or Cymbalta™ deficiency!

Depression may involve a neurotransmitter deficiency, such as low serotonin or norepinephrine, but that is just the chemical basis or representation of depression rather than a cause. (It's like saying you have a fever because your temperature is high.) Neurotransmitter deficiency is not a cause but just a way of explaining what is going on in molecular terms. You still have to identify the reasons why the person's serotonin is low; they could have used it up through ongoing emotional or psychological stress, become depleted due to a diet that is low in tryptophan, have genetic difficulty in manufacturing neurotransmitters like the common MTHFR mutations, or be deficient in vitamin B-6 for example.

Though it is not addressing underlying causes, it is very helpful to supplement with nutrients to increase the neurotransmitters in need. Methylfolate, B-12, B-6 and magnesium are helpful in every case. Taking 5-HTP is helpful in the case of low serotonin, which is an issue in almost every case of depression. Add tyrosine if norepinephrine is needed; these folks will usually experience melancholy, a lack of motivation, and may have widespread pain issues. Those with low dopamine will have lots of trouble with mental focus and concentration; they will need tyrosine (the precursor for both norepinephrine and dopamine) and also iron supplementation.

The place where conventional medicine and I tend to agree on this subject is in the psychological causes of depression. I find that some people have no identifiable physiological issue where I can help intervene: they don't respond to vitamin D or thyroid replacement, they don't have elevated heavy metals or other potential toxins, they don't have any apparent food allergies, their other relevant hormones seem normal, and so on. In that event, we often focus on the psychological, emotional, and energetic aspects of their issues.

Since depression is, in a practical sense, a psychological symptom, it can certainly have purely psychological causes. Past traumatic events, major ongoing life stressors and causes of sadness, hopelessness, and grief are all possible causes. If someone comes in with this sort of history and experience, I may look at this route of investigation and treatment first, rather than testing for physiological causes. I am likely to have them supplement with items such as vitamin D and 5-HTP as well, to assist in their recovery. Those things will need to be supported to improve the person's resilience and adaptability. Adrenal support with adaptogenic herbs, and sometimes the hormones cortisol or DHEA can be helpful as well.

Physiological issues can still be very relevant even when people have a history of abuse, major stress, or psychological trauma; we shouldn't just jump to blaming depression on an abusive childhood for example. Many completely happy people have similar experiences, so why can some people cope better than others? The answer may lie in nutrient or hormone reserves or other physiological factors, so those fundamental factors should not be ignored even in the presence of obvious psychological factors. Giving those people vitamin D, fish oil, 5-HTP, methylfolate, and appropriate hormone therapy like thyroid or DHEA can still be very important. (That's why it's called "integrative medicine.")

I suggest some interventions to address the psychological and energetic components of depression, anxiety, or other psychiatric mood disturbances. Counseling is a good idea for many, though it is often difficult to find a good counselor for a given individual, so you may have to keep trying different ones until you "click" with somebody. Specific forms of psychotherapy, such as cognitive-behavioral therapy, are particularly effective, and exercise is of course essential.

Electro-convulsant therapy, or ECT, is still the most effective medical intervention for severe depression (Lee, 2012), and it is performed in a very safe and comfortable manner these days. (Get those images from *One Flew Over the Cuckoo's Nest* out of your head.) All the energetic therapies mentioned in the previous chapter (e.g., qi gong, bioelectric machines, Reiki, acupuncture) should also be considered. In my opinion we should use all of these tools along with or as a replacement for pharmaceuticals if possible.

Drug therapy for mental illness is one of the most heavily used medication classes in our culture. There are many drugs to choose from, and the response varies by individual, so move on to the next one right away if one causes unpleasant side effects or doesn't seem to have an effect in a reasonable amount of time (a week or two). Psychiatrists and other providers are now throwing all sorts of drugs, including antipsychotics and mood stabilizers, at patients with "treatment-resistant" depression now. (Perhaps they are resistant to medication because the drugs don't represent appropriate "treatment" for these folks.) Learn about all the potential side effects and drug interactions of your prescription so you know what to expect.

Avoid using drug therapy for too long, as these medications have not been studied for longer than a year of use, and most have not been studied for more than six months. My sister specializes in research and has been published over 70 times in the psychology literature. She ran the journal club for the psychiatry residents at UMASS medical school at one point and was horrified at this realization, and also the fact that the doctors did not see bothered by it. We don't know the long-term effects of drug therapies on the brain, and there are concerns about increased suicide or homicide risk in the short term. We don't know if there could be increased risk of dementia and other cognitive problems in the long term. Don't rely on the drugs alone, and don't take them for longer than a year if you can help it.

That said, depression is a difficult and potentially life-threatening problem, for which I often cannot find a treatable physiologic basis. I still end up keeping some people on their medications for long stretches because they become so symptomatic when they try to stop them. This is most often because they have stressful life factors that do not change. It is an admittedly difficult problem, but that doesn't mean we should give up. These are most often people who haven't tried the other treatments that may help; taking a pill every day is certainly the *easiest* thing to do; therefore, it is too often the only thing people stick with. I prescribe these drugs because it's my job to help in whatever way I can, but I almost never feel that drugs are the best choice.

Autism

Autistic spectrum disorders are a very important example of how changes in the modern environment have created a major physiological problem. This is *not a psychiatric disorder*, as it was thought to be fifty years ago; it is a multisystem disintegration of normal physiology, with the most significant factor being brain inflammation. Most of the inflammation for many of these kids originates in the gut, so food allergies, dysbiosis, and basic nutrition are very important. Heavy metals and other toxins are important for some as well, while chronic or recurring infections are more important for others.

Autism is a manifestation of a wide array of environmental afflictions intertwined with an individual's genetics, nutritional status, and immune system. Autism is a very complex issue, but it has great potential for improvement in most cases. It is an excellent example of a chronic condition that involves every aspect of health and integrative medicine described in this book. If someone in your family has an autism-related issue, seek out a provider trained by the Defeat Autism Now! (DAN) or Autism Research Institute (ARI) organizations. Also connect with TACA (Talk About Curing Autism) at www.tacanow.org/

Fibromyalgia and Chronic Fatigue Syndromes

The diagnosis of "fibromyalgia" in my view epitomizes the ignorance and lack of persistence that are so rampant in conventional medicine. If a patient comes in complaining of serious chronic fatigue, mental suppression or "brain fog," and random widespread muscle or joint pains, don't you think there's probably something *physically* wrong? However, when a conventional physician has done all the physiological tests he or she knows how to do, and all the tests are "normal," the physician decides there must not be anything *really* wrong with the patient and labels the problem something like "fibromyalgia" or "chronic fatigue syndrome." Conventional medicine agrees on some basic diagnostic criteria and pawns these diagnoses off on the public as if they were actual disease conditions.

To make things worse, most providers consider fibromyalgia primarily a psychiatric disorder and brush these patients off with a prescription for counseling, mild exercise, and an antidepressant. Some providers will put these patients on painkillers, which can create a whole new problem for them. Television commercials now promote certain drugs for the pain symptoms, telling people: "The pain of fibromyalgia is caused by *overactive nerves.*" Well, why the hell are they overacting? That's not a *cause*; it's a made-up explanation of the physiology that doesn't even make sense! You could say that about seizures and it would be far truer.

I have seen many patients who have been diagnosed with "fibromyalgia" by other physicians, rheumatologists, and even big ivory-tower medical facilities like the Mayo Clinic (shameful!). In my opinion, this is plain laziness; these symptoms always have a cause, and the physician has to keep looking until he or she finds it. The most common causes I find in my practice include thyroid deficiency, adrenal deficiency, vitamin D deficiency, gluten sensitivity, yeast hypersensitivity, food allergies, heavy metals and other toxins, iron deficiency, Lyme disease or other chronic occult infections, and vitamin B-12 deficiency. They often have more than one of these contributing factors present. There are so many options here it takes me a while to exhaust the possibilities, and I rarely have to look beyond this list.

Doctors have created other "functional disorders" as well; conditions that they decide are discrete disorders that must have psychiatric underpinnings because they can't determine the physiological causes. Examples include "irritable bowel syndrome," "multiple chemical sensitivity syndrome," "migraine," "premenstrual dysphoric disorder," endometriosis, interstitial cystitis, and ADHD. In my opinion we must do better than that; we must keep looking scientifically into other possibilities. We must think outside the proverbial "box". The box is tiny and stifling.

SECTION V

SUMMARY

This final section may serve as a synopsis of the majority of the book, a refresher or reminder as to the highlights of the book, or a guide and checklist for you to keep handy and refer to in your daily life.

There are two general instances to consider here:

1. Those who are generally in good health and would like to maintain optimal health and wellness, with the longest life span they can attain.

2. Those with some sort of illness or medical complaints.

For the generally fit and healthy person the focus should be on maintaining a healthy lifestyle and internal environment, including ongoing detoxification measures. The more proactive folks may choose to do biochemical evaluations of their individual functional nutritional status, toxin levels, hormone levels, and even some relevant genetic mutations if desired to optimize their long-term health. Most ill people were healthy at one point; it's conceivable their illnesses could have been avoided with optimized biochemistry.

The following outline begins with things relevant to everyone. For those with illness I have included a section of the outline to help direct your efforts at solving a health problem as well.

Part I – Things for Everyone

- Diet and Nutrition
  o Healthy whole foods only (no processed or devitalized foods)
  o Organic or wild foods only, especially animal products
  o Lots of organic fruits and vegetables (no pesticides, fungicides…)
  o High intake of omega-3 fats, preferably from animal products (low-mercury wild fish and seafood, grass-fed beef or wild game)
  o High intake of other healthy fats (coconut oil, olive oil, grass-fed butter)
  o Daily intake of "super foods" with healthy phytonutrients
    · Dark berries and fruits like blueberries, pomegranate, acai, blackberry, prunes and others
    · Broccoli sprouts, watercress
    · Broccoli and other cruciferous vegetables
    · Raw garlic, onions
    · Olives, purple or green
    · Tomatoes, preferably cooked with olive oil
    · Apples, apple cider vinegar
    · Kale, spinach, other dark leafy green vegetables
    · Cilantro, basil, oregano and other herbs
    · Green tea (organic only)
    · Curry (coconut milk, turmeric and other spices)
    · Dark organic chocolate
    · Grass-fed butter, chia seeds, walnuts for healthy oils
    · Wild game, Pacific salmon, squid and shellfish
    · Organic red wine or sake without sulfites (up to 10 oz per day)
    · Fermented foods (kefir, kimchi, tempeh, miso…)
  o Pure filtered water at ½ to 1 gallon per day
  o Raw unrefined sea salt in liberal amounts (1/8-1/2 tsp daily)
  o Supplements as needed (doses for adults):

- Vitamin D 5,000iu or more daily, often up to 10,000iu daily or 50,000iu twice per week. Use D3, cholecalciferol, only. Consider laboratory guidance.
- Iodine 5,000-12,500mcg daily, or possibly kelp
- Magnesium 500+mg, Zinc 25-50mg, Se 200-300mcg (totals) inclusive with a multi-mineral daily
- Toxin-free Fish oils with EPA totaling at least 800mg daily
- Possibly Folic acid (methylfolate preferred) 400mcg or more daily
- B complex vitamin (preferably with active forms of vitamins)
- Vitamin C 1,000mg or more daily
- Glutathione precursors (N-acetyl cysteine mainly – 600mg+ daily)
- Any others which seem necessary

- Exercise
  o Find something you enjoy if possible
  o You need to break a sweat and get your heart rate up
  o Do something to stimulate your muscles; not "cardio"
  o Try to get in 10-15 minutes of exercise every day
  o Try not to overdo it. Listen to your body. Stimulate muscle growth, but don't tear it down.
  o Interval training is best; try the P.A.C.E. program (Dr. Al Sears)
  o MAKE the time – don't wait to "find" the time

- Managing microorganisms
  o Practice good oral hygiene
    - Get a water pick and use it twice a day, after brushing
    - Consider iodine or silver in your water pick
  o Avoid prescription antibiotics unless they are truly necessary
    - Be sure to use them when serious infection is present
  o Maintain proper gut flora
    - Eat fermented foods with live bacterial cultures
    - Take a high-quality, broad spectrum probiotic regularly
    - Eat foods with healthy fibers that nourish the right

gut bacteria: bananas, tomatoes, Jerusalem artichoke, onions, chicory root and jicama
- o Keep your immune system strong
  - · Avoid toxins as much as possible
  - · Get adequate rest
  - · Control stress
  - · Take your vitamins (D especially, also A and C)
  - · Consider adaptogenic or tonic herbs for those with demanding lifestyles (see below)
- • Energetic wellness and controlling stress
  - o Positive thinking and visualization
  - o Avoid negative thinking and feelings toward self and others
  - o Mindfulness, meditation or prayer
  - o Energetic exercise (yoga, tai chi, qi gong)
  - o Mild to moderate physical exercise
  - o Play time
  - o Make time for yourself (take the time)
  - o Energy therapies (acupuncture, Reiki, bio-energetic machines)
- • Detoxification (an ongoing need for everyone)
  - o Avoiding toxins in the first place
    - · Eat and drink organic beverages and foods only
    - · Avoid all plastic containers for beverages or foods with a liquid component
    - · Avoid city water supplies, and test your well water. Filter water for drinking and cooking if needed. Consider filtering city water to your shower as well, if you are very sensitive to chemicals
    - · Phthalate-free cosmetics and personal care products
    - · Nontoxic home materials (tile or wood floors, granite or other solid material countertops, low-VOC paint...)
    - · Protective gear at work if there are toxic exposures
    - · Move away from metropolitan areas if possible, or at least away from the busiest traffic areas, factories, power plants, etc.
  - o Adequate nutrient intake (healthy whole-food diet)
  - o Super foods – get some every day (see list above)

- o Regular mild to moderate exercise (stimulates circulation, lymphatic drainage, sweating)
- o Sauna, Epsom salt baths or other "heat purification"
- o Consider milk thistle, marshmallow, dandelion and other herbs
- o Amino acids essential to detoxification:
  - · N-Acetyl Cysteine 600mg daily, or more
  - · Taurine 200mg daily, or more
  - · Glycine 200mg daily, or more
  - · Alpha-Lipoic Acid 150-300mg daily
  - · Clear yeast and balance gut flora before taking NAC or Taurine
- o B complex vitamins, Magnesium, Folate
- Changing the world
  - o It's everyone's job; don't just sit and wait for it to happen
  - o You have far more power than you realize; complacency results in movement further down the spiral
  - o Don't wait until half of all children born develop autism or other developmental disorders and half of healthy young adults are infertile, because by then it's too damn late
  - o Our government is clearly not taking steps to ensure the health of future generations or our planet – and don't expect the government to fix it
  - o Use the power of your dollar to "vote" every day about how you want things to be; buy organic foods and locally grown organic produce, products without harmful chemicals, recycled products, promote alternative energy and environmental safety
  - o Purchase items that travel the shortest distances - buy local whenever possible
  - o Reduce, reuse, recycle
  - o Spread awareness, starting with yourself

Part II – For Those With Problems

- Address everything above as best you can, especially personal stress
- Solving an illness problem
    - Try to make your diet perfect based on the principles above
        · Get junk or processed foods, sugar and excessive carbs out totally
        · Avoid all gluten and dairy strictly
        · Eat the super foods in larger amounts, every day
        · Drink plenty of clean water
            - Consider trying ionized alkaline water
        · Avoid alcohol and coffee. Green tea is okay as a source of caffeine
        · Avoid any unnecessary medications (prescription or OTC)
    - Take all appropriate supplements discussed above
        · Vitamin D, Iodine, Fish Oil, Magnesium, Vitamin C, B complex...
        · Amino acids for detox
        · Minerals (high-range zinc, selenium, magnesium)
    - Get adequate physical exercise
        · Ease into it if you are in poor health
    - Try to get enough sleep
        · Review the sleep hygiene issues
        · Melatonin, 5-HTP, GABA, Taurine, Theanine...
    - Pay more attention to your "energetic" needs
        · Positive visualization, mindfulness
        · Yoga, tai chi, qi gong
        · Pray, meditate, scrap book, socialize...
        · Get adequate time for yourself
        · Reduce stress as much as possible; take care of yourself
        · Consider bio-energetic analysis (Indigo Machine, others)
    - Consider or investigate possible infectious causes, or imbalances of your normal gut flora
        · Think about events prior to your symptoms and whether infection could have been a trigger or chronic presence

- Tick bites
- Acute illnesses
- Dental infections, gum disease
o Try some herbal and alternative remedies for possible infections:
  · Colloidal Silver
  · Olive Leaf extract, grapefruit seed extract, extra vitamin D for viruses
  · Wormwood (Artemesia) for intestinal worms
  · Neem for parasites
  · Various herbs for yeast (berberine, walnut, pau d'arco, caprylic acid, Oregon grape root, oregano...)
    - Don't forget you must also go completely off sugar and all grains!
    - Herbals may not be strong enough for some of you, so see if your primary care provider is willing to prescribe some nystatin and/or fluconazole, if you are not successful with herbals alone
o Take probiotics for decreased gut inflammation and overall improved immune system balance
  · Multiples different types of bacteria: Bifidus species, Lactobacillus species, Streptococcus species
  · At least 25 billion live organisms (cfu's) per day
  · Saccharomyces boulardii yeast
- Consider and self-investigate for environmental or allergic causes
  o Are your symptoms specific to certain places or exposures?
  o Are your symptoms still present when you go on vacation?
  o Do your symptoms occur only during certain times of the year?
  o Consider indoor airborne allergens
    · Pay attention to mold, dust, and animal exposures/reactions
    · Get a good air cleaner system
    · Remove old carpeting, cover mattresses and pillows
    · Remove any mold possible

- Vinegar and lemon juice (never use bleach), ozone
- o Consider food allergies
  - Keep a food and activity/location diary while tracking your symptoms every day
  - Try avoiding the most common allergenic foods for at least a few weeks
    - Wheat (all gluten-containing grains actually), dairy products, corn, soy and eggs
  - Consider getting food allergy/sensitivity testing
- o Consider chemical toxicity, sensitivity or allergy
  - Try avoiding all household and workplace chemicals for at least a couple weeks
    - Use an ozone generator (carefully) to decontaminate indoor environments (including your car)
  - Avoid all food-borne chemicals, additives, plastics…
    - Go to only organic, whole foods
  - Carefully review all possible side effects of any medications (prescription or OTC) you may be taking
    - Stop any non-essential medications, herbs, or other supplements
  - Follow all above recommendations on systemic detoxification
  - Consider heavy metals testing, of your water supply and your self
  - Test your house or workplace for carbon monoxide, radon, toxic molds, possibly EMF and other toxic entities
- If you suspect an autoimmune component to your illness symptoms, follow all the recommendations here and seek experienced consultation
- Consider hormonal deficiencies, imbalances (review the relevant chapters in section IV)
  - o Do you have symptoms of adrenal or thyroid deficiency?
    - Try herbal adaptogens or tonics:
      - Rhodiola
      - Siberian ginseng (eleutherococcus)
      - Ashwagandha

- Korean Ginseng
- Cordyceps
- Schizandra
- Maca
- Rhemannia

o Are symptoms consistent with androgen (testosterone, DHEA) deficiency?

o Are symptoms consistent with progesterone or estrogen deficiency? Estrogen/Progesterone imbalance?

o Are symptoms timed with your menstrual cycle?

o Did symptoms start after a major hormonal change like pregnancy or menopause, or appear gradually with aging?

o Seek the help of a practitioner with advanced training and experience in bio-identical hormone therapy

- Consider structural problems, especially if your symptoms involve localized or regional pain or physical dysfunction

o Find a good osteopathic or chiropractic practitioner

- Hyperbaric oxygen should be considered in certain instances; this is of particular concern if problems involve mental or cognitive function problems, behavioral or emotional problems of any sort.

o History of traumatic or stressful birth, with the possibility of low oxygen for more than a minute

o History of head trauma or repeated concussions

o History of near-drowning, carbon monoxide poisoning or other causes of asphyxia

o Drug poisoning affecting the brain, including illicit or prescription drugs, anesthesia during surgery

o Stroke

o Dementia

o Autism

o Seriously evaluate psychological and energetic factors

· Take a hard look at all of your personal and professional relationships

- · Look at your own views of yourself and your outlook on life
- · Pay special attention to psychological and energetic self-care
- · Look into mindfulness meditation, positive visualization
  - – Change the way you react to your world, if you can't change your world
- · Consider formal psychological counseling, spiritual consultation, or whatever else appeals to you in this area
- o If you get to this point and aren't better, you may need some additional help
- Seeking effective health care
  - o Feel free to do your own research all along as well
    - · Bring all your own ideas, the reasons why, and make sure your ideas are heard and considered
  - o Ask people you know and trust about good practitioners
  - o Find a practitioner with an integrative philosophy and practice style
  - o Make sure you are listened to and the plan makes sense to you
  - o Ask lots of questions – bring a list to every appointment
  - o Always bring a list of medications and supplements you are currently taking as well
  - o Form a collaborative relationship with your providers
    - · Don't let them take a paternalistic, dictatorial stance over you
    - · Make sure your concerns are addressed, and your ideas are respected
  - o Be actively engaged and proactive in your own care
  - o If you don't like a particular practitioner, find a different one
  - o See as many providers as you need – gather multiple opinions and sources of information and make your own decisions about health

o You may be stuck with a bad provider due to location or insurance rules; keep doing your own research and see if you can educate them in the process

o Do what you think is best even if your provider doesn't agree, if they can't really explain their opinion and convince you their plan is the best one

o Don't accept "because it isn't the standard of care" or "because I don't know anything about it and it's probably dangerous" or other biased philosophies like that

CLOSING REMARKS/EPILOGUE

This book has been admittedly long and dense, but hopefully not too ponderous to get through. It has taken me more than three years to write it with the limited and sporadic time I've had, but I feel it has been worth the effort because I think there is at least one useful insight for everyone.

Over the years it took me to write this book I myself learned a great deal more about health and healing, both through clinical practice and actively researching for the book. This forced me to repeatedly go back and add information to the book where appropriate or change something for which I had acquired a new understanding or opinion. This could have gone on potentially forever. Every time I looked for new current research there was something relevant just published within the recent few months.

It occurred to me I would never feel truly satisfied with this book and it was bound to have some misinformation in it no matter how hard I tried, because new information is always coming out. At some point I had to stop changing and adding content and decide I was finished. I have finally cut the umbilical cord and delivered it for you to read.

A key point to make here is you should not take anything in this book (or any other book on health and medicine) as gospel; I certainly don't mean to present my ideas as such. I came to realize long ago that I would never feel like I truly *knew* anything with certainty; and I have realized that attitude makes me a better healer. I try to avoid becoming so bound to my own beliefs, theories or ideas that I fail to hear what the individual in front of me is saying. I believe everyone else should do the same, especially other medical providers.

The points here are: "knowledge" in medicine will never be truly complete or correct, "opinion" is or at least should be a fluid concept if one continues to learn, "truth" is an extremely elusive quarry, what you *think* or *believe* should never be confused with the *truth*, and ideal health is an ever-moving target. It also means you should view yourself in a unique light; don't expect to respond the same as someone else did to any given therapy and don't believe you have the same problem as another person just because your symptoms sound similar.

Begin down the path toward solving your own health riddle and keep your eyes and ears open along the way. The most important thing is to treat everyone as an individual and pay far more attention to actual results and outcomes than to expectations and assumptions.

Remember that doctors and other health care practitioners are *human* and have the inherent faults of ego and narrow mindedness common to our species; they may have extreme biases and arrogance that can be a major barrier to your success. Get as many opinions and as much information about your health issues you need to make your choices; don't just take any doctor's or other practitioner's word for anything. Be proactive and strong; make sure your practitioners know they are working for *YOU*.

Medicine and health are truly consumer-driven industries. Use the power of your choices and your dollar to help move medical care in the right direction. Use your dollar to help move the food industry, auto industry, tech industries and chemical industries toward a safer and healthier environment for you and all our generations to come.

Lastly, if you meet me at some point and ask me something, don't be too surprised if I give you a different answer than this book provided. I am a different practitioner and healer every year, hopefully a better one.

References

Abdel-Fattah, K., et al – <u>Serum pattern of thyroxine (T4), 3,3',5-triiodothyronine (T3) and 3,3',5'-triiodothyronine (rT3) in fed and fasted cocks following TRH stimulation</u> – *Zentralblatt fur Veterinarmedizin* – July 1991;38(6):401-8

Abegaz, E. and Bursey, R. – <u>Formaldehyde, aspartame, migraines: a possible connection</u> – *Dermatitis* – May-June 2009;20(3):176-7

Abol-Enein, H., et al. – <u>Ionized alkaline water: new strategy for management of metabolic acidosis in experimental animals</u> – *Therapeutic Apheresis and Dialysis* – June 2009;13(3):220-4

Abramson, J. – *Overdosed America: The Broken Promises of American Medicine* – HarperCollins Publishers Inc., New York – 2004

Adams, S., et al. – <u>Dietary cadmium and risk of invasive postmenopausal breast cancer in the VITAL cohort</u> – *Cancer Causes Control* – April 20, 2012 (Epub ahead of print)

Akinbami, L., et al. – <u>Trends in athma prevalance, health care use, and mortality in the United States, 2001-2010</u> – *NCHS Data Brief* – May 2012;(94):1-8

Albizzati, A., et al. – Normal concentrations of heavy metals in autistic specrum disorders – *Minerva Pediatrica* – February 2012;64(1):27-31

Albrecht, T. and Taylor, A. – Physical activity in patients with advanced-stage cancer: a systematic review of the literature – *Clinical Journal of Oncology Nursing* – June 1, 2012;16(3):293-300

Alonso-Magdalena, P. – Endocrine disruptors in the etiology of type 2 diabetes mellitus – *Nature Reviews: Endocrinology* – June 2011; 7(6):346-53

American Academy of Pediatrics Committee on Environmental Health Policy Statement – *Toxic Effects of Indoor Molds (RE9736)* – American Academy of Pediatrics - 1998

Anandan, C., et al. – Omega 3 and 6 oils for primary prevention of allergic disease: systematic review and meta-analysis – *Allergy* – June 2009;64(6):840-8

Anderson, J.L., et al. – Relation of vitamin D deficiency to cardiovascular risk factors, disease status, and incident events in a general healthcare population – *American Journal of Cardiology* – October 1, 2010;106(7):963-8

Andriankaja, O., et al. – Association between periodontal pathogens and risk of nonfatal myocardial infarction – *Community Dental and Oral Epidemiology* – April 2011; 39(2):177-85

Angell, M. – Former editor in chief of the New England Journal of Medicine – November 26, 2002 interview on *Frontline*, PBS network – interview available at www.pbs.org/wgbh/pages/frontline/shows/other/interviews/angell.html

Annesi, J. and Vaughn, L. – Relationship of exercise volume with change in depression and its association with self-efficacy to control emotional eating in severely obese women – *Advances in Preventive Medicine* – March 14, 2011 (epub);2011:514271

Antoniades, C., et al. – <u>MTHFR 677 C>T Polymorphism reveals functional importance for 5-methyltetrahydrofolate, not homocysteine, in regulation of vascular redox state and endothelial function in human atherosclerosis</u> – *Circulation* – May 12, 2009;119(18):2507-15

Antonsson, A., et al. – <u>Prevalence and stability of antibodies to the BK and JC polyomaviruses: a long term longitudinal study of Australians</u> –*The Journal of General Virology* – July 2010;91(Pt 7):1849-53

Alderman, M, et al. – *Lancet* – 351:781-778, 1998 – cited information on sodium consumption and mortality – presentation of Dr. Stephen Hoption-Cann; IFM spring 2007 conference

Arnst, C. – <u>Study Links Medical Costs and Personal Bankruptcy</u> – *Bloomberg Businessweek* (online journal) – ePublished June 4, 2009

Arshi, S., et al. – <u>Vitamin D serum levels in alleric rhinitis: any difference from the normal population?</u> – *Asia Pacific Allergy* – January 2012;2(1):45-8

Asensi, M, et al. – <u>Inhibition of cancer growth by resveratrol is related to its low bioavailability</u> – *Free Radical Biology and Medicine* – August 2002;33(3):387-98

Aslanyan, G., et al. – <u>Double-blind, placebo-controlled, randomised study of single dose effects of ADAPT-232 on cognitive functions</u> – *Phytomedicine* – June 2010;17(7):494-9

Backes, J.M., et al – <u>Effects of once weekly rosuvastatin among patients with a prior statin intolerance</u> – *American Journal of Cardiology* – August 1, 2007;100(3):554-5

Bager, P., et al. – <u>Symptoms after ingestion of pig whipworm Trichuris suis eggs in a randomized placebo-controlled double-blind clinical trial</u> – *PloS One* – 2011;6(8):e22346

Baggerly, L., et al. – <u>Vitamin D and pancreatic cancer risk – no U-shaped curve</u> – *Anticancer Research* – March 2012;32(3):981-4

Bahceciler, N. and Cobanoglu, N. – <u>Subcutaneous versus sublingual immunotherapy for allergic rhinitis and/or asthma</u> – *Immunotherapy* – June 2011;3(6):747-56

Bain, J. – <u>Testosterone and the aging male: to treat or not to treat?</u> – *Maturitas* – May 2010;66(1):16-22

Ballard-Barbash, R., et al. – <u>Physical activity, biomarkers, and disease outcomes in cancer survivors: a systematic review</u> – *Journal of the National Cancer Institute* – June 6, 2012;104(11):815-40

Baral, V., et al. – <u>Colloidal silver for lung disease in cystic fibrosis</u> – *Journal of the Royal Society of Medicine* – July 2008;101 Supplement 1:S51-2

Barnes, B. and Galton, L. – *Hypothyroidism: The Unsuspected Illness* – Copyright 1976 by Broda Barnes and Lawrence Galton; also published in Toronto, Canada by Fitzhenry & Whiteside Limited

Barr, L., et al. – <u>Measurement of paraben concentrations in human breast tissue at serial locations across the breast from axilla to sternum</u> – *Journal of Applied Toxicology* – March 2012;32(3):219-32

Barrager, E., et al. – <u>A multicentered, open-label trial on the safety and efficacy of methylsulfonylmethane in the treatment of seasonal allergic rhinitis</u> – *Journal of Alternative and Complementary Medicine* – April 2002;8(2):167-73

Basnet, P. and Skalko-Basnet, N. – <u>Curcumin: an anti-inflammatory molecule from a curry spice on the path to cancer treatment</u> – *Molecules* – June 3, 2011;16(6):4567-98

Baur, J., et al. – <u>Resveratol improves health and survival of mice on a high-calorie diet</u> – *Nature* – November 2006;444(7117):337-42

Bazile, A., et al. – Periodontal assessment of patients undergoing angioplasty for treatment of coronary artery disease – *Journal of Periodontology* – June 2002;73(6):631-6

Bergkvist, C., et al. – Occurrence and levels of organochlorine compounds in human breast milk in Bangladesh – *Chemosphere* – April 30, 2012 (Epub ahead of print)

Bertoglio, K., et al. – Pilot study of the effect of methyl B12 treatment on behavioral and biomarker measures in children with autism – *Journal of Alternative and Complementary Medicine* – May 2010;16(5):555-60

Bisht, S. and Maltra, A. – Systemic delivery of curcumin: 21st century solutions for an ancient conundrum – *Current Drug Discovery Technologies* – September 2009;6(3):192-9

Bixquert-Jimenez, M. – Treatment of irritable bowel syndrome with probiotics. An etiopathogenic approach at last? – *Revista de Espanola Enfermedades Digestivas* (Spain) – August 2009;101(8):553-64

Bjuresten, K., et al. – Luteal phase progesterone increases live birth rate after frozen embryo transfer – *Fertility and Sterility* – February 2011;95(2):534-7

Bland, J., et al. – *Clinical Nutrition: A Functional Approach* – Institute for Functional Medicine – 1999 (2nd edition revised in 2004)

Blum, A. – When "More doctors smoked Camels" Cigarette advertising in the journal – *Social Medicine* – Vol 5, No 2 (2010)

Boggs, D., et al. – Fruit and vegetable intake in relation to risk of breast cancer in the Black Women's Health Study – *American Journal of Epidemiology* – December 1, 2010;172(11):1268-79

Bolton, P. and Budgell, B. – Visceral responses to spinal manipulation –

Journal of Electromyography and Kinesiology – March 20, 2012 (Epub ahead of print)

Bonefeld-Jorgensen, E., et al. – <u>Perfluorinated compounds are related to breast cancer risk in Greenlandic Inuit: a case control study</u> – *Environmental Health* – October 6, 2011;10:88

Bosch, B., et al. – <u>Human chorionic gonadotropin and weight loss. A double-blind, placebo-controlled trial</u> – *South African Medical Journal* – Februar 17, 1990;77(4):185-9

Bosso, J.A. and Drew, R.H. – <u>Application of antimicrobial stewardship to optimise management of community acquired pneumonia</u> –*International Journal Clinical Practice* – July 2011; 65(7): 775-83

Bouchard, M., et al. – <u>Attention-deficit/hyperactivity disorder and urinary metabolites of organophosphate pesticides</u> – *Pediatrics* – June 2010;125(6):e1270-7

Brasky, T., et al. – <u>Non-steroidal anti-inflammatory drugs and small cell lung cancer risk in the VITAL study</u> – *Lung Cancer* – May 16, 2012 (Epub ahead of print)

Broder, K. – <u>Growing Controversy over Use of Medtronic's Infuse for Bones</u> – Article on www.allgov.com - June 30, 2011

Brown, D. – <u>Life expectancy in the U.S. varies widely by region, in some places is decreasing</u> – *The Washington Post National* – June 14, 2011

Brown, R., et al – <u>Artificial sweeteners: a systematic review of metabolic effects in youth</u> – *International Journal of Pediatric Obesity* – August 2010;5(4):305-12

Brownstein, D. – *Iodine: Why You Need It, Why You Can't Live Without It* – Medical Alternatives Press – Michigan - 2004

Brownstein, D. – *Overcoming Arthritis* – Medical Alternatives Press – Michigan - 2001

Brownstein, D. - *Salt Your Way to Health* – Medical Alternatives Press – Michigan - 2006

Bush, R., et al. – <u>Prevalence of sensitivity to sulfiting agents in asthmatic patients</u> – *The American Journal of Medicine* – November 1986;81(5):816-20

Bywater, R. – <u>Identification and surveillance of antimicrobial resistance dissemination in animal production</u> – *Poultry Science* – April 2005;84(4):644-8

Cain, A. and Karpa, K. – <u>Clinical utility of probiotics in inflammatory bowel disease</u> – *Alternative Therapies in Health and Medicine* – January-February 2011;17(1):72-9

Calvey, H., et al. – <u>A new prognostic index in surgery and parenteral feeding: the ratio of T3 and reverse T3 in serum</u> – *Clinical Nutrition* – August 1986;5(3):145-9

Campbell, T.C. – *The China Study: The Most Comprehensive Study of Nutrition Ever Conducted* – BenBella Books – Dallas, TX - 2006

Cani, P. and Delzenne, N. – <u>The role of the gut microbiota in energy metabolism and metabolic disease</u> – *Current Pharmaceutical Design* – 2009;15(13):1546-58

Cannon, S., et al. – <u>Epidemic kepone poisoning in chemical workers</u> – *American Journal of Epidemiology* – June 1978;107(6):529-37

Carek, P., et al. – <u>Exercise for the treatment of depression and anxiety</u> – *International Journal of Psychiatry in Medicine* – 2011;41(1):15-28

Caress, S. and Steinemann, A. – <u>A review of a two-phase population study</u>

of multiple chemical sensitivities – *Environmental Health Perspective* – September 2003;111(12):1490-7

Castanon-Cervantes, O., et al. – Dysregulation of inflammatory responses by chronic circadian disruption – *Journal of Immunology* – November 15, 2010;185(10):5796-805

Castro-Costa, E., et al. – Association between sleep duration and all-cause mortality in old age: 9-year follow-up of the Bambui Cohort Study, Brazil – *Journal of Sleep Research* – June 2011;20(2):303-10

Catling, L.A., et al. – A systematic review of analytical observational studies investigating the association between cardiovascular disease and drinking water hardness – *Journal of Water Health* – December 2008;6(4):433-42

Cattabiani, C., et al. – Relationship between testosterone deficiency and cardiovascular risk and mortality in adult men – *Journal of Endocrinological Investigation* – January 2012;35(1):104-20

Centre for Clinical Practice at NICE (National Institute for Health and Clinical Excellence – UK) – Respiratory Tract Infections – Antibiotic Prescribing: Prescribing of Antibiotics for Self-Limiting Respiratory Tract Infections in Adults and Children in Primary Care – July 2008

Cesarone, M., et al. – Prevention of venous thrombosis in long-haul flights with Flite Tabs: the LONFLITE-FLITE randomized, controlled trial – *Angiology* – September-October 2003;54(5):531-9

Chamie, K., et al. – Agent Orange exposure, Vietnam War veterans, and the risk of prostate cancer – *Cancer* – November 1, 2008;113(9):2464-70

Chan, J., et al. – Water, other fluids, and fatal coronary heart disease: The Adventist Health Study – *American Journal of Epidemiology* – February 2002;155(9):827-33

Chang, A., et al. – Tai chi Qigong improves lung functions and activity tolerance in COPD clients: a single blind, randomized controlled trial – *Complementary Therapies in Medicine* – February 2011;19(1):3-11

Chang, C., et al. – Cancer risk associated with insulin glargine among adult type 2 diabetes patients – a nationwide cohort study (Taiwan) – *PloS One* – 2011;6(6):e21368

Chelleng, P., et al. – Risk factors for cancer of the nasopharynx: a case-control study from Nagaland, India – *National Medical Journal of India* – Jan-Feb 2000;13(1):6-8

Chen, P., et al. – Pharmacological ascorbate induces cytotoxicity in prostate cancer cells through ATP depletion and induction of autophagy – *Anticancer Drugs* – April 2012;23(4):437-44

Christiani, D. – Combating Environmental Causes of Cancer – *New England Journal of Medicine* – March 3, 2011; 364:791-793

Clair, E., et al. – A glyphosate-based herbicide induces necrosis and apoptosis in mature rat testicular cells in vitro, and testosterone decrease at lower levels – *Toxicology In Vitro* – March 2012;26(2):269-79

Claus, E., et al. – Dental x-rays and risk of meningioma – *Cancer* – April 10, 2012 (Epub ahead of print)

Cohen, H., et al. – *American Journal of Medicine* – 2006; 119:275 - cited information on sodium consumption and mortality – presentation of Dr. Stephen Hoption-Cann; IFM spring 2007 conference

Cohen, M. and Bendich, A. – Safety of pyridoxine – a review of human and animal studies – *Toxicology Letter* – December 1986; 34(2-3):129-39

Colborn, T., et al. – *Our Stolen Future* – Penguin Books – New York – 1997

Compare, D., et al. – Risk factors in gastric cancer – *European Review for Medical and Pharmacological Sciences* – April 2010;14(4):302-8

Connett, P. – *The Case Against Fluoride* – Chelsea Green Publishing Company – Vermont – 2010

Cooke, M. – American Medical Education 100 Years after the Flexner Report – *New England Journal of Medicine* - vol 355; 9-28-2006

Cordain, L. – *The Paleo Diet: Lose Weight and Get Healthy by Eating the Foods You Were Designed to Eat* – John Wiley & Sons, Inc. – Hoboken, NJ – 2002 S-III, p 19

Correa, D., et al. – Antigens and antibodies in sera from human cases of epilepsy or taeniasis from an area of Mexido where Taenia solium cysticercosis is endemic – *Annals of Tropical Medicine and Parasitology* – January 1999;93(1):69-74

Cowan, L., et al. – Secular trends in the prevalence of HIV infection among a population of males with hemophilia, 1988-1997: the Oklahoma Hemophilia Surveillance System – *Journal of the Oklahoma State Medical Association* – September 1999;92(9):462-7

Crinnion, W. – Chlorinated pesticides: Threats to health and importance of detection – *Alternative Medicine Review* – 2009: vol 14, #4

Cudowski, B. and Kaczmarski, M. – Atopy patch test in the diagnosis of food allergy in children with atopic eczema dermatitis syndrome – *Roczniki Akademii Medycznej w Bialymstoku* (Polish) – 2005;50:261-7

Damyanov, C., et al. – Low-dose chemotherapy with insulin (insulin potentiation therapy) in combination with hormone therapy for treatment of castration-resistant prostate cancer – *ISRN Urology* (Bulgaria) – May 8, 2012 (Epub)

Darnall, B., et al. – Pilot study of inflammatory responses following a negative imaginal focus in persons with chronic pain: analysis by sex/ gender – *Gender Medicine* – June 2010;7(3):247-60

De Benoist, B., et al. – Prevalence of iodine deficiency worldwide – *The Lancet* – November 29, 2003;362(9398):1859-60

Del Razo, L., et al. – Exposure to arsenic in drinking water is associated with increased prevalence of diabetes: a cross-sectional study in the Zimapan and Lagunera regions in Mexico – *Environment and Health* – August 24, 2011;10:73

Demoor-Goldschmidt, C., et al. - Breast cancer after radiotherapy: Risk factors and suggestion for breast delineation as an organ at risk in the prepubertal girl – *Cancer Radiotherapy* – April 2012;16(2):140-51

DeNoon, D. – Does Fluoridation Up Bone Cancer Risk? – *WebMD Health News* – April 6, 2006 - (Original research study reviewed was the doctoral thesis of Elise Bassin, DDS completed in 2001)

Derry, D. – *Breast Cancer and Iodine* – Trafford Publishing - 2001

Dhawan, K. and Sharma, A. – Prevention of chronic alcohol and nicotine-induced azospermia, sterility and decreased libido, by a novel tri-substituted benzoflavone moiety from Passiflora incarnata Linnaeus in healthy male rats – *Life Science* – November 15, 2002;71(26):3059-69

Dinan, T. and Cryan, J. – Regulation of the stress response by the gut microbiota: implications for psychoneuroendocrinology – *Psychoneuroendocrinology* – April 4, 2012 (Epub ahead of print)

Dong, J. and Qin, L. – Soy isoflavones consumption and risk of breast cancer incidence or recurrence: a meta-analysis of prospective studies – *Breast Cancer Research and Treatment* – January 2011;125(2):315-23

Drinkard, J. – <u>Drugmakers go furthest to sway Congress</u> – *USA Today* – 4/25/2005, post on www.usatoday.com

Duggal, J., et al. – <u>Effect of niacin therapy on cardiovascular outcomes in patients with coronary artery disease</u> – *Journal of Cardiovascular Pharmacology and Therapeutics* – June 2010;15(2):158-66

Elhkim, M., et al. – <u>New considerations regarding the risk assessment on Tartrazine: An update on toxicological assessment, intolerance reactions and maximum theoretical daily intake in France</u> – *Regulatory Toxicology and Pharmacology* – April 2007;47(3):308-16

Eliason, A., et al. – <u>Urinary estrogens and estrogen metabolites and subsequent risk of breast cancer among premenopausal women</u> – *Cancer Research* – February 1, 2010;72(3):696-706

Elliott, P. and Jirousek, M. – <u>Sirtuins: novel targets for metabolic disease</u> – *Current Opinion in Investigational Drugs* – April 2008;9(4):371-8

Eltholth, M., et al. – <u>Contamination of food products with Mycobacterium avium subspecies paratuberculosis: a systematic review</u> – *Journal of Applied Microbiology* – October 2009;107(4):1061-71

Emoto, M. – *The Hidden Messages in Water* – Simon & Schuster - 2005

Engdahl, W. – *Seeds of Destruction: The Hidden Agenda of Genetic Manipulation* – Global Research - 2007

Ertugrul, D., et al – <u>STATIN-D Study: Comparison of the influences of Rosuvastatin and Fluvastatin Treatmet on the Levels of 25 Hydroxyvitamin D</u> – *Cardiovascular Therapy* – March 27, 2010

Ezzati, M, et al – <u>The Reversal of Fortunes: Trends in County Mortality and Cross-County Mortality Disparities in the United States</u> – *PloS Medicine* – April 22, 2008 – PloS Med 5(4): e66

Fallon, S. – *Nourishing Traditions* – NewTrends Publishing – Washington, D.C. – 1999

Fallon, S. and Enig, M. – *The Ploy of Soy* – Weston Price Foundation – September 27, 1995

FDA Consumer Magazine (no specific author named) – Study Shows St. John's Wort Ineffective for Severe Depression– May-June 2002; 36(3):8

Fielding, J., et al. – Increases in plasma lycopene concentration after consumption of tomatoes cooked with olive oil – *Asia Pacific Journal of Clinical Nutrition* – 2005;14(2):131-6

Fleet, J.C. – Dietary selenium repletion may reduce cancer incidence in people at high risk who live in areas with low soil selenium – *Nutrition Review* – July, 1997;55(7):277-9

Flueckiger, J., et al. – Microfabricated formaldehyde gas sensors – *Sensors* (Basel, Switzerland) – 2009;9(11):9196-215

Fox, R., et al. – Intradermal testing for food and chemical sensitivities: a double-blind controlled study – *Journal of Allergy and Clinical Immunology* – May 1999;103(5 Pt 1):907-11

Frikke-Schmidt, H. and Lykkesfeldt, J. – Role of marginal vitamin C deficiency in atherogenesis: in vivo models and clinical studies – *Basic and Clinical Pharmacology and Toxicology* – June 2009; 104(6):419-33

Fu, S. and Kurzrock, R. – Development of curcumin as an epigenetic agent – *Cancer* – October 15, 2010;116(20):4670-6

Fujiki, H. and Suganuma, M. – Green tea: An effective synergist with anticancer drugs for tertiary cancer prevention – *Cancer Letter* – May 21, 2012 (Epub ahead of print)

Gal-Tanamy, M., et al. – <u>Vitamin D: an innate antiviral agent suppressing hepatitis C virus in human hepatocytes</u> – *Hepatology* – November 2011;54(5):1570-9

Gallicchio, L. and Kalesan, B. – <u>Sleep duration and mortality: a systematic review and meta-analysis</u> – *Journal of Sleep Research* – June 2009;18(2):148-58

Gammon, C. – <u>Weed-Whacking Herbicie Proves Deadly to Human Cells</u> – *Scientific American* – June 23, 2009

Gardener, H., et al – <u>Mediterranean-style diet and risk of ischemic stroke, myocardial infarction, and vascular death: the Northern Manhattan Study</u> – *American Journal of Clinical Nutrition* – November 9, 2011

Gellad, W., et al – <u>What if the Federal Government Negotiated Pharmaceutical Prices for Seniors? An Estimate of National Savings</u> – *Journal of General Internal Medicine* – Sept 2008; 23(9): 1435-40

Genuis, S. – <u>Elimination of persistent toxicant from the human body</u> – *Human and Experimental Toxicology* – January 2011;30(1):3-18

Genuis, S. – <u>Human Detoxification of Perfluorinated Compounds</u> – *Public Health* – July 2010;124(7):367-75

George, O., et al. – <u>Neurosteroids and cholincergic systems: implications for sleep and cognitive processes and potential role of age-related changes</u> – *Psychopharmacology (Berlin)* – June 2006;186(3):402-13

Gerber, R. – *Vibrational Medicine* – Bear & Company - 2001

Gilbert, R., et al. – <u>Predictors of 25-hydroxyvitamin D and its association with risk factors for prostate cancer: evidence from the Prostate Testing for Cancer and Treatment Study</u> – *Cancer Causes and Control* – April 2012;23(4):575-88

Glerach, G., et al. – Coffee intake and breast cancer risk in the NIH-AARP diet and health study cohort – *International Journal of Cancer* – August 16, 2011

Goralczyk, R – Beta-carotene and lung cancer in smokers: review of hypotheses and status of research – *Nutrition and Cancer* – 2009; 61(6): 767-74

Gove, W. – Sleep deprivation: a cause of psychotic disorganization – *American Journal of Sociology* – March 1970;75(5):782-99

Govett, G., et al. – Chlorinated pesticides and cancer of the head and neck: a retrospective case series – *European Journal of Cancer Prevention* – July 2011;20(4):320-5

Gracely, R., et al. – Clinicians' expectations influence placebo analgesia – *Lancet* – January 5, 1985;1(8419):43

Grandjean, P., et al. – Serum vaccine antibody concentrations in chilren exposed to perfluorinated compounds – *JAMA* – January 25, 2012;307(4):391-7

Grant, W. – An ecological study of cancer incidence and mortality rates in France with respect to latitude, an index for vitamin D production – *Dermatoendocrinology* – April 2010;2(2):62-7

Greenway, F. and Bray, G. – Human chorionic gonadotropin (HCG) in the treatment of obesity: a critical assessment of the Simeons method – *The Western Journal of Medicine* – December 1977;127(6):461-3

Grigor'ev, IuG. – [The probability of developing brain tumours among users of cellular telephones (scientific information to the decision of the International Agency for Research on Cancer (IARC) announced on May 31, 2011)] (Russian) – *Radiatsionnaia Biologiia, Radioecologiia* – Sept-Oct;51(5):633-8

Grimes, D.S. – Are statins analogues of vitamin D? – *Lancet* – July 1, 2006;368(9529):83-6

Groff, J. – *Advanced Nutrition and Human Metabolism, Third Edition* – Wadsworth/Thomson Learning – Belmont, CA – 2000

Guarda-Nardini, L., et al. - Myofascial pain of the jaw muscles: comparison of short-term effectiveness of botulinum toxin injections and fascial manipulation technique – *Cranio* – April 2012;30(2):95-102

Gunturu, K., et al. – Ayurvedic herbal medicine and lead poisoning – *Journal of Hematology and Oncology* – December 20, 2011;4:51

Guo, Y., et al. – Phthalate metabolites in urine from China, and implications for human exposures – *Environment International* – July 2011;37(5):893-8

Hallmann, E. – The influence of organic and conventional cultivation systems on the nutritional value and content of bioactive compounds in selected tomato types – *Journal of the Science of Food and Agriculture* – February 20, 2012 (Epub)

Harch, P. – *The Oxygen Revolution* – Hatherleigh Press – New York – 2007

Hardell, L., et al. – Long-term use of cellular phones and brain tumours: increased risk associated with use for > or = 10 years – *Occupational and Environmental Medicine* – September 2007;64(9):626-32

Harrabin, R. – China building more power plants – *BBC News* – Tuesday, June 19, 2007

Harrison, R. and Page, J. – Multipractitioner Upledger CranioSacral Therapy: descriptive outcome study 2007-2008 – *Journal of Alternative and Complementary Medicine* – January 2011;17(1):13-7

Havas, M. and Olstad, A. – Power quality affects teacher wellbeing and student behavior in three Minnesota schools – *The Science of the Total Environment* – September 1, 2008;402(2-3):157-62

Heidari, B., et al. – Association between nonspecific skeletal pain and vitamin D deficiency – *International Journal of Rheumatic Diseases* – October 2010;13(4):340-6

Hemmingsen, B., et al. – Intensive glycemic control for patients with type 2 diabetes: systematic review with meta-analysis and trial sequential analysis of randomised clinical trials – *British Medical Journal* – November 24, 2011;343:d6898

Hendler, S. (chief editor) – *PDR For Nutritional Supplements* – Thomson PDR – Montvale, NJ – 2001

Hewison, M. – Vitamin D and immune function: autocrine, paracrine or endocrine? – *Scandinavian Journal of Clinical and Laboratory Investigation, Supplementum* – April 2012;243:92-102

Hitchcock, S. – *Geography of Religion* – National Geographic Society – Washington, D.C. - 2004

Hites, R., et al. – Global assessment of organic contaminants in farmed salmon – *Science* – 2004; 303, p226-229.

Hoffman, C., et al. – Effectiveness of mindfulness-based stress reduction in mood, breast- and endocrine-related quality of life, and well-being in stage 0 to III breast cancer: a randomized, controlled trial – *Journla of Clinical Oncology* – April 20, 2012;30(12):1335-42

Hoifodt, R., et al. – Effectiveness of cognitive behavioural therapy in primary health care: a review – *Family Practice* – October 2011;28(5):489-504

Holloway, E., et al. – Diagnosing and managing food allergy in children – *Practitioner* – June 2011;255(1741):19-22

Holmberg, I., et al. – 25-Hydroxylase activity in subcellular fractions from human liver. Evidence for the different rates of mitchondrial hydroxylation of vitamin D2 and D3 – *Scandinavian Journal of Clinical and Laboratory Investigation* – December 1986;46(8):785-90

Holmes, H. – *The Well-Dressed Ape* – Random House – New York - 2008

Holohan, C., et al. – Wine consumption and 20-year mortality among late-life moderate drinkers – *Journal on Studies of Alcohol and Drugs* – January 2012;73(1):80-8

Holohan, C., et al. – Late-life alcohol consumption and 20-year mortality – *Alcoholism, Clinical Experience and Research* – November 2010;34(11):1961-71

Holy, J. – Chlorpropham [isopropyl N-(3-chlorophenyl) carbamate] disrupts microtubule organization, cell division, and early development of sea urchin embryos – *Journal of Toxicology and Environmental Health* – June 26, 1998;54(4):319-33

Hong, P. and Li, J. – Lack of evidence for a role of xenotropic murine leukemia virus-relate virus in the pathogenesis of prostate cancer and/or chronic fatigue syndrome – *Virus Research* – July 2012;167(1):1-7

Hoption-Cann, S. – lecture at the spring 2007 IFM (Institute for Functional Medicine) conference, symposium on thyroid and adrenal disorders

Houssen, M., et al. – Natural anti-inflammatory products and leukotriene inhibitors as complementary therapy for bronchial asthma – *Clinical Biochemistry* – July 2010;43(10-11):887-90

Hyman, M. – *Ultrametabolism* – Atria Books – New York - March 2008

Hypericum Depression Trial Study Group – <u>Effect of Hypericum perforatum (St. John's wort) in major depressive disorder: a randomized controlled trial</u> – *JAMA* – April 10, 2002; 287(14): 1807-14

Ikeda, Y., et al. – <u>Intake of fermented soybeans, natto, is associated with reduced bone loss in postmenopausal women: Japanese Population-Based Osteoporosis (JPOS) Study</u> – *The Journal of Nutrition* – May 2006;136(5):1323-8

Janssen, S. (MD, PhD, MPH) – staff scientist for the National Resources Defense Council, associate clinical professor for the University of California, San Francisco - March 2010 presentation in Girdwood, Alaska for the Alaska Academy of Family Physicians

Jarvis, D.C. – *Folk Medicine* – Fawcett Crest - 1985

Jeffries, W.M. – *Safe Uses of Cortisol* – Charles C. Thomas Publisher, Ltd. - 1996

Jepson, B. – *Changing the Course of Autism: A Scientific Approach for Parents and Physicians* – Sentient Publications – Boulder, CO – 2007

Jett, D. – <u>Neurotoxic pesticides and neurologic effects</u> – *Neurology Clinics* – August 2011;29(3):667-77

Jin, Y. – <u>3,3'-Diindolylmethane inhibits breast cancer cell growth via miR-21-mediated Cdc25A degradation</u> – *Molecular and Cellular Biochemistry* – December 2011;358(1-2):345-54

Johnson, S., et al. – <u>Diminished Use of Osteopathic Manipulative Treatment and its Impact on the Uniqueness of the Osteopathic Profession</u> – *Academic Medicine* – 2001 – 76 (8): 821-8

Jones, David (editor) – *Textbook of Functional Medicine* – Institute for Functional Medicine – Gig Harbor, WA - 2005

Joshi, A., et al. – Fish intake, cooking practices, and risk of prostate cancer: results from a multi-ethnic case-control study – *Cancer Causes and Control* – March 2012;23(3):405-20

Julin, B., et al. – Dietary cadmium exposure and risk of postmenopausal breast cancer: a population-based prospective cohort study – *Cancer Research* – March 15, 2012;72(6):1459-66

Kalliomaki, M., et a. – Probiotics in primary prevention of atopic disease: a randomised placebo-controlled trial – *Lancet* – April 7, 2001;357(9262):1076-9

Katan, M. – [How much vitamin B6 is toxic?] (Dutch) – *Nederlands Tijdschrift voor Geneeskunde* – November 12, 2005;149(46):2545-6

Kelkel, M., et al. – Antioxidant and anti-proliferative properties of lycopene – *Free Radical Research* – August 2011;45(8):925-40

Kemnitz, J. – Calorie restriction and aging in nonhuman primates – *Institute of Laboratory Animal Resources Journal* – February 8, 2011;52(1):66-77

Kew, M. – Hepatocellular carcinoma in developing countries: Prevention, diagnosis and treatment – *World Journal of Hepatology* – March 27, 2012;4(3):99-104

Khoo, A., et al. – Translating the role of vitamin D(3) in infectious diseases – *Critical Reviews in Microbiology* – February 5, 2012 (Epub ahead of print)

Khosro, S., et al. – Night work and inflammatory markers – *Indian Journal of Occupational and Environmental Medicine* – January 2011;15(1):38-41

Kim, J., et al., - Fermented and non-fermented soy food consumption and gastric cancer in Japanese and Korean populations: a meta-analysis of observational studies – *Cancer Science* – January 2011;102(1):231-44

Kim, L., et al. – Treatment of seasonal allergic rhinitis using homeopathic preparation of common allergens in the southwest region of the US: a randomized, controlled clinical trial – *The Annals of Pharmacotherapy* – April 2005;39(4):617-24

King, M.C. – Quoted by Dr. Jeffrey Bland at the Institute for Functional Medicine cancer conference, May 2010 – article in *Science* - 2003; 302:643-50

Kingsolver, B. – *Animal, Vegetable, Miracle* – HarperCollins Publishers – 2007

Klanicova, B., et al. – Mycobacterium avium subsp. paratuberculosis survival during fermentation of soured milk products detected by culture and quantitative real time PCR methods – *International Journal of Food Microbiology* – May 1, 2012 (Epub ahead of print)

Koh, E., et al. – Effect of organic and conventional cropping systems on ascorbic acid, vitamin C, flavonoids, nitrate and oxalate in 27 varieties of spinach – *Journal of Agricultural and Food Chemistry* – March 28, 2012;60(12):3144-50

Koninkx, J. and Malago, J. – The protective potency of probiotic bacteria and their microbial products against enteric infections-review – *Folia Microbiologica* – 2008;53(3):189-94

Kosiewicz, M., et al. – Gut microbiota, immunity, and disease: a complex relationship – *Frontiers in Microbiology* – 2011;2:180

Kotecha, D., et al. – Five-minute heart rate variability can predict obstructive angiographic coronary disease – *Heart* – March 2012;98(5):395-401

Kramer, M. – <u>Sleep loss in resident physicians: the cause of medical errors?</u> – *Frontiers in Neurology* – October 20, 2010;1:128

Kulis, M., et al. – <u>Pioneering immunotherapy for food allergy: clinical outcomes and modulation of the immune response</u> – *Immunology Research* – April 2011;49(1-3):216-26

Kuntsevich, V., et al. – <u>Mechanisms of yogic practices in health, aging, and disease</u> – *Mount Sinai Journal of Medicine* – Sept-Oct 2010;77(5):559-69

Kushi, L.H., et al. – <u>Health implications of Mediterranean diets in light of contemporary knowledge</u> – *American Journal of Clinical Nutrition* – June 1995; 61(6 Suppl): 1407S-1415S

Kuznik, F. – <u>Spider plants and clean air</u> – *National Wildlife Federation* (online reference) – June 1, 1999

Lai, C.C., et al. – <u>Correlation between antimicrobial consumption and resistance among Staphylococcus aureus and enterococci causing healthcare-associated infections at a university hospital in Taiwan from 2000 to 2009</u> – *European Journal of Clinical Microbiology and Infectious Disease* – February 2011; 30(2): 265-71

Lansdown, A. – <u>Silver in health care: antimicrobial effects and safety in use</u> – *Current Problems in Dermatology* – 2006;33:17-34

Laura, A., et al. – <u>Vitamin D2 is much less effective than vitamin D3 in humans</u> – *The Journal of Clinical Endocrinology and Metabolism* – November 1, 2004;89(11):5387-91

Le Couteur, D.G. – <u>Pesticides and Parkinson's Disease</u> – *Biomed Pharmacotherapy* – April 1999;53(3):122-30

Lee, D.H., et al. – <u>Polychlorinated Biphenyls and Organochlorine Pesticides in Plasma Predict Development of Type 2 Diabetes in the Elderly:</u>

The Prospective Investigation of the Vasculature in Uppsala Seniors (PIVUS) study – *Diabetes Care* – August 2011; 34(8):1778-84

Lee, J. – *Hormone Balance Made Simple* – Warner Books – New York – 2006

Lee, J. – *What Your Doctor May Not Tell You About Menopause* – Warner Books – New York - 2004

Lee, J., et al. – The role of transcranial magnetic stimulation in treatment-resistant depression: A review – *Current Pharmaceutical Design* – June 6, 2012 (Epub ahead of print)

Lee, W. – Acetaminophen and the U.S. Acute Liver Failure Study Group: lowering the risks of hepatic failure – *Hepatology* – July 2004;40(1):6-9

Li, Y., et al. – Overprescribing in China, driven by financial incentives, results in very high use of antibiotics, injections and corticosteroids – *Health Affairs (Millwood)* – May 2012;31(5):1075-82

Li, Y., et al. – Prevalence and severity of gingivitis in American adults – *American Journal of Dentistry* – February 2010;23(1):9-13

Li, Y., et al. – Sulforaphane, a dietary component of broccoli/broccoli sprouts, inhibits breast cancer stem cells – *Clinical Cancer Research* – May 1, 2010;16(9):2580-90

Libby, P. and Aikawa, M. – Vitamin C, collagen, and cracks in the plaque – *Circulation* – March 26, 2002; 105(12):1396-8

Lindsted, K., et al. – Body mass index and patterns of mortality among Seventh-day Adventist men – *International Journal of Obesity* – June 1991;15(6):397-406

Lippman, S., et al. – Effect of Selenium and Vitamin E on Risk of Prostate

Cancer and Other Cancers (SELECT trial) – *Journal of the American Medical Association (JAMA)* – January 2009; 301(1): 39-51

Liu, P., et al. – A double-blind, placebo-controlled, randomized clinical trial of recombinant human chorionic gonadotropin on muscle strength and physical function and activity in older men with partial age-related androgen deficiency – *Journal of Clinical Endocrinology and Metabolism* – July 2002;87(7):3125-35

Lizer, M., et al. – Comparison of the frequency of the methylenetetrahydrofolate reductase (MTHFR) C677T polymorphism in depressed versus nondepressed patients – *Journal of Psychiatric Practice* – November 2011;17(6):404-9

Lloyd, A., e al. – Coherence training in children with attention-deficit hyperactivity disorder: cognitive functions and behavioral changes – *Alternative Therapies in Health and Medicine* – July-August 2010;16(4):34-42

Lopez-Garcia, E., et al. – Coffee consumption and mortality in women with cardiovascular disease – *American Journal of Clinical Nutrition* – July 2011;94(1):218-24

Lubinsky, M. – Hypothesis: Estrogen related thrombosis explains the pathogenesis and epidemiology of gastroschisis – *American Journal of Medical Genetics* – March 1, 2012 (Epub ahead of print)

Luke, J. – Fluoride deposition in the aged human pineal gland – *Caries Research* – March-April 2001;35(2):125-8

Luque, A., et al. – Early atherosclerotic plaques show evidence of infection by Chlamydia pneum. – *Frontiers in Bioscience (Elite Edition)* – June 1, 2012;4:2423-32

Ly, N., et al. – Gut microbiota, probiotics, and vitamin D: interrelated exposures influencing allergy, asthma, and obesity? – *Journal of Allergy and Clinical Immunology* – May 2011;127(5):1087-94

Ma, L., et al. – <u>Lutein and zeaxanthin intake and the risk of age-related macular degeneration: a systematic review and meta-analysis</u> – *British Journal of Nutrition* – September 8, 2011:1-10

Maggi, M. and Corona, G. – <u>Love protects lover's life</u> – *The Journal of Sexual Medicine* – April 2011;8(4):931-5

Magnus, M., et al. – <u>Delivery by Cesarean section and early childhood respiratory symptoms and disorders: the Norwegian mother and child cohort study</u> – *American Journal of Epidemiology* – December 1, 2011;174(11):1275-85

Malagoli, C., et al. – <u>Risk of hematological malignancies associated with magnetic fields exposure from power line: a case-control study in two municipalities of northern Italy</u> – *Environmental Health* – March 30, 2010;9:16

Malinowska, E., et al. – <u>Assessment of fluoride concentration and daily intake by human from tea and herbal infusions</u> – *Food Chemical and Toxicology* – March 2008;46(3):1055-61

Manfo, F., et al. – <u>Effects of maneb on testosterone release in male rats</u> – *Drug and Chemical Toxicology* – April 2011;34(2):120-8

Maniscalco, B. and Taylor, K. – <u>Calcification in coronary artery disease can be reversed by EDTA-tetracycline long-term chemotherapy</u> – *Pathophysiology* – October 2004;11(2):95-101

Marco, H., et al. – <u>Diagnostic accuracy of skin prick testing in children with tree nut allergy</u> – *The Journal of Allergy and Clinical Immunology* – June 2006;117(6):1506-1508

Marconett, C., et al. – <u>Indole-3-carbinol downregulation of telomerase gene expression requires the inhibition of estrogen receptor-alpha and Sp1 transcription factor interactions within the hTERT promoter and mediates the G1 cell cycle arrest of human breast cancer cells</u> – *Carcinogenesis* – September 2011:32(9):1315-23

Margheri, M., et al. – Combined effects of melatonin and all-trans retinoic acid and somatostatin on breast cancer cell proliferation and death: molecular basis for the anticancer effect of these molecules – *European Journal of Pharmacology* – April 15, 2012;681(1-3):34-43

Maslanyj, M., et al. – Investigation of the sources of residential power frequency magnetic field exposure in the UK Childhood Cancer Study – *Journal of Radiological Protection* – March 2007;27(1):41-58

Masters, K. and Spielmans, G. – Prayer and health: review, meta-analysis, and research agenda – *Journal of Behavioral Medicine* – October 2007;30(5):447

Matsunaga, M., et al. – Association between perceived happiness levels and peripheral circulating pro-inflammatory cytokine levels in middle-aged adults in Japan – *Neuro Endocrinology Letters* – 2011;32(4):458-63

Mazur, P., et al. – Nï -homocysteinyl-lysine isopeptide is associated with progression of peripheral artery disease in patients treated with folic acid – *European Journal of Vascular and Endovascular Surgery* – March 19, 2012 (Epub)

Messamore, E. – Niacin subsensitivity is associated with functional impairment in schizophrenia – *Schizophrenia Research* – March 22, 2012 (Epub ahead of print)

McCann, S., et al. – Dietary intakes of Total and Specific Lignans Are Associated with Clinical Breast Tumor Characteristics – *The Journal of Nutrition* – November 23, 2011 (Epublication, ahead of print)

McCraty, R. – Coherence: Bridging personal, social and global health – *Alternative Therapies in Health and Medicine* – July/August 2010; 16(4):10-24

McGee, C. – *Heart Frauds* – Picadilly Books, Ltd. – Colorado Springs, CO - 2007

McGill, H., et al. – <u>Origin of atherosclerosis in childhood and adolescence</u> – *American Journal of Clinical Nutrition* – November 2000;72(5 Suppl):1307S-1315S

Meggs, W. – presentation on <u>Outdoor Air Pollution</u> - lecture section from *The Diagnosis and Treatment of Chemical Sensitivities* course syllabus – The American Academy of Environmental Medicine – 2008. Original citation of interest (diesel exhaust exposure inducing inhalant allergy) came from the *Journal of Allergy and Clinical Immunology* 1999; 104:1183-88 (cited in Dr. Meggs' lecture slides)

Meier, C., et al. – <u>Use of depot medroxyprogesterone acetate and fracture risk</u> – *Journal of Clinical Endocrinology and Metabolism* – November 2010;95(11):4909-16

Mendoza, R., et al. – <u>No biological evidence of XMRV in blood or prostatic fluid from prostate cancer patients</u> – *PloS One* – 2012;7(5):e36073 (Epub May 16, 2012)

Mensching, D., et al. – <u>The feline thyroid gland: a model for endocrine disruption by polybrominated diphenyl ethers (PBDEs)?</u> – *Journal of Toxicology and Environmental Health. Part A* – 2012;75(4):201-12

Mikirova, N., et al. – <u>Effect of weight reduction on cardiovascular risk factors and CD34-positive cells in circulation</u> – *International Journal of Medical Sciences* – 2011;8(6):445-52

Miklossy, J. – <u>Emerging roles of pathogens in Alzheimer disease</u> – *Expert Reviews in Molecular Medicine* – September 20, 2011;13:e30

Miles, E. and Calder, P. – <u>Influence of marine n-3 polyunsaturated fatty acids on immune function and a systematic review of their effects on clinical outcomes in rheumatoid arthritis</u> – *British Journal of Nutrition* – June 2012;107 Suppl 2:S171-84

Million, M., et al. – <u>Comparative meta-analysis of the effect of Lactobacillus</u>

species on weight gain in humans and animals – *Microbial Pathogenesis* – May 24, 2012 (Epub ahead of print)

Minaev, S., et al. – Polyenzymatic therapy in prevention of adhesive processes in the abdominal cavity in children – *Vestnik Khirurgii Imeni, I. I. Grekova* – 2006;165(1):49-54

Mitrou, P., et al. – Mediterranean dieatary pattern and prediction of all-cause mortality in a U.S. population – *Archives of Internal Medicine* – 2007;167:2461

Monti, D., et al. – Phase I evaluation of intravenous ascorbic acid in combination with gemcitabine and erlotinib in patients with metastatic pancreatic cancer – *PloS One* – 2012;7(1) – Epub January 17, 2012-04-07

Mora-Ripoll, R. – The therapeutic value of laughter in medicine – *Alternative Therapies in Health and Medicine* – November-December 2010;16(6):56-64

Morgentaler, A., et al. – Testosterone therapy in men with untreated prostate cancer – *Journal of Urology* – April, 2011;185(4):1256-60

Mozzon, M. – Resveratrol content in some Tuscan wines – *Italian Journal of Food Science* – (1996);8(2):145-52

Muczynski, V., et al. – Effect of mono-(2-ethylhexyl) phthalate on human and mouse fetal testis: in vitro and in vivo approaches – *Toxicology and Applied Pharmacology* – May 15, 2012;261(1):97-104

Mudrak, J. - Switzerland's Lotschental Yesterday and Today - *Price-Pottenger Nutrition Foundation Newsletter* - winter 2008-9, vol 32, #4

Mueck, A. – Postmenopausal hormone replacement therapy and cardiovascular disease: the value of transdermal estradiol and micronized progesterone – *Climacteric* – April 2012;15 Suppl 1:11-7

Mulligan, T. - Prevalence of hypogonadism in males aged at least 45 HIM study - *International Journal of Clinical Practice* – 2006, 60; (7): 762

Murray, C.W., et al. – US Food and Drug Administration's Total Diet Study: dietary intake of perchlorate and iodine – *Journal of Exposure Science and Environmental Epidemiology* – November, 2008;18(6):571-80

Na, X. and Kelly, C. – Probiotics in clostridium difficile infection – *Journal of Clinical Gastroenterology* – November 2011;45 Supple:S154-8

Nachman, K., et al. – Arsenic species in poultry feather meal – *Science and the Total Environment* – February 15, 2012;417-418:183-8

Nakagawa, Y., et al. – Chlorpropham induces mitochondrial dysfunction in rat hepatocytes – *Toxicology* – August 5, 2004;200(2-3):123-33

Nakagawa, Y., et al. – Biotransformation of chlorpropham (CIPC) in isolated rat hepatocytes and xenoestrogenic activity of CIPC and its metabolites by in vitro assays – *Xenobiotica* – March 2004;34(3):257-72

Ng, T.-P., et al. – Curry Consumption and Cognitive Function in the Elderly – *American Journal of Epidemiology* – 2006, vol. 164, No. 9

Nitika, et al. – Physico-chemical characteristics, nutrient composition and consumer acceptability of wheat varieties grown under organic and inorganic farming conditions – *International Journal of Food Sciences and Nutrition* – May 2008;59(3):224-45

Novati, A., et al. – Chronic partial sleep deprivation reduces brain sensitivity to glutamate N-methyl-d-aspartate receptor-mediated neurotoxicity – *Journal of Sleep Research* – June 14, 2011 (Epub)

Nuvolone, D., et al. – Short-term association between ambient air pollution and risk of hospitalization for acute myocardial infarction : results of the cardiovascular risk and air pollution in Tuscany (RISCAT) study – *American Journal of Epidemiology* – July 1, 2011;174(1):63-71

Obrenovich, M., et al. – Altered heavy metals and transketolase found in autistic spectrum disorder – *Biological Trace Element Research* – December 2011;144(1-3):475-86

Okyay, P., et al. – Intestinal parasites prevalence and related factors in school children, a western city sample—Turkey – *BMC Public Healh* – December 22, 2004;4:64

Oschmann, J. – *Energy Medicine: The Scientific Basis* – Elsevier Limited – 2000

Ozdemir, O. – Any benefits of probiotics in allergic disorders? – *Allergy Asthma Proceedings* – March-April 2010;31(2):103-11

Palatnik, A., et al. – Double-blind, controlled, crossover trial of inositol versus fluvoxamine for the treatment of panic disorder – *Journal of Clinical Psychopharmacology* – June 2001:21(3):335-9

Parikh, A., et al. – Association between a DASH-like diet and mortality in adults with hypertension: findings from a population-based follow-up study. – *American Journal of Hypertension* – April 2009 – 22(4):409-16

Park, A. – America's Health Checkup – article in *TIME* magazine - December 1, 2008; p41

Parnell, J. and Reimer, R. – Prebiotic fiber modulation of the gut microbiota improves risk factors for obesity and the metabolic syndrome – *Gut Microbes* – January-February 2012;3(1):29-34

Paro, R., et al. – The fungicide mancozeb induces toxic effects on mammalian granulosa cells – *Toxicology and Applied Pharmacology* – April 15, 2012;260(2):155-61

Pashikanti, L. and Von Ah, D. – <u>Impact of early mobilization protocol on the medical-surgical inpatient population: an integrated review of literature</u> – *Clinical Nurse Specialist* – March-April 2012;26(2):87-94

Patel, K. – <u>Food Pollution</u> – lecture section from *The Diagnosis and Treatment of Chemical Sensitivities* course syllabus – The American Academy of Environmental Medicine Instructional Courses- 2008

Peeters, R., et al. – <u>Serum 3,3',5'-triiodothyronine (rT3) and 3,5,3'-triiodothyronine/rT3 are prognostic markers in critically ill patients and are associated with postmortem tissue deiodinase activities</u> – *Journal of Clinical Endocrinology and Metabolism* – August 2005;90(8):4559-65

Pellacani, C., et al. – <u>Synergistic interactions between PBDEs and PCBs in human neuroblastoma cells</u> – *Environmental Toxicology* – March 20, 2012 (Epub ahead of print)

Peng, J., et al. – <u>Fucoxanthin, a marine carotenoid present in brown seaweed and diatoms: metabolism and bioactivities relevant to human health</u> – *Marine Drugs* – October 10, 2011;9(10):1806-28

Pereira, F., et al. – <u>Vitamin D and colon cancer</u> – *Endocrine Related Cancer* – March 1, 2012 (Epub ahead of print)

Pestana, S., et al. – <u>Safety of ingestion of yellow tartrazine by double-blind placebo controlled challenge in 26 atopic adults</u> – *Allergologia et Immunopathologia* – May-June 2010;38(3):142-6

Pfeiler, G., et al. – <u>Vaginal estriol to overcome side-effects of aromatase inhibitor in breast cancer patients</u> – *Climacteric* – Jun 2011;14(3):339-44

Phipps, K., et al. – <u>Prevalence and severity of dental caries among American Indian and Alaska Native preschool children</u> – *Journal of Public Health Dentistry* – April 20, 2012 (Epub ahead of print)

Pierce, E. – <u>Ulcerative colitis and Crohn's disease: is Mycobacterium avium subspecies paratuberculosis the common villain?</u> – *Gut Pathology* – December 17, 2010;17;2(1):21

Pitchford, P. – *Healing With Whole Foods* – North Atlantic Books – Berkeley - 2002

Plantinga, T., et al. – <u>Human genetic susceptibility to Candida infections</u> – *Medical Mycology* – June 4, 2012 (Epub ahead of print)

Pohl, H., et al. – <u>Metal ions affecting the neurological system</u> – *Metal Ions in Life Sciences* – 2011;8:247-62

Pollan, M. – *Omnivore's Dillema* – The Penguin Press – New York - 2006

Pottenger, F. – *Pottenger's Cats: A Study in Nutrition* – Price-Pottenger Nutrition Foundation, Inc. - 1983

Poudyal, H., et al. – <u>Lipid redistribution by alpha-linolenic acid-rich chia seed inhibits stearoyl-CoA desaturase-1 and induces cardiac and hepatic protection in diet-induced obese rats</u> – *The Journal of*

Nutritional Biochemistry – March 22, 2011 (Epub ahead of print)

Pozzoni, P., et al. – <u>Saccharomyces boulardii for the prevention of antibiotic-associated diarrhea in adult hospitalized patients: a single-center, randomized, double-blind, placebo-controlled trial</u> – *American Journal of Gastroenterology* – June 2012;107(6):922-31

Price, L., et al. – <u>Fluoroquinolone-resistant Campylobacter isolate from conventional and antibiotic-free chicken products</u> – *Environmental Health Perspectives* – May 2005;113(5):557-60

Price, W. – *Nutrition and Physical Degeneration* – The Price-Pottenger

Nutrition Foundation, Inc. – La Mesa, CA – 2006 (originally in 1939)

Prossin, A., et al. – Association of plasma interleukin-18 levels with emotion regulation and μ-opioid neurotransmitter function in major depression and healthy volunteers – *Biological Psychiatry* – April 15, 2011;69(8):808-12

Qu, L., et al. – Human herpesvirus 8 genomes and seroprevalence in United States blood donors – *Transfusion* – May 2010;50(5):1050-6

Radlovic, N., et al. – Vitamin D in the light of current knowledge – *Srp Arh Celok Lek* (Serbian journal) – Jan-Feb 2012;140(1-2):110-4

Raffone, E., et al. – Insulin sensitizer agents alone and in co-treatment with r-FSH for ovulation induction in PCOS women – *Gynecological Endocrinology* – April 2010;26(4):275-80

Randolph, T. – *Environmental Medicine: Beginnings and Bibliographies of Clinical Ecology* – Clinical Ecology Publications – Fort Collins, CO – 1987.

Raynaud, J., et al. – Prostate cancer risk in testosterone-treated men - *Journal of Steroid Biochemistry and Molecular Biology* – December 2006; 102(1-5):261-6

Rea, W. – *Chemical Sensitivity, vol I* – CRC Press – 1992

Reeves, J. – The rise and fall of food minerals – *Nutrition and Health* – 2011:20(3-4):209-29

Rhoades, D.R., et al – Speaking and interruptions during primary care office visits – *Family Medicine* – July-August 2001; 33(7):528-32

Riedl, B. – Still at the Federal Trough: Farm subsidies for the rich and famous shattered records in 2002 – *Heritage Foundation* – April 30, 2002 – cited in Wikipedia article on farm subsidies

Righi, E., et al. – Trihalomethanes, chlorite, chlorate in drinking water and risk of congenital anomalies: A population-based case-control study in Northern Italy – *Environmental Research* – May 9, 2012 (Epub ahead of print)

Riley, K., et al. – Early life linguistic ability, late life cognitive function, and neuropathology: Findings from the Nun Study – *Neurobiology of Aging* – 2005; 26(3):341-347

Rocas, I., et al. – Microorganisms in root canal-treated teeth from a German population – *Journal of Endodontics* – August 2008;34(8):926-31

Roine, P, et al. – *Lancet* – 1958;2:173 – derived from presentation by Stephen Hoption-Cann, PhD at the spring 2007 IFM conference, symposium on thyroid and adrenal disorders

Rooks, M. and Garrett, W. – Bacteria, food, and cancer – *F1000 Biology Reports* – 2011;3:12

Rossmann, J. – Ask the Experts: Why do jets leave a white trail in the sky? – *Scientific American* – November 19, 2011 (online)

Rostom, A., et al. – Use of Aspirin and NSAIDs to prevent colorectal cancer – *US Preventive Services Task Force Evidence Synthesis* – March 2007

Rowe, K.S. and Rowe, K.J. – Synthetic food coloring and behavior: a dose response effect in a double-blind, placebo-controlled, repeated-measures study – *Journal of Pediatrics* – November 1994;125(5 Pt 1):691-8

Ruiter, R., et a. – Risk of cancer in patients on insulin glargine and other insulin analogues in comparison with those on human insulin:

results from a large population-based follow-up study – *Diabetologia* – January 2012;55(1):51-62

Rusyn, I. and Corton, J. – Mechanistic considerations for human relevance of cancer hazard of di)2-ethylhexyl) phthalate – *Mutation Research* – December 20, 2011 (Epub ahead of print)

Sager, A. and Socolar, D. – 61 Percent of Medicare's New Prescription Drug Subsidy is Windfall Profit to Drug Makers – Boston University School of Public Health, private publication – October 31, 2003 – Health Reform Program website: www.healthreformprogram.org

Sakurai, Y., et al. – Prevalence and risk factors of allergic rhinitis and cedar pollinosis among Japanese men – *Preventive Medicine* – July-August 1998;27(4):617-22

Salazar, C., et al. – Association between oral health and gastric precancerous lesions – *Carcinogenesis* – February 2012;33(2):399-403

Sathyapalan, T. and Dixit, S. – Radiotherapy-induced hypopituitarism: a review – *Expert Review of Anticancer Therapy* – May 2012;12(5):669-83

Sahlen, A., et al. – Effects of prolonged exercise on left ventricular mechanical synchrony in long-distance runners: importance of previous exposure to endurance races – *Journal of the American Society of Echocardiography* – September 2010;23(9)977-84

St. Louis, V., et al. – Differences in mercury bioaccumulation between polar bears (*Ursus maritimus*) from the Canadian high- and sub-Arctic – *Environmental Science & Technology* – July 15, 2011;45(14):5922-8

Sang, Z., et al. – Thyroid dysfunction during late gestation is associated with excessive iodine intake in pregnant women – *Journal of Clinical Endocrinology and Metabolism* – June 5, 2012 (Epub ahead of print)

Saporta, D. – Efficacy of sublingual immunotherapy versus subcutaneous injection immunotherapy in allergic patients – *Journal of Environmental and Public Health* – (Epub) February 20, 2012

Schencking, M., et al. – Intravenous vitamin C in the treatment of shingles: Results of a multicenter prospective cohort study – *Medical Science Monitor* – April 1, 2012;18(4):CR215-224

Schiapparelli, P., et al. – Non-pharmacological approach to migraine prophylaxis: part II – *Neurological Sciences* – June 2010;31 Suppl 1:S137-9

Schroeter, H., et al. – Recommending flavanols and procyanidins for cardiovascular health: current knowledge and future needs – *Molecular Aspects of Medicine* – December 2010;31(6):546-57

Schwartz, A., et al. – Inhibition of tumor development by dehydroepiandrosterone and related steroids – *Toxicologic Pathology* – 1986;14(3):357-62

Science Daily, Science News (www.sciencedaily.com) – St. John's Wort Ineffective for Depression, Study Finds – Apiril 10, 2002

Sears, A. – *PACE: The 12-Minute Fitness Revolution for Weight Loss* – Wellness Research and Consulting, Inc. – Royal Palm Beach, Fl – 2010

Sears, B. – *The Anti-Inflammation Zone* – Harper Collins Publishers – New York - 2005

Seeger, H. and Mueck, A. – Are the progestins responsible for breast cancer risk during hormone therapy in the postmenopause? Experimental vs. clinical data – *Journal of Steroid Biochemistry and Molecular Biology* – March 2008;109(1-2):11-5

Seifert-Klauss, V. and Prior, J. – Progesterone and bone: actions promoting bone health in women – *Journal of Osteoporosis* – October 31, 2010;2010:845180

Seitz, H., et al. – Epidemiology and pathophysiology of alcohol and breast cancer: Update 2012 – *Alcohol and Alcoholism* – March 29, 2012 (Epub ahead of print)

Seltzer, J. – Health effects of mold in children – *Pediatric Clinics of North America* – April 2007;54(2):309-33

Shaffer, M. – Waste Lands: The Threat of Toxic Fertilizer – *Toxics Policy Advocate, CALPIRG Charitable Trust* – The State PIRG's – May 3, 2001

Shekelle, R.B., et al – Dietary vitamin A and risk of cancer in the Western Electric study – *Lancet* – November 28, 1981; 2(8257): 1185-90

Shen, Y., et al. – Boswellic acid induces epigenetic alterations by modulating DNA methylation in colorectal cancer cells – *Cancer Biology and Therapy* – May 1, 2012;13(7) (Epub ahead of print)

Sheth, F., et al. – Sister chromatid exchanges: A study in fluorotic individuals of North Gujurat – *Fluoride* – 1994;27:215-219

Siddique, S., et al. – Levels of dechlorane plus and polybrominated diphenylethers in human milk in two Canadian cities – *Environment International* – February 2012;39(1):50-5

Singer, F. and Oberleitner, H. – Drug therapy of activated arthrosis. On the effectiveness of an enzyme mixture versus diclofenac – *Wiener Medizinische Wochenschrift* – 1996;146(3):55-8

Singh, P., et al. – Inhibition of autophagy stimulates molecular iodine-induced apoptosis in hormone independent breast tumors – *Biochemical and Biophysical Research Communications* – November 11, 2011;415(1):181-6

Smeds, A., et al. – <u>Quantification of a Broad Spectrum of Lignans in Cereals, Oilseeds, and Nuts</u> – *Journal of Agricultural and Food Chemistry* – 2007;vol 55(4):1337-46

Smith, J. – *Genetic Roulette: The Documented Health Risks of Genetically Engineered Foods* – Yes! Books – May 2007

Smith, J. and Bimbaum, J. – <u>Drug Bill Demonstrates Lobby's Pull</u> – *Washington Post* – Friday, January 12, 2007

Smith, R. – <u>Medical Journals Are an Extension of the Marketing Arm of Pharmaceutical Companies</u> – *PloS Medicine* – May 17, 2005 – PloS Med 2(5): e138.

Sohrabi, M., et al. – <u>Living near overhead high voltage transmission power line as a risk factor for childhood acute lymphoblastic leukemia: a case-control study</u> – *Asian Pacific Journal of Cancer Prevention* – 2010;11(2):423-7

Souyri, C., et al. – <u>Severe necrotizing soft-tissue infections and nonsteroidal anti-inflammatory drugs</u> – *Clinical and Experimental Dermatology* – May 2008;33(3):249-55

Srinivasan, V., et al. – <u>Therapeutic actions of melatonin in cancer: possible mechanisms</u> – *Integrative Cancer Therapies* – September 2008;7(3):189-203

Stanchina, M., et al. – <u>The influence of white noise on sleep in subjects exposed to ICU noise</u> – *Sleep Medicine* – September 2005;6(5):423-8

Starfield, B. – <u>Is US health really the best in the world?</u> – *Journal of the American Medical Association* – July 26, 2000;284(4):483-5

Starr, M. – *Hypothyroidism Type 2* – Mark Starr Trust - 2005

Stehr-Green, P.A. – <u>Demographic and seasonal influences on human serum pesticide residue levels. – *Journal of Toxicology and Environmental Health* – 1989; 27:405-21

Steinemann, A. – Fragranced consumer products and undisclosed ingredients – *Environmental Impact Assessment Review* – January 2009;29(1):32-38

Strohle, A. – Physical activity, exercise, depression and anxiety disorders – *Journal of Neural Transmission* – June 2009;116(6):777-84

Strong, T. – *Expecting Trouble: What Expectant Parents Should Know About Prenatal Care in America* – New York University Press - 2002

Stumpf, W. – Drugs in the brain; cellular imaging with receptor microscopic autoradiography – *Progress in Histochemistry and Cytochemistry* – March 2012;47(1):1-26

Sufrin, C.B. and Ross, J.S. – Pharmaceutical industry marketing: understanding its impact on women's health" – *Obstetrics and Gynecology Survey* – September 2008; 63(9):585-96

Sulforaphane Glucosinolate Monograph – (no single author listed) – *Alternative Medicine Review* – December 2010; vol 15, #4

Sumi, H., et al. – Enhancement of the fibrinolytic activity in plasma by oral administration of nattokinase – *Acta Haematologica* – 1990;84(3):139-43

Sun-Edelstein, C. and Mauskop, A. – Role of magnesium in the pathogenesis and treatment of migraine – *Expert Reviews in Neurotherapeutics* – March 2009;9(3):369-79

Suzuki, M., et al. – Implications from and for food cultures for cardiovascular disease: longevity – *Asia Pacific Journal of Clinical Nutrition* – 2001;10(2):165-71

Takaishi, H., et al. - Anti-high mobility group box 1 and box 2 non-histone chromosomal proteins (HMGB1/HMGB2) antibodies and anti-Saccharomyces cerevisiae antibodies (ASCA): accuracy in differentially diagnosing UC and CD and correlation with inflammatory bowel disease phenotype – *Journal of Gastroenterology* – May 30, 2012 (Epub ahead of print)

Tanaka, T., et al. – Congener-specific polychlorinated biphenyls and the prevalence of diabetes in the Saku Control Obesity Program (SCOP) – *Endocrine Journal* – 2011;58(7):589-96

Taylor, G. – Periodontal treatment and its effects on glycemic control: a review of the evidence – *Oral Surgery, Oral Medicine, Oral Pathology, Oral Radiology and Endodontics* – March 1999;87(3):311-6

Thein, D. and Hurt, W. – Lysine as a prophylactic agent in the treatment of recurrent herpes simplex labialis – *Oral Surgery, Oral Medicine, and Oral Pathology* – December 1984;58(6):659-66

Thomas, G., et al. – Vitamin D levels predict all-cause and cardiovascular disease mortality in subjects with the metabolic syndrome: The Ludwigshafen Risk and Cardiovascular Health (LURIC) study – *Diabetes Care* – March 7, 2012 (Epub ahead of print)

Tilg, H., et al. – Gut, inflammation and osteoporosis: basic and clinical concepts – *Gut* – May 2008;57(5):684-94

Toth, P. and Maki, K. – A commentary on the implications of the ENHANCE Trial: Should ezetimibe move to the "Back of the Line" as a therapy for dyslipidemia? – *Journal of Clinical Lipidology* – October 2008;2(5):313-7

Traish, A., et al. – Testosterone Deficiency – *American Journal of Medicine* – July 2011;124(7):578-87

Tufano, A., et al. – The infection burden in atherothrombosis – *Seminars in Thrombosis and Hemostasis* – June 2, 2012 (Epub ahead of print)

Turan, V., et al. – <u>The effects of steroidal estrogens in ACI rat mammary carcinogenesis: 17-beta-estradiol, 2-hydroxyestradiol, 4-hydroxyestradiol, 16alpha-hydroxyestradiol, and 4-hydroxyestrone</u> – *Journal of Endocrinology* – October 2004;183(1):91-9

Uchiyama, K., et al. – <u>N-3 polyunsaturated fatty acid diet therapy for patients with inflammatory bowel disease</u> – *Inflammatory Bowel Disease* – October 2010;16(10):1696-707

Ursinyova, M., et al. – <u>The relation between human exposure to mercury and thyroid hormone status</u> – *Biological Trace Element Research* – March 18, 2012 (Epub ahead of print)

Van Nimwegen, F., et al. – <u>Mode and place of delivery, gastrointestinal microbiota, and their influence on asthma and atopy</u> – *Journal of Allergy and Clinical Immunology* – November 2011;128(5):948-55

Veerappan, G., et al. – <u>Probiotics for the treatment of inflammatory bowel disease</u> – *Current Gastroenterology Reports* – May 13, 2012 (Epub ahead of print)

Vicente-Barrero, M., et al. – <u>The efficacy of acupuncture and decompression splints in the treatment of temporomandibular joint pain-dysfunction syndrome</u> – *Medicina Oral, Patologia Oral y Cirugia Bucal* – May 1, 2012 (Epub ahead of print)

Vidal, J. – <u>Dust storms spread deadly diseases worldwide</u> – *The Observer* – September 27, 2009

Villarruz, M., et al. – <u>Chelation therapy for atherosclerotic cardiovascular disease</u> – *Cochrane Database of Systematic Reviews* – 2002;(4):CD002785

Viswanatha Swamy, A. and Patil, P. – <u>Effect of some clinically used proteolytic enzymes on inflammation in rats</u> – *Indian Journal of Pharmaceutical Sciences* – January 2008;7(1):114-7

Waite, K. – <u>Blackley and the development of hay fever as a disease of civilization in the nineteenth century</u> – *Medical History* – April 1995;39(2):186-96

Wallinga, D. – "Mercury from chlor-alkali plants: measured concentrations in food product sugar." – *Environmental Health* – January 2009; 8:2

Wang, C. – <u>Tai chi and rheumatic diseases</u> – *Rheumatic Disease Clinics of North America* – February 2011;37(1):19-32

Warnock, D., et al. – <u>Toxic gas generation from plastic mattresses and sudden infant death syndrome</u> – *Lancet* – December 9, 1995;346(8989):1516-20

Watanabe, T. – <u>Effect of alkaline ionized water on reproduction in gestational and lactational rats</u> – *Journal of Toxicological Sciences* – May 1995;20(2):135-42

Watanabe, T., et al. – <u>Influence of alkaline ionized water on rat erythrocyte hexokinase activity and myocardium</u> – *Journal of Toxicological Sciences* – May 1997;22(2):141-52

Watanabe, T., et al. – <u>Degradation of myocardiac myosin and creatine kinase in rats given alkaline ionized water</u> – *Journal of Veterinary Medical Science (Japan)* – February 1998;60(2)245-50

Watanabe, T., et al. – <u>Influences of alkaline ionized water on milk electrolyte concentrations in maternal rats</u> – *Journal of Toxicological Sciences* – December 2000;25(5):417-22

Waterman, B., et al. – <u>Low back pain in the United States: incidence and risk factors for presentation in the emergency setting</u> – *The Spine Journal* – January 2012;12(1):63-70

Weber, R., et al. – <u>Dioxin- and POP-contaminated sites—contemporary and future relevance and challenges: overview on background aims</u>

and scopes of the series – *Environmental Science and Pollution Research International* – July 2008;15(5):363-93

Weigert, G., et al. – Effects of lutein supplementation on macular pigment optical density and visual acuity in patients with age-related macular degeneration – *Investigative Ophthalmology and Visual Science* – October 17, 2011;52(11):8174-8

West, D., et al. – Antibody responses of healthy infants to concurrent administration of a bivalent haemophilus influenzae type b-hepatitis B vaccine with diphtheria-tetanus-pertussis, polio and measles-mumps-rubella vaccines – *BioDrugs* – 2001;15(6):413-8

Whitehouse, C., et al. – The potential toxicity of artificial sweeteners – *AAOHN Journal* – June 2008;56(6):251-9

Williams, R. – *Nutrition Against Disease* – Pitman Publishing Corporation – New York - 1971

Wilson, D. – Harvard Medical School in Ethics Quandry – *New York Times* – March 3, 2009

World Cancer Research Fund – research review on processed meats and pancreatic cancer – first printed in *The Holistic Dental Digest PLUS* – March/April 2008 – sourced from the *Price-Pottenger Journal of Health and Healing* – summer 2008; vol 32, #2, p20

World Health Organization (WHO) – The World Health Report, 2000 – 2000

Wright, B., et al. – A comparison of urinary mercury between children with autism spectrum disorders and control children – *PloS One* – 2012;7(2):e29547

Writing Group for the Women's Health Initiative Investigators – Risks and benefits of estrogen plus progestin in healthy postmenopausal women:

principal results from the Women's Health Initiative Randomized Controlled Trial – *JAMA* – 2002;288(3):321-333

Wu, F. – Mycotoxin reduction in Bt corn: potential economic, health, and regulatory impacts – *Transgenic Research* – 2006;15:277-89

Yamagashi, S., et al. – Kinetics, role and therapeutic implications of endogenous soluble form of receptor for advanced glycation end products (sRAGE) in diabetes – *Current Drug Targets* – October 2007;8(10):1138-43

Yan, L. and Spitznagel, E. – Soy consumption and prostate cancer risk in men: a revisit of a meta-analysis – *American Journal of Clinical Nutrition* – April 2009;89(4):1155-63

Yang, Q. – Gain weight by "going diet?" Artificial sweeteners and the neurobiology of sugar cravings: Neuroscience 2010. – *Yale Journal of Biological Medicine* – June 2010; 83(2): 101-8

Yeh, G., et al. – Tai chi exercise in patients with chronic heart failure: a randomized clinical trial – *Archives of Internal Medicine* – April 25, 2011;171(8):750-7

Youngster, I., et al. – Probiotics and the immunological response to infant vaccinations: a prospective, placebo controlled pilot study – *Archives of Disease in Childhood* – April 2011;96(4):345-9

Youssef, D., et al. – Antimicrobial implications of vitamin D – *Dermatoendocrinology* – October 2011;3(4):220-9

CPSIA information can be obtained at www.ICGtesting.com
Printed in the USA
LVOW12s2112230914

405488LV00003B/6/P